ALLE ZEIT WACH
1842

Transluminal Coronary Angioplasty and Intracoronary Thrombolysis

Coronary Heart Disease IV

Edited by

M. Kaltenbach A. Grüntzig K. Rentrop W.-D. Bussmann

Contributors

M. Amor K. Bachmann L.G. Bentivoglio P.C. Block T. Bonzel
K. Breddin W.-D. Bussmann G. Dorros H.J. Engel E.O. Feigl
M.C. Fishbein G.C. Friesinger W.F.M. Fulton M.I.H. El Gamal
W. Ganz A. Grüntzig G. Heyndrickx M. Hofmann W. Huhmann
M. Kaltenbach K.R. Karsch K.M. Kent H. Klepzig Jr. G. Kober
K.H. Leitz J.R. Margolis D. Mathey K. Mathias H.C. Mehmel
W. Merx B.J. Messmer J. Meyer M. Mock W. Porstmann
W. Rafflenbeul K.P. Rentrop W. Rutsch T.J. Ryan A. Ryzlewicz
M. Schartl A.D. Schmidt-Moritz K. Schnellbacher R. Schröder
F. Schwarz P.W. Serruys W. Seyferth U. Sigwart K. Silberbauer
H. Smith R. Sörensen Th.A. Sos S.H. Stertzer M. Stolte
V. Tilsner D.O. Williams E. Zeitler

With 210 Figures

Springer-Verlag Berlin Heidelberg New York 1982

Professor Dr. Martin Kaltenbach
Abteilung für Kardiologie, Zentrum der Inneren Medizin
Klinikum der Johann Wolfgang Goethe-Universität
Theodor-Stern-Kai 7, 6000 Frankfurt/Main 70, FRG

Andreas Roland Grüntzig, M.D.
Professor of Medicine, Emory University
School of Medicine, Department of Medicine
1364 Clifton Road, Atlanta, Georgia 30322, USA

Klaus Peter Rentrop, M.D.
Associated Professor of Medicine
Division of Cardiology, Mount Sinai Medical Center
One Gustave L. Levy Place, New York, N.Y. 10029, USA

Professor Dr. Wulf-Dirk Bussmann
Abteilung für Kardiologie, Zentrum der Inneren Medizin
Klinikum der Johann Wolfgang Goethe-Universität
Theodor-Stern-Kai 7, 6000 Frankfurt/Main 70, FRG

ISBN-13: 978-3-642-68360-2 e-ISBN-13: 978-3-642-68358-9
DOI: 10.1007/978-3-642-68358-9

Library of Congress Cataloging in Publication Data
Main entry under title: Transluminal coronary angioplasty and intracoronary thrombolysis. Bibliography: p. Includes index. 1. Coronary arteries--Surgery--Congresses. 2. Coronary heart disease--Surgery--Congresses. 3. Cardiac catheterization--Congresses. 4. Angiocardiography--Congresses. 5. Fibrinolysis--Congresses. I. Kaltenbach, Martin. II. Amor, M. [DNLM: 1. Angioplasty-Transluminal--Congresses. 2. Fibrinolysis--Congresses. 3. Coronary disease--Therapy--Congresses. W3 C09988A 4th 1981c / WG 300 C825 1981] RD598.T64 1982 617'.412059 82-5440

Softcover reprint of the hardcover 1st edition 1982

2127/3140-543210

Dedicated to Werner Porstmann

Prof. Dr. sc. med.
† April 5, 1982

Werner Porstmann, who contributed to this book, performed pioneering work in the fields of cardiology and radiology. His achievements were milestones in transluminal angioplasty and in nonoperative occlusion of the persistent ductus arteriosus. We will remember him as an ingenious and outstandingly inventive cardiologist, and a most honored colleague.

Preface

This volume contains the proceedings of the Fourth International Symposium on Coronary Heart Disease, held in Frankfurt/Federal Republic of Germany. In 1970, when the first symposium was held, the whole range of diagnostic and therapeutic measures was covered, but since then interest in coronary heart disease has increased so considerably that the fourth symposium was restricted to only two therapeutic aspects, angioplasty and intracoronary thrombolysis. It can be noted with pleasure that European cardiologists, namely Andreas Grüntzig and Peter Rentrop, have made essential contributions to the applicability of these modes of treatment.

When angioplasty was first discussed at the Third International Symposium (*Coronary Heart Disease*, Stuttgart, 1978) a great deal of astonishment was expressed. Today the procedure has gained an important place in the treatment of angina pectoris. The proportion of candidates for coronary surgery in whom angioplasty can be attempted instead of operation is around 10%, in certain subgroups even higher. The most remarkable finding of our 5-year experience with angioplasty are the extremely good long-term results. Recurrences happen in about 15%–20% of cases within the first 3 months; after this period of time, recurrences are very unusual and mostly due to progression of the disease at other sites. Angioplasty has thus also contributed to our understanding of the dynamics of the atherosclerotic process.

Long-term success in angioplasty appears more likely in "old" atheromas with a tendency towards organization than in "fresh" atheromas with predominant proliferation. If the coronary arterial lumen is reopened by angioplasty when the atherosclerotic process has changed from proliferation to organization, a long-term improvement can be achieved.

It can be extrapolated from the results available today, that the importance of coronary angioplasty as therapeutic tool will grow even further.

After long experience in peripheral arteries, Andreas Grüntzig has applied angioplasty to renal, abdominal, and coronary arteries, and several contributions to the book show the application to extracranial cerebral arteries.

The second part of the volume is dedicated to intracoronary thrombolysis. The role of coronary thrombosis in the evolution of myocardial infarction has been a subject of controversy for many years. A final judgement was particularly difficult since results could only be analysed post mortem.

In the studies inaugurated by Peter Rentrop involving intracoronary lysis of thrombi and careful angiographic controls, it has been shown that intracoronary thrombosis is present in most patients with transmural myocardial infarction. The amount of coronary arterial lumen narrowing created by thrombosis, however, varies considerably from patient to patient, and therefore intracoronary thrombolysis results in varying degrees of restoration of lumen. Intracoronary thrombolysis has already contributed to the basic understanding of human myocardial infarction, but it may be concluded from the results documented here that the therapeutic role of this intervention is not yet fully defined and has to be established with further carefully designed studies.

It is my hope that this volume will contribute to better understanding of both topics covered and thus to better treatment for our patients. I express my gratitude to all who have helped in the preparation, in particular to Mrs. Kratzenberg, Mrs. Glücklich, Dr. Bussmann, Dr. Schrey, and Mr. Gücker, as well as to Springer-Verlag.

Frankfurt a.M., September 1982 M. Kaltenbach

Contents

List of Senior Authors

Amor, M., M.D., Cliniques de Maladies cardiovasculaires, C.H.U. Hôpital de Brabois, 54500 Vandoeuvre Les Nancy, France

Bachmann, K., Prof. Dr. med., Medizinische Universitäts-Poliklinik, Östliche Stadtmauerstraße 29, 8520 Erlangen, FRG

Bentivoglio, L.G., M.D., Medical College of Pennsylvania, 3300 Henry Avenue, Philadelphia, PA 19129, USA

Block P.C., M.D., Prof. of Medicine, Director, Cardiac Catheterization Laboratory, Massachusetts General Hospital, Boston, MA 02114, USA

Bonzel, T., Dr. med., Medizinische Universitätsklinik, Kardiologie, Hugstetter Straße 55, 7800 Freiburg i. Br., FRG

Breddin, K., Prof. Dr. med., Abteilung für Angiologie, Zentrum der Inneren Medizin, Klinikum der Johann-Wolfgang-Goethe-Universität, Theodor-Stern-Kai 7, 6000 Frankfurt/Main 70, FRG

Bussmann, W.-D., Prof. Dr. med., Abteilung für Kardiologie, Zentrum der Inneren Medizin, Klinikum der Johann-Wolfgang-Goethe-Universität, Theodor-Stern-Kai 7, 6000 Frankfurt/Main 70, FRG

Dorros, G., M.D., F.A.C.C., Medical College of Wisconsin, Suite 930, 811 East Wisconsin Avenue, Milwaukee, WI 53202, USA

Engel, H.J., Prof. Dr. med., Kliniken der Freien Hansestadt Bremen, Zentralkrankenhaus „Links der Weser", Medizinische Klinik (Bereich Kardiologie), Senator-Weßling-Straße 1, 2800 Bremen 61, FRG

Feigl, E.O., M.D., Prof., University of Washington, School of Medicine, Department of Physiology and Biophysic, SJ-40, Seattle, WA 98195, USA

Fishbein, M.C., M.D., Department of Pathology, Cedars-Sinai Medical Center, 8700 Beverly Boulevard, Los Angeles, CA 90048, USA

Friesinger, G.C., M.D., Prof. of Medicine, Director, Division of Cardiology, Department of Medicine, Vanderbilt University, Nashville, TN 37232, USA

Fulton, W.F.M., M.D., Prof., University Department of Materia Medica, Stobhill General Hospital, Glasgow G21 3UW, Scotland

El Gamal, M.I.H., M.D., Catharina Ziekenhuis, Department of Cardiology, Michelangelolaan 2, Postbus 13 50, 5602 ZA Eindhoven, The Netherlands

Ganz, W., M.D., Prof. of Medicine, Cedars-Sinai Medical Center, 8700 Beverly Boulevard, Los Angeles, CA 90048, USA

Grüntzig, A., M.D., Prof. of Medicine, Emory University School of Medicine, Department of Medicine, 1364 Clifton Road, Atlanta, GA 30322, USA

Heyndrickx, G.R., M.D., Department of Cardiology, Akademisch Ziekenhuis, De Pintelaan 185, 9000 Gent, Belgium

Hofmann, M., Dr. med., Medizinische Klinik der Ruprecht-Karls-Universität, Abteilung Innere Medizin III (Kardiologie), Bergheimer Straße 58, 6900 Heidelberg, FRG

Huhmann, W., Priv.-Doz. Dr. med., Städtische Kliniken Fulda, Medizinische Klinik I, Pacelliallee 4, 6400 Fulda, FRG

Kaltenbach, M., Prof. Dr. med., Abteilung für Kardiologie, Zentrum der Inneren Medizin, Klinikum der Johann-Wolfgang-Goethe-Universität, Theodor-Stern-Kai 7, 6000 Frankfurt/Main 70, FRG

Karsch, K.R., Dr. med., Medizinische Klinik der Universität, Abt. III, Kardiologie, Otfried-Müller-Straße, 7400 Tübingen, FRG

Kent, K.M., M.D., Head, Cardiovascular Diagnosis, Department of Health, Education and Welfare, National Institute of Health, Bethesda, MD 20014, USA

Klepzig, H., Jr., Dr. med., Abteilung für Kardiologie, Zentrum der Inneren Medizin, Klinikum der Johann-Wolfgang-Goethe-Universität, Theodor-Stern-Kai 7, 6000 Frankfurt/Main 70, FRG

Kober, G., Prof. Dr. med., Abteilung für Kardiologie, Zentrum der Inneren Medizin, Klinikum der Johann-Wolfgang-Goethe-Universität, Theodor-Stern-Kai 7, 6000 Frankfurt/Main 70, FRG

Leitz, K.H., Prof. Dr. med., Abteilung Koronarchirurgie, Medizinische Einrichtungen der Universität Göttingen, Robert-Koch-Straße 40, 3400 Göttingen, FRG

Margolis, J.R., M.D., Cardiovascular Laboratory, South Miami Hospital, 7400 SW 62 Ave., Miami, FL 33143, USA

Mathey, D., Prof. Dr. med., Universitätsklinik Eppendorf, II. Medizinische Klinik, Kardiologie, Martinistraße 52, 2000 Hamburg 20, FRG

Mathias, K., Priv.-Doz. Dr., Zentrum Radiologie, Abteilung Röntgendiagnostik, Klinikum der Albert-Ludwigs-Universität, Hugstetterstraße 55, 7800 Freiburg i. Br., FRG

Mehmel, H.C., Priv.-Doz. Dr. med., Abteilung Innere Medizin III – Kardiologie –, Medizinische Klinik der Ruprecht-Karls-Universität, Bergheimer Straße 58, 6900 Heidelberg, FRG

Merx, W., Prof. Dr. med., Abteilung Innere Medizin I der Rheinisch-Westfälischen Technischen Hochschule, Goethestraße 27–29, 5100 Aachen, FRG

Messmer, B.J., Prof. Dr. med., Abteilung für Herz- und Gefäßchirurgie, Klinikum der Rheinisch-Westfälischen Technischen Hochschule, Goethestraße 27–29, 5100 Aachen, FRG

Meyer, J., Prof. Dr. med., Abteilung Innere Medizin I der Rheinisch-Westfälischen Technischen Hochschule, Goethestraße 27–29, 5100 Aachen, FRG

Mock, M., M.D., Cardiovascular Division, Mayo Clinic, Rochester, MN 55901, USA

Porstmann, W., Prof. Dr. med., Abteilung für Kardiovaskuläre Diagnostik, Bereich Medizin (Charité) der Humboldt-Universität zu Berlin, Schumannstraße 20–21, DDR-1040 Berlin

Rafflenbeul, W., Dr. med., Abteilung für Kardiologie, Medizinische Hochschule Hannover, Department für Innere Medizin, Karl-Wiechert-Allee 9, 3000 Hannover 61, FRG

Rentrop, K.P., M.D., Prof., Mount Sinai Hospital, Department of Cardiology, 1 Gustave L. Levy Place, New York, N.Y. 10029, USA

Rutsch, W., Ass. Prof. Dr. med., Abteilung Innere Medizin, Kardiologie, Klinikum Charlottenburg der Freien Universität Berlin, Spandauer Damm 130, D-1000 Berlin 19

Ryan, T.J., M.D., Prof. of Medicine, Section of Cardiology, Boston University School of Medicine, 75 East Newton Street, Boston, MA 02118, USA

Ryzlewicz, A., Dr. med., Abteilung Innere Medizin – Kardiologie/Pulmologie –, Freie Universität Berlin, Klinikum Charlottenburg, Spandauer Damm 130, D-1000 Berlin 19

Schartl, M., Dr. med., Abteilung Kardiologie, Klinikum Charlottenburg der Freien Universität Berlin, Spandauer Damm 130, D-1000 Berlin 19

Schmidt-Moritz, A.D., Dr. med., Abteilung für Kardiologie, Zentrum der Inneren Medizin, Klinikum der Johann-Wolfgang-Goethe-Universität, Theodor-Stern-Kai 7, 6000 Frankfurt/Main 70, FRG

Schnellbacher, K., Dr. med., Benedikt-Kreutz-Rehabilitationszentrum für Herz- und Kreislaufkranke Bad Kronzingen e.V., Südring 15, 7812 Bad Krozingen, FRG

Schröder, R., Prof. Dr. med., Abteilung für Innere Medizin mit Schwerpunkt Kardiologie/Pneumologie, Medizinische Klinik und Poliklinik, Klinikum Steglitz der Freien Universität Berlin, Hindenburgdamm 30, D-1000 Berlin 45

Schwarz, F., Priv.-Doz. Dr. med., Medizinische Universitätsklinik, Abteilung Innere Medizin III, Kardiologie, Bergheimer Straße 58, 6900 Heidelberg, FRG

Serruys, P.W., M.D., Academisch Ziekenhuis Dijkzigt, Thoraxcenter, Postbus 1738, 3000 DR Rotterdam, The Netherlands

Seyferth, W., Dr. med., Radiologisches Zentrum, Abteilung Diagnostik, Klinikum Nürnberg, Flurstraße 17, 8500 Nürnberg, FRG

Sigwart, U., M.D., Hôpital Cantonal Universitaire, Département de Cardiologie des Services de Médicine et de Chirurgie, 1011 Lausanne, Switzerland

Silberbauer, K., Dr. med., II. Medizinische Universitätsklinik, Garnisongasse 13, 1090 Wien, Austria

Smith, H.C., M.D., Cardiovascular Division, Mayo Clinic, Rochester, MN 55901, USA

Sörensen, R., Dr. med., Abteilung für Röntgendiagnostik und chirurgische Klinik, Klinikum Steglitz der Freien Universität Berlin, Hindenburgdamm 30, D-1000 Berlin 45

Sos, Th.A., M.D., Division of Cardiovascular Radiology, The New York Hospital, Cornell Medical Center, 525 East 68th Street, New York, N.Y. 10021, USA

Stertzer, S.H., M.D., F.A.C.C., Chief, Hemodynamics Laboratory, Lenox Hill Hospital, 130 East 77th Street, New York, N.Y. 10021, USA

Stolte, M., Prof. Dr. med., Pathologisches Institut, Städtische Krankenanstalten, Kulmbacher Str. 23, 8580 Bayreuth, FRG

Tilsner, V., Prof. Dr. med., II. Medizinische Universitätsklinik des Universitäts-Krankenhauses Eppendorf, Abteilung Kardiologie, Martinistraße 52, 2000 Hamburg 20, FRG

Williams, D.O., M.D., Division of Cardiology, Rhode Island Hospital, Brown University, Providence, Rhode Island 02902, USA

Zeitler, E., Prof. Dr. med., Radiologisches Zentrum, Abteilung Diagnostik, Klinikum Nürnberg, Flurstraße 17, 8500 Nürnberg, FRG

Transluminal Angioplasty.
Development and Experiences

Percutaneous Transluminal Angioplasty

A. Grüntzig

Emory University School of Medicine, Department of Medicine, 1364 Clifton Road, Atlanta, Georgia 30322, USA

Atherosclerosis is a progressive disease for which there is still no cure. Progression of the disease may be favorably influenced by reducing the risk factors, and the sense of well-being enhanced with physical exercises. Often we are unable to control the symptoms (e.g., hypertension, angina pectoris, or intermittent claudication) and are therefore compelled to consider surgical treatment even though it is known to be only palliative.

Besides operative bypass techniques, percutaneous transluminal angioplasty (PTA) of coronary, renal, and peripheral arteries is now available. Percutaneous dilatation, first described by Charles Dotter and Melvin Judkins in their visionary communication in 1964 [1], has attracted more and more physicians throughout the world in the past years.

In most centers involved in the procedure, the dilatation is done with a double-lumen balloon catheter [2] that is introduced under local anesthesia at the groin and advanced into the different vessel areas. The balloon is filled with a contrast medium mixture and inflated to 4–10 atm. With this overpressure the atherosclerotic material is compressed and dislodged into the vessel wall, thereby partly disrupting and dissecting the intima and overstretching the media. The "controlled injury" is repaired and the inner surface of the vessel wall is smoothed in the follow-up period. The hospitalization period is only about 3–4 days. The socioeconomic and psychological advantages of the method are obvious.

General prerequisites of the application of PTA are as follows:

Results of previous invasive and noninvasive testing of the potential candidate for the procedure are shown to and discussed with the cardiac or vascular surgeon. This is important not only for goodwill and cooperation in the hospital, but also in case of complication. If the surgeon was informed about the case, the appropriate operative treatment can be performed immediately.

The possible benefits and risks of the procedure and alternative treatments available are explained to the patients. After informed consent is obtained, the procedure is performed when the surgeon, anesthesiologist, and operating room with cardiopulmonary bypass equipment are available. This is not necessary in the case of PTA of peripheral arteries. The physician starting with PTA today should be trained by centers that already have gained experience with the technique.

There are no general contraindications for the application of the technique. In proposed PTA of coronary arteries, a short history of angina pectoris is important. If

Transluminal Coronary Angioplasty and
Intracoronary Thrombolysis. Ed. by Kaltenbach et al.

the history of pain goes back for more than a year, the stenosis is most likely hardened or calcified and passage of the coronary dilatation catheter might not be possible. In case of femoropopliteal obstructions, calcifications are not so important because the antegrade puncture at the groin and the straight vessel vacilitate longitudinal force and the passage through the stenosis or occlusion.

Coronary Arteries

The indications for coronary dilatation and the success rate which can be expected are briefly as follows. The ideal candidate should have a proximal discrete stenosis, not longer than 15 mm, located in the left anterior descending, left circumflex, or right coronary artery. The patient should have clinical symptoms that compromise his quality of life and the disease should be unsatisfactorily controlled with beta-blocking agents and nitrates. The myocardial ischemia should be proven by stress test with electrocardiogram recording or thallium-201 scintigraphy. Failing medical therapy and disabling angina pectoris necessitates consideration of a blood flow augmentation procedure. The patients are therefore candidates for coronary bypass surgery. If these circumstances and anatomic conditions are given, the dilatation can be performed. These rules apply because in case of complications surgery will have been indicated for clinical reasons as well.

Since September, 1977 [4] we have had 750 cases. We were able to pass the lesion and achieve angiographic, hemodynamic, and clinical success in 630 (84%). In 6% of the cases, emergency aortocoronary bypass operations were required due to reclosure of the stenosis. The overall myocardial infarction rate (Q wave criteria) was 3%. In the follow-up period of the Swiss series (mean 24 months, range 12–48 months), 25% recurrences occured, most of which had a second dilatation. The overall continuing patency was therefore 85%.

Renal Artery Stenosis

The results of renal artery dilatation in patients with uncontrolled hypertension are very promising [5]. Percutaneous transluminal angioplasty can be done in case of discrete stenosis either of atherosclerotic or fibromuscular origin. Since 1977 we have done this in 50 patients, of whom ten had fibromuscular stenosis. According to our follow-up data (mean follow-up time, 11 months), we were able to cure the hypertension in 38%, to improve it in 37%, and could not influence the disease in 25%. The definitions of cured, improved, and unimproved are taken from Maxwell et al. [4].

Iliac and Femoropopliteal Arteries

Candidates for PTA of pelvic and leg arteries are patients with intermittent claudication, rest pain, and/or ischemic ulcer. In addition to stenoses, total occlusions can be recanalized. However, the occlusion should not exceed 10 cm, otherwise it becomes too difficult to pass the lesion [3]. Starting with Dotter's original technique in 1971, we modified the catheter in 1974 and treated 600 cases until 1980. In case of femoropopliteal obstructions, we could achieve a primary success rate of 84% and a patency rate over 3 years of 70%. In the case of iliac stenoses, the primary success rate was 92% with a long-term patency of 83%.

The results described indicate that PTA is a complement, and in properly selected cases an alternative, to reconstructive surgery. At present, this fact is still not widely accepted in the medical community. The current interest in PTA is an encouraging sign that it might become one of the standard treatments of arterial obstructive disease in the 1980s.

References

1. Dotter CT, Judkins MP (1964) Transluminal treatment of arteriosclerotic obstruction: description of a new technic and a preliminary report of its application. Circulation 30:654–670
2. Grüntzig A (1976) Die perkutane Rekanalisation chronischer arterieller Verschlüsse (Dotter-Prinzip) mit einem neuen doppel-lumigen Dilatationskatheter. Fortschr Roentgenstr 124:80–86
3. Grüntzig A (1977) Die perkutane transluminale Rekanalisation chronischer Arterienverschlüsse mit einer neuen Dilatationstechnik. G Witzstrock, Baden-Baden
4. Grüntzig A, Senning A, Siegenthaler W (1979) Nonoperative dilatation of coronary artery stenosis: Percutaneous transluminal coronary angioplasty (PTCA). N Engl J Med 301:61–68
5. Kuhlmann U, Vetter W, Furrer J, Lütolf U, Siegenthaler W, Grüntzig A (1980) Renovascular hypertension: Treatment by percutaneous transluminal dilatation. Ann Intern Med 92:1–6
6. Maxwell MH, Bleifer KH, Franklin SS, Varady P, Deegan C (1972) Cooperative study of renovascular hypertension: demographic analysis of the study. JAMA 220:1195

Transluminal Coronary Angioplasty: Results, Complications, Follow-up, and Consideration of Extension of Indications. An Analysis of 409 Procedures

S.H. Stertzer*, R.K. Myler, E. Wallsh, M.S. Bruno

St. Mary's and Lenox Hill Hospitals, San Francisco, California
and New York, New York

This communication represents the combined clinical experience in percutaneous transluminal coronary angioplasty (PTCA) collated from St. Mary's Hospital in San Francisco and the Lenox Hill Hospital Medical Center in New York. It represents all cases attempted in the 3 year period from 1 March 1978, and is the original block of PTCA material performed in the United States.

Table 1. Clinical data of patients selected for PTCA

Attempts	409
Patients	386
Male	317
Female	69
Mean age and range (years)	53 (26–82)
Functional classification	386
Class I	1 (0.2%)
Class II	159 (41%)
Class III	176 (46%)
Class IV	50 (13%)
Coronary disease	386
Single	241 (62%)
Multiple	113 (29%)
S/P CABG	32 (8%)
Vessels attempted	409
LCA	19 (5%)
LAD	272 (67%)
LCFX	19 (5%)
RCA	86 (21%)
SVG	13 (3%)

409 attempts at PTCA are described herein. Table 1 summarizes the patients' clinical data. The series consisted of 386 patients (317 male and 69 female). The mean age of all patients undergoing the procedure was 53 years. The largest group of

* Hemodynamics Laboratory, Lenox Hill Hospital, 130 East 77 th Street, New York, N.Y. 10021, USA

Transluminal Coronary Angioplasty and
Intracoronary Thrombolysis. Ed. by Kaltenbach et al.

176 subjects (46%) were in Canadian Heart Association Class III in terms of their anginal symptoms. Although 241 patients (62%) were afflicted solely with single-vessel disease, 145 (37%) of the series suffered from multivessel coronary artery disease, or had already undergone previous coronary bypass graft surgery. Two-thirds of the patients had left anterior descending coronary artery dilatations, but 86 (21%) had right coronary artery angioplasty; 19 (5%) underwent left main coronary dilatations, and 32 (8%) had left circumflex or saphenous vein dilatations. Twenty-three patients (6%) underwent multiple dilatations during the same procedure.

Figure 1 depicts a flow sheet of the overall angioplasty results. Of the 409 attempts in 386 patients, 303 lesions were passed, a 78% passage of lesion rate. The passage of lesion rate depends on the experience of the operator as well as upon the selection of the cases to be dilated. The more sagaciously a lesion is chosen for angioplasty, the safer the procedure and the more felicitous the result.

Primary angiographic success was obtained in 269 patients, representing 89% of the lesions passed and 70% of the total attempts. There were 19 cases of primary failure, where despite the lesion passage, the stenosis was too inflexible to yield to pressure of at least 6 atm. Fifteen instances (4.9%) of abrupt reclosure were also experienced in the 303 cases where the lesion was passend and the balloon inflated.

Among 99 patients (24%) where the lesion was not passed, 76 underwent elective coronary bypass graft surgery whereas 22 elected to continue medical therapy.

The data in Table 2 break down the passage of lesion rate and primary success rate into the yearly statistics for the first 36 months of the combined PTCA expe-

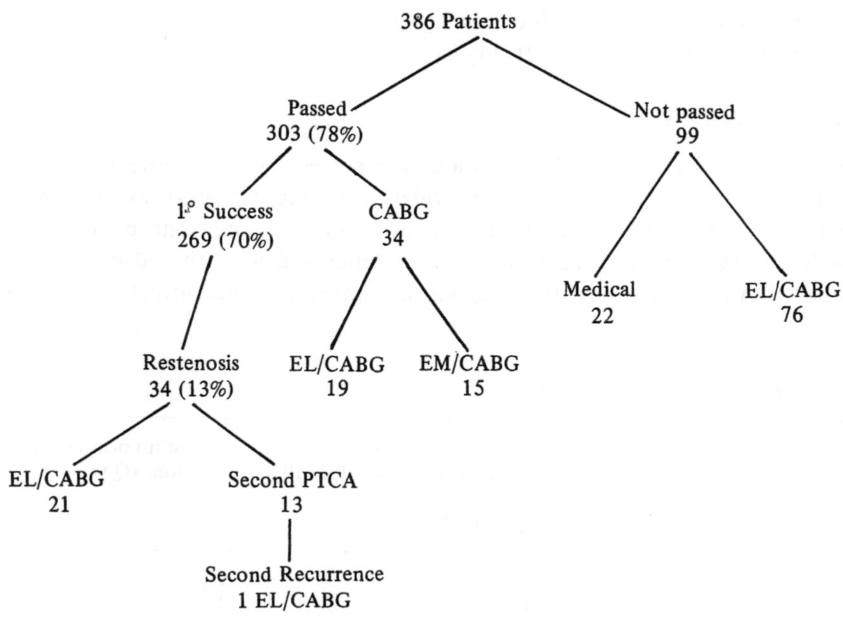

Fig. 1. Overall results of PTCA. EL/CABG, elective coronary artery bypass graft; EM/CABG, emergency coronary artery bypass graft

Table 2. Passage of lesion rate and primary success rate in the 3 years of PTCA

Year	No. of patients	Passage of lesion rate (%)	Primary[a] success rate (%)
First	56	61	50
Second	94	73	63
Third	230	86	73
Total	380	303 (78%)	269 (71%)

[a] Defined as > 20% reduction in % diameter stenosis
15 cases: (abrupt reclosure/need for EM/CABG)
19 total: (to "hard" to change diameter stenosis > 20%)

rience in the two centers. The passage of lesion rate rose sequentially from 61% to 86% during the period of observation. Correspondingly, the primary success rate (defined as greater than 20% reduction in the diameter of the stenosis as calculated by the method of Gruntzig) rose 23% over the 36 month working period.

It is of interest that independent data from the first 1000 National Heart, Lung, and Blood Institute (NHLBI) Registry cases show a distinct learning curve, wherein 60–75 cases must be performed by an angiographer before the success rate rises significantly and the complication rates fall to acceptable clinical levels.

Tables 2–4 permit analysis of the major complications of angioplasty:

1. Failure to cross and dilate
2. Abrupt reclosure sequelae:
   a) Myocardial infarction (CPK-MB or new Q wave)
   b) Emergency coronary bypass graft surgery
   c) Death
3. Recurrence (restenosis)

Complications of PTCA have been variously reported by many investigators at different levels of experience, and within widely differing complexities of lesions. In the San Francisco and New York series considered here, only one patient died within 24 h of PTCA from an accident directly connected with the adverse consequences of a PTCA attempt in the catheterization laboratory. Consequently, the recorded

Table 3. Complications in 3 years of PTCA

Year of PTCA	No. of deaths	No. of emergency coronary ortery bypass grafts	No. of CPK-MB	No. of myocardial infarctions (Q wave)
First	1	5	4	2
Second	0	5	3	1
Third	0	4	3	3
Total 409 attempts 386 patients	1 (0.2%)	14 (3.4%)	10 (2.4%)	6 (2%)

Table 4. Primary successes, recurrences, and deaths in PTCA. (Observation period 1–36 months)

Outcome	No. of patients	Remarks
Death (n = 386)	6 (1.5%)	Three patients died, after emergency bypass surgery, 2 after elective bypass surgery, and one in a car accident *not* directly connected with the adverse consequences of a PTCA attempt.
Recurrences (n = 269)	34 (13%)	Five recurrences were only partial. Twenty-one patients elected for surgery, 13 for repeated PTCA.
Success (n = 269)	247 (92%)	Total includes 12 patients who had a second PTCA

immediate mortality for PTCA as shown in Table 3 is 0.2%, or one direct fatality in 409 attempts on 386 patients. Table 3 further summarizes the emergency coronary bypass surgery rate and the myocardial infarction rate. There were 14 instances of emergency coronary bypass surgery equally distributed throughout the 3 years of PTCA activity. This represents an overall incidence of 3.4% and compares favorably with the NHLBI series of 1000 cases, where the cumulative emergency surgery rate was 5.3%. The CPK-MB elevations which were only noted in emergency coronary bypass surgery, also occurred with equal distribution over the 36 month period, and were discovered in a total of ten patients, or 2.4% of the entire series. New Q waves were seen in six patients over a 3 year period in both institutions, representing electrocardiographic evidence of infarction in 1.5% of the subjects.

Follow-up data in 269 cases where primary success was achieved is summarized in Table 4. There were six deaths in the entire series of 386 patients, representing a 1.5% mortality rate for the period under study. As previously mentioned, five of these deaths were not directly connected with the catheterization laboratory, and two were not direct sequelae of the PTCA procedure itself.

There were 34 instances (13%) of restenosis at the site of a previously successful dilatation. Five of these were partial recurrences, and 29 represented a virtual total return to the original obstructive lesion. Thirteen of these patients underwent a successful second dilatation attempt, and twelve of them remain clinically well after the repeat procedure. Twenty-one patients declined a second procedure and underwent elective coronary bypass graft surgery. The recurrence rate in the original PTCA series of 269 successful cases is 13%, some 7% lower than is presently being experienced in the NHLBI series in general.

When the successful redilatations are added to the sustained successes, a total of 247 patients remain clinically benefited from PTCA in the follow-up range from 1 week to 36 months. This 92% overall continued clinical success rate compares favorably with the 83% success rate recorded at 12 months in the NHLBI follow-up series.

In virtually all of the recurrences, the restenosis could be documented within 6 months after the PTCA procedure.

Extension of PTCA to the left main coronary artery was performed under separate protocol in 19 patients. There was a 100% passage of lesion rate, corresponding to the obvious accessibility of the main stem stenosis. No complications were observed in those cases where the main stem was protected by the presence of collateral circulation, or by a previously inserted bypass graft. In those cases where the main stem was unprotected, urgent surgery was required onces secondary to bradycardia and mild hypotension. This patient survived a double bypass graft, so that mortality in the combined San Francisco and New York serien for main stem disease remains at nil. It is, however, much too premature to include main stem PTCA in the routine armamentarium of all interventional cardiac laboratories. Not only because of its potential danger, but also because of an approximate 30% recurrence rate, left main stem PTCA should still be considered an investigative procedure.

Tandem lesions in the left anterior descending coronary artery do not appear to affect the risk of PTCA materially when the lesions are carefully selected. Calcified, tubular stenoses which are eccentrically located tend to compromise PTCA results.

Turning from the left to the right coronary, or vice versa, during the same procedure for multiple dilatations has been accomplished with success, especially from the brachial approach, yet is too premature to be considered routine. Finally, all multi vessel PTCA attempts (as well as PTCA in patients who have had previous coronary bypass surgery) must be considered in light of the potential risk incurred by abrupt reclosure. If the remainder of the patent circulation is not judged adequate by the cardiologist and surgeon to support the patient from the hemodynamics laboratory to the operating room, then PTCA should not be attempted.

As the technology of the Gruntzig method progresses over the next few years, combined perhaps with the use of streptokinase (in impending infarction), it is expected that the passage of lesion rate will increase, and the percentage of primary success in angioplasty will continue to rise in experienced laboratories.

References

1. Gruntzig A (1978) Transluminal dilatation of coronary artery stenosis. Lancet 1:263
2. Gruntzig AR et al. (1977) Coronary transluminal angioplasty. Circulation [Suppl] 84:55–56
3. Gruntzig AR, Senning A, Siegenthaler WE (1979) Nonoperative dilatation of coronary artery stenosis percutaneous transluminal coronary angioplasty. N Engl J Med 301:61–68
4. Stertzer SH, Myler RK, Bruno MS, Wallsh E (1979) Transluminal coronary artery dilatation. Pract Cardiol 5:25–32
5. Stertzer SH, Myler RK, Wallsh E, Bruno MS, DePasquale NP (1980) Dilatation of obstructed coronaries by percutaneous transluminal angioplasty. J Cardiovasc Med 5:1059–65

The National Heart, Lung, and Blood Institute Percutaneous Transluminal Coronary Angioplasty Registry: The First 1116 Cases

M.B. Mock*, K.M. Kent, L.G. Bentivoglio, P.C. Block, M. Bourassa, M.J. Cowley, K. Detre, G. Dorros, J. Gosselin, A. Grüntzig, R.K. Myler, J. Simpson, S.H. Stertzer, D.O. Williams, S.M. Mullin, B. Costa, H. Mitchell, and Participating Medical Centers**

* Department of Health, Education and Welfare, National Institute of Health, Bethesda, Maryland 20014, USA

Introduction

In 1977 Dr. Andreas Gruntzig first used the selective coronary catheter as a therapeutic tool in treating an obstructed coronary artery [1, 2]. Percutaneous transluminal coronary angioplasty (PTCA) was readily accepted as an alternative therapeutic approach to the more invasive coronary artery bypass operation in treating patients with ischemic heart disease.

In 1979 the National Heart, Lung, and Blood Institute (NHLBI) initiated a registry for patients treated with PTCA [3]. The concept and goals of a PTCA registry and the data that would be collected were discussed at a workshop on PTCA held at the National Institutes of Health in June 1979 [5]. The objective of this central registry is to provide a current, comprehensive profile of this new therapeutic procedure. The registry permits prompt identification of any untoward effects associated with PTCA and facilitates the location of investigators who are using PTCA so that they can be informed early of the incidence of serious and fatal complications. Through the central registry, both the advantages and the limitations of PTCA can be evaluated in a timely manner. The results of the first 631 patients in the registry have previously been reported [4].

** Rhode Island Hospital, Milwaukee Lutheran Hospital, Medical College of Pennsylvania, St. Mary's Hospital (San Francisco), The National Heart, Lung, and Blood Institute, Stanfort University Hospital, St. Joseph's Hospital (Atlanta), Medical College of Virginia, Massachusetts General Hospital, Albany Medical College, University of Massachusetts, Hospital of the University of Pennsylvania Medical Center, Dr. David M. Brotman Hospital (Culver City, California), Long Island Jewish Hospital, Mayo Clinic, Mt. Carmel Medical Center, Long Beach Memorial Hospital Medical Center, University of California, Davis, Presbyterian University of Pennsylvania Medical Center, University Hospital (Aachen, West Germany), Boston University Hospital, University of Frankfurt (West Germany), St. Luke's Episcopal Hospital/Texas Heart Institute, University of Michigan Medical Center, Emory University Hospital, Detroit Osteopathic Hospital, St. Luke's Hospital/Mid-American Heart Institute, Providence Medical Center, VA Medical Center-University Hospital (Gainesville), George Washington University, Northwestern Hospital (Minnesota), South Miami Hospital, Miami Heart Institute, St. Luke's Hospital (Milwaukee), VA Medical Center/University of Arkansas, Montreal Heart Institute, Scott and White Clinic, University of Wisconsin Hospital, St. Mary's Hospital (Madison, Wisconsin), University Hospital Medical Center (Augusta), Baylor University Medical Center (Dallas), Medical Center del Oro, Hahnemann Hospital, Straub Clinic and Hospital, Gundersen Clinic/LaCrosse Lutheran Hospital, Deborah Heart and Lung Center, St. Anthony Hospital System, The Christ Hospital, Ochsner Clinic, St. Francis Hospital (Wichita), Lubbock General Hospital

Transluminal Coronary Angioplasty and
Intracoronary Thrombolysis. Ed. by Kaltenbach et al.

Methods

Centers participating in the registry submit a protocol and then on standardized registry forms clinical, laboratory, and angiographic information is recorded on all patients who have PTCA and consent to be registered. The registry forms are filled out on the basis of a manual of operations provided to each investigator. Computer-generated numerical labels are supplied to each center. These labels provide a means of identifying the patients while maintaining confidentiality. Follow-up information is forwarded on registry patients annually. The centers are regularly provided with a list of the numbers of patients requiring follow-up before the follow-up is due. All forms are edited before they are entered into the databank, and the participating investigator is contacted about any item on the form in question.

Results

By February 1981, 1116 patients from 69 centers were entered in the registry.

Seventy-six percent of the patients were male. The patients' average age was 51.6 years. Forty-six percent were employed full-time at baseline evaluation (Table 1).

Two definitions of stenosis were employed. Definition 1 was reduction of vessel diameter by 70% or more, and definition 2 was reduction of vessel diameter by 50% or more. An analysis of risk factors for CAD revealed that 35% of the patients were currently smoking cigarettes, and 36% had formerly smoked cigarettes. Twenty-five

Table 1. Baseline characteristics by vessel disease (definition 2, 50%)

	Vessel disease				
Characteristics	Minimal	Single	Multiple	Left main	Total
	(*n* = 17)	(*n* = 852)	(*n* = 215)	(*n* = 27)	(*n* = 1116)
Sex					
Male	58.8	75.6	81.4	81.5	76.5
Female	35.3	22.7	16.7	18.5	21.7
Unknown	5.9	1.5	1.9	0	1.6
Age					
< 30	0	0.2	0	0	0.2
30–39	11.8	10.2	5.6	11.1	9.3
40–49	29.4	30.4	29.8	37.0	30.4
50–59	35.3	39.4	40.0	25.9	39.1
60–69	23.5	15.7	20.0	14.8	16.8
70–79	0	2.1	3.3	7.4	2.4
Unknown	0	1.9	1.4	3.7	1.9
Employment status					
Full-time	47.1	46.9	43.3	40.7	46.0
Part-time	0	4.8	5.6	0	4.7
Retired (age)	11.8	7.3	15.8	18.5	9.4
Retired (ill health)	11.8	6.6	2.3	7.4	5.8
Other	17.6	10.4	10.7	3.7	10.4
Unknown	11.8	7.3	15.8	18.5	9.4

percent of the patients had a history of a cholesterol level greater than 250 mg/dl, and 8% had a history of diabetes. Twenty-eight percent had a history of hypertension, 32% had a family history of premature coronary artery disease, and 25% had a history of a previous myocardial infarction.

Ninety-six percent of the patients presented with chest pain. Thirty-nine percent were Class III angina and 23% Class IV angina by the Canadian Heart Classification. Twenty-nine percent had had their baseline level of symptoms for less than a month (Table 2). The mean duration of angina was 4 months.

The majority of the patients (78%) had single vessel disease and 19.3% had double or triple vessel disease. Only 2.4% had left main coronary disease (Table 3). The ejection fraction was greater than 70% in 27% of the patients and less than 30% in 6% of the patients.

The most frequent obstructive lesion in which dilatation was attempted was the left anterior descending (63%). Lesions in the right coronary artery were attempted in 23% of the patients, lesions in the circumflex artery in 5%, lesions in the left main in 2%, lesions in a bypass graft in 3%, and in 5% of the patients multiple lesions were attempted (Table 4).

Table 2. Distribution of baseline symptom characteristics by vessel disease (definition 2, 50%)

	Vessel disease				
	Minimal (n = 17)	Single (n = 852)	Multiple (n = 215)	Left main (n = 27)	Total (n = 1116)
Predominant symptom					
Chest pain	94.1	97.4	93.0	96.3	96.5
Heart failure	0	0.1	0	0	0.1
Arrhythmia	0	0.2	0	0	0.2
Asymptomatic	0	0.4	2.8	0	0.8
Other	5.9	0.9	3.7	3.7	1.6
Unknown	0	0	0	0	0
Canadian Heart Classification					
I	11.8	2.7	0.5	0	2.3
II	23.5	32.3	24.2	14.8	30.2
III	35.3	38.8	39.5	55.6	39.2
IV	17.6	21.2	27.4	25.9	22.7
Unrelated to exertion	0	0.6	0	0	0.4
Not applicable	0	1.9	0.5	0	1.5
Unknown	5.9	1.8	1.4	0	1.7
Duration of present level of symptoms (months)					
⩽ 1	41.2	29.1	30.7	18.5	29.3
2	17.6	18.2	12.6	14.8	17.0
3	5.9	14.7	15.8	3.7	14.4
4–5	17.6	12.8	13.0	0	12.6
6–11	5.9	13.7	13.5	22.2	13.8
12–23	5.9	5.5	4.2	25.9	5.7
24–35	0	0.7	0.5	3.7	0.8
⩾ 36	0	0.5	0	0	0.4
Unknown	5.9	4.8	9.8	11.1	5.9
Range 1–60					
Average 4.02					

Table 3. Number of vessels diseased (n = 1116)

Definition 1 (70%)	Number of patients	Proportion of total (%)
Minimal	77	6.9
1	906	81.2
2	80	7.2
3	21	1.9
LMCA	27	2.4
Unknown	5	0.4
	1116	100.0
Definition 2 (50%)		
Minimal	17	1.5
1	852	76.3
2	174	15.6
3	41	3.7
LMCA	27	2.4
Unknown	5	0.4
	1116	100.0

Table 4. Dilatation by vessels diseased (definition 2, 50%)

	Vessel disease				
Dilatation attempted	Minimal (n = 17)	Single (n = 852)	Multiple (n = 215)	Left main (n = 27)	Total (n = 1178)
Single RCA	35.3	20.1	34.4	0	22.7
Single LMCA	5.9	0	0	62.0	1.6
Single LAD	47.1	71.4	38.6	11.0	63.2
Single CX	5.9	3.5	9.8	3.0	4.7
Single BG	5.9	2.1	4.7	3.0	2.7
Miltiple	0	2.9	12.1	18.0	5.0
Unknown	0	0	0	0	0

The overall success rate, based on at least a 20% decrease in the degree of coronary stenosis, was 62%. Evaluated by vessel, this ranged from 66% in the left anterior descending coronary artery to 33% in the circumflex artery (Table 5).

The most frequent reason cited for an unsuccessful dilatation was "too tight a stenosis", whereas the most frequent reason for the inability to dilate a lesion in which the catheter could be passed was "too rigid a lesion" (Table 6).

Four hundred and thirty-nine nonexclusive complications were reported in 216 patients (19%). The type and frequency are listed in Table 7. Of the total registry patients, myocardial infarction occurred in 4.4% during the in-hospital period. In-hospital mortality was 1.3%; 0.7% in patients without previous coronary artery bypass

Table 5. Results of dilatation (definition 2, 50%)

Dilatation successful	Vessel disease Minimal (*n* = 17)	Single (*n* = 852)	Multiple (*n* = 215)	Left main (*n* = 27)	Total (*n* = 1178)
Single RCA	66.7	57.3	50.0	0	55.7
Single LMCA	0	0	0	70.0	68.6
Single LAD	75.0	69.2	49.4	33.0	66.4
Single CX	0	40.0	28.6	0	33.3
Single BG	100.0	66.7	60.0	0	61.3
Multiple	0	48.0	46.2	40.0	45.9
Unknown	0	0	0	0	0

Table 6. Reasons for unsuccessful dilatation, by vessel disease (definition 2, 50%)

	n = No. of unsuccessful dilatations			Vessel disease	
	Minimal (*n* = 2)	Single (*n* = 128)	Multiple (*n* = 60)	Left main (*n* = 3)	Total (*n* = 193)
Inability to pass only					
Inability to enter ostium of CA	0	8	5	0	13
Inability to enter ostium of BG	0	1	0	0	1
Too tight stenosis	2	72	36	1	111
Too sharp bend	0	28	11	1	40
Technical failure	0	4	2	0	6
Other	0	24	8	1	33
	2	137	62	3	204
Inability to dilate only	(*n* = 2)	(*n* = 57)	(*n* = 27)	(*n* = 4)	(*n* = 90)
Rigidity of lesion	2	40	23	4	69
Technical failure	0	3	0	0	3
Other	0	14	5	0	19
	2	57	28	4	91
Both Inability to Pass and Inability to Dilate	1	16	11	1	29
Total number of reasons found	6	228	117	9	360

graft surgery, and 8.1% in patients with previous coronary artery bypass graft surgery (Table 8). Emergency coronary artery bypass graft surgery was performed on 6.6% of the patients during the initial hospitalization.

Seventy-five percent of the patients with a follow-up reported after PTCA had no further therapeutic procedure.

Table 7. Complications in hospital

Complication	Time after PTCA In Lab.	< 24 h	24 h–1 Wk	> 1 Wk	Total
Coronary spasm	47	0	0	0	47
Prolonged angina	62	13	7	0	82
Myocardial infarction	19	27	3	0	49
Excessive blood loss	6	3	0	0	9
Pseudoaneurysm	0	0	1	0	1
Coronary embolization	3	0	0	0	3
Ventricular fibrillation	15	2	1	0	18
Ventricular tachycardia	4	2	0	0	6
Hypotension	17	6	0	0	23
Bradycardia	13	2	0	0	15
Coronary occlusion	50	0	0	0	50
Prolonged symptoms	0	0	0	0	0
Arterial thrombosis					
Requiring surgery	0	4	4	0	8
Resulting in loss of limb	0	0	0	0	0
Death	3	17	1	2	13
Other	27	8	3	3	41
Emergency bypass surgery	0	0	0	0	74
Totals	266	84	20	5	439

Table 8. Deaths: clinical summary

Age/sex		No. of Vessels diseased	Previous CABG	Vessel dilatation attempted	CABG	Complications
Deaths directly related to PTCA						
39	F	2	–	LAD	Emergency	LM dissection
42	M	3	+	LM	No	Angina: "spasm"
56	M	1	–	LAD	Emergency	Angina, Postoperative MI
64	F	1	–	CIRC	Emergency	Hypotension, LM thrombus
40	F	1	–	LAD	Emergency	LM dissection
Deaths probably related to PTCA						
49	F	1	+	DIAG	Elective	Dissection, arrest: induction
49	F	1	0	RCA	Emergency	"Spasm" postoperatively
55	M	1	0	RCA	Emergency	"Spasm" 9 h after operation
62	M	2	+	RCA graft (not entered)	Elective	Hypotension: induction
54	M	1	0	LAD	Emergency	Respiratory failure 14 days after operation
57	M	3	+	LAD	Elective	Postoperative MI
Deaths probably unrelated to PTCA						
56	F	3	+	RCA	Elective	RV perforation
46	M	3	0	LAD-CIRC	Elective	Disseminated intravascular coagulation

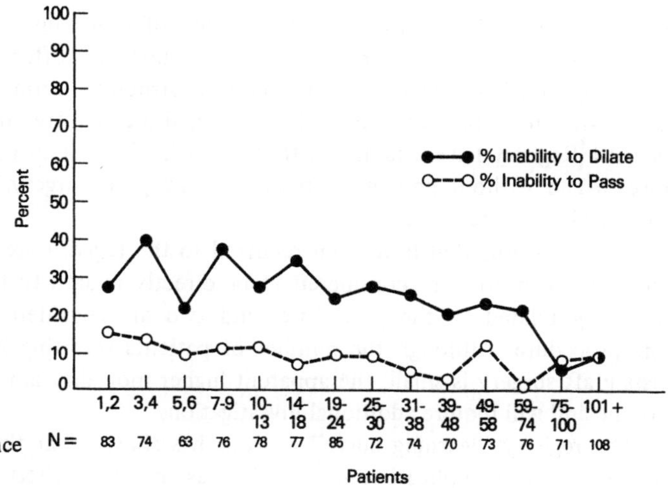

Fig. 1. The learning experience of dilatation

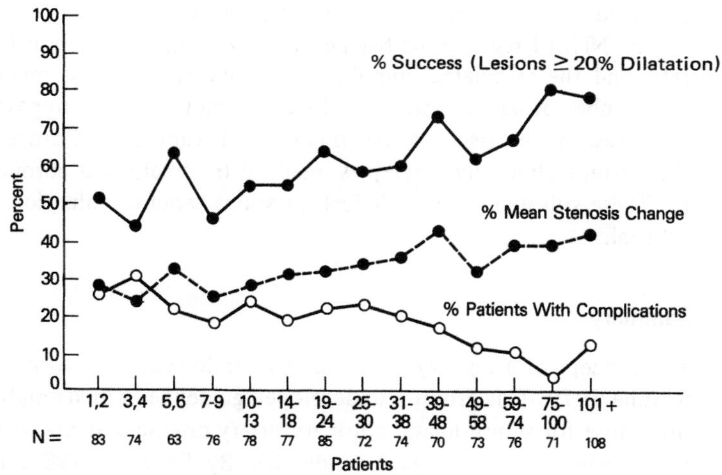

Fig. 2. The learning experience based on outcome

An analysis based on time of performance of PTCA was done to determine learning experience. Figure 1 shows the learning experience of dilatation, and Fig. 2 shows the learning experience based on outcome.

Discussion

Coronary heart disease is the predominant form of heart disease in the Western World, and most symptomatic patients can be shown to have an obstruction in a coronary artery. Since the introduction of the coronary artery bypass operation for the treatment of obstructive coronary artery disease, the annual number of these operations performed has been increasing steadily. Currently, over 110,000 such operations are performed each year in the United States alone, at a cost of approximately one billion dollars per year. Percutaneous transluminal coronary angioplasty offers a less invasive and less costly approach to treating symptomatic obstructive coronary disease in certain patients who have failed to respond to maximal medical treatment. The data from the NHLBI Registry have established that the risk of PTCA in patients with single vessel disease and without previous coronary bypass graft surgery is equivalent to that for primary bypass graft surgery.

The 13 deaths that have been reported to the registry are summarized in Table 8. Five of the deaths are considered to be directly related to the PTCA procedure, six probably related to the procedure, and two are considered probably unrelated to the procedure. Although the number of patients receiving PTCA after previous bypass graft surgery is small, the apparent higher mortality among these patients is worrisome and will require additional investigation.

The registry "learning curve" analysis has shown that the success rate is increasing while the complication rate is decreasing. The registry experience has enabled those angiographers adopting the technique to gain from the large prior experience collected, analyzed, and reported by the registry.

The NHLBI registry has been extremely valuable in demonstrating the early success rate, and the associated complications such as mortality, myocardial infarction, and the number of patients who require emergency coronary bypass surgery. It is not likely to resolve the issue of the long-term efficacy of this procedure in comparison to the current alternative therapies, medical treatment and coronary bypass graft surgery. These still unanswered clinical questions require evaluation in a randomized clinical trial.

Summary

The concept of a registry for PTCA was endorsed by a workshop held at the NHLBI in June 1979. This group also developed guidelines which emphasized the value of the procedure for symptomatic coronary artery disease patients with single vessel obstructive disease.. who are surgical candidates. By February 1981, 1116 patients from 69 centers were enrolled in the registry.

The mean age was 51.6 years and the mean duration of angina was 4 months. Seventy-eight percent of the patients had single vessel disease, 19.3% had double or triple vessel disease and 2.4% had left main disease.

Percutaneous transluminal coronary angioplasty was considered successful if at least a 20% decrease in degree of coronary stenosis was obtained. Overall, 61.9% of the stenosed lesions were successfully treated.

In the in-hospital period, 1.3% of the patients died; 0.7% of those without previous coronary artery bypass graft surgery and 8.1% of those with previous coronary artery bypass graft surgery. Myocardial infarction occurred in 4.4% of the patients in the in-hospital period. Emergency coronary artery bypass graft surgery was performed on 6.6% of the patients during the initial hospitalization.

Seventy-five percent of the patients with a follow-up reported after PTCA had no further therapeutic procedure. Four percent underwent repeat PTCA and 14% had late coronary artery bypass graft surgery.

The cooperation of a large number of centers from the United States, Canada, and Europe has permitted a timely evaluation of the safety and efficacy of a new procedure for treating obstructive coronary disease and has permitted an evaluation of a learning curve for the technique. Another workshop on the technique was planned for June 1981 at the National Institutes of Health in Bethesda, Maryland, United States of America, to review the status of the registry and to reevaluate the current indications for PTCA.

References

1. Gruntzig AR, Turina MI, Schneider JA, (1976) Experimental percutaneous dilatation of coronary artery stenosis. Circulation [Abstr] 54:81
2. Gruntzig AR, Senning A, Silgenthaler WE (1979) Non-operative dilatation of coronary artery stenosis. Percutaneous transluminal coronary angioplasty. N Engl J Med 301:61–68
3. Levy RI, Mock MB, Willman VL, Frommer PL (1979) Percutaneous transluminal coronary angioplasty. N Engl J Med 301:301–103
4. NHLBI (to be published) Report on Percutaneous transluminal coronary angioplasty. Circulation
5. US Dept HEW (1980) Proceedings of the workshop on percutaneous transluminal coronary angioplasty. NIH Publ 80:2030

Immediate and Late Results of Percutaneous Transluminal Coronary Angioplasty

W. Porstmann, A.R. Parsi, P. Romaniuk, H.J. Pech, H. Eger

Institute of Cardiovascular Diagnostic, Humboldt University, Charité, Schumannstr., Berlin

Percutaneous transluminal angioplasty (PTA) is intimately linked with the name of CT Dotter [1]. In the late 1960s we introduced with good results our caged balloon (to treat occlusions of pelvic and lower extremity arteries) [5]. The development of newer types of catheter by Dr. Grüntzig has resulted in a major breakthrough and the present significance of PTA [3]. He was the first to dilate a coronary stenosis successfully [2]. Although more than a thousand patients worldwide have so far been treated by percutaneous transluminal coronary angioplasty (PTCA), it is still a method that must be used with great caution if it is not going to fall into disrepute [4, 6]. Only a prolonged period of objective analysis of all results will allow us do define more clearly its indications and contraindications. During the last 2 1/2 years we have applied PTCA only 40 times. We have selected patients who would otherwise have had to undergo bypass procedures.

Thirty-seven patients were identified presenting indications for PTCA according to our approach. They were among 826 patients who had undergone coronarography for ischemic heart disease during the previous 2 1/2 years, an incidence of 5%. Grüntzig's stringent criteria must be considered as an ideal model: we did not apply a number of them. Primarily we based ourselves on the clinical presence of angina pectoris refractory to medication in combination with a single centrally located coronary artery stenosis. In only one-third of our patients was the duration of angina pectoris less than a year. The mean duration of angina pectoris of all treated patients was 2 1/2 years. The higher incidence of good results was in the group of patients with a short history, but our results are primarily good in 50% of patients with a longer history.

Seventeen of 37 patients had a history of infarcts. Twenty-two revealed kinetic disturbances at ventriculography. The mean age of all patients was 47 1/2 years. All these figures indicate the great difficulty in trying to adhere to the initial stringent criteria.

From October 1978 to the end of April 1981 we had 15 failures and 22 successful interventions. In three patients we performed a second successful PTCA. Two patients, after initially good clinical and morphologic results, required bypass operation 3 and 5 months later respectively. One patient died 4 months after a second PTCA, the exact cause of death being unknown. From the 22 patients who underwent a primary procedure, with a mean follow-up period of 15 months (2–29 months), there remains a group of 19 with a good result of PTCA judged by subjective and objective criteria. In this group no new infarcts have developed. We are trying to find an explanation for

Transluminal Coronary Angioplasty and
Intracoronary Thrombolysis. Ed. by Kaltenbach et al.

the relatively high incidence of primary failures (one-third) in spite of a stringent consideration of morphologic indications.

We did not sufficiently consider and appreciate tortuosities in the immediate vicinity of a stenosis. They present one of the main obstacles. Fequently they can only be recognized in an angulated projection.

In individual instances we attempted to enter stenotic areas located too far peripherally and with too narrow a lumen, usually without success.

Calcifications within the area of stenosis present a major obstacle. Eccentric stenoses can be dilated – in our experience stenoses of the LAD directly behind the origin of an open side branch result in failure in all cases. The balloon catheter will always enter the side branch. We consider this anatomic constellation as an absolute contraindication. Stenotic lesions within a vascular portion devoid of side branches, however, can be catheterised.

A seemingly good coronarographic documentation of a stenosis cannot by itself be accepted as a guarantee that it can be passed. We must anticipate the possible presence of fibrotic narrowing preventing successful dilatation. In such a situation only the attempt to dilate will give the answer.

One observation of a 48-year-old man with severe angina pectoris and a filiform left stem stenosis should be emphasized. We could not insert the diagnostic catheter into the left ostium. The guidewire, however, slipped through this extremly stenotic portion. In this situation we pressed special diagnostic catheters with tapered ends, sizes 7–10, over the guidewire and through the stenotic lesion. Subsequently balloon dilatation could be performed. It is thus possible to alter a stenotic lesion from impassable to passable for a balloon catheter. Dotter's old concept of dilatation still has its significance today.

A special problem is the recognition of coronary spasms. These are frequently located in the vicinity of true organic lesions. Errors are known from bypass surgery. PTCA frequently leads to spasms within the abnormal arterial segment despite generous application of nitroglycerin. We have observed several instances of initially extreme stenoses subsequent to PTCA being relieved by nitroglycerin. Differentiation between spasms and anatomic narrowing under the conditions of PTCA is truly an important and as yet unsolved problem. So far we do not have any personal experience in the dilatation of bypass stenosis.

Some Comments on Pressure Readings

For the evaluation of the results of PTCA neither determination of the pressure gradient nor percentage evaluation of the degree of stenosis can serve as reliable parameters. The decisive factor must remain influence on the patient's symptoms. We thus have to ascertain the complete disappearance or decline of symptoms of angina pectoris, a decreased need for nitroglycerin, an improved stress tolerance, and finally local improvements at subsequent coronarography and ventriculography.

A Final Word on Complications

Among our 37 patients one died 6 months after PTCA. In three patients we observed occlusion of the LAD or the RCA during PTCA, resulting in an infarct. These patients were immediately operated upon. Dissection of one LAD later resulted in occlusion but this without clinical signs of a new infarct. The majority of patients with a primarily unsuccessful PTCA, but not all, were operated on at a later time. On the basis of the postulates of Grüntzig and experience gained by others as well as our own, we are definitely of the opinion that without sufficient surgical back-up, promptly available, performance of PTCA cannot be justified.

In conclusion, we can state that:

1. In individual selected patients PTCA offers a true alternative to bypass surgery.
2. Of the patients conforming to the presently accepted indications for coronarography, from 5% to a maximum of 10% are amenable to PTCA.
3. Long-term follow-up, up to 29 months confirms that a prolonged good result is possible.

To arrive at a definitive evaluation, however, longer follow-up periods are required.

References

1. Dotter CT, Judkins MP (1964) Transluminal treatment of arteriosclerotic obstruction. Circulation 30:654–670
2. Grüntzig AR (1978) Transluminal dilatation of coronary artery stenosis. Lancet 1:263
3. Grüntzig A, Hopff H (1974) Perkutane Rekanalisation chronischer arterieller Verschlüsse mit einem neuen Dilatationskatheter. Modifikation der Dotter-Technik. Dtsch Med Wochenschr 99:2502–2510
4. Kaltenbach M, Kober G, Scherer D (1980) Mechanische Dilatation von Koronararterienstenosen (Transluminale Angioplastie). Z Kardiol 69:1–10
5. Porstmann W (1973) Ein neuer Korsett-Ballon-Katheter zur transluminalen Rekanalisation nach Dotter unter Berücksichtigung von Obliterationen an den Beckenarterien. Radiol Diagn (Berl) 14:239–244
6. Porstmann W, Parsi AR, Romaniuk P, Pech HJ (1979) Die perkutane transluminale Koronar-Angioplastik – ein Katheterverfahren zur Behandlung singulärer Koronararterienstenosen. Dtsch Gesundheitswes 34:1224–1229

Transluminal Coronary Angioplasty: Transbrachial Approach and Prevention of Thromboembolic Complications*

M. Kaltenbach, G. Kober, D. Scherer

Department of Cardiology, Zentrum der Inneren Medizin, Klinikum der Johann Wolfgang Goethe-Universität, Theodor-Stern-Kai 7, 6000 Frankfurt a.M. 70, FRG

Starting in October 1977, transluminal coronary angioplasty (TCA) [1] was performed predominantly using the transbrachial approach [2]. This approach was preferred because at the end of the procedure the brachial artery can be closed with sutures. Therefore even with intensive antithrombotic medication no danger of arterial bleeding exists; reversal of heparin effect by administration of protamine sulfate is not necessary. Prophylaxis of thromboembolic complications was considered essential because after creating a "controlled intimal injury" of a coronary artery the tendency to thrombotic reocclusion must be considered as critical.

Methods

Catheters

Preshaped French 8 catheters were used. The catheters for the right coronary artery were applied in three different sizes, for the left coronary artery in five different sizes, according to the individual patient (Fig. 1).[1]

Prevention of Thromboembolism

At the beginning of the procedure heparin was given via the brachial artery in a dose of 100 U/kg body wt. If the procedure exceeded 1 h, half this dose was given hourly. In addition to heparin, the patients received 1.5 g acetylsalicylic acid/day, including the days before, during, and after the procedure. Instead of a second bolus injection, more recently a continuous infusion 4000 U/h trough a Y connection of the guiding catheter was used.

---

* This study was supported by the Bundesministerium für Forschung und Technologie with grant NT/A – MT 0316 – 01 ZJ 0496.

[1] The catheters are commercially available from Schneider-Medintag, Zürich, Witkonerstr. 289, CH 8047 Zürich/Switzerland.

Transluminal Coronary Angioplasty and Intracoronary Thrombolysis. Ed. by Kaltenbach et al.

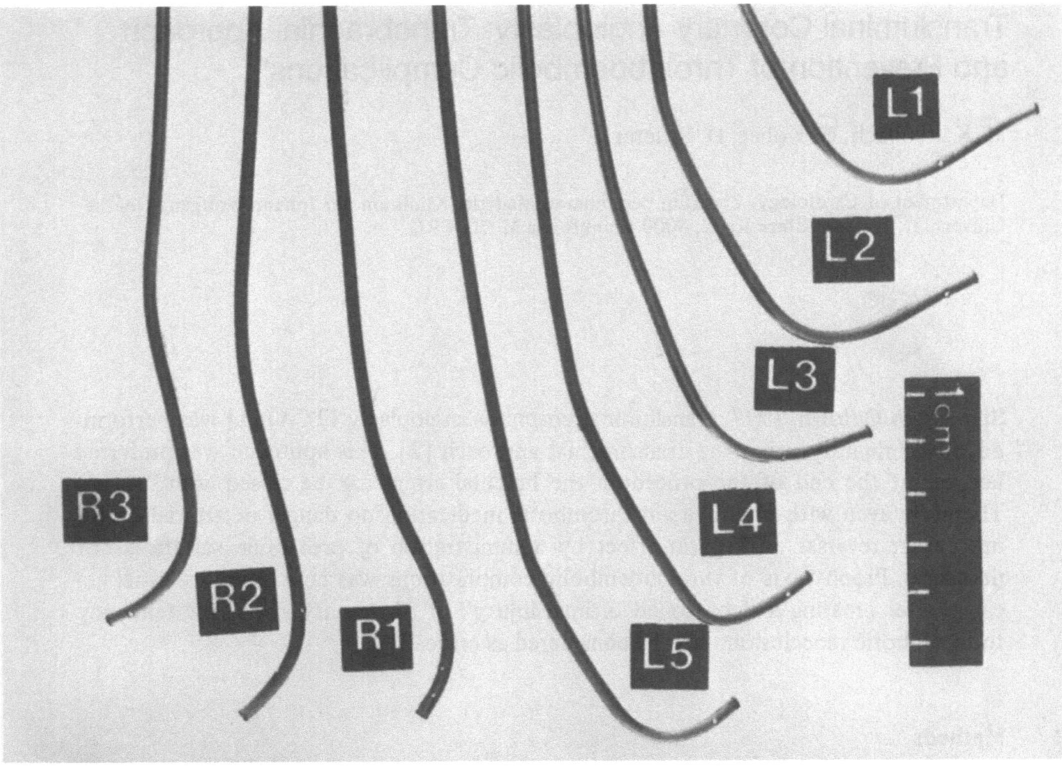

Fig. 1. Preshaped guiding catheters for the transbrachial approach in three sizes for the right and in five sizes for the left coronary artery

Prevention of Coronary Artery Spasm

After left ventricular pressure measurements and a preliminary coronary arteriogram the patient received nitroglycerin as well as nifedipine. Nitroglycerin was administered intracoronarily in a dose of 1.5 mg, nifedipine sublingually in a dose of 2 × 10 mg or intracoronarily in a dose of 0.1 mg. After this medication the coronary arteriogram was repeated. TCA was only performed if after the coronary dilating medication a high-grade (⩾ 70%) stenosis remained.

Long-term Treatment

The patients were kept on acetylsalicylic acid 1.5 g/day as antithrombotic medication; no Coumadin was given. In addition a medication for the prophylaxis of coronary artery spasm was maintained, consisting of isosorbide dinitrate orally 120 mg/day plus verapamil orally 480 mg/day or nifedipine orally 60 mg/day.

Beta-blockers were considered contraindicated. No digitalis was administered.

Localization of Stenosis, Extent of Coronary Artery Disease, Patients

The attempted stenosis was localized in the LAD in 96 instances, in the RCA in 34, in an aortocoronary bypass in seven and in the circumflex branch in five; 107 patients presented with single-vessel disease, 28 with double- and 17 with triple-vessel disease. Age ranged from 30 to 65 years with a mean of 48 years; 83% were male, and 17% female.

Results

From October 1977 to May 1981 152 attempts were performed. The transbranchial approach was used 148 times and the transfemoral approach four times. In 105 attempts the stenosis was passed with the balloon catheter; in 87 of these attempts a successful dilatation of the stenosis was achieved. In 47 attempts the stenosis was not passed with the balloon catheter. In 21 of these it could not be reached, either because the guiding catheter could not be selectively positioned or stabilized in the ostium, or because the corresponding coronary branch could not be selectively catheterized. In 14 instances the balloon catheter was advanced to the attempted stenosis, but could not be passed through. Usually, the wire tip and the hole for pressure measurements entered the stenosis but the hull of the balloon did not pass. In the 12 other unsuccessful attempts, the anatomy of the attempted stenosis had changed since the first arteriogram from which the indication for the procedure was made: in four instances a coronary spasm appeared to be the predominant mechanism for the stenosis, in the other eight instances the high-grade stenosis had progressed to total occlusion since the first arteriogram. The mean interval between the two arteriograms was 3 months (Fig. 2).

Successful Attempts

In 87 attempts the stenosis was successfully dilated ($\geqslant$ 20%). The stenosis diameter, judged on the projection with the highest degree of obstruction, was reduced on average from 80% to 40%. This reduction in stenosis diameter corresponds to an ninefold increase in the obstructed vessel cross-sectional area. Applying the law of Hagen and Poiseuille, an increase in coronary flow as great as 81-fold can be calculated if constant perfusion pressure is assumed. (Fig. 3).

Functional results of dilatation were uniformly in good agreement with the angiographic success. Besides subjective improvement in anginal pain, patients displayed loss of ST depression in the exercise electrocardiogram and normalization of thallium-201 scan and nuclear ventriculography during exercise [3].

Impressive results were achieved in all regions of the coronary arteries, as shown by a few examples:

Figure 4 shows the coronary arteriogram of a 48-year-old male with high-grade left main stenosis who suffered from severe angina at exercise and at rest. After successful dilatation the symptoms disappeared. The coronary arteriogram 1 year after TCA showed normal coronary arteries with no remaining stenosis in the left main stem.

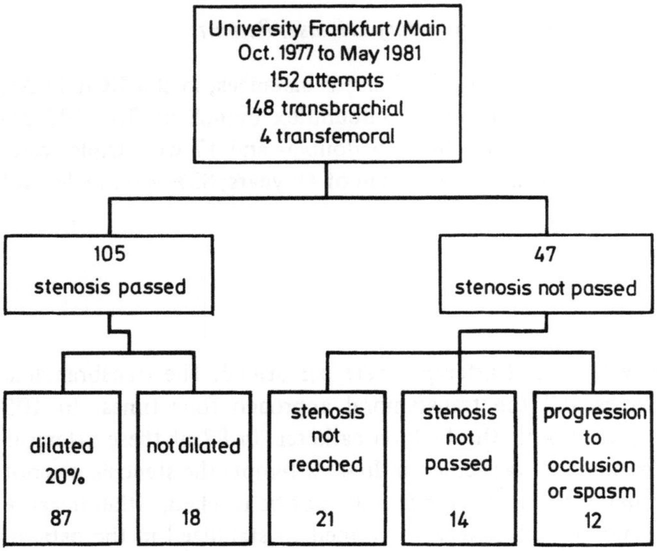

Fig. 2. Results of the first 152 TCA attempts 300 procedures were performed by June 1982

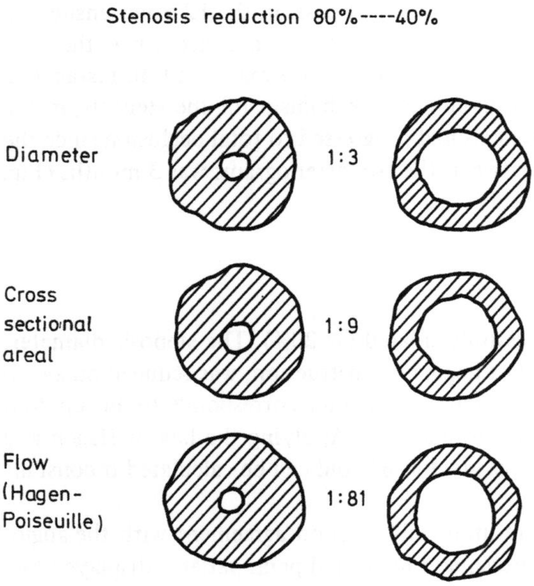

Fig. 3. Average stenosis reduction in 87 successful PTCA procedures from 80% to 40%, showing the corresponding increase in diameter, cross-sectional area, and flow

In Fig. 5 a high-grade distal RCA stenosis from another 48-year-old man is shown. The exercise electrocardiogram reveals ischemic ST depression which occurred together with typical exertional angina. TCA was performed with the balloon catheter advanced through the whole length of the RCA. After successful dilatation the patient be-

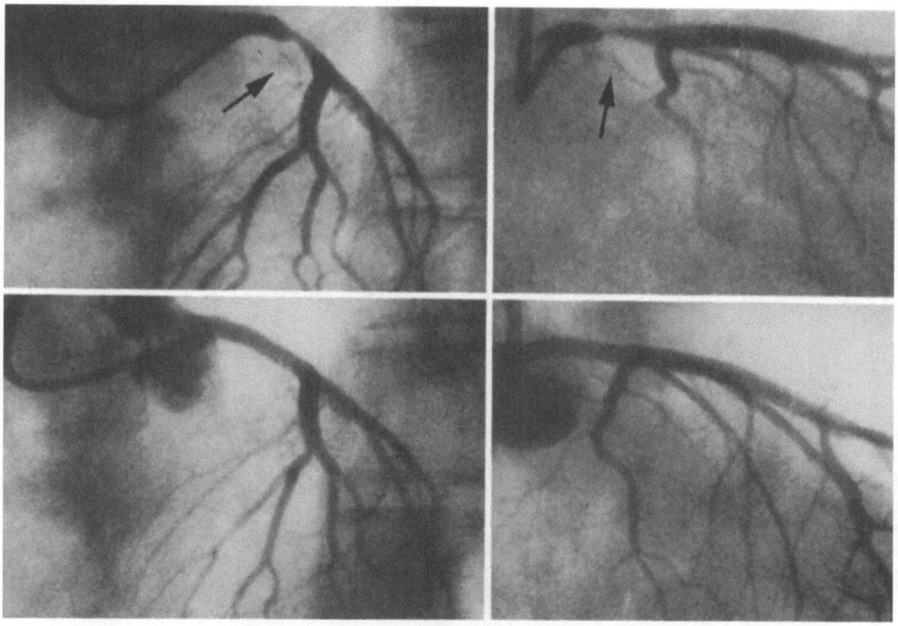

Fig. 4. Ei. T., 48-year-old man. Left main stenosis with severe angina. After TCA complete release of symptons. Normal coronary arteriogram 1 year after TCA *(bottom)*

came symptom-free and the exercise electrocardiogram normalized completely even at a very high level of exercise. The control arteriogram 1 year after TCA shows only very little remaining stenosis at the site of dilatation. This result was confirmed by a third angiogram 3 years after TCA.

Totally occluded vessels were seldom approached. In the patient illustrated in Fig. 6, a very fresh occlusion was apparent from the patient's history and the previous arteriogram. The balloon catheter was easily advanced through the obstruction and the vessel could be reopened. The control arteriogram showed a good result and the left cineventriculogram revealed a normalization of left ventricular contraction in the diaphragmatic wall, which was akinetic before. A few weeks later, however, anginal symptoms reappeared. A second control arteriogram showed restenosis but no occlusion and unimpaired left ventricular function. In this instance, no redilatation was attempted; the patient received an aortocoronary bypass without further difficulties. Up to 1982 8 patients with total obstructions were attempted. In 50% the procedure was successful.

The patient whose arteriogram is shown in Fig. 7 had severe triple-vessel disease with occlusion of the RCA and LAD and high-grade CX stenosis. Coronary surgery with a bypass to LAD and CX was performed. The patient became symptom-free. Half a year later, however, severe angina reoccurred; the control arteriogram revealed an occluded CX bypass. Successful dilatation of the CX stenosis was performed. The patient experienced dramatic improvement which 2 years later is still completely maintained.

The patient shown in Fig. 8 also had severe triple-vessel disease; despite occlusion of all the three coronary branches left ventricular function was well conserved. After

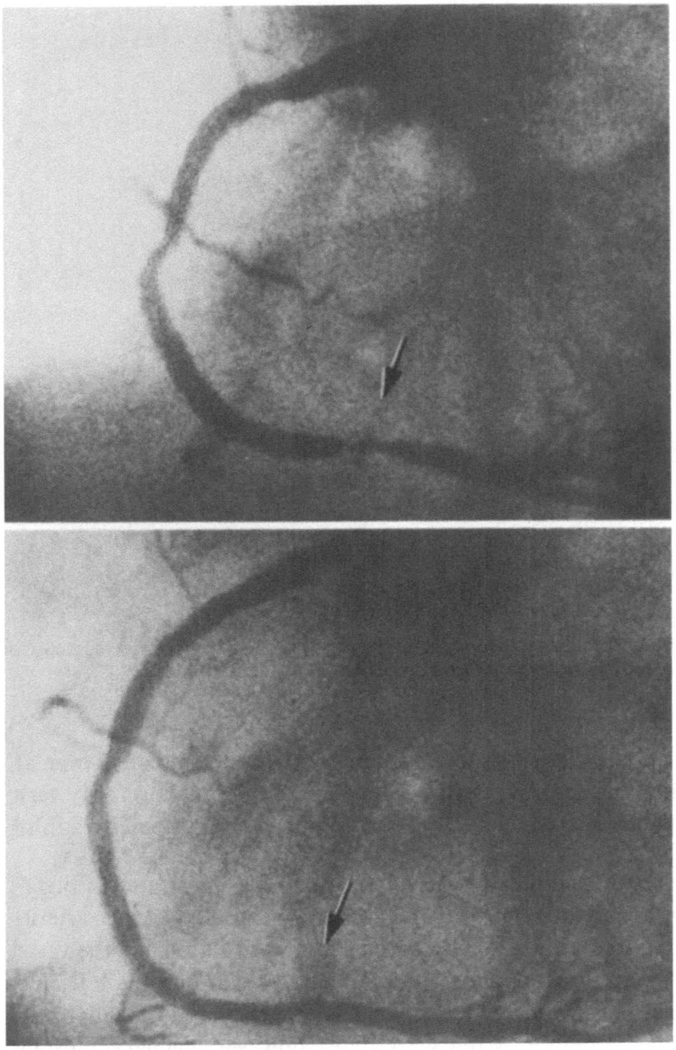

Fig. 5a

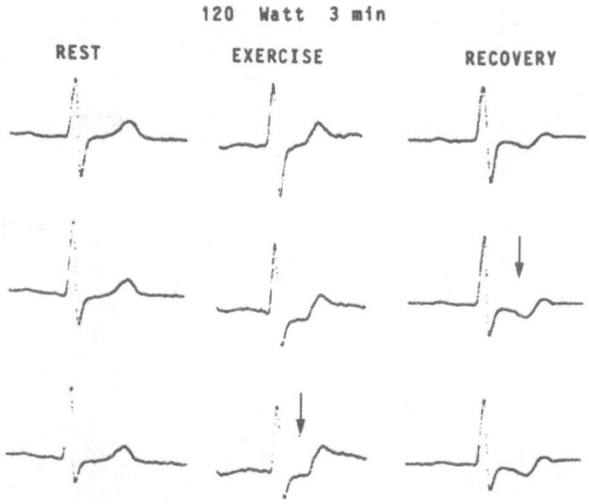

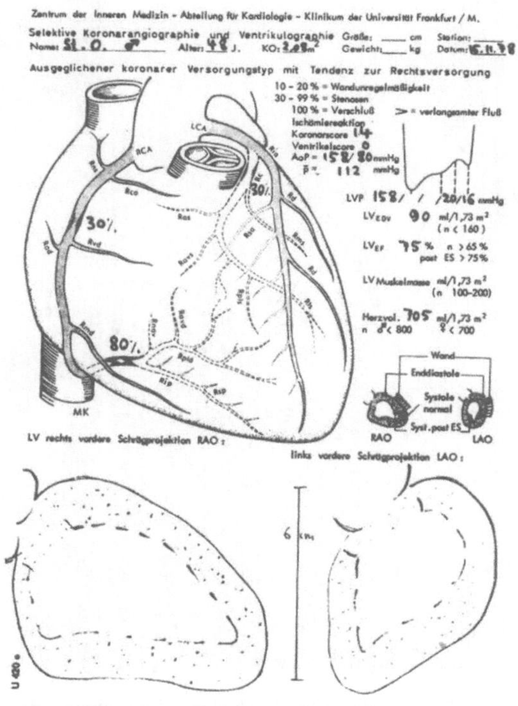

Fig. 5 b

Fig. 5a, b. St. O., 48-year-old man. Isolated severe stenosis in the distal part of the RCA. One year after successful angioplasty the stenosis has almost disappeared (*bottom*). Complete release from preexisting stress angina (see ECG)

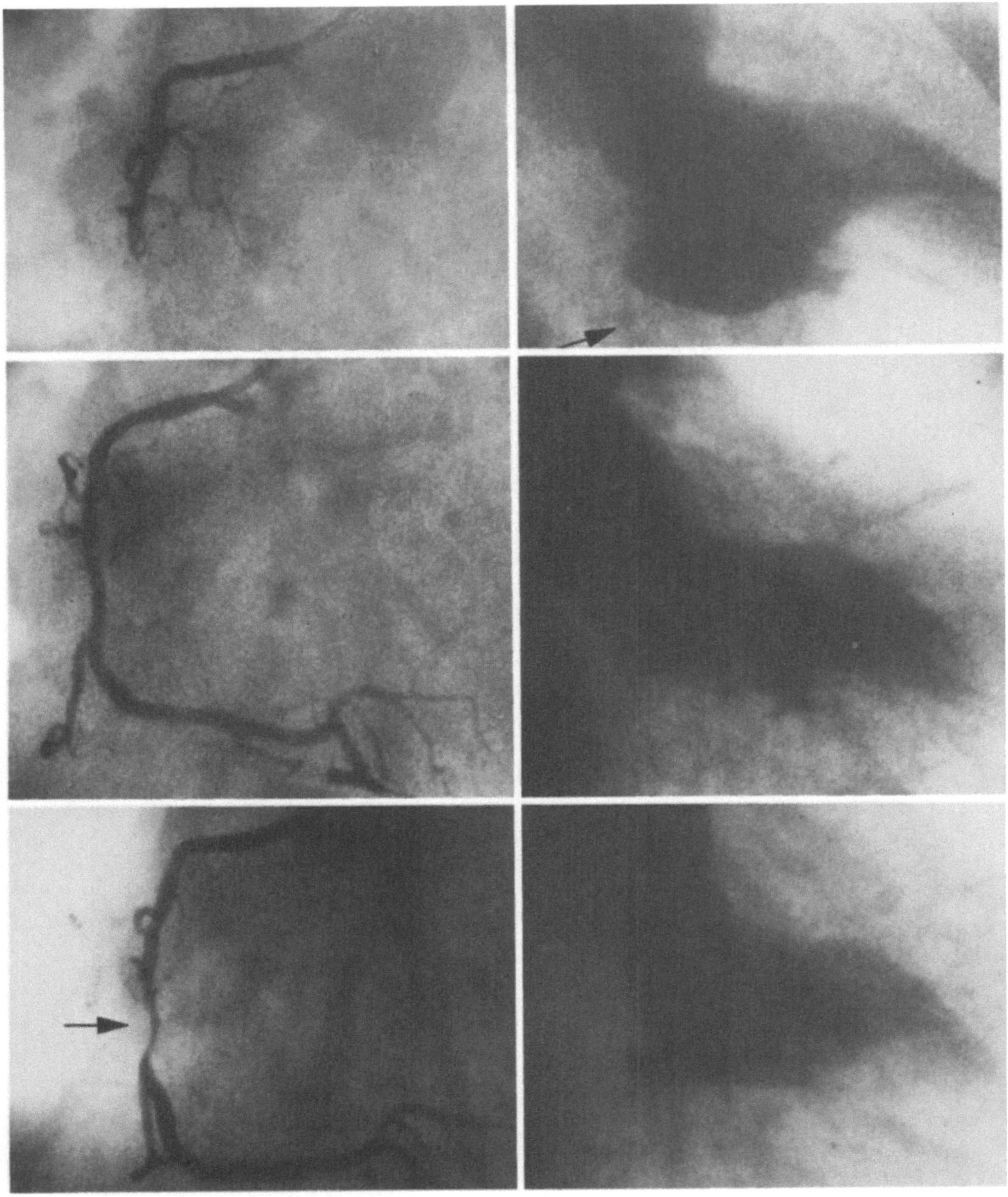

Fig. 6. G. 52-year-old man. Occlusion of dominant RCA with akinesis in the diaphragmatic wall of the left ventricle (*rop, arrow*). Six weeks after PTCA (*middle*) open RCA, normalization of left ventricular contraction. Some weeks later reoccurrence of angina with RCA restenosis. Aortocoronary bypass grafting was performed.

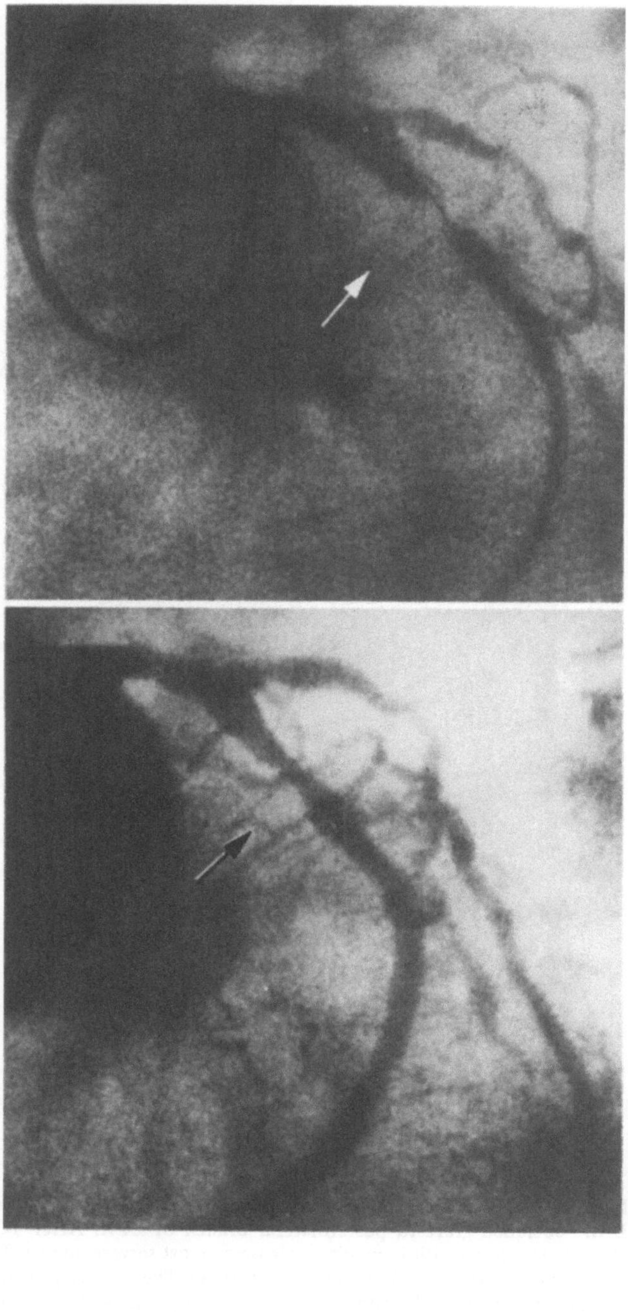

Fig. 7a

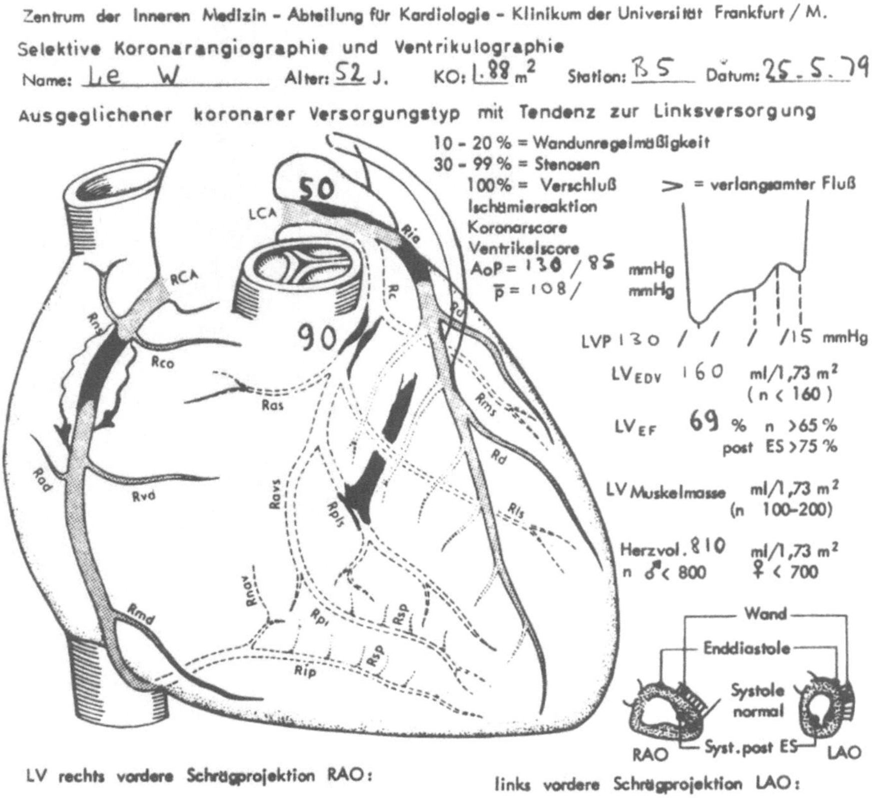

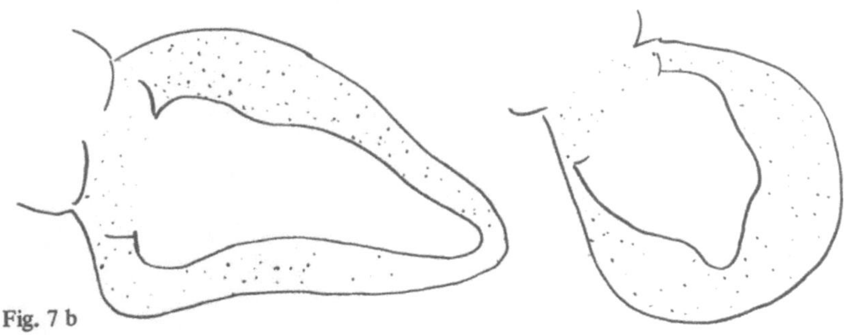

Fig. 7 b

Fig. 7a, b. Le. F. 53-year-old man. Severe stenosis in LCX. Open aortocoronary bypass graft to LAD, occluded graft to posterolateral branch of LCX. After TCA significant dilatation of LCX stenosis (*bottom*) with immediate release of most servere angina. This patient developed recurrence of angina pectoris in 1982 (3 years after TCA). The coronary arteriogram showed the dilated vessel completely open at the site of TCA; however, a new stenosis in the distal RCX was present. A second TCA was successfully performed, after which the patient became again symptom-free

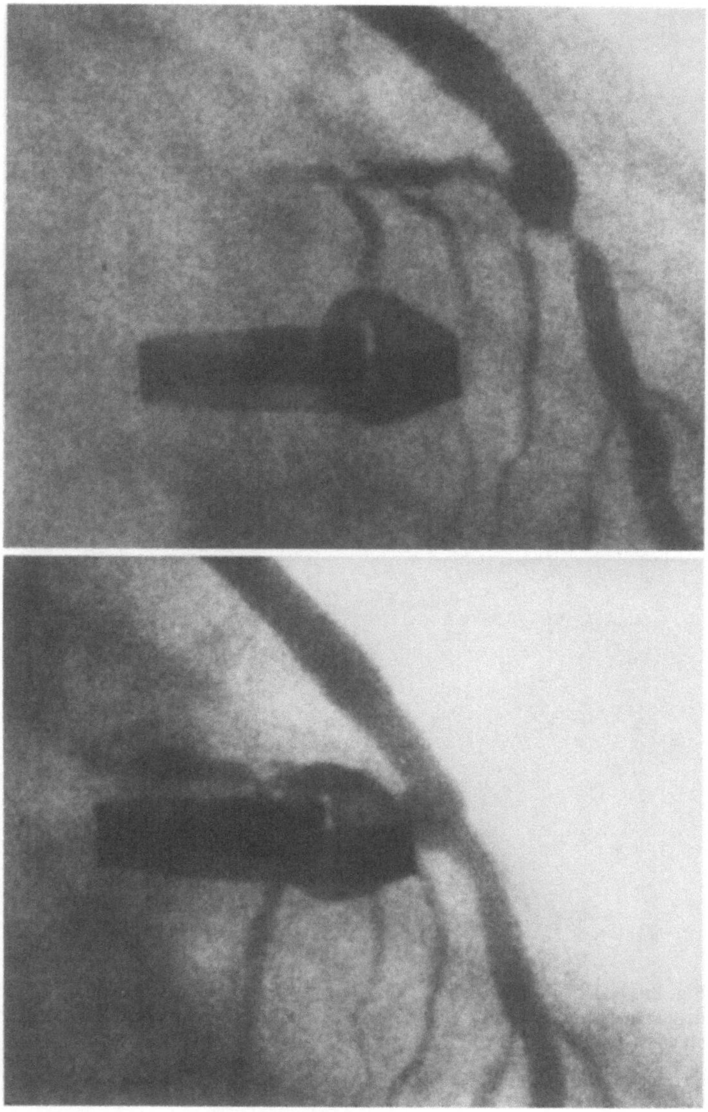

Fig. 8a

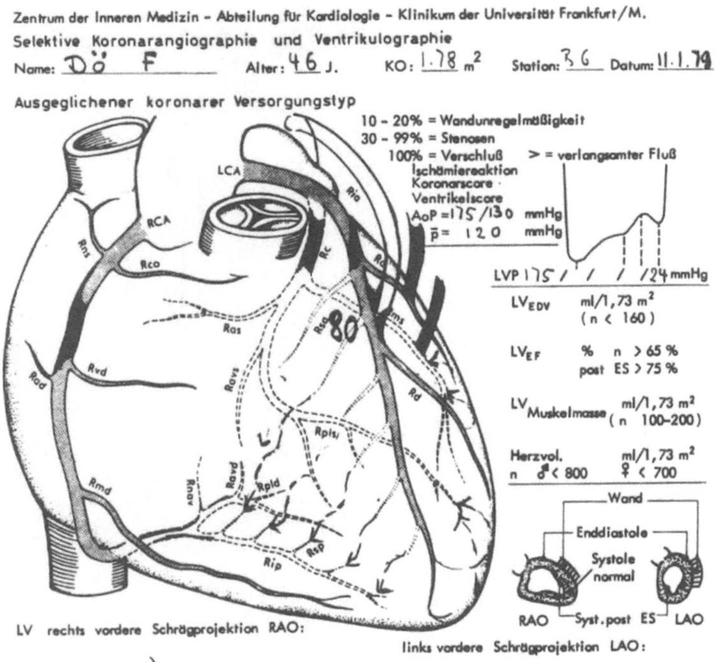

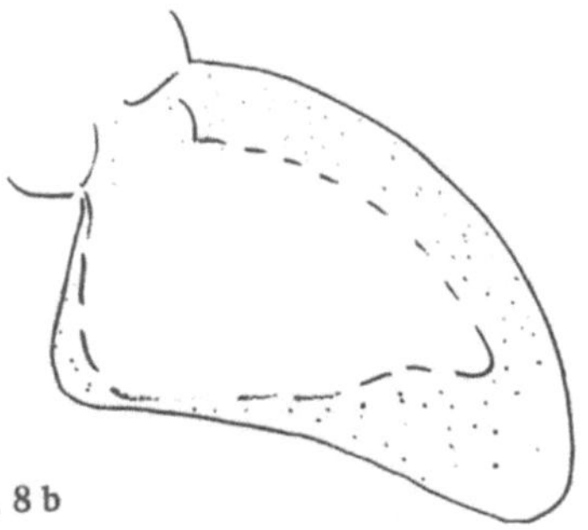

Fig. 8 b

Fig. 8a, b. Dö. F. 46-year-old man. Severe stenosis in aortocoronary bypass to LAD at the site of distal anastomosis. After successful TCA in the 1 year control angiogram *(bottom, a)* no more stenosis

surgery the patient's symptoms improved; several months later however, deterioration was apparent. The arteriogram revealed occluded bypasses to a diagonal and marginal branch, the LAD bypass showed critical stenosis at the site of distal anastomosis. This stenosis was successfully dilated. The patient improved remarkably. The control arteriogram 1 year after dilatation showed no more stenosis, the patient remained stable and has remained so for more than 2 years now.

In Fig. 9 a high-grade LAD stenosis is shown. In this patient the electrocardiogram during exercise with a load of only 50 watts performed over 2.5 min revealed marked ST elevation with severe angina. After successful dilatation anginal pain disappeared and the exercise electrocardiogram normalized.

In Fig. 10 the findings in a 46-year-old man with subtotal LAD stenoses are shown. He had severe exertional angina. Radionuclide ventriculography revealed during 90 watts a decrease of ejection fraction from 67% to 45%. After successful dilatation

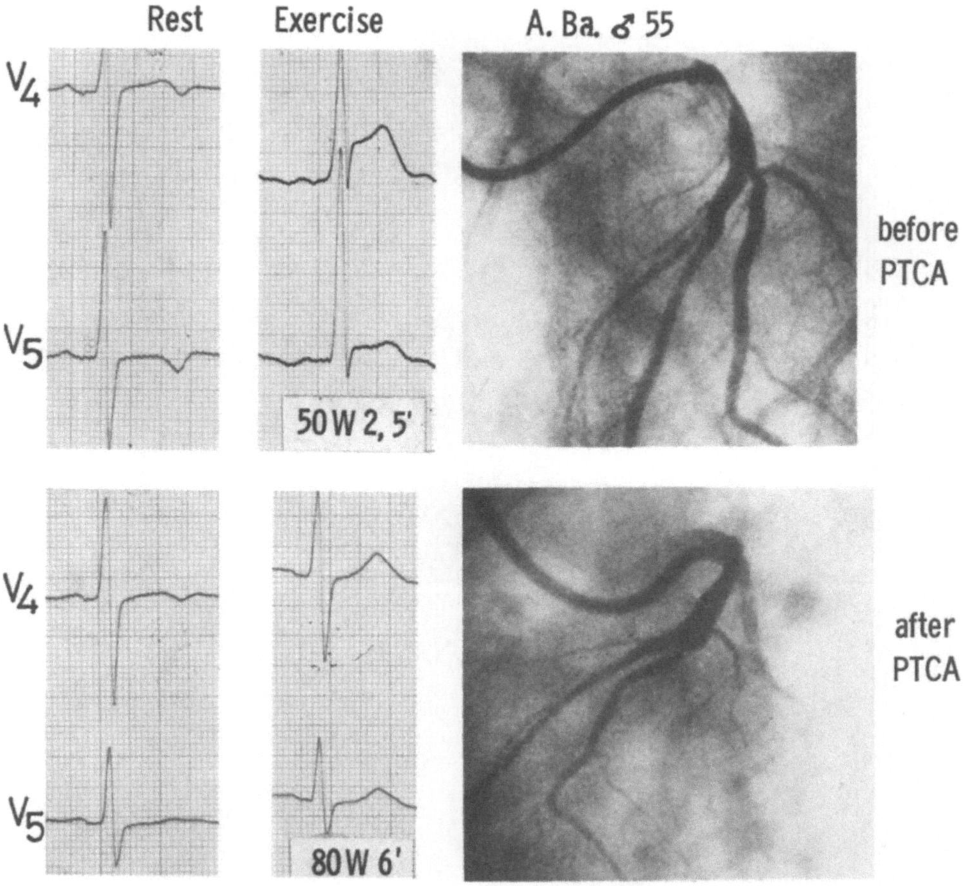

Fig. 9. A. Ba. 55-year-old man. Proximal LAD stenosis. Before TCA severe angina with ischemic ST elevation in stress ECG. After TCA higher stress over a longer period of time can be performed without ST alterations

during exercise, ejection fraction remained unchanged. Exercise with 150 watts, which now also could be performed, led to an increase of ejection fraction from 66% to 69%. The preexisting collaterals from the RCA to the LAD region had completely disappeared as a consequence of elevated coronary perfusion pressure in the LAD.

Long-term Results and Recurrences

After successful TCA the patients were kept on a daily medication of 1.5 g acetylsalicylic acid and 120 mg isosorbide dinitrate. In addition 480 mg verapamil or 60 mg nifedipine was administered.

Fifty-five of the 87 patients had a control arteriogram at an average of 3 months after TCA; 13 had an additional arteriogram at an average of 12 months after TCA. One patient had only the late follow-up angiogram. Thus a total of 56 patients were

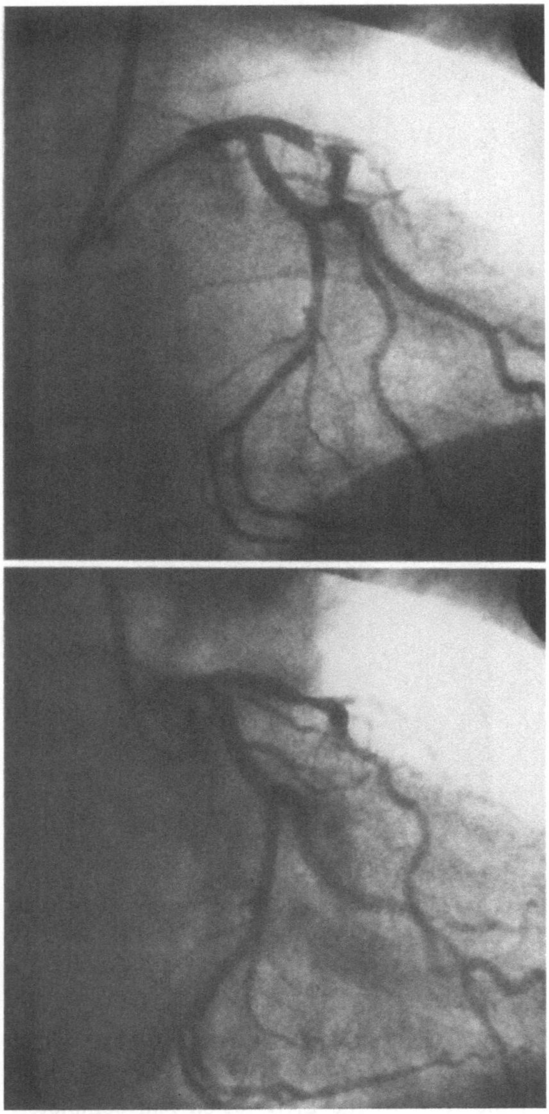

Fig. 10a

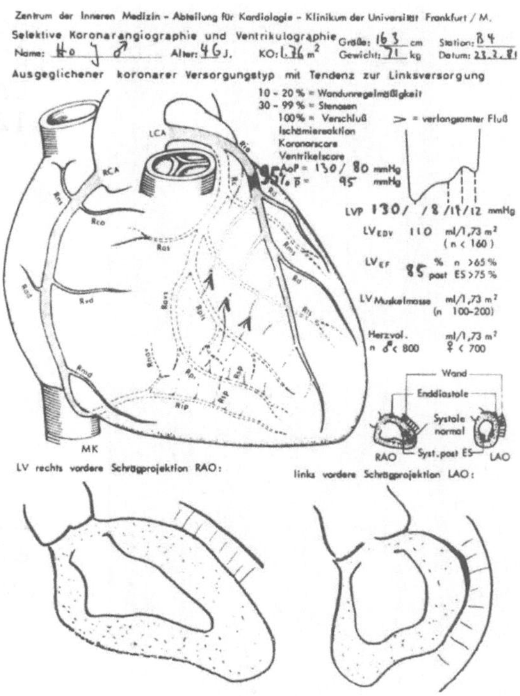

Ho. J. 46 ♂ Radionuclide ventriculography (EF%)

	Rest	90 W	150 W
Before TCA	67	45	
After TCA	66	65	69

Fig. 10b

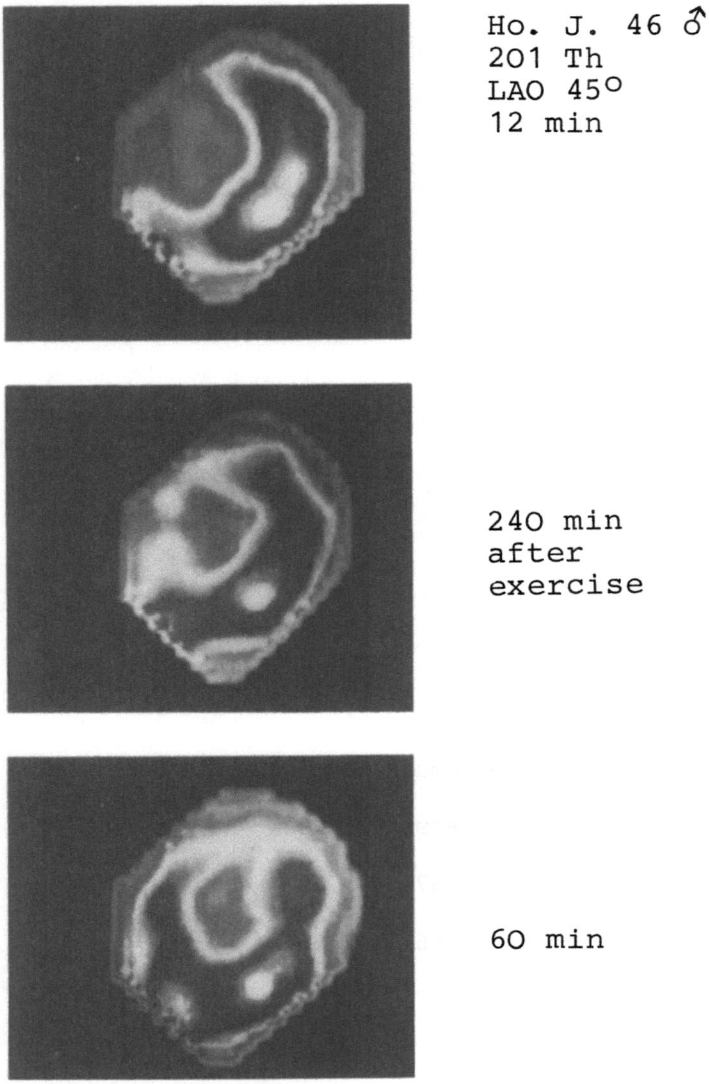

Fig. 10a–c. Ho. J. 46-year-old man. Subtotal occlusion of proximal LAD. After TCA in radionuclide ventriculography significant increase of ejection fraction during exercise. Thallium-201 scan with anteroseptal filling defect and redistribution was completely normalized

angiographically controlled. In the first 3 months eight recurrences were seen, while in the later arteriograms no recidivations occurred. Thus from control arteriograms in 56 patients eight recidivations occurring within the first 3 months were encountered, a recurrence rate of 14%. Long-term observations of all 87 patients, including the 56 with control arteriograms as well as the 31 without control arteriograms, over a period of 15 months showed a total of 11 patients with recurring symptoms. From these findings a recurrence rate of 13% can be derived.

Complications

Immediate surgery, i.e., surgery within 12 h of TCA, was performed in seven patients. In four of them this was considered an emergency procedure. Twice coronary artery dissection was created, twice severe anginal pain occurred in patients in whom TCA could not be accomplished: at the end of the procedure the attempted high-grade stenosis in one instance had progressed to a subtotal stenosis, in the other patient a subtotal stenosis had progressed to total occlusion. Surgery in all seven patients was performed without complications. Intraoperatively, sequelae of the procedure were only detectable in one patient: the RCA showed a dissecting aneurysm. In all 152 attempts no deaths, myocardial infarctions, or other severe complications occurred. It seems important to mention that in no case was acute reocclusion after successful dilatation observed. Intraoperatively, no fresh thrombi were detected in the bypassed vessels.

Discussion

Our results are in good agreement with those obtained from the NHLBI registry [4]. The patients treated in Frankfurt, however, had a higher proportion of double- and triple-vessel disease. The recurrence rate appears no higher in our series receiving acetylsalicylic acid than in patients receiving Coumadin. Most remarkably, in no instance was evidence found of coronary thrombus formation after TCA. No thrombi were seen in seven patients operated on after TCA, nor was there any secondary (thrombotic) reocclusion after successful dilatation. From postmortem findings collected in the NHLBI registry it is apparent that sudden reocclusion after successful TCA does occur and can be the result of coronary thrombosis. Sigwart [5] has shown successfull thrombolysis with intracoronary streptokinase in such a situation. Lichtlen (1981, personal communication) has seen one case of extensive occluding coronary thrombosis after primary successful dilatation. The absence of thromboembolic complications (including myocardial infarctions) in our series is ascribed to the protocol, which includes high dose acetylsalicylic acid administered in addition to heparin, and to the fact that in no case had protamine sulfate to be administered after TCA. The application of such a protocol therefore may increase the safety of the procedure. Presumably this refers not only to coronary but also to other arteries.

Summary

152 attempts of coronary angioplasty are reported. Successful dilatation was achieved in 87 patients, with a reduction on average from 80% to 40% stenosis diameter.

Recurrence rate over 15 months observations was 14%. Complications were four emergency operations.

No deaths and no myocardial infarctions were encountered. The low complication rate in regard to myocardial infarction and the lack of intracoronary thrombosis is ascribed to a protocol which includes high dose (1.5 g/day) acetylsalicylic acid administered in addition to heparin.

Addendum. Up to June 1982 the total number of TCA procedures was 300. With further experience the success rate has increased to 75%.

Acknowledgment. Surgery was performed by Drs. Satter and Krause. We are greatly indebted to them for their support.

References

1. Grüntzig A (1978) Transluminal dilatation of coronary artery stenosis. Lancet 1:263
2. Kaltenbach M, Kober G, Scherer D (1981) Mechanische Dilatation von Koronararterienstenosen. Z Kardiol 69:1–10
3. Klepzig H, Scherer D, Kober G et al. (1982) Myocardial function before and after transluminal coronary angioplasty. In: this book p. 53–63
4. Mock MB, Kent KM et al. The National Heart, Lung, and Blood Institute percutaneous transluminal coronary angioplasty registry: the first 1116 cases. In: this book p. 11–19
5. Sigwart U, Essinger A, Grbic M et al. (1980) Emergency reopening of right coronary occlusion after angioplasty using guide wire and thrombolysis. In: this book p. 151–154

Treatment with Platelet Function Inhibitors

H.K. Breddin

Department of Internal Medicine, J.W. Goethe-University, Division of Angiology,
6000 Frankfurt a.M., FRG

Acetylsalicylic acid (ASA) was the first drug, to be tested in a variety of diseases for its antithrombotic effect. In man, single doses of 100 mg ASA and more inhibit platelet aggregation for several days by inhibiting platelet cyclooxygenase. This effect leads to the inhibition of thromboxane A_2 formation in the platelets [5].

Following the concept of an important role of the prostaglandin metabolism in regulation of blood-vessel wall interactions, Moncada and Vane suggested the use of very small doses of ASA, in the range of 100–200 mg/day, in future clinical trials to test its antithrombotic effect. It was their hypothesis that in higher doses ASA inhibits prostacyclin formation in the vessel wall as well as thromboxane A_2 formation in the platets, and that the antithrombotic effect of ASA might be reduced thereby. This concept was based on the assumption that the antithrombotic effect of ASA is closely related with the inhibition of thromboxane A_2 formation in the platelets and therefore with the inhibition of platelet aggregation.

Several animal studies by different investigators are not compatible with this concept [2, 4, 6, 10, 11]. In these studies ASA in doses of 1–10 mg/kg, sufficient to inhibit cyclooxygenase in the platelets, had little if any antithrombotic effect, but higher doses up to 100 mg/kg were more effective in inhibiting experimental thromboses.

Pietsch et al. [9] noticed that after IV injection of 500 or 1000 mg ASA, the spontaneous platelet shape change after blood sampling was inhibited for 6–8 h.

A new test system studies the extent to which platelets can be stimulated by tissue extracts in venous blood, directly after blood sampling, and how fast stimulated platelets are transformed back into the disk form. In this test system 250 mg ASA inhibit platelet stimulation for about 6 h. The maximum inhibiting effect was observed 4 h after ingestion. This inhibitory effect was most pronounced 6 h after oral intake of 500 mg ASA. The initial values were reached within 10–14 h.

In this test system dipyridamole was as effective as ASA but the effect of single doses of 75 or 150 mg lasted for only 6 h. The maximal inhibitory effect was reached 2–4 h after ingestion of the drugs. The combination of both drugs did not prolong the duration of the stimulation inhibiting effect of ASA alone.

Clinical trials on the effect of ASA have usually been performed with daily doses ranging between 900 and 1500 mg/day and in combination with dipyridamole in a dose of 3 × 75 mg/day. If ASA is administered in doses of less than 1 g/day, platelet stimulation and also platelet adhesiveness are not continuously inhibited during a 24-h period. For the same reasons, 3 × 300 mg are likely to be more effective than

Transluminal Coronary Angioplasty and
Intracoronary Thrombolysis. Ed. by Kaltenbach et al.

2 × 500 mg. If the inhibition of platelet stimulation is partly or mainly responsible for the antithrombotic action of both drugs, the dosage for continuous inhibition during a 24-h period has to be much larger than the doses which are needed to inhibit platelet aggregation. There are now several arguments against the concept that the antithrombotic effect of ASA is caused by the inhibition of cyclooxygenase alone:

1. In most of the clinical trials in which an antithrombotic effect of ASA has been made likely doses of 900–1500 mg/day have been administered.
2. Several investigators have reported a dose-dependent increase of the antithrombotic effect of ASA in animal models.
3. ASA prolongs the bleeding time, and inhibits platelet shape change and tissue extract induced platelet shape change as well as platelet adhesiveness dose dependently for a much shorter period than platelet aggregation.
4. The total absence of cyclooxygenase in platelets and in the vessel wall leads to a mild bleeding tendency and not to thrombosis, as has been shown by Pareti et al. [7].

Further studies with drugs which inhibit either aggregation or stimulation should verify which effects are important for an antithrombotic effect or if all inhibitory effects contribute to an inhibition of thrombus formation.

The different results in two large clinical trials on the effect of ASA in the prevention of death and/or recurrent infarction after a first myocardial infarct [1, 8] can also possibly be explained by dose differences between these two studies. In AMIS [1], patients in the ASA group received 2 × 500 mg daily, while in the persantin-aspirin reinfarction study [8], patients in the ASA and ASA + Persantingroups received 3 × 300 mg daily. If the effect of ASA on platelet stimulation and adhesion is a contributing factor in the action of this drug, 3 × 300 mg will result in an inhibition of stimulation for about 14–16 of 24 h, while 2 × 500 mg are effective for only 10–12 h/day.

From this point of view ASA should be administered in a slowly absorbed form, and combinations of ASA and dipyridamole might also be more effective if the absorption of both drugs is retarded to result in a more continuous inhibition of platelet adhesiveness and platelet stimulation. For the clinical use of ASA, it should be administered in a dose of 3 × 500 mg daily if the usual preparations are prescribed or 2 × 750 mg daily if a slowly absorbed form is used, e.g., Monobeltin. In future clinical trials it should be ascertained that the ASA preparation and dosage leads to a continuous inhibition of platelet stimulation and adhesiveness.

Sulfinpyrazone is a mild antiaggregatory drug, which does not inhibit platelet adhesiveness or platelet stimulation. This drug has not been effective as an antithrombotic in the Canadian study [3]. Its effects after fresh myocardial infarction are currently under debate. If the positive effect which was observed during the first months after a fresh myocardial infarct is confirmed, it is likely that this beneficial effect is not caused by the antiaggregating properties of this drug.

References

1. Aspirin Myocardial Infarction Study Research Group (1980) A randomised, controlled trial of aspirin in persons recovered from myocardial infarction. JAMA 243:661–669
2. Busse WD, Seuter F (1981) Erfahrungen mit Azetylsalizylsäure, Dipyridamol und Sulfinpyrazon in verschiedenen Tiermodellen. In: Breddin K, Gross D, Rotter W (eds) Thrombosemodelle am Tier. Prostaglandine und Thrombogenese. FK Schattauer, Stuttgart New York, pp 157–172
3. Canadian Cooperative Study Group (1978) A randomized trial of aspirin and sulfinpyrazone in threatened stroke. New Engl J Med 299:53–59
4. Haarmann W (1981) Erfahrungen mit Azetylsalizylsäure, Dipyridamol und Sulfinpyrazon in verschiedenen Tiermodellen. In: Breddin K, Gross D, Rotter W (eds) Thrombosemodelle am Tier. Prostaglandine und Thrombogenese. FK Schattauer, Stuttgart New York, pp 173–188
5. Hamberg MJ, Svensson B, Samuelson B (1974) Mechanism of the antiaggregating effect of aspirin in human platelets. Lancet I:223–224
6. Melzer G (1981) Erfahrungen mit Azetylsalizylsäure, Dipyridamol und Sulfinpyrazon in verschiedenen Tiermodellen. In: Breddin K, Gross D, Rotter W (eds) Thrombosemodelle am Tier, Prostaglandine und Thrombogenese. FK Schattauer, Stuttgart New York, pp 193–200
7. Pareti FJ, Smith JB, D'Angelo A, Mari D, Capitano A, Manucci PM (1980) Congenital deficiency of platelet thromboxane and vascular wall prostacyclin in a patient with aspirin like syndrome. In: Deutsch E, Lechner K (eds) Fibrinolyse, Thrombose, Haemostase, FK Schatauer, Stuttgart New York, pp 619–622
8. Persantin-Aspirin Study Research Group (1980) Persantin and aspirin in coronary heart disease. Circulation 62:449–461
9. Pietsch U, Lippmann M, Scharrer I, Breddin K (1977) Neue Befunde zur Wirkung von Azetylsalizylsäure. Die Hemmwirkung auf den Formwandel der Thrombozyten und ihre Bedeutung für die Dosierung als Antithrombotikum. In: Alexander K, Cachovan M (eds) Diabetische Angiopathien. Witzstrock G, Baden-Baden Köln New York, pp 348–351
10. Seuter F (1976) Inhibition of platelet aggregation by acetylsalicylic acid and other inhibitors. Haemostasis 5:85–95
11. Weichert W, Wiedemann R, Breddin K (1981) Versuche zur Standardisierung eines Tiermodells. Erzeugung Laser-induzierter Thromben im Rattenmesenterium. In: Breddin K, Gross D, Rotter W (eds) Thrombosemodelle am Tier, Prostaglandine und Thrombogenese. FK Schattauer, Stuttgart New York, pp 117–124

Functional Results of TCA

Effects of Percutaneous Transluminal Coronary Angioplasty on Myocardial Function During Exercise

K.M. Kent, R.O. Bonow, D.R. Rosing, L.C. Lipson, C.L. McIntosh, S. Bacharach, M. Green, S.E. Epstein

Cardiology Branch, Nuclear Medicine, Surgery Branch, NHLBI, Clinical Center, NIH, Bethesda, MD 20205, USA

To determine if the angiographic improvement of coronary arterial stenoses following percutaneous transluminal coronary angioplasty (PTCA) leads to augmentation of functionally important myocardial blood flow, the effects of PTCA on exercise induced myocardial dysfunction were examined. Since most patients undergoing PTCA had single-vessel disease and normal ventricular function at rest, the transient exercise-induced abnormalities of left ventricular function would be expected to improve if PTCA enhanced the capacity of the coronary artery to perfuse the myocardium during increased oxygen requirement. A consecutive series of patients undergoing PTCA who had coronary artery disease without associated cardiac abnormalities and without severe left ventricular dysfunction at rest were evaluated with radionuclide ventriculograms at rest and during exercise before, several days after, and 6 months after PTCA.

Methods

Between February 1979 and April 1980 PTCA was performed in 90 patients at the National Institutes of Health (NIH); 69 were men and 21 were women, with an average age of 51 years (range 31–72 years). Four patients were excluded from the study because of associated coexistent mitral stenosis in addition to valvular, primary myocardial disease or ventricular aneurysms. Seventy-one patients had single-vessel coronary artery disease, 13 had multivessel disease and in two patients PTCA was performed in a bypass graft.

The procedure initially described by Gruntzig [5] was followed with catheters of the Gruntzig design (Gruntzig Dilica, USCI, Billerica, MA) or the Simpson-Roberts catheters (Advanced Catheter Company, Santa Clara, CA). Thirty-four patients were receiving verapamil at the time of the early postprocedure study, but no patient was taking verapamil or any other cardiac medication at the time of the 6-month study. All patients received aspirin 300 mg q.d. and dipyrimadole 50 mg t.i.d. for 1 day before and 6 months after PTCA.

Prior to the procedure, 24 h after discontinuation of beta-blocking agents and 8 h after any nitrates, 62 patients underwent radionuclide ventriculography at rest and during exercise. The remaining patients had or developed rest angina during the withdrawal of beta-blocking agents and/or nitrates and were not exercised.

Transluminal Coronary Angioplasty and Intracoronary Thrombolysis. Ed. by Kaltenbach et al.

Radionuclide cineangiography was performed as previously described [1, 2, 3, 4]. Twenty mCi technetium red blood cells with ^{99m}Tc in vivo labeled is administered i.v. After equilibration of the tracer in the blood pool, with the patient in the supine position, an Anger camera is positioned over the patient's chest in a modified left anterior oblique (LAO) position to isolate the left ventricle from other cardiac structures. Electrocardiographic gating is employed in the organization of scintigraphic data into a series of images that span the average cardiac cycle. The data are then displayed in two formats. In the first, images are displayed in rapid-sequence endless-loop movies so that wall motion can be evaluated qualitatively [1]. Sequential end-diastolic and end-systolic frames can also be analyzed. In the second format, function of the inferior and anterobasal walls (not border forming in this LAO projection) are evaluated by examining the difference image, created by subtracting the end-systolic from the end-diastolic image [4]. With this latter technique, wall motion abnormalities of the non-border-forming areas can be assessed qualitatively. In the present study, a central defect in the difference image area is interpreted as abnormal motion of the inferior or anterobasal wall. Global ventricular function is assessed by determining ejection fraction, which is calculated from the ratio of radioactive emissions (counts after background correction) collected from the left ventricle (LV):

$$\text{Ejection fraction} = \frac{\text{end diastolic LV counts} - \text{end systolic LV counts}}{\text{end diastolic LV counts}}$$

After studies are performed at rest, imaging is repeated during maximal supine bicycle exercise. Exercise work loads, initially 25 watts, are increased stepwise in 25 watt increments every 2 minutes until angina pectoris, dyspnea, or fatigue of moderate severity necessitates terminating the test. Imaging is begun shortly after the exercise starts, but only those portions of the data series occurring during maximal exercise encompassing the final 2 minutes of the test are selected for analysis of regional contractile function and ejection fraction.

All patients in whom PTCA was successful (> 20% increase in lumen diameter) had radionuclide ventriculography at rest and exercise 1–14 days following the procedure. The same exercise protocols for the radionuclide studies were followed after PTCA. In addition to repeating the maximal exercise level achieved before PTCA, patients also exercised after PTCA to their new (invariably higher) symptom-limited exercise level. In addition, 19 patients have been followed at least 6 months after successful PTCA and have had repeat radionuclide ventriculography at 6 months.

Results

In 57 of the 86 patients (67%), PTCA resulted in a 20% or greater increase in vessel diameter at the site of the stenosis. In the remaining 29 patients, either the stenosis could not be crossed with the balloon catheter [19] or no change in the angiographic appearance of the stenosis occurred after balloon inflation. In the 57 patients who had successful dilatation, the average stenosis was 76% ± 3% prior to the procedure and was reduced to 28% ± 4% after balloon inflation. Initially there was an average gradient of 60 ± 4 mmHg across the stenosis; this fell to 20 ± 2 mmHg following the successful procedure. Three serious complications resulted from PTCA in the total group of 86 patients: one patient sustained an acute myocardial infarction 12 h after an unsuccessful procedure; one patient had coronary dissection following balloon inflation which resulted in occlusion of the artery; and one patient had coronary artery dissection and occlusion in attempting to cross the stenosis. Emergency coronary bypass operation was successfully performed in the latter two patients; there was no subsequent evidence of myocardial infarction as determined by ECG, enzymes, or radionuclide studies.

Myocardial Function Patients with Successful Angiographic Result

Radionuclide ventriculography was performed at rest and during supine bicycle exercise prior to the procedure in 42 of the patients in whom PTCA was angiographically successful (prior to PTCA ventricular tachycardia terminated exercise in one patient before sufficient counts were obtained for analysis). Ejection fraction averaged 55% ± 2% at rest and 50% ± 4% (NS) during symptom-limited exercise (Fig. 1). Ejection fraction fell by 5% or more in 13 patients, did not change in 23, and increased by more than

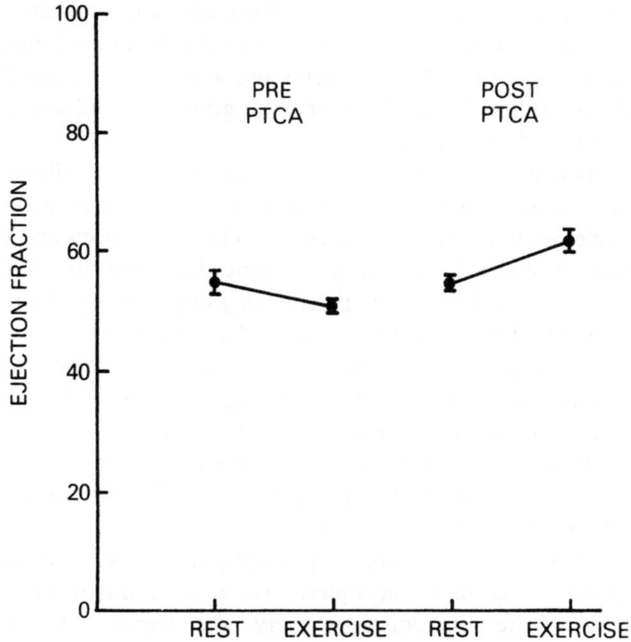

Fig. 1. Ejection fraction (%) determined by radionuclide ventriculography at rest and during exercise before and after PTCA (mean ± standard error)

Myocardial Function Before and After Transluminal Coronary Angioplasty

H. Klepzig jr., D. Scherer, G. Kober, F.D. Maul, N. Kanemoto, R. Standke, G. Hör, M. Kaltenbach

Department of Cardiology and General Nuclear Medicine, Zentrum der Inneren Medizin, J.W. Goethe-Universität, Theodor-Stern-Kai 7, 6000 Frankfurt a.M., FRG

In selected cases transluminal coronary angioplasty (TCA) may represent an effective alternative to bypass surgery in the treatment of coronary heart disease [2, 3, 4, 9, 15].

The purpose of this study was to compare the improvement of myocardial function and perfusion after successful TCA with the results after bypass operation by means of exercise ECG, thallium myocardial scintigraphy and equilibrium radionuclide ventriculography.

Methods

Forty-eight patients with coronary heart disease (mean age 51 years) were investigated: 36 patients with successful TCA, i.e., reduction of the stenosis by at least 20% (group 1); six patients with successful aortocoronary bypass operation (group 2); and six patients with TCA attempts, in whom the coronary artery stenosis could not be reached or crossed by the balloon catheter and who remained angiographically unchanged after the procedure (group 3). Patients in group 3 served as controls for the reproducibility of the applied methods.

In group 1, 29 of 36 patients had single-vessel disease, five patients had double-vessel disease, and two patients had triple-vessel disease. In group 2, three patients had single-vessel disease, one patient main branch stenosis and two patients triple-vessel disease. In group 3, four of six patients had single-vessel disease and two patients had double-vessel disease. Ten patients in group 1, two patients in group 2, and one patient in group 3 had had previous myocardial infarctions.

In group 1 TCA was successful in 27 LAD stenoses, in eight stenoses of the right coronary artery and in one distal bypass stenosis. On average coronary diameter narrowing was reduced from 84% ± 8.4% to 43% ± 13.7% (Fig. 1). In group 2 three patients received one aortocoronary bypass, the three other patients two grafts each. Five grafts were implanted into the LAD, two into the left circumflex artery and two into the right coronary artery.

Six weeks after surgery angiography showed all grafts open with a good blood flow. In group 3, coronary angioplasty was unsuccessful in three LAD stenoses and three stenoses of the right coronary artery. The degree of the stenoses, which could not be passed by the balloon catheter, remained angiographically unchanged at 82% on average before and after the procedure.

Transluminal Coronary Angioplasty and
Intracoronary Thrombolysis. Ed. by Kaltenbach et al.

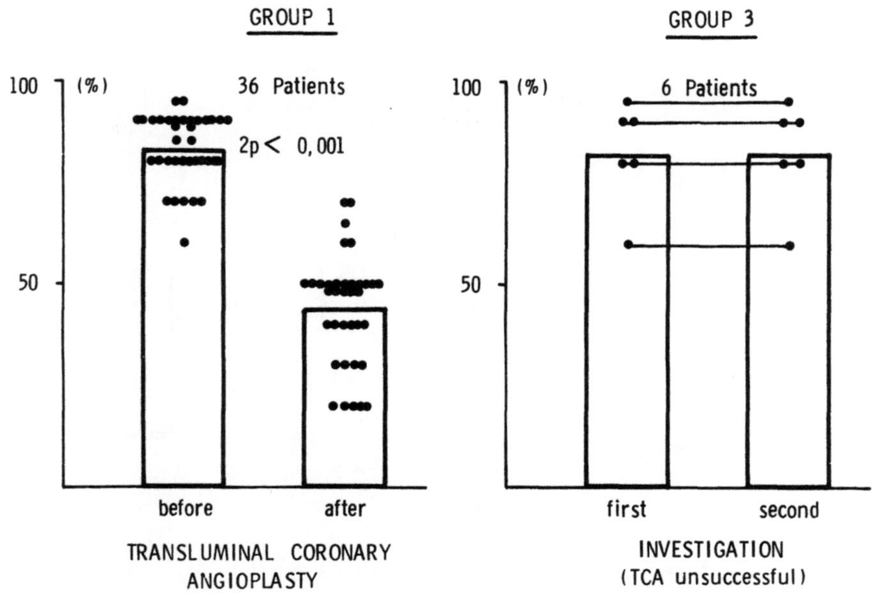

Fig. 1. Degree of stenosis

Forty-six of the 48 patients underwent repeated exercise ECG. 26 were studied twice by thallium-201 myocardial scintigraphy during exercise, and in 38 equilibrium radionuclide ventriculography at rest and during exercise was performed before and after therapeutic intervention.

In patients with successful TCA (group 1) and unsuccessful TCA (group 3) the second tests were performed within a week of the intervention. In patients with bypass grafts (group 2) the second tests were performed 6 weeks after surgery. The tests prior to intervention were always carried out within a week before TCA.

The exercise ECG was quantified by means of quotient ("ischemia score") consisting of ST depression (mm × 100), work load (watts), and duration of exercise (min) (Fig. 2).

Thallium-201 myocardial scintigraphy was performed as an early scan between 5 and 30 minutes after completion of exercise, and as a delayed scan 1 h and 3–4 h (average 3.5 h) after exercise. The reduction in thallium activity in the region of interest in the scan acquired immediately after exercise was quantified by means of the myocardial perfusion index, which is the ratio between the rates of counts in the minimum and maximum perfusion areas [5, 6, 7].

The redistribution of thallium into the ischemic defects was quantified by means of the ratio between the increase of washout-corrected thallium activity in the delayed scans and the maximum thallium activity in the scans, acquired immediately after exercise [6]. If large ischemic defects appeared in the myocardial scintigraphy, several areas from each patient were included in the calculations.

Equilibrium radionuclide ventriculography was performed at rest and during supine bicycle ergometry. Ventricular function was expressed in terms of global ejection frac-

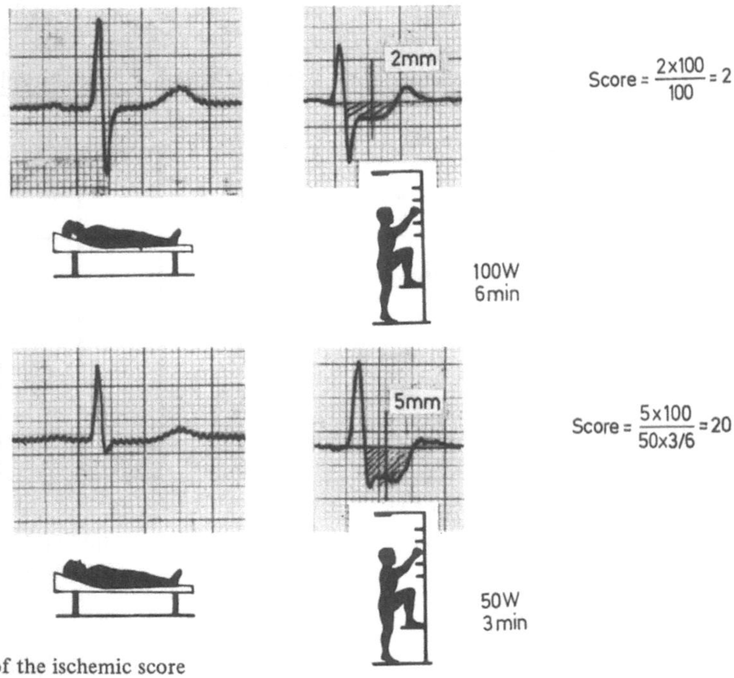

Fig. 2. Calculation of the ischemic score

tion and maximal systolic volume change as a fraction of end-diastolic volume [1]. Global ejection fraction values greater than 55% were judged normal.

Significance of differences was calculated for results containing more than 20 values by means of Student's t test.

Results

Repeated exercise ECG quantified by means of the described index showed marked improvement after successful coronary angioplasty. The index dropped significantly from 2.4 to 0.36 after TCA, and from 3.8 to 0 after aortocoronary bypass operation. No differences appeared in the control group (4.5 to 4.5) (Fig. 3).

Myocardial perfusion index derived from thallium-201 scan showed significant improvement after TCA from 69% ± 9.1% to 82% ± 9.3%, and after aortocoronary bypass operation from 74% to 82%; again, no difference was noted in the control group (72% to 72%) (Fig. 4).

Corresponding to the improved myocardial perfusion a reduction of redistribution of thallium-201 was seen after TCA and aortocoronary bypass operation. (Group 1: 1 h, from 3.1% ± 5.6% to 0.9% ± 1.5%; 3.5 h, from 9.8% ± 8% to 3.3% ± 4.6%. Group 2: 1 h, from 2.2% to 1.4%; 3.5 hours, from 7.5% to 4.2%.) Redistribution factors remain pathological in patients with unsuccessful TCA (1 h, 3.6% and 3.0%; 3.5 hours, 5.4% and 5.6%) (Fig. 5).

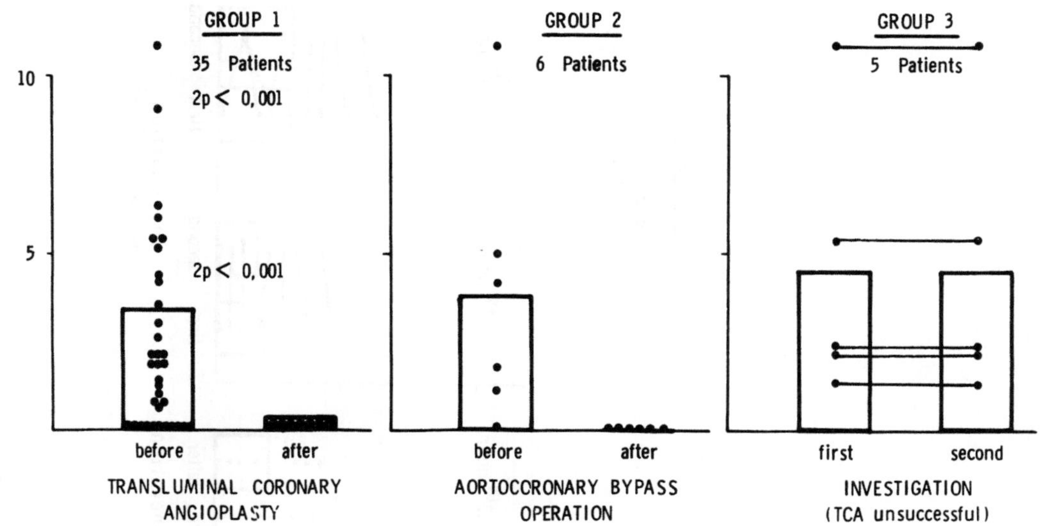

Fig. 3. Exercise ECG: ischemia score

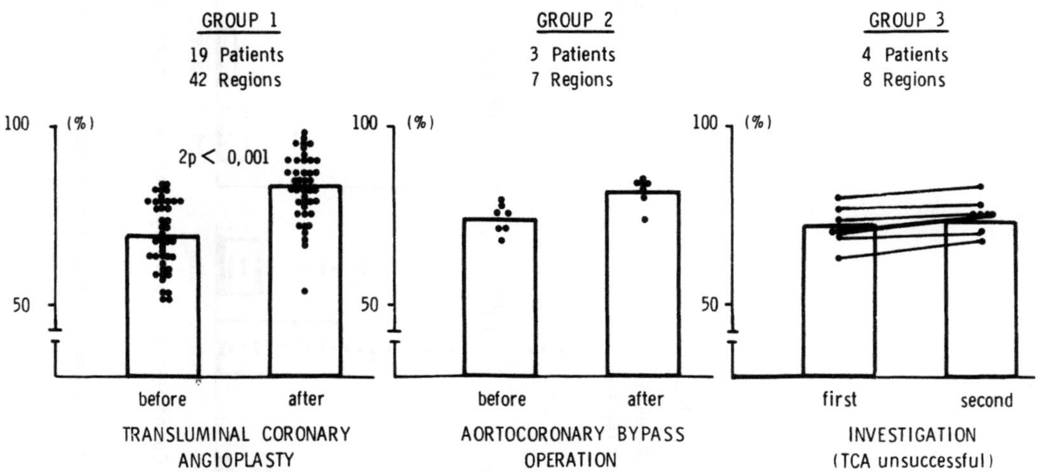

Fig. 4. Thallium-201 myocardial scintigraphy: index for myocardial perfusion

Ejection fraction of the left ventricle increased significantly after successful TCA and aortocoronary bypass operation at rest and during exercise. (Group 1: rest, from 46% ± 9.9% to 52% ± 9.3%; exercise, from 41% ± 11.5% to 49% ± 10.6%. Group 2: rest, from 38% to 46%: exercise, from 36% to 44%.) No significant changes appeared in the control group (rest, from 47% to 47%; exercise, from 43% to 43%) (Fig. 6).

Improvement of left ventricular function is also demonstrated by maximal systolic volume change as a fraction of end-diastolic volume. After successful TCA and after aortocoronary bypass operation contractility showed a significant increase at rest and during exercise. (Group 1: rest, 2.6 ± 0.7/sec to 3.2 ± 1.4/sec; exercise, from 2.8 ± 0.9/

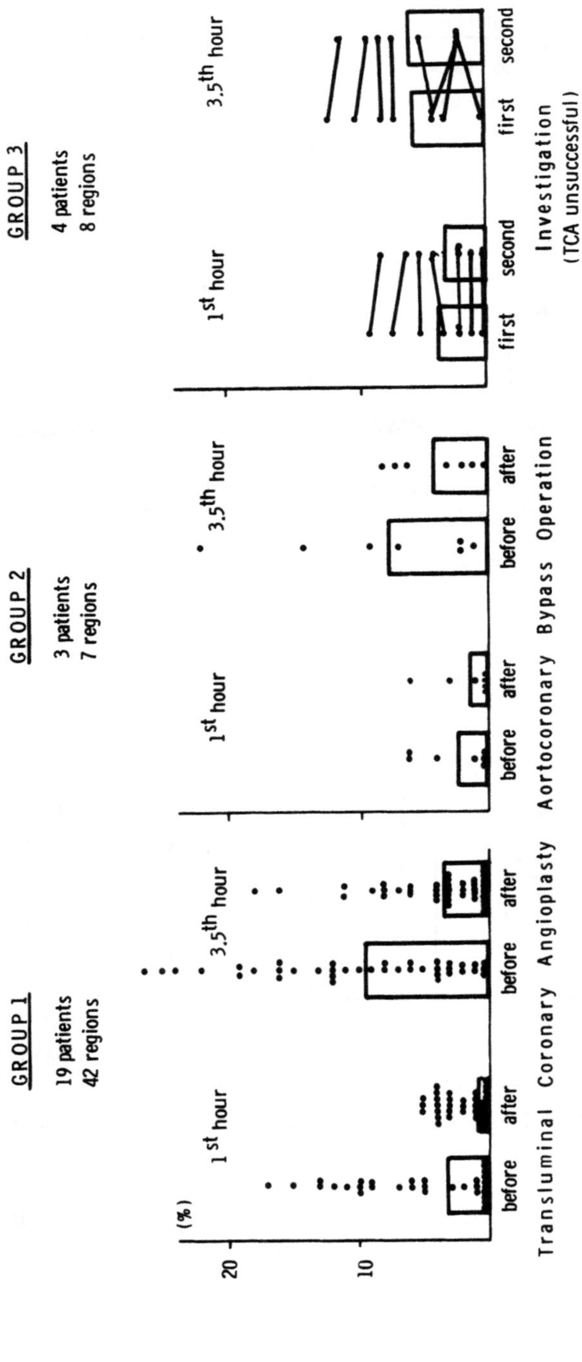

Fig. 5. Thallium-201 myocardial scintigraphy: redistribution factors

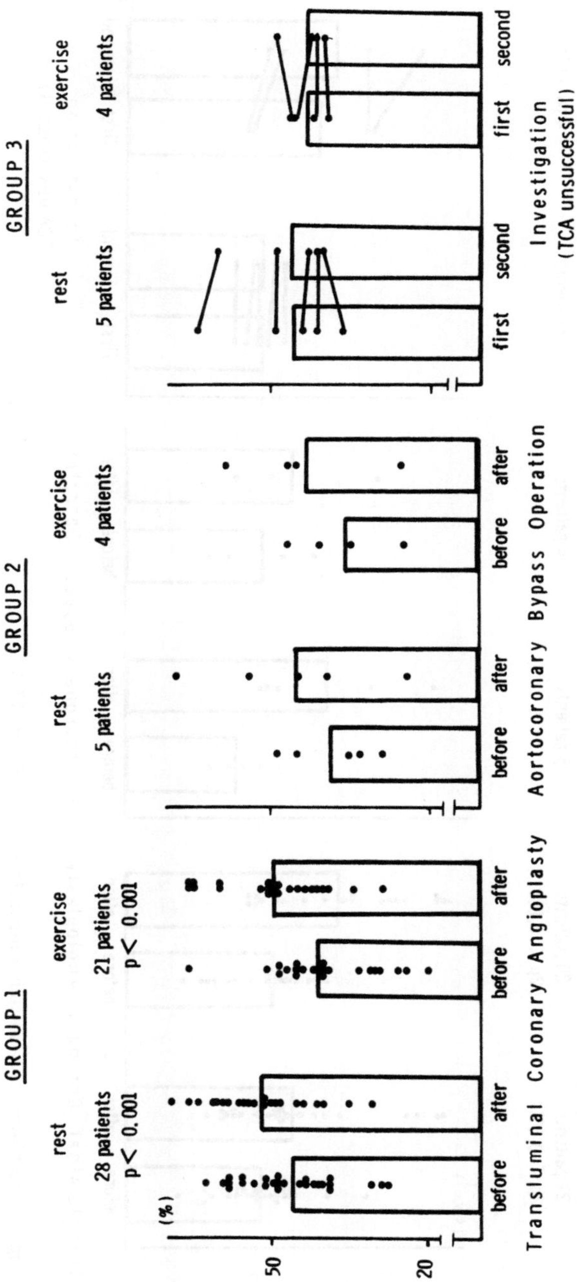

Fig. 6. Equilibrium radionuclide ventriculography: ejection fraction

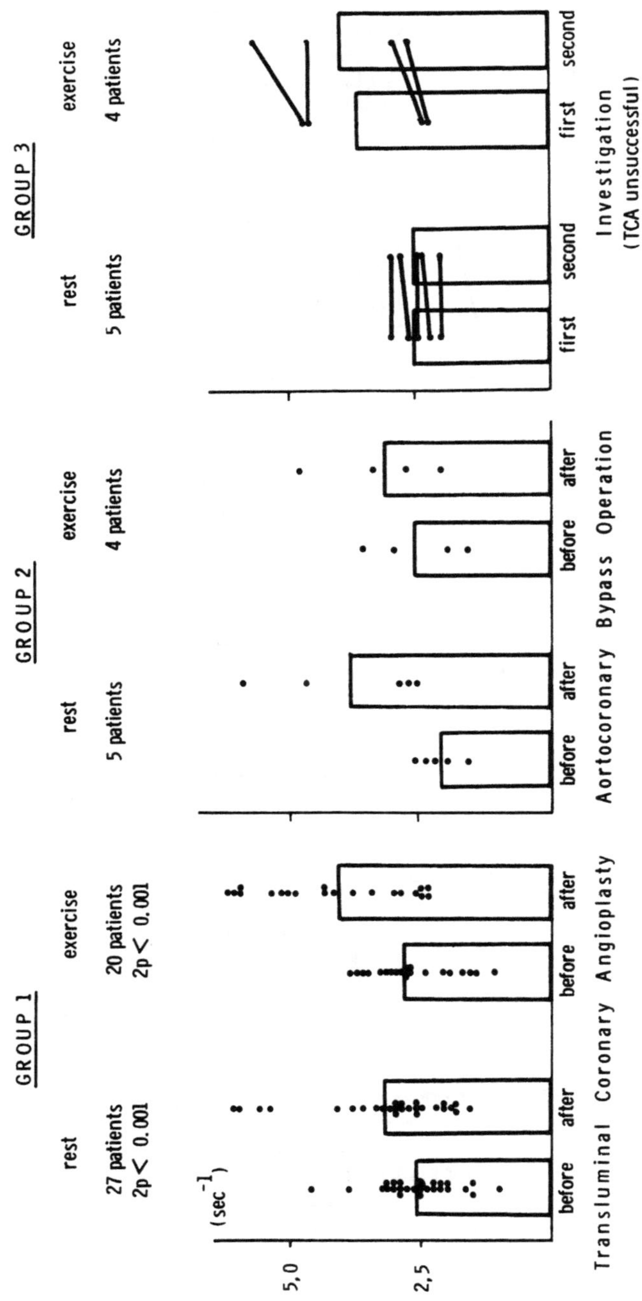

Fig. 7. Equilibrium radionuclide ventriculography: –dV/dt/EDV

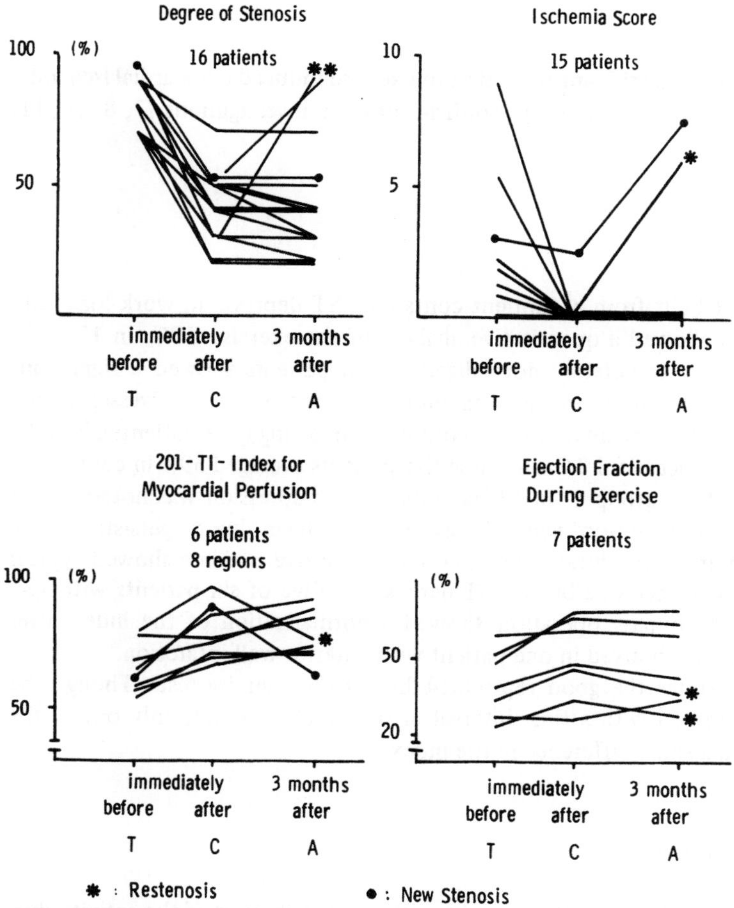

Fig. 8. Three months follow-up

sec to 4.1 ± 1.4/sec. Group 2: rest, from 2.2/sec to 2.6/sec; exercise, from 3.8/sec to 3.3/sec.) Only slight differences were seen in the control group (rest, 2.6/sec and 2.7/sec; exercise, 3.6/sec and 4.1/sec) (Fig. 7).

Sixteen of 36 successfully dilated patients were reinvestigated after 3 months (Fig. 8). In 13 of these patients the degree of narrowing in the control angiography remained unchanged in comparison to the result immediately after TCA; exercise ECG, myocardial perfusion index, and ejection fraction during exercise also showed no significant differences.

Two patients showed severe restenosis (Fig. 8). Correspondingly, functional deterioration was observed in the exercise ECG, perfusion index, and ejection fraction. The restenosis in one of these patients could be dilated successfully again; the other underwent aortocoronary bypass operation. A third patient developed a new stenosis distal to the successfully dilated narrowing as a result of progression of coronary heart disease. He also showed significant deterioration in comparison to the results immediately after successful TCA (Fig. 8).

Discussion

Successful TCA effects a significant reduction of exercise-induced myocardial ischemia. The results, demonstrated in the study, confirm previous investigations [7, 8, 10, 11, 12, 14].

Exercise ECG

The described index built from a quotient containing ST depression, work load, and duration of exercise allowed a quantitative analysis of the exercise ECG. In 17 of 35 patients the index was completely normalized. Seven patients showed a significant decrease. It was not normalized in these patients due to coronary multivessel disease (two patients) or insufficient dilatation of coronary narrowing (five patients). The degree of stenosis after successful TCA in these five patients averaged 59% in contrast to 43% in all 36 patients of group 1. In 11 patients no ST depression was noted before and after successful intervention, which in six cases had been due to persisting ST/T alterations after anterior wall infarctions. The remaining five patients showed typical exericse-induced angina pectoris but no ST depression. Five of six patients with successful aortocoronary bypass operation showed a normalization of the index after surgery. No change was observed in one patient with anterior wall infarction.

Group 3 demonstrates the good reproducibility of the exercise tests. Though the two tests were performed with a time interval of one week or more, only one of the five patients showed a small difference in the index.

Thallium-201 Scintigraphy

Defects in thallium-201 fixation after exercise with a redistribution of the activity during the following hours is a sensitive parameter of exercise-induced myocardial ischemia [5, 6]. If a myocardial scar is excluded the increase in thallium-201 perfusion index represents an improved coronary blood flow during exercise after successful coronary angioplasty and aortocoronary bypass operation.

In group 1 normalization was shown in 33 of 42 analyzed regions. A distinct increase, but not a complete normalization of perfusion index, was observed in five patients (eight regions) in whom TCA was performed in the vessel responsible for a transmural myocardial infarction.

In group 2 perfusion index was normalized in six of seven regions; only one patient with an anterior wall infarction showed a distinct increase but not a normalization. In group 3 average values were identical before and after the intervention, though slight deviations were observed in some individuals. The results reflect a good reproducibility of this method.

Corresponding to the improved thallium-201 fixation after successful intervention, thallium redistribution also showed a significant decrease in both groups. Though in group 1 perfusion index remained pathological in nine of 42 regions, the redistribution factor showed a decrease or were apparently normalized in the same patients. In these regions the lenght of observation (on average 3.5 h) might have been too short; a significant redistribution of thallium-201 might have been observed several hours later.

In group 2 reduction of thallium-201 redistribution also indicates improved myocardial perfusion. Again, only slight differences were noted in group 3.

Radionuclide Ventriculography

In contrast to other authors [13] a significant increase in ejection fraction and maximum systolic volume change as a fraction of end-diastolic volume already at rest after successful transluminal angioplasty was observed. However, coronary narrowing in these patients was distinctly higher than in other studies. It appears possible that improved contraction at rest was due to a reduction of latent myocardial ischemia. In group 1 ejection fraction at rest was normalized in 14 patients with single-vessel disease. In seven patients contraction remained pathological because of myocardial infarctions or coronary multivessel disease. They as well as the remaining seven patients showed only slight differences at rest.

A normal increase during exercise (over 4%) was observed only in three patients in group 1. This result points to a reduced left ventricular function in supine position even after successful TCA.

Results in group 2 were comparable with these in group 1. Ejection fraction showed some increase at rest in four of five patients, complete normalization in two patients. During exercise three of four patients showed a normal increase, only one patient with a large myocardial infarction remaining unchanged. Again, only slight differences were observed in group 3.

Although patients from groups 1 and 2 were not completely comparable, demonstrated results derived from three independent methods repeatedly performed during exercise show that TCA can achieve an improvement of myocardial function and perfusion comparable to that of aortocoronary bypass operation.

In conclusion, exercise ECG, radionuclide ventriculography, and thallium-201 myocardial scintigraphy demonstrate marked improvement of myocardial function after TCA. Repeated studies in patients with unsuccessful TCA show excellent reproducibility of the methods. By 1982 further improvement of scintigraphic analysis of left ventricular function was obtained by computerized calculation of regional ejection fraction, thallium-201 filling-in and redistribution (G. Hör et al.: Congress on Nuclear Medicine, Vienna, 1982).

References

1. Adam WE, Tarkowska A, Bittner F, Stauch M, Geffers H (1979) Equilibrium (gated) radionuclide ventriculography. Cardiovasc Radiol 2:161
2. Grüntzig A (1978) Transluminal dilatation of coronary artery stenoses. Lancet 1.263
3. Grüntzig A, Schneider J (1977) Die perkutane Dilatation chronischer Koronarstenosen. Experiment und Morphologie. Schweiz Med Wochenschr 107:1588
4. Grüntzig A, Hirzel H, Gattiker R, Turina M, Myler R, Kaltenbach M (1978) Die perkutane transluminale Dilatation chronischer Koronarstenosen. Schweiz Med Wochenschr 108:1721

5. Hör G (1979) 201-Thallium-Myokardszintigraphie. II. Klinik und Sensitivität. Nuklearmedizin 2:12
6. Hör G, Sebening H, Sauer E et al. (1979) 201-Tl-redistribution analysis in early and delayed myocardial scintigrams of patients with coronary heart disease. Eur J Nucl Med 4:343
7. Hör G, Kanemoto N, Standke R et al. (1980) Transluminale Angioplastik: Erfolgskontrolle durch Verfahren der Nuklearmedizin nach nicht-operativer Dilatation kritischer Koronararterienstenosen. Herz 5:168
8. Kaltenbach M (1979) Transluminal angioplasty of coronary artery stenoses. Circulation [Abstr] 60:264
9. Kaltenbach M, Kober G, Satter P, Krause E (1979) Koronarchirurgie versus Ballondilatation. Z Kardiol 68:692
10. Kaltenbach M, Kober G, Scherer D (1980) Mechanische Dilatation von Koronararterienstenosen. Z Kardiol 69:1
11. Kanemoto N, Kaltenbach M, Klepzig H Jr, Standke R, Maul FD, Hör G (1980a) Radionuclide evaluation of transluminal coronary angioplasty. Z Kardiol [Abstr] 69:230
12. Kanemoto N, Hör G, Kaltenbach M, Maul FD, Standke R, Klepzig H Jr (1980) Noninvasive assessment of left ventricular performance following transluminal coronary angioplasty. Circulation [Abstr] 62:218
13. Kent KM, Bonow RO, Rosing DR et al. (1982) Effects of percutaneous transluminal coronary angioplasty on myocardial function during exercise. In: Kaltenbach M, Bussmann W-D, Grüntzig A, Rentrop K (eds) Coronary heart disease. Springer, Berlin Heidelberg New York
14. Klepzig H Jr, Scherer D, Kober G et al. (1980) Ergebnisse der transluminalen koronaren Angioplastie. Z Kardiol [Abstr] 69.701
15. Satter P (1979) Transluminale Katheterdilatation von Koronararterienstenosen: eine Alternative zur Koronarchirurgie? Dtsch Med Wochenschr 104:1687

Interest of Radionuclide Methods for the Assessment of the Results of Percutaneous Transluminal Coronary Angioplasty

M. Amor, N. Danchin, J.-P. Godenir, A. Bertrand, M. Cuilliere, F. Cherrier

Clinique des maladies cardio-vasculaires
C.H.U. de Nancy-Brabois, 54500 Vandoeuvre les Nancy, France

Percutaneous transluminal coronary angioplasty (PTCA) is a new therapeutic technique in ischemic heart disease, used mostly in patients with single-vessel disease. At present, medical management is still considered as more advisable in these patients, unless they remain symptomatic. Some consider that prompt surgery is indicated in patients with a very proximal lesion of the LAD.

Percutaneous transluminal coronary angioplasty might be an interesting alternative in patients with proximal single-vessel disease, provided the consequences of the stenosis and the potential benefits of its relief by PTCA can be estimated. Furthermore, because it is a new method, repeated evaluation of its results is necessary. Therefore, we feel that radionuclide techniques are particularly appropriate, in order to evaluate myocardial perfusion and left ventricular function. We wish to report here our preliminary results on the interest of isotopic methods in the assessment and follow-up of patients undergoing PTCA.

Material

Between April 1980 and March 1981, 31 PTCAs were performed in patients with single-vessel disease whose mean age was 49 ± 10 years; All stenoses were judged as 70% or higher by several independent and well-trained observers. Nine PTCAs were unsuccessful: in four cases the lesion was impossible to pass, three patients had obstruction of a coronary artery, and two developed recurrence of stenosis. Among the 22 successful PTCAs, 18 patients had a stenosis of the LAD and 4 had a stenosis of the right coronary artery.

Twelve patients presented with New York Heart Association (NYHA) class IV angina, five with NYHA class I to III, and four with Prinzmetal's angina. One patient was free of angina but had suffered a recent anterior myocardial infarction.

Ten patients had a normal ECG at rest, ten showed anterior ischemia and two had an image of anterior myocardial infarction. In patients who could undergo an exercise test before PTCA, two showed a marked ST segment depression.

Transluminal Coronary Angioplasty and
Intracoronary Thrombolysis. Ed. by Kaltenbach et al.

Protocol and Methods

The following protocol was used:

Before PTCA:
When an exercise test was considered possible (eight patients, NYHA class I to III): thallium-201 myocardial scintigraphy at maximal exercise in the morning and exercise radionuclide angiography (RNA) in the afternoon.

When an exercise test was not possible (14 patients, NYHA class IV): thallium-201 scintigraphy and RNA at rest on the same day.

After PTCA:
All patients underwent exercise thallium-201 scintigraphy and radionuclide angiography 8 days after PTCA.
These investigations were repeated in the five patients followed up for 6 months or more.

In most patients, PTCA was performed using Gruntzig's method, 24 h after isotopic investigations.

Myocardial scintigraphy was performed after an injection of 2 mCi thallium-201 in four views (anteroposterior, LAO 45°, LAO 60°, and left lateral). Exercise scintigraphy was performed after an injection of thallium at maximal exercise and redistribution was studied 4 h later in the two views showing the defects most clearly during exercise. Several independent observers reviewed the scans and calculated the number of cold spots in the LAO 45° and anteroposterior views. Each image was divided into three sectors (Figs. 1, 2).

Multiple-gated equilibrium scintigraphy was performed after an injection of 30 mCi technetium 99m labeled red blood cells [5]. The angiography is performed in the LAO view and global ejection fraction (GEF) is determined from the end-diastolic and end-systolic frames, according to a method previously reported [1].

Regional wall motion was analyzed according to our method [3]; the left ventricle is divided into 16 angular sectors, around the center of gravity of the end-diastolic frame and the ejection fraction of each sector is determined. A sector is considered as asynergic when its regional ejection fraction (REF) is 0.45 or less. The number of asynergic sectors was determined in each patient (Fig. 4). This RNA is performed at rest, on exercise, and during recovery. The patient is placed in a supine position; a first scintigram is performed at rest, a second when he has reached maximal heart rate and a third 2 minutes after the end of exercise.

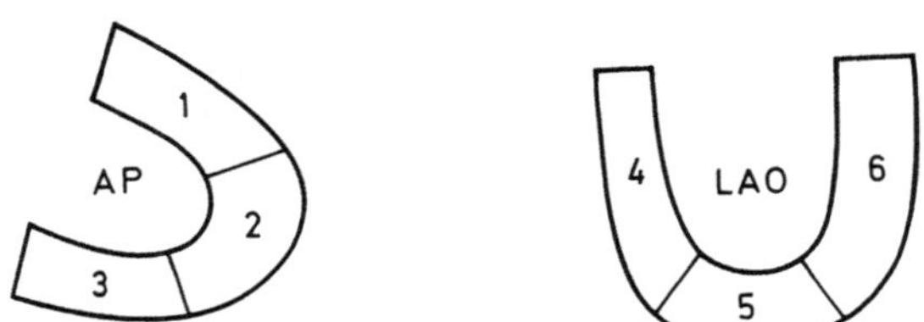

Fig. 1. Anteroposterior (AP) and left anterior oblique (LAO) views divided into six sectors

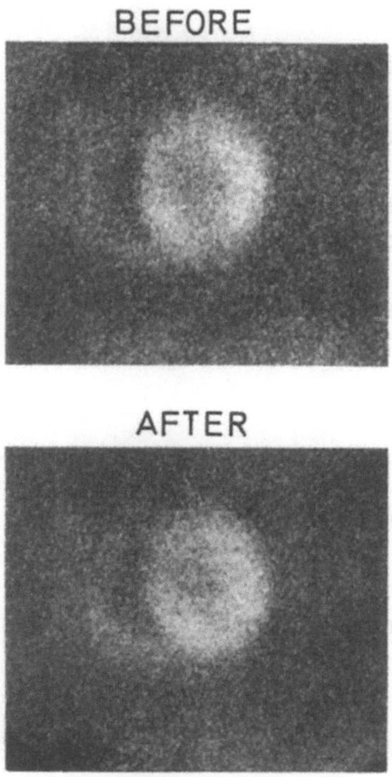

Fig. 2. Patient with a RCA stenosis. *Top:* Before PTCA, there is a cold spot in the inferior sector and the right ventricle is not visualized. *Bottom:* after PTCA, the cold spot disappears and the right ventricle is clearly visualized

Statistical analysis used Student's paired test and the results are given in terms of mean ± standard deviation.

Results

Myocardial Scintigraphy

Before PTCA, the 14 patients with rest studies there was an average of 0.78 ± 1.3 cold spots and myocardial imaging was abnormal in four patients. In the eight patients with exercise studies, there were 2.23 ± 1.6 cold spots on exercise and 0.08 ± 0.02 cold spots on redistribution. Six cold spots were located in the septal sector, four in the apical sector, and two in the inferior sector. Exercise thallium imaging was abnormal in seven patients.

After PTCA, exercise myocardial scintigraphy performed in all 22 patients showed a normal scan in 21 cases; one patient had persistent cold spots corresponding to a previous anterior myocardial infarction (Fig. 2).

Radionuclide Angiography

In the 14 patients with rest studies before PTCA, global ejection fraction (GEF) was 66% ± 9% and was not significantly different after PTCA. The number of asynergic sectors did not change and remained less than one on average.

When exercise studies were possible, GEF at rest and after PTCA remained stable (59.2% ± 11% and 63.4% ± 7%). In contrast, GEF on exercise increased markedly and significantly after PTCA (54% ± 6% and 72% ± 11%); during recovery GEF was 64% ± 8% before and 73% ± 3% after PTCA (Figs. 3, 4).

Similarly, the number of asynergic sectors during exercise decreased after PTCA, as shown in Table 1.

Follow-up

Five patients underwent coronary arteriography and isotopic studies after 6 months; in four of them, the angiographic result remained stable (Table 2). In four patients, there was no cold spot on thallium scans. In one patient with a previous anterior myocardial infarction, a cold spot was still noted. RNA showed unchanged results.

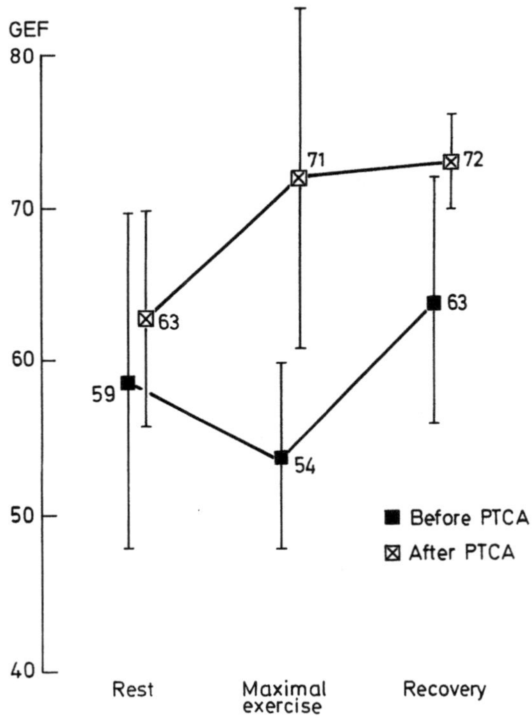

Fig. 3. Evolution of global ejection fraction (GEF) at rest, maximal exercise, and recovery states before and after PTCA

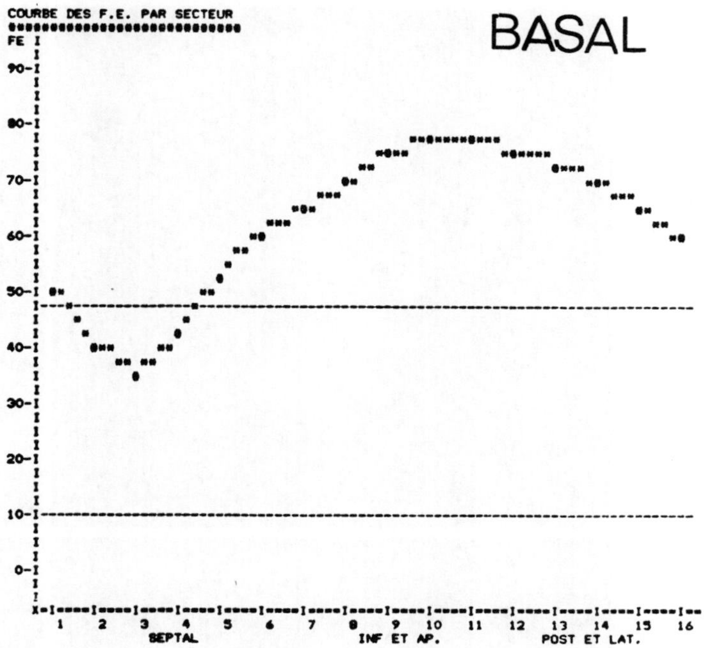
COURBE DES F.E. PAR SECTEUR
BASAL
FE
90-
80-
70-
60-
50-
40-
30-
20-
10-
0-
1 2 3 4 5 6 7 8 9 10 11 12 13 14 15 16
SEPTAL
INF ET AP.
POST ET LAT.

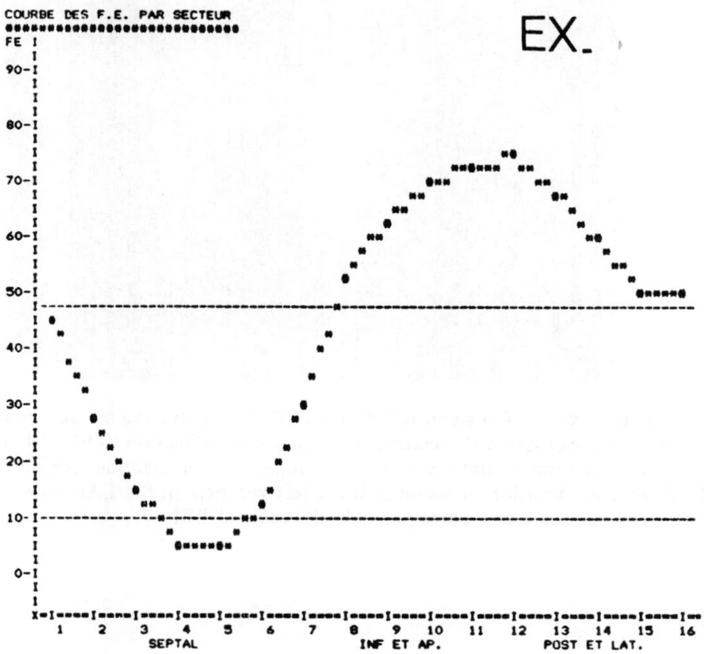
COURBE DES F.E. PAR SECTEUR
EX
FE
90-
80-
70-
60-
50-
40-
30-
20-
10-
0-
1 2 3 4 5 6 7 8 9 10 11 12 13 14 15 16
SEPTAL
INF ET AP.
POST ET LAT.

Fig. 4a

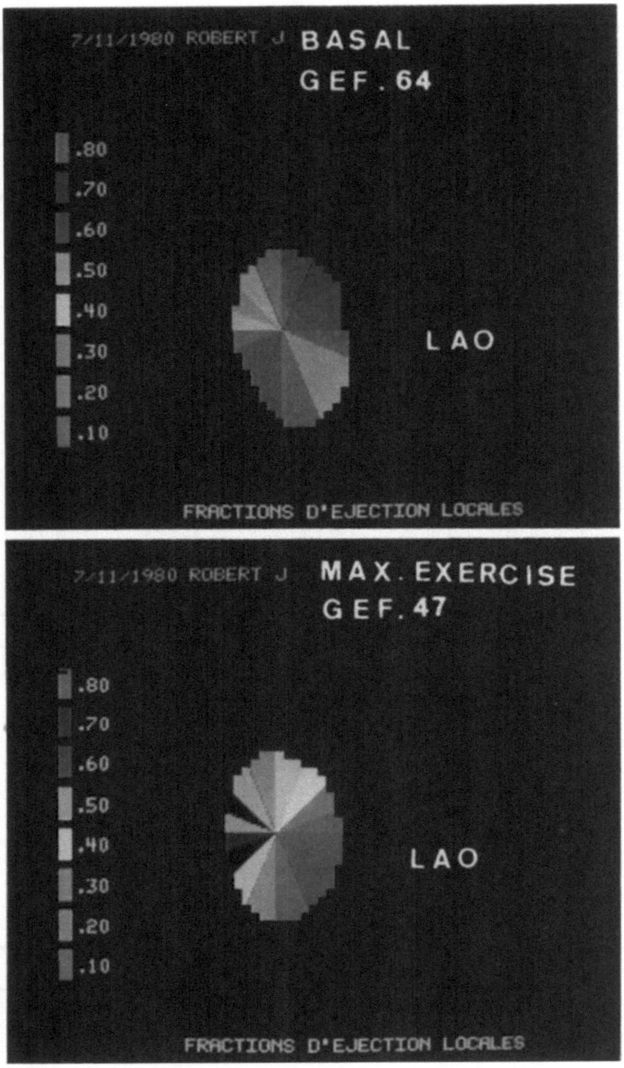

Fig. 4b

Fig. 4a, b. An example of a patient with LAD stenosis before PTCA. It appears as a severe hypokinesia in septal sectors at maximal exercise with decrease of global ejection fraction (0.64–0.47). *Top:* basal state. ***Bottom:*** maximal exercise state. **a** curve of regional ejection fraction (REF) of each sector (ordinate, REF; abscissa, location of sectors). **b** the left ventricle in the LAO view is divided into 16 sectors. The color of each sector corresponds to the value of REF

Table 1. Exercise RNA results before and after PTCA and mean number of dyskinetic sectors in eight cases

	Global ejection fraction (%)			Mean number of dyskinetic sectors		
Time of RNA	Rest	Maximal exercise	Recovery state	Rest	Maximal exercise	Recovery state
Before PTCA	59.2 ± 11	54 ± 6	64 ± 3	4	5	3
After PTCA	63.4 ± 7	72 ± 11	73 ± 3	3	1	0
P	NS	< 0.001	< 0.001	NS	< 0.001	< 0.001

Table 2. Exercise RNA 8 days and 6 months after PTCA: global and local study in eight patients

	Global ejection fraction			Mean number of dyskinetic sectors		
Time of RNA	Rest	Maximal exercise	Recovery state	Rest	Maximal exercise	Recovery state
Eight days after PTCA	72.8 ± 6	76 ± 8	76 ± 8	0	0	0
Six months after PTCA	63.6 ± 5	72 ± 6	76 ± 6	0	0	0

Unsuccessful Cases

Among the nine unsuccessful cases, there were:

Three patients who had had myocardial infarctions; one lateral, one small anteroseptal, and one large anterior. In this large infarction, there was a decrease in GEF from 47% to 32% and 2 months later GEF was 34%.

Two patients who underwent surgery for LAD stenoses.

Four patients with no further procedure who did not have a myocardial infarction and whose GEF remained stable. In one patient GEF remained normal 11 months later.

One death in the catheterization laboratory immediately after PTCA. At autopsy, we found two small thrombi in the LAD.

Discussion

Thallium-201 myocardial scintigraphy is the best present non-invasive method to study myocardial perfusion, and shows ischemic or infarcted areas [6, 7]. Exercise RNA proves useful in order to study wall motion abnormalities induced by abnormal coronary perfusion [4]. Recent reports [2] have shown the interest of coupling both methods for the diagnosis of myocardial ischemia and for the evaluation of its detrimental effects on ventricular function.

Usually, PTCA is performed in patients with single-vessel disease and unimpaired left ventricular function at rest, as confirmed by RNA. Indeed, perfusion defects and wall motion abnormalities are only apparent during exercise. The beneficial effects of PTCA do not appear on our rest studies, but exercise studies show that myocardial perfusion improves and that wall motion abnormalities induced by exercise decrease or disappear.

Furthermore, isotopic methods allow for repeated evaluation and follow-up of these patients. Thus, isotopic techniques could predict the good result in all patients whose result proved satisfactory at a 6 months follow-up coronary angiogram.

Finally, these methods may be helpful in the initial choice of therapy: to the therapeutic PTC is indicated in cases of regressive cold spot during redistribution and/or of wall motion abnormalities appearing or increasing during exercise RNA.

References

1. Amor M, Karcher G, Bertrand A, Hocquard C, Cherrier F, Faivre G (1981) Une nouvelle méthode isotopique des fractions d'éjection locales. Arch Mal Coeur 74:1121
2. Elkayam U, Weinstein M, Berman D et al. (1981) Stress thallium-201 myocardial scintigraphy and exercise technetium ventriculography in the detection and location of chronic coronary artery disease: Comparison of sensitivity and specificity of these noninvasive tests alone and in combination. Am Heart J 101:657
3. Ethevenot G, Amor M, Karcher G, Bertrand A (1981) Comparaison de deux méthodes volumétriques angiographique et isotopique d'étude de la contractilité locale. Arch Mal Coeur 74:1367
4. Leppo JA, Scheuer J, Pohost GM, Freeman LM, Strauss HW (1980) The evaluation of ischemic heart disease. Semin Nucl Med 10:115
5. Pavel DG, Zimmer AM, Patterson VN (1977) In vivo labeling of red blood cells with 99 m Technetium. J Nucl Med 18:305
6. Pohost GM, Alpert NM, Ingwall JS, Strauss HW (1980) Thallium redistribution: mechanisms and clinical utility. Semin Nucl Med 10:70
7. Wackers FJT (1980) Thallium 201 Myocardial scintigraphy in acute myocardial infarction and ischemia. Semin Nucl Med 10:127

Parameters of Left Ventricular Contractility After Transluminal Coronary Angioplasty

U. Sigwart, M. Grbic, J.-L. Rivier, H. Sadeghi

Centre Hospitalier Universitaire Vaudois, 1011 Lausanne, Switzerland

Introduction

The anatomical aspects of transluminal coronary angioplasty with balloon catheters have been the subject of several publications [2, 3, 4]. The functional results of the procedure have been studied noninvasively by bicycle ergometry and measurement of ejection fraction during exercise with gated blood-pooling techniques using radioisotopes [5, 6]. We have attempted to follow left ventricular function measured by contractility parameters before and after successful angioplasty with the help of invasive techniques during cardiac catheterization.

Material and Method

A study protocol was approved by the hospital ethics committee. Nine consecutive patients presenting with high-grade proximal stenosis of the left anterior descending coronary artery who had positive exercise ECG, angina pectoris refractory to standard therapy, and who were willing to participate were admitted to the study.

All medication, including beta-blockers and nitrates, was discontinued 1 day prior to standard left and right heart catheterization. A double-tip manometer (Millar 771) was employed in the left ventricle and aorta, as well as a Swan-Ganz thermodilution catheter in the pulmonary artery. The pressures were recorded on a Hewlett-Packard 6800 A optical recorder and cardiac output was measured with a Roche ECG triggered automatic injector. After a resting period, measurements were obtained during dynamic bicycle exercise in the supine position until a heart rate of approximately 120–130/min was obtained or until the patient experienced angina pectoris with ECG changes. The patients were then allowed a recovery period during which measurements were continued. When the resting heart rate had again been reached, an isoproterenol infusion was begun with dose increments being given every minute until the exercise heart rate was reached.

The calculations were carried out with the help of a Numonics graphics analyzer, the data being interpreted by calculating the mean and the standard error and the statistical analysis being performed with the paired t test.

One day after this investigation, balloon angioplasty of the stenosed coronary artery was performed employing standard techniques [2, 3, 4]. A good functional result of

Transluminal Coronary Angioplasty and
Intracoronary Thrombolysis. Ed. by Kaltenbach et al.

the dilatation was judged upon reduction of the transstenotic pressure gradient. The patients were discharged on regular anticoagulation and readmitted 6 months later for an identical study.

Results

There was no significant difference in heart rate before and after angioplasty within the different study conditions. Before angioplasty the heart rate increased with exercise from 69.3 ± 2.7 to 120.0 ± 2.1 beats/min; after angioplasty, an increase from 69.1 ± 1.4 to 125.7 ± 1.4 beats/min was seen. The heart rate during isoproterenol infusion did not differ significantly from the exercise heart rate (120.7 ± 3.4 beats/min before and 125.1 ± 2.8 beats/min after angioplasty).

The cardiac index was found to be normal in all patients at rest. With exercise it increased significantly but the increase was more pronounced after angioplasty (Fig. 1). This improvement was highly significant ($P < 0.001$). During isoproterenol infusion the cardiac index did not change significantly after angioplasty.

Pulmonary artery pressures at rest were normal even before angioplasty. With exercise, the mean pulmonary artery pressure rose from 15.9 ± 0.8 to 41.7 ± 1.4 mmHg. After angioplasty, it increased with exercise only to 27.1 ± 1.5 mmHg. No significant increase was observed during isoproterenol infusion.

An impressive reduction of left ventricular end-diastolic pressure (LVEDP) during exercise became evident after angioplasty (Fig. 2). Before balloon dilatation LVEDP increased with exercise from 12.1 ± 0.7 to 33.8 ± 1.6 mmHg; after angioplasty an average rise during exercise to 19.2 ± 0.5 mmHg was seen. This difference was highly significant ($p < 0.001$). No significant change was noted during isoproterenol infusion.

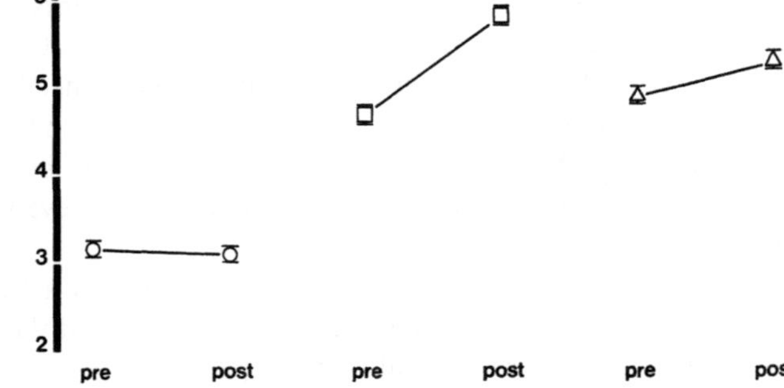

Fig. 1. Cardiac index (CI) at rest (*R*), with exercise (*E*), and with isoproterenol (*I*) before and 6 months after successful coronary angioplasty

LVEDP

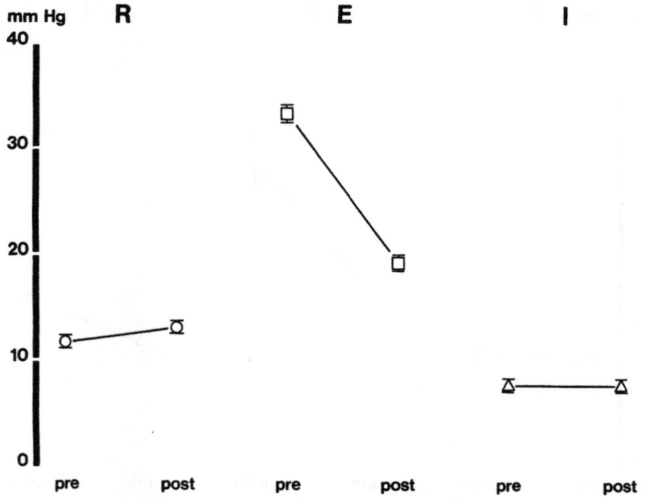

Fig. 2. Left ventricular end-diastolic pressure (*LVEDP*) at rest (*R*), with exercise (*E*), and with isoproterenol (*I*) before and 6 months after successful coronary angioplasty

Also the systolic arterial pressure failed to show any significant difference before and after coronary angioplasty.

As to the contractility parameters, it was found that the maximum rate of left ventricular pressure rise (dP/dt max) at rest was within the normal range in all patients before and after the angioplasty. With exercise dP/dt max increased from 2181 ± 209 mmHg/sec before angioplasty to 2419 ± 244 mmHg/sec after angioplasty (Fig. 3);

DP/DT max

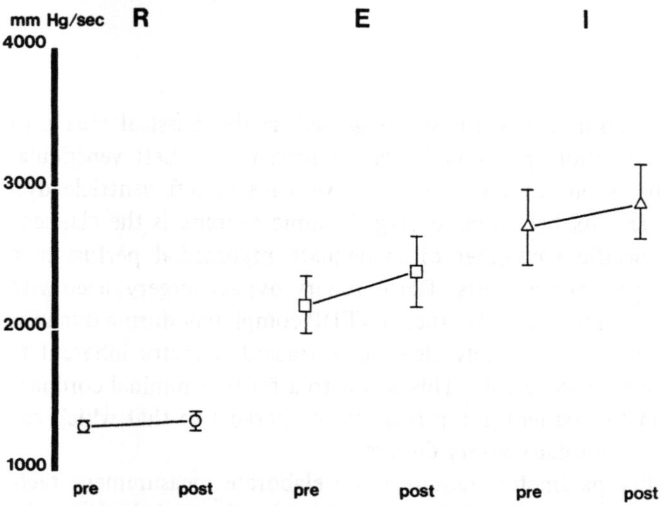

Fig. 3. Maximal rate of left ventricular pressure rise (*dP/dt max*) at rest (*R*), with exercise (*E*), and with isoproterenol (*I*) before and 6 months after successful coronary angioplasty

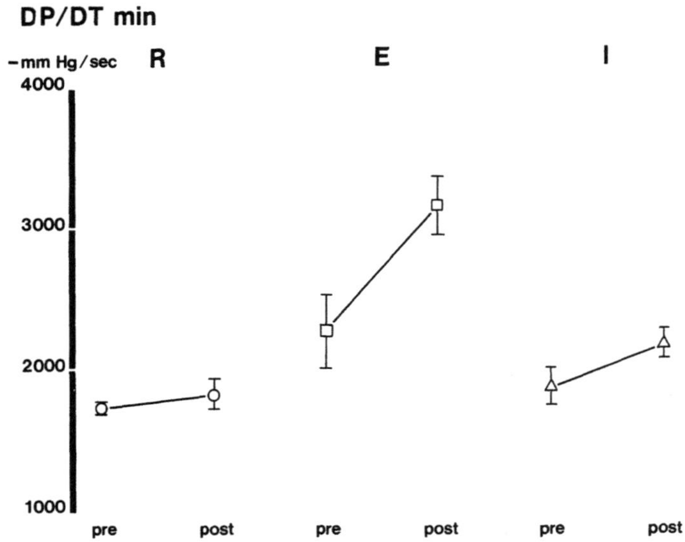

Fig. 4. Maximal rate of left ventricular pressure fall (*dP/dt min*) at rest (*R*), with exercise (*E*), and with isoproterenol (*I*) before and 6 months after successful coronary angioplasty

the paired t test revealed this difference to be significant ($p < 0.05$). No substantial difference with isoproterenol was noted before and after angioplasty.

The maximum rate of left ventricular pressure fall (dP/dt min) normalized at rest in the majority of patients; the difference, however, was not statistically significant. With exercise, dP/dt min changed from -2307 ± 260 mmHg/sec before to -3154 ± 200 mmHg/sec after angioplasty ($p < 0.001$). Also with isoproterenol an augmentation from -1874 ± 134 to -2166 ± 108 mmHg/sec was measured ($p < 0.05$) (Fig. 4).

Discussion

Left ventricular pressure measurements are still regarded as the classical means of estimating left ventricular function, particularly with interventions. Left ventricular end-diastolic pressure remains one of the most sensitive signs of left ventricle dysfunction due to ischemia and its behaviour during dynamic exercise is the classical, highly sensitive, but nonspecific parameter of inadequate myocardial perfusion in coronary disease. In our experience patients after coronary bypass surgery, even with single-vessel disease, have failed to normalize their LVEDP completely during dynamic exercise. The reason for this is not entirely clear; an extracardiac factor inherent to the surgical procedure may play some role. This is not so after transluminal coronary angioplasty. The LVEDP in this patient group is quite comparable to that which can be seen in individuals without coronary artery disease.

The so-called contractility parameters require more elaborate measurement techniques. Their merit in detecting myocardial abnormalities is undisputed. In particular dP/dt max and dP/dt min are considered highly sensitive reflections of myocardial performance during systole [1, 9] and diastole [7, 8]. Similar but less pronounced changes of these parameters have been noted in coronary heart disease during isoproterenol infusion [1].

In our group of patients with subtotal proximal stenosis of the left anterior descending coronary artery, these parameters were highly abnormal before transluminal angioplasty when the patient underwent exercise or was subjected to isoproterenol infusion. Six months after the procedure, no residual signs of myocardial functional abnormalities due to ischemia could be observed. In view of the astonishing anatomical results of coronary angioplasty and the impressive subjective improvement, these findings are neither unexpected nor surprising. The objective measurement of left ventricular contractility and relaxation recorded directly in the left ventricle without distortion by residual medication is, however, a reassuring and comforting detail in the appreciation of this highly innovative and fascinating method of treating coronary disease. In practice noninvasive techniques to estimate myocardial function and left ventricular performance, together with stress testing and the patients' history, may eventually be sufficient to estimate accurately the long-term results of transluminal angioplasty.

Summary

In order to study the effects of transluminal coronary angioplasty, nine patients were studied using left and right heart catheterization and high-fidelity pressure recording 1 day before and 6 months after successful coronary angioplasty. Left ventricular contractility was measured at rest, during isoproterenol infusion, and with dynamic bicycle exercise. Only patients with high-grade stenosis of the left anterior descending coronary artery were included.

A significant improvement in the parameters of left ventricular function was found. After successful coronary angioplasty LVEDP at exercise became normal (33.8 ± 1.6 mmHg). There was a significant increase in dP/dt max during exercise after angioplasty ($p < 0.05$). At rest or with isoproterenol dP/dt max was not significantly affected before and after angioplasty; dP/dt min was augmented significantly during exercise ($p < 0.001$) and also at rest ($p < 0.05$). Improvement of left ventricular function appears to reflect the success of transluminal coronary angioplasty. Noninvasive determination of left ventricular function may help to estimate the success of transluminal coronary angioplasty.

References

1. Grassi de Gende AO, Perez Alzueta AD, Cingolani HE (1977) Effect of isoproteronol on relation between maximal rate of contraction and maximal rate of relaxation. Am J Physiol 2:H 404
2. Grüntzig AR (1977) Die perkutane transluminale Rekanalisation chronischer Arterienverschlüsse mit einer neuen Dilatationstechnik. G. Witzstrock, Baden-Baden
3. Grüntzig AR (1978) Transluminal dilatation of coronary-artery stenosis. Lancet 1:263
4. Grüntzig AR, Senning A, Siegenthaler WE (1979) Non-operative dilatation of coronary artery stenosis. N Engl J Med 301:61–68
5. Hirzel HP, Nuesch K, Grüntzig A, Luetolf UM (1981) Short and long term changes in myocardial perfusion following percutaneous transluminal coronary angioplasty assessed by thallium-201 exercise scintigraphy. Circulation 63:1001–1007

6. Hör G, Kanemoto N, Standke R, Maul FD et al. (1980) Transluminal angioplasty: control of efficiency by nuclear medical methods after non-operative dilatation of critical coronary artery stenoses. Herz 5:168–173
7. Lewis BS, Gotsman MS (1980) Current concepts of left ventricular relaxation and compliance. Am Heart J 99:101
8. Papapietro SE, Coghlan HC, Zissermann D, Russel RO, Rackley CE, Rogers WJ (1979) Impaired maximal rate of left ventricular relaxation in patients with coronary artery disease and left ventricular dysfunction. Circulation 59:894
9. Rutishauser W, Amende J, Mehmel H (1972) Comparison of left ventricular dynamics in normals and patients with ischemic heart disease at rest, during pacing and exercise. Eur J Clin Invest 2:304

Dynamic Changes in Left Ventricular Geometry and Pressure During Coronary Artery Occlusion in Man

L.G. Bentivoglio, M.J. Barrett, N.M. Wolf, S.G. Meister

Medical College of Pennsylvania, 3300 Henry Avenue, Philadelphia, PA 19129, USA

Analysis of the early left ventricular geometry and hemodynamic response to the abrupt occlusion of a major coronary artery has not been feasible in man thus far.

Percutaneous transluminal coronary angioplasty (PTCA), however, has now provided a unique opportunity to study the time course of these variables during the sudden, transient interruption of coronary flow in the balloon occlusion sequence.

We have studied the dynamic changes in left ventricular (LV) geometry by two-dimensional echocardiography (2D Echo) in ten patients and the concurrent LV hemodynamic abnormalities in five patients during PTCA limited to the anterior descending artery.

The patients were imaged by 2D Echo in the apical four-chamber or the apical long-axis view using a Varian phased-array sector scanner. The geometry changes were described quantitatively as fractional shortening abnormalities of the short axis chords expressed as percentage of control.

The left ventricular end-diastolic pressure (LVEDP) was measured directly in three patients with an indwelling 8F pigtail catheter and indirectly with a 7F Goodale Lubin catheter, in one patient as left atrial (LA) pressure following accidental penetration in this chamber through a patent foramen ovale and in one patient as wedge pressure. The transducers were Statham P 23 Db strain gauges. The LVEDP was measured at the peak of the R wave on the ECG and the LA and wedge pressures at the peak of their "a" wave. The Echo and hemodynamic measurements were made with the patient lying in a 30–40° RAO position. Wall geometry and pressure changes were expressed as percentage of the control value which was taken as 100%.

Figure 1 shows the mean fractional chord shortening changes in ten patients and the mean LVEDP changes in five patients following balloon inflation. Reduction of left ventricular segmental shortening begins immediately upon interruption of flow, with a monotonic drop which reaches its nadir just after the balloon is deflated. The return of flow is followed by the rapid improvement of contractility which recovers completely, and rebounds slightly at 30 s, that is 18 s after flow resumes.

At variance with the geometry changes, the LVEDP rise shows a lag of 6 s after the beginning of balloon inflation, and its fall shows an 8 s lag following balloon deflation, with a pressure peak at 21 s. At 30 s the LVEDP is still significantly elevated at a time when segmental wall motion has fully recovered, and does not fall back to normal till about 10 s later. A 20 s rebound follows, with a pressure drop which is more pronounced and prolonged than the contractility rebound. The changes are statistically significant for both parameters.

Transluminal Coronary Angioplasty and
Intracoronary Thrombolysis. Ed. by Kaltenbach et al.

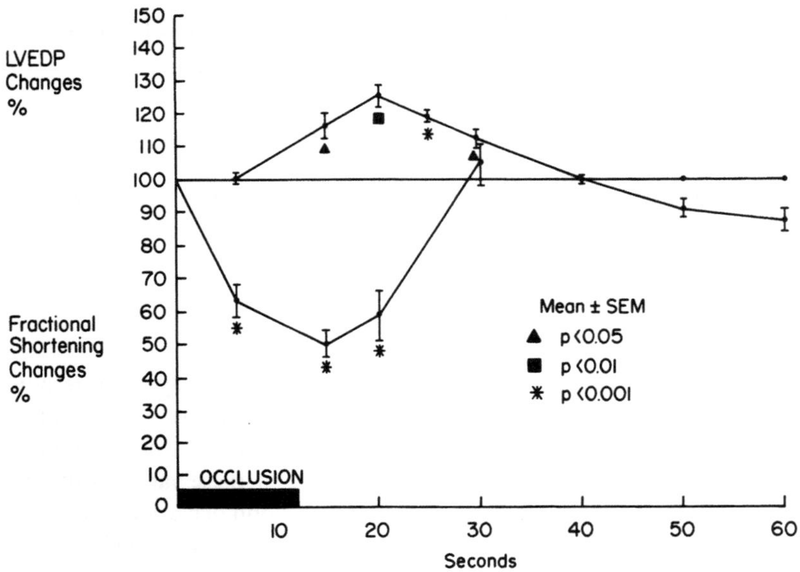

Fig. 1. Dynamic changes in left ventricular geometry and pressure during coronary artery occlusion in man: mean fractional chord shortening changes in ten patients (*lower curve*) and mean LVEDP changes in five patients (*upper curve*)

The time lag between these two variables is not surprising in that segmental shortening is a systolic phenomenon while LVEDP is a diastolic event not necessarily related to the former.

The loss of wall motion presumably stems directly from the O_2 deficiency which accompanies the interruption of flow, with exhaustion of ATP and ischemia-mediated blockage of its resynthesis from ADP. The rise of end-diastolic pressure, on the other hand, may relate to a variety of factors. LVEDP may increase because of a gain in end-diastole volume (EDV) and the resultant pressure along the normal diastolic compliance curve. This volume gain may have three causes: (1) a reduction of heart rate (HR) with the consequent increase in filling time in the face of stable afterload and venous return, resulting in increased EDV and EDP; (2) an increase in afterload and therefore in end-systolic volume, EDV, and EDP if HR and venous return are unchanged; and (3) an increase in venous return. Any of these three factors could be triggered by a hypothetical coronary stretch reflex from the inflating balloon. However, our data show only insignificant and random changes in HR and aortic pressure during and after balloon inflation, and change in venous return is unlikely. Furthermore, the LVED area, measured from 2D images, does not appear to increase during or after balloon inflation. One is left with two other possible explanations: an apparent reduction of true diastolic compliance, that is increased EDP despite unchanged EDV due to transiently altered characteristics of the parallel elastic system, or persistence of residual systolic actin-myosin interaction at end-diastole, superimposed on unaltered diastolic compliance. These two mechanisms have been postulated and seemingly demonstrated by some authors as a result of ischemia.

In conclusion, we have observed a reduction in LV segmental wall motion immediately after coronary artery occlusion in man, followed by a rise in LV filling pressure. Both variables return to normal upon reinstitution of coronary blood flow but the hemodynamics again lay behind the wall motion.

Salutory Effect of Percutaneous Transluminal Coronary Angioplasty on Coronary Circulatory Dynamics

D.O. Williams, R.S. Riley, A.K. Singh, K.S. Korr, A.S. Most

Division of Cardiology, Department of Medicine, Section of Cardiovascular Thoracic Surgery, Department of Surgery, Rhode Island Hospital, Brown University, Providence, Rhode Island 02902, USA

Introduction

Percutaneous transluminal coronary angioplasty (PTCA) has been demonstrated to reduce the extent of coronary artery narrowing as judged angiographically in a large population of symptomatic patients with coronary artery disease [3]. In addition, noninvasive nuclear tests have suggested that coronary blood flow to previously ischemic myocardium may be increased [2]. However, no data are yet available directly assessing the effect of angiographically successful PTCA on coronary blood flow. Thus, the goal of this investigation was to measure coronary blood flow and myocardial metabolism directly to test the hypothesis that angiographically successful PTCA corrects abnormal coronary dynamics and myocardial ischemia resulting from significant coronary artery stenosis.

Methods

In designing an appropriate investigation to test the hypothesis of this investigation, three criteria must be satisfied: (1) patients with coronary artery stenosis selected as candidates for PTCA should demonstrate abnormal coronary circulatory responsiveness prior to PTCA; (2) PTCA must then be performed successfully according to angiographic criteria; and (3) patients should then be reassessed to determine whether previously observed abnormal coronary responsiveness has been corrected.

The initial study population consisted of ten patients with isolated left anterior descending coronary artery stenosis. In nine of these patients, a thermodilution catheter was successfully placed into the coronary sinus and advanced to the point where the catheter tip was located at the junction of the anterior interventricular and great cardiac veins. In all nine patients, great cardiac vein flow and blood content of lactate and oxygen, in arterial and great cardiac vein samples, were first determined at a paced heart rate ten beats per minute (bpm) greater than the resting heart rate and then during rapid atrial pacing. The end point for pacing was development of angina pectoris of moderate severity or second degree AV block. Then PTCA was attempted and was successful in seven of the nine patients. The pre-PTCA pacing protocol was then repeated in these seven successfully dilated patients at a time remote from the injection of radiographic contrast material or administration of nitroglycerin. No patient received a calcium antagonist. These seven patients formed the study group.

Transluminal Coronary Angioplasty and
Intracoronary Thrombolysis. Ed. by Kaltenbach et al.

We performed PTCA as previously described [1] using preformed guiding catheters, Gruntzig balloon dilating catheters, and a pneumatic inflation device (USCI Cardiology and Radiology Products, Billerica, Massachusetts). A no. 20 cannula was placed in the left brachial artery for pressure monitoring and blood sampling. A similar cannula was inserted into a left anticubital vein for intravenous fluid and drug administration. Leads II and V_5 of the electrocardiogram were continuously monitored. In patients in whom lesions were successfully crossed, initial balloon inflation pressure was 3.5–4.0 atm. Balloon inflations were repeated until improvement in the transstenotic gradient was observed. Maximal balloon inflation pressure was 6 atm.

Assessment of regional coronary blood flow and myocardial metabolism was performed as previously described [4]. Intravascular pressures, great cardiac vein flow, and the electrocardiogram were recorded simultaneously on a multichannel recorder (Hewlett Packard model 8890A). Oxygen content was analyzed utilizing a Lex-O_2-Con TL Analyzer (Lexington Instruments, Lexington, Massachusetts). Lactate concentration was determined by a photometric technique (Calbiochem-Bering Corporation, LaJolla, California). Coronary stenoses were quantitated in at least two views utilizing an optical comparator with a 10-mm reticle. The extent of reduction in lumen diameter was expressed as an average of the measured stenoses in the two views. The initial transstenotic pressure gradient was determined by comparing mean pressure recorded from the dilating catheter tip proximal and distal to the stenosis as the catheter traversed the lesion. The post-PTCA gradient was obtained during the pullback of the dilating catheter across the dilated segment. Rate pressure product, an index of myocardial oxygen demand, was calculated as a product of peak systolic arterial blood pressure (mmHg) and heart rate (bpm). Regional myocardial oxygen consumption was determined as the product of great cardiac vein flow (ml/min) and the difference in oxygen content of the paired arterial and great cardiac vein blood samples (cc O_2/100 ml blood divided by 100). Regional coronary vascular resistance (units) was calculated by dividing mean arterial blood pressure by great cardiac vein flow. Myocardial lactate extraction was calculated as the difference between arterial and great cardiac vein lactate concentrations divided by the arterial lactate concentration.

Repeated observations were analyzed by two-way analysis of variance. Individual patients were considered as a second factor to remove interpatient differences. Significant differences between specific means were determined by the Newmann Keuls multiple comparison test. Significance of paired observations was assessed by Student's t test.

Results

All patients had significant coronary stenosis (> 50% diameter reduction). Coronary spasm was excluded by demonstrating the persistence of lesions angiographically during the hypotensive phase following sublingual nitroglycerin administration. Vessel stenosis in these successfully dilated patients was reduced from 74% ± 14% to 35% ± 12% ($P < 0.001$). This reduction in the extent of coronary obstruction was associated with a decline in the mean pressure gradient across the stenosis from 72 ± 13 mmHg to 25 ± 12 mmHg ($P < 0.001$). In the two patients in whom PTCA was unsuccessful, failure was due to inability to reach the stenosis in one and to cross the stenosis in the other.

The effects of PTCA on regional coronary blood flow and myocardial metabolism are shown in Table 1. Prior to PTCA heart rate was increased from 81 ± 7 bpm to 148 ± 17 bpm ($P < 0.001$) with atrial pacing. Angina pectoris developed in five of the seven patients. Great cardiac vein flow, myocardial oxygen consumption, and coronary vascular resistance were unchanged during pacing. Myocardial lactate extraction, however, which was normal at rest, fell from 28% ± 25% to 3% ± 18% ($P < 0.01$) during pacing (Fig. 1).

Following PTCA, both control and paced heart rates and rate pressure products were not significantly different from pre-PTCA values. Great cardiac vein flow at rest was unchanged. During atrial pacing, however, great cardiac vein flow increased significantly ($P < 0.01$) following PTCA compared to resting values and pre-PTCA paced values. Regional myocardial oxygen consumption also increased significantly during rapid atrial pacing following PTCA. Coronary vascular resistance now decreased significantly with pacing. Lactate extraction, normal at rest following PTCA, now remained normal during rapid pacing. Typical angina pectoris was not noted in any of the patients, although one patient complained of a nonspecific chest pain during pacing after angioplasty.

Discussion

Prior to PTCA, in the presence of proximal flow-limiting coronary stenosis, coronary blood flow failed to increase and coronary vascular resistance did not decline in re-

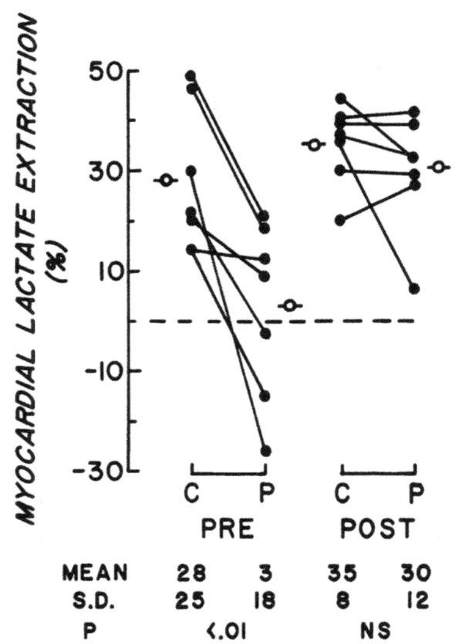

Fig. 1. Effect of successful PTCA on myocardial lactate metabolism. *Pre*, before PTCA; *Post*, after PTCA; *C*, control heart rate; *P*, rapid pacing. *Dashed line* indicates zero extraction Values *above the line* represent extraction, *below the line* lactate production

Table 1. The effects of PTCA on regional coronary blood flow and myocardial metabolism

	Before PTCA			After PTCA		
	Control	Pacing	Change (%)	Control	Pacing	Change (%)
Heart rate (bpm)	81 ± 7	148 ± 17[a]	83 ± 26	78 ± 7	141 ± 20[a]	71 ± 25
Rate pressure product (mmHg/min)	12.0 ± 1.3	21.5 ± 5[a]	78 ± 31	11.2 ± 1.7	19.3 ± 4.3[a]	72 ± 30
Great cardiac vein flow (ml/min)	104 ± 27	131 ± 44	28 ± 40	106 ± 29	174 ± 68[a,b]	64 ± 46[b]
Coronary vascular resistance (units)	1.09 ± 0.25	0.94 ± 0.29	−12 ± 24	0.98 ± 0.31	0.67 ± 0.23[a,b]	−30 ± 20[b]
Myocardial oxygen consumption (cc O_2/min)	15.2 ± 4.1	19.2 ± 5.6	35 ± 45	12.6 ± 3.1	21.4 ± 5.6[a]	70 ± 50[b]
Lactate extraction (%)	28 ± 25	3 ± 18[a]	−25 ± 17	35 ± 8	30 ± 12	− 5 ± 12[b]

Values are mean ± standard deviation
[a] $P < 0.05$ compared to control
[b] $P < 0.05$ compared to pre-PTCA

sponse to rapid atrial pacing. This observation suggests that coronary resistance vessels were maximally dilated at rest and incapable of responding to the added metabolic vasodilatory stimulus of rapid pacing. Coronary blood flow was thus inadequate to meet myocardial oxygen needs and consequently lactate extraction fell, an indication of anerobiosis.

PTCA resulted in a relief of the proximal coronary stenosis. Thus resistance vessels were no longer maximally dilated to maintain basal flow requirements. With vasodilatory reserve restored, rapid atrial pacing resulted in a decrease in coronary vascular resistance and an increase in coronary blood flow commensurate with myocardial oxygen demand. Aerobic metabolism was preserved, as reflected by preservation of lactate extraction. These data indicate that the improved clinical course observed in these angina patients who underwent successful dilatation could be attributed to improved coronary blood flow and myocardial metabolism.

Summary

Although ample evidence indicates that PTCA can relieve angiographic coronary obstruction, few data are available regarding the impact of successful PTCA on the flow dynamics of the coronary circulation. Thus, changes in regional coronary blood flow, coronary vascular resistance, and myocardial metabolism were assessed at rest and during pacing tachycardia in seven patients who underwent angiographically successful PTCA. Significant increases in coronary blood flow and myocardial oxygen consumption, a decrease in coronary vascular resistance and preservation of lactate extraction during pacing resulted from successful PTCA. These results indicate that prior to PTCA, coronary vascular resistance vessels were maximally dilated at rest to compensate for the proximal flow-limiting stenosis. Additional vasodilatation in response to pacing stress was not possible and anerobic metabolism was observed. Proximal coronary stenosis was relieved by PTCA such that resistance vessels were no longer maximally dilated to maintain basal flow requirements. Vasodilatory reserve was restored permitting coronary flow to increase during pacing and aerobic myocardial metabolism to be preserved. Relief of angina pectoris in patients undergoing PTCA may be attributed to improved coronary blood flow and myocardial metabolism.

Acknowledgment. The authors acknowledge the assistance of Karen Jessop, John Larney, Christine Abatiello, Katherine Seropian, Thomas DeVona and the staff of the Cardiovascular and Cardiac Research Laboratories.

References

1. Gruntzig A, Senning A, Siegenthaler W (1979) Nonoperative dilation of coronary artery stenosis. New Engl J Med 301:61
2. Hirzel H, Nuesch K, Gruntzig A, Luetoff U (1981) Short and long term changes in myocardial perfusion after percutaneous transluminal coronary angioplasty assessed by Thallium-201 exercise scintigraphy. Circulation 63:1001
3. Kent K, Banka L, Bentivoglio L et al. (1980) Percutaneous transluminal coronary angioplasty (PTCA): update from the NHLBI registry. Circulation [Suppl] 62:160
4. Williams D, Riley R, Singh A, Most A (1980) Restoration of normal coronary hemodynamics and myocardial metabolism after percutaneous transluminal coronary angioplasty. Circulation 62:653

Overview

A. Grüntzig

Emory University School of Medicine, Department of Medicine, 1364 Clifton Road, Atlanta, Georgia 30322, USA

In the four years since the introduction of the technique of percutaneous transluminal coronary angioplasty, the involvement of professionals around the world has led to many significant observations and technical advances.

Large scale studies such as that presented by Stertzer from New York and Myler from San Francisco have confirmed the applicability of the technique as well as its success. Their primary success rate as well as the meticulous recording of results are to be applauded. These investigators are advancing into further frontiers of PTCA, such as main stem stenosis, tandem lesions of the left anterior descending, and multivessel attempts in the same session.

Porstmann has outlined the results from East Berlin of 37 patients undergoing PTCA. His presentation points out some explanations for angioplasty failures due to vessel anatomy. He cites tortuosity, distal location of stenoses, calcification and side branches as potential problems in proper positioning of the balloon catheter. Bonzel from Freiburg attempts to alleviate these problems somewhat by pointing out the advantages of using biplane isocentric coronary angiography in interventional therapy in order to maximize information and minimize risk.

Mock and Kent, from Bethesda, Md., summarize the results of PTCA compiled by the NIH PTCA registry in their presentation which reveals a 62% primary success rate from 69 centers. They point out the presence of a learning curve in the instigation of this procedure by an individual or institution.

Methodology is constantly a subject for debate. This is illustrated in the two papers submitted by Kaltenbach from Frankfurt. In the first communication the use of the transbrachial approach is defended by the claim of a reduction of arterial bleeding at the puncture site in the face of therapy aimed at reduction of thromboembolic complication. Kaltenbach also proposes in his second communication the use of longer inflation times in order to maximize fluid expression from an atherosclerotic lesion. The results of postmortem studies on human iliac arteries suggest a significant role for fluid extraction especially in the case of nonorganized thrombi. A comparison of follow up results of lesions of comparable age dilated with a more standard inflation time versus the proposed inflation time of up to one minute would provide a clinical confirmation of this interesting conclusion especially if conducted as randomized prospective study.

Such studies are also urgently needed in the area of the use of anticoagulants after PTCA. Such an investigation comparing the results of the administration of low dose aspirin to that of coumadin is currently underway in Atlanta. Breddin introduces expe-

Transluminal Coronary Angioplasty and
Intracoronary Thrombolysis. Ed. by Kaltenbach et al.

rimental results and physiological therories to support the employment of high dose aspirin as adjunctive therapy. He cites inhibition of platlet stimulation as the primary mechanism responsible for the drug's antithrombotic effect and thus claims that much larger doses must be used in order to achieve this effect uniformly in a 24 hour period. Criticisms of this paper include the contention that aspirin exerts its effect for the entire life of the platelet thus rendering larger doses unnecessary as well as the fear that larger aspirin doses might in fact activate an opposing platelet system via prostacycline thereby negating the antithrombotic effect. Clinical studies are needed to settle this question.

Many investigators are anxious to determine the best objective method available to assess the benefit of a therapeutic procedure. PTCA is no exception. Klepzig illustrates the beneficial result of dilatation on myocardial function and perfusion by analyzing exercise testing, thallium myocardial scintigraphy, and equilibrium radionuclide ventriculography. Amor claims thallium 201 myocardial scintigraphy to be the best noninvasive method available to assess myocardial perfusion. He reports improvement with exercise only. Technicium radionuclide ventriculograms were used by Kent to reveal similar results which correlated with studies of coronary bypass surgery. Sigwart from Lausanne used invasive techniques to confirm the results of noninvasive studies, but his results show that patients post PTCA normalize completely LVEDP after the procedure as opposed to patients with single vessel disease who have undergone bypass grafting. Williams from Rhode Island illustrated the salutory effect of PTCA on coronary circulation dynamics in his study concluding that the relief of angina pectoris after this procedure may be secondary to improved coronary blood flow and myocardial metabolism. He used pacing stress before and after PTCA accompanied by measurements of coronary blood flow, myocardial oxygen consumption, coronary vascular resistance, and degree of aeorbic metabolism to form the basis for this conclusion. Bentivoglio from Philadelphia, however, studied the dynamic changes in left ventricular geometry and pressure during the procedure itself which inevitably involves coronary occlusion. He observed that hemodynamic effects such as increase in LVEDP lag behind the decrease in wall motion seen on coronary occlusion using 2-D echocardiography. He did not, however, control his results for degree of initial stenosis.

The clinical results are themselves the basis for the procedure. Grüntzig's results illustrate that a primary success rate of 84% can be achieved for coronary dilatation and a 84% rate for ilio-femoral occlusions. Long term patency is shown to be between 80 and 85% for these two lesions. In addition, it is possible to cure or improve hypertension in 60 to 80% of cases of renovascular hypertension by relief of renal artery stenosis. In summary, approximately 60% of all patients who actually undergo the procedure will derive long term benefit from the efforts of doctor and patient.

Grüntzig's presentation also indicates the number of technical advancements which are continuing to be made in this field. The use of nitroglycerine injection proximal to the stenosis, French 8 catheters, G rather than DG catheters, and improved guiding systems all combine to form the basis of an even more effective procedure as angioplasty takes its place in the therapy of atherosclerotic disease in the 1980's.

Successful and Unsuccessful TCA

Unsuccessful Percutaneous Transluminal Coronary Angioplasty: Identification of Remedial Causes

D.O. Williams, R.S. Riley, A.K. Singh, A.S. Most

Division of Cardiology, Department of Medicine, Section of Cardiovascular Thoracic Surgery, Department of Surgery, Rhode Island Hospital, Brown University, Providence, Rhode Island 02902, USA

Introduction

Percutaneous transluminal coronary angioplasty (PTCA) is a new innovative technique that directly reduces the extent of coronary artery stenosis, enhances myocardial blood flow, and relieves anginal symptoms and myocardial ischemia [1, 2]. Coronary artery bypass graft surgery (CABG) also relieves angina pectoris by increasing coronary blood flow. Distinct potential advantages of PTCA compared to CABG are the nonoperative nature of the procedure, with attendant reduction in patient morbidity and possibly mortality, and a reduction of cost to the health care system. One relative disadvantage of PTCA, compared to CABG, is that a successful angioplasty cannot be prospectively assured in any given patient. In fact, data from 1000 patients voluntarily entered into the National Heart, Lung, and Blood Institute PTCA Registry indicate that only 62% of attempts are successful. Enhanced success could potentially result if specific reasons for failure were identified and then scrutinized to determine if correctable factors are present. With this objective in mind, we have reviewed the details of 23 consecutive unsuccessful angioplasty attempts taken from a total group of 50 patients who underwent the procedure.

Methods

The records of 50 patients who underwent attempted PTCA from November of 1978 to May 1981 at Rhode Island Hospital were reviewed. Patients in whom the procedure was considered unsuccessful (less than 20% decrease in the angiographic degree of stenosis) were assessed according to a stepwise analysis of the PTCA procedure. We considered PTCA as a composite of five separate procedures: (1) positioning the guiding catheter at the appropriate coronary orifice, (2) entering the stenotic vessel with the dilating catheter, (3) reaching the stenosis with the dilating catheter, (4) crossing the stenosis and positioning the dilating catheter so that the balloon straddles the stenosis, and (5) dilating the stenosis following balloon inflation. Finally, patients were also reviewed in whom PTCA was successful but in whom one or more of these reasons for failure were encountered. In these cases attention is focused on measures taken which contributed to a successful outcome.

Transluminal Coronary Angioplasty and Intracoronary Thrombolysis. Ed. by Kaltenbach et al.

Table 1. Reasons for unsuccessful PTCA

Reason for failure	No of unsuccessful procedures	Proportion of all PTCA attempts (%)	Proportion of unsuccessful PTCA attempts (%)
Unable to position guiding catheter	1	2	4
Unable to enter stenotic vessel	3	7	13
Unable to reach lesion	6	14	26
Unable to cross lesion	11	30	48
Unable to dilate	2	8	9

Results

In 23 patients, PTCA was unsuccessful. A tabulation of these patients according to which step of the PTCA procedure was responsible for failure is shown in Table 1. Inability to cross a stenosis was the most frequent cause, responsible for nearly half of all failures. Furthermore, 30% of attempts to pass all lesions, including successfully dilated patients and those unsuccessfully dilated patients in whom the dilating catheter reached the stenosis, were unsuccessful. Inability to reach a stenosis was the second most common cause for failure but its incidence was half that of inability to cross a stenosis. Inability to properly position the guiding catheter, enter the stenotic vessel, or cause an effective dilatation following balloon inflation were infrequent reasons for failure; each occurred in 8% or less of total attempts.

Since inability to cross a stenosis was by far the most common reason for failure, this aspect of PTCA was evaluated further. In ten of these unsuccessful procedures the wire guide of the dilating catheter could be advanced into the lumen of the stenosis, and the tip of the dilating catheter traversed the stenosis in six, as demonstrated by the recording of a poststenotic intracoronary pressure and injection of contrast through the dilating catheter. Failure in these latter patients was clearly attributable to the added dimensions of the deflated balloon.

To further evaluate those factors which might be responsible for failure in passing a stenosis, all patients with this reason for failure were compared to successfully dilated patients in term of the degree of coronary stenosis (Fig. 1). Several observations are evident. First, all patients in whom the stenosis could not be traversed demonstrated high-grade coronary stenosis. All but one patient had at least 90% stenosis. Less tight lesions were uniformly crossed. Thus the degree of coronary narrowing appears to influence the ability to cross the stenosis. Importantly, not all tight lesions were impassable: at least half of the successfully dilated patients demonstrated lesions of severe narrowing, suggesting that some other factor, for example, the rigidity of the lesion, may influence passability.

Of patients in whom PTCA was successful, five had subtotal stenoses that could not be passed with the standard dilating catheter system. In each of these, attempts to

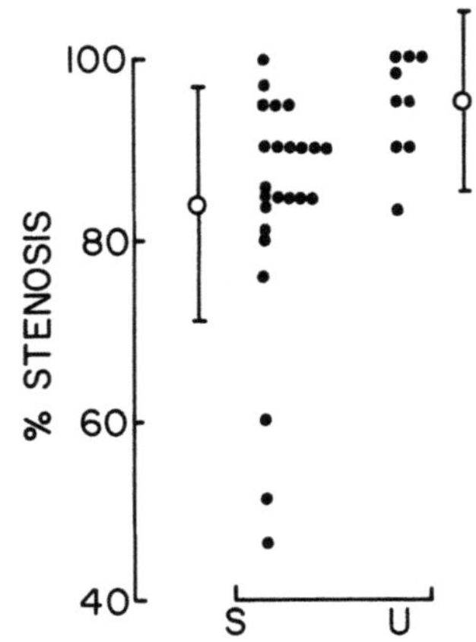

Fig. 1. Severity of coronary narrowing for each patient (*closed circles*) undergoing attempted PTCA. *S*, successful PTCA; *U*, unsuccessful PTCA. *Open circles*, mean ± 1 SD

cross the lesion with a lower profile catheter (Model DG 20-20, USCI Cardiology and Radiology Products) proved successful.

Discussion

Operator skill, performance characteristics of the radiologic equipment and catheter system, and patient pathoanatomy can all potentially influence the likelihood of successful PTCA. In this investigation most lesions were reached with a dilating catheter, but many could not be crossed because of the severity of stenosis and relative size of the dilating catheter. Potential solutions to this problem are to develop catheters of smaller dimensions or to exclude patients with very severe stenoses. Early, limited experience utilizing a low-profile catheter system indicates that a substantial proportion of patients may be successfully treated in whom PTCA would have been unsuccessful because of the severity of the stenosis.

In conclusion, a significant proportion of attempted coronary angioplasty procedures are unsuccessful. Inability to cross a stenosis is the most common reason for failure. Many "tight" lesions can be successfully crossed, however, suggesting a second factor, for example lesion "rigidity", as a determinant of success. Lesions that are both tight and rigid may be successfully dilated with a small diameter catheter. Such advances may have the greatest potential impact on improving the likelihood of successful PTCA.

Summary

Percutaneous transluminal coronary angioplasty is a new innovative technique which permits direct relief of proximal coronary artery stenosis. One relative disadvantage. compared to coronary bypass surgery, is that successful PTCA cannot be prospectively assured in any given patient. Enhanced success may result, however, if correctable factors responsible for failure can be identified. We have reviewed results of attempted

PTCA in 50 patients and focused upon 23 in whom it was unsuccessful. Inability to (a) properly position the guiding catheter, (b) enter the stenotic vessel, and (c) dilate a stenotic segment once crossed were infrequent causes of failure. The most frequent cause of failure was inability to advance the dilating catheter across the stenosis when it was reached. In each patient in whom this occurred, high-grade coronary stenosis was present. In a subset of successfully dilated patients, intial attempts to cross a high-grade stenosis with the standard dilating catheter system were unsuccessful. Use of a lower profile dilating catheter resulted in successful angioplasty.

In this investigation, a significant proportion of attempted coronary angioplasty procedures were unsuccessful. Inability to cross a stenosis was the most common reason for failure. Such lesions may potentially be successfully dilated with a low-profile catheter. Such advances may have the greatest potential impact on improving the likelihood of successful PTCA.

Acknowledgment. The authors wish to acknowledge the assistance of Karen Jessop, Jack Larney, Christine Abatiello, and Katherine Seropian.

References

1. Gruntzig AR, Senning A, Siegenthaler WE (1979) Nonoperative dilation of coronary artery stenosis. N Engl J Med 301:61
2. Williams DO, Riley RS, Singh AK, Most AS (1980) Restoration of normal coronary hemodynamics and myocardial metabolism after percutaneous transluminal coronary angioplasty. Circulation 62:653

Criteria for Primary Success and Long-term results. Analysis of 152 Consecutive Transluminal Coronary Angioplasties*

G. Kober, D. Scherer, R. Koch, S. Dowinsky, M. Kaltenbach

Zentrum der Inneren Medizin, Abteilung für Kardiologie, Klinikum der Johann-Wolfgang-Goethe-Universität, 6000 Frankfurt a.M., FRG

Between October 1977 and May 18, 1981, 152 attempts at transluminal coronary angioplasty (TCA) were carried out at our institution. The results of these procedures are the subject of this presentation. It should be emphasized that patients were not selected on the basis of findings which suggested a high probability of success. Only a number of patients with fluoroscopically visible calcifications in the region of the stenosis were excluded. The total also includes those cases in which TCA had been planned but in whom the indication was no longer evident at routine angiography immediately before the procedure. An example of this would be progression of coronary disease with vessel occlusion following the original angiogram or a confirmed proclivity toward marked vasospasm.

Methods

The procedure was performed in the vast majority of patients (148) by the transbrachial method. In four cases a femoral approach was employed; twice during the introductory phase of the technique and twice because of spasm in the narrow brachial artery of two female patients.

The technical details of the transbrachial approach and accompanying medication have been published elsewhere. All procedures were performed at a second sitting following evaluation of the initial diagnostic angiogram. Prior to TCA, the stenotic coronary vessel was again visualized in several planes before and after the administration of nitroglycerin and nifedipine. The degree of stenosis was estimated in percentage terms on the basis of the plane which displayed maximal luminal reduction. Following dilatation, reangiography was carried out employing identical projections.

Dilatation was considered technically successful if the degree of luminal narrowing was decreased by 20% or more.

Pressures were measured continuously via the balloon catheter, which provides lower than actual levels but nonetheless gives evidence of stenosis severity and the success of dilatation. The transstenotic pressure gradient was measured prior to dilatation during advancement of the catheter and after dilatation during catheter pullback.

The total complication rate includes all patients subjected to catheterization for an attempt at TCA. Not excluded were 11 of 152 patients in whom angioplasty was not attempted at recatheterization because of vessel spasm or occlusion subsequent to the initial catheterization.

*With the support of the Bundesministerium für Forschung und Technologie, Bonn (Kz 01Z J 049 – ZA/NT)

Transluminal Coronary Angioplasty and
Intracoronary Thrombolysis. Ed. by Kaltenbach et al.

The rate of technical success was calculated on the basis of those patients in whom the guiding catheter was introduced into the vascular system for the purpose of TCA. Failures were classified according to cause. They were individually attributable to inability to stabilize the guiding catheter in the coronary ostium, to enter the stenotic vessel or cross the stenosis, and finally to dilate the stenotic segment despite balloon inflation.

Results

Figure 1 shows an improving success rate in terms of the number of TCA attempts, calculated on the basis of groups of 50 consecutive procedures. Whereas the primary success rate for the first 50 patients was 52%, a success rate of 71% was achieved in the most recent 50 cases.

Figure 2 shows that the initially high rate of technically unsuccessful procedures was influenced considerably by failure to position the guiding catheter at the coronary ostium. Subsequent modification of the guiding catheters has virtually eliminated this problem. With increasing experience, the stenotic segments could almost always be reached. A slight increase has been noted in stenoses which, once reached, could not be crossed. This is attributed to a chance selection of patients with tight stenoses.

A decrease has occured in stenoses which could not be dilated after inflation of the balloon. The reason for this lies in the recently increasing frequency (4–8 times) and duration (up to 90 s, according to tolerance) of dilatation maneuvers.

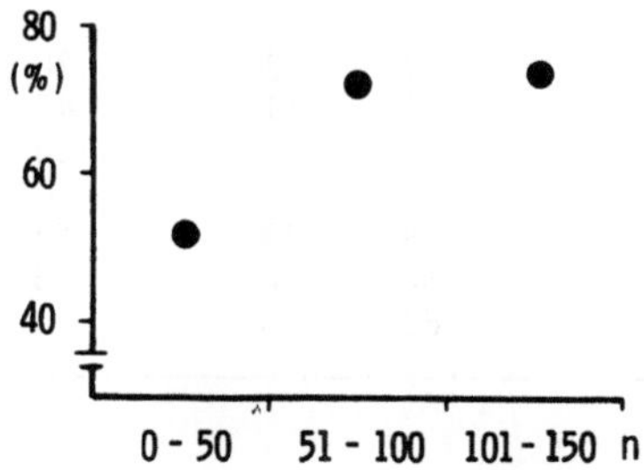

Fig. 1. Increasing rate of technically successful TCA for the first, second, and third groups of 50 patients

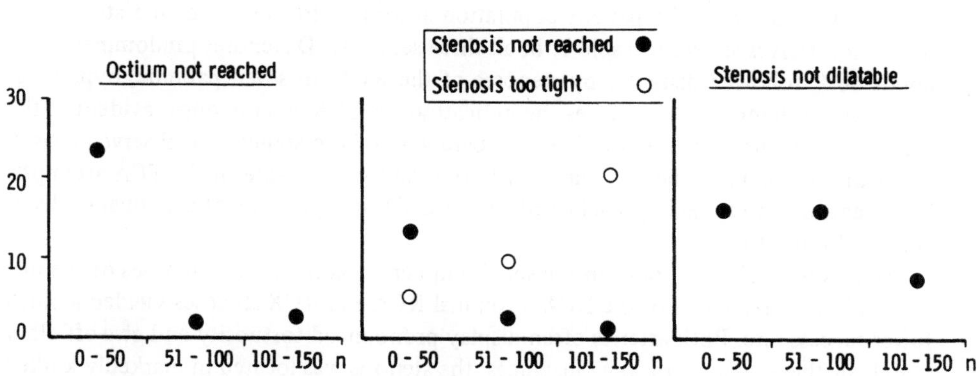

Fig. 2. Causes of technical failures in 150 TCA attempts

Table 1. Site of stenosis in 152 TCA attempts divided into groups of 50 consecutive cases (Oct. 1977 – May 1981)

Site	Cases 0–50	51–100	101–152
LMCA	5	0	2
LAD	29	30	29
RCA	13	11	8
RCX	2	0	4
Bypass	1	2	4
No indication (Progression, Spasm)	0	7	5

LMCA, left main; LAD, left anterior descending; RCA, right coronary; RCX, circumflex artery

Table 2. Success Rate of TCA related to case history in 97 stenoses crossed in native vessels

History	No. of patients	Immediate success rate (%)	Success rate at 3 months No. of patients	%	Success rate at 1 year No. of patients	%
Angina pectoris at rest only	1	100	1	–	–	–
Angina pectoris on exposure to cold	5	60	1	–	–	–
Angina pectoris of effort	63	87	29	69	14	64
Angina pectoris during rest and effort	25	80	14	57	5	20
History ⩽ 6 months	52	87	25	52	11	45
History > 6 months	45	78	20	75	8	63
Women	19	84	8	50	–	–
Men	78	83	37	68	18	56
Age < 50 years	65	86	29	66	16	63
> 50 years	32	75	16	63	3	–

The distribution of the patient population according to the site of the stenosis selected for TCA is shown in Table 1. In all three series, LAD stenoses predominate with about 60%, followed distantly by stenoses of the RCA. In seven patients, bypass stenoses were attempted. In 12 cases the indication for TCA was no longer evident at the time of the planned procedure due to progression of the stenosis or observed spasm.

Figure 3 illustrates the regional distribution and success rate of the TCA attempts. The greatest success rate was achieved in the LAD, independent of proximal or distal stenosis localization.

Results were also favorable in the small number of patients with stenoses of the medial and distal segments of the RCA. Proximal RCA and RCX stenoses yielded a much lower success rate. Both arteries often display pronounced tortuosity and give off other vessels in these regions. In some instances, the stenosis was located in markedly kinked segments.

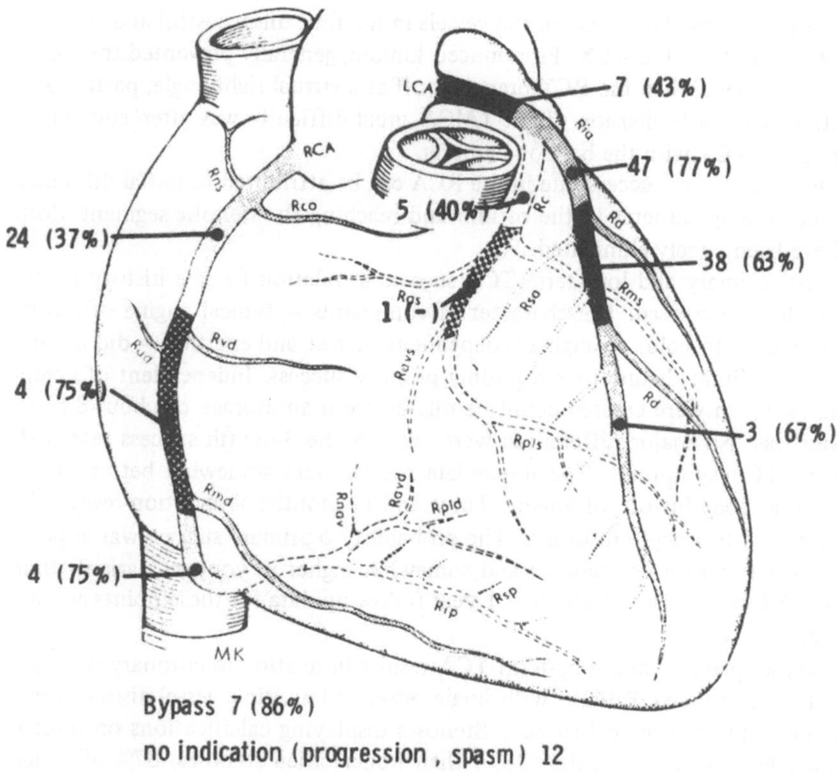

Fig. 3. Regional distribution and success rate in 152 TCA attempts

Table 3. Success rate of TCA related to coronary morphology in 97 stenoses crossed in native vessels

	No. of patients	Immediate success rate (%)	Success rate at 3 months No. of patients	%	Success rate at 1 year No. of patients	%
Single-vessel disease	76	83	35	63	15	60
Multiple-vessel disease	21	81	10	70	4	25
Calcification not present	89	87	43	65	19	53
Calcification present	8	38	2	50	–	–
Discrete (no calcification)	45	87	20	75	9	66
	6	100	3	100	2	50
	20	90	10	50	3	100
Tubular (< 10 mm)	18	78	10	50	5	0

Figure 4 summarizes the course of the vessels in the four unsuccessful and two successful TCA attempts in the RCX. Pronounced kinking generally prevented the stenosis from being crossed. When the RCX branched off at a virtual right angle, particularly in conjunction with early division of the LMCA, great difficulty was often encountered in entering the RCX with the balloon catheter.

In addition, the lower success rate in the RCA can be attributed to initial difficulty in placing the guiding catheter in the ostium and reaching the stenotic segment. Both problems have been largely eliminated.

Table 2 lists primary and long-term TCA success in relation to case history for 97 stenoses which were crossed. The character of complaints – typical angina of effort, angina on exposure to cold, or angina independent of rest and exertion – did not demonstrate any definite distinctions regarding primary success. Independent of symptoms, stenoses which were crossed could be dilated from an average of about 80% to 40% or even less. No major differences were seen in the 3-month success rate with respect to pre-TCA symptoms. The immediate results were somewhat better with a short rather than long history of angina. Three and 12 months observation reveals the opposite in regard to long-term results. The probability o primary success was approximately the same in men and women and somewhat higher in younger patients than in those over 50 years of age. Sufficient 1 year follow-up data for these points are not yet available.

Table 3 shows primary and long-term TCA results in relation to coronary morphology in 97 stenoses crossed. Patients with single-vessel and multiple-vessel disease showed comparable rate of technical success. Stenoses displaying calcifications on fluoroscopy yielded less favorable results (38%) than noncalcified stenoses, 87% of which could be dilated. No difference in primary success was noted between the various types of discrete stenoses and tubular narrowing. Due to the limited number of patients followed up, coronary morphology also does not yet provide any reliable predictors of long-term success.

Table 4. Success rate of TCA related to hemodynamics

		Immediate success		No success	≤ Immediate 3 months n	(%)	1 year n	(%)
Mean gradient pre TCA (mmHg)	(n = 64)	53 (0–90)		41 (0–70)				
Peripheral pressure post TCA		n	%					
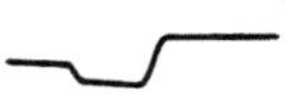	(n = 50)	41	(82)		14	64	4	25
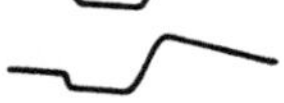	(n = 7)	7	(100)		4	50	–	–

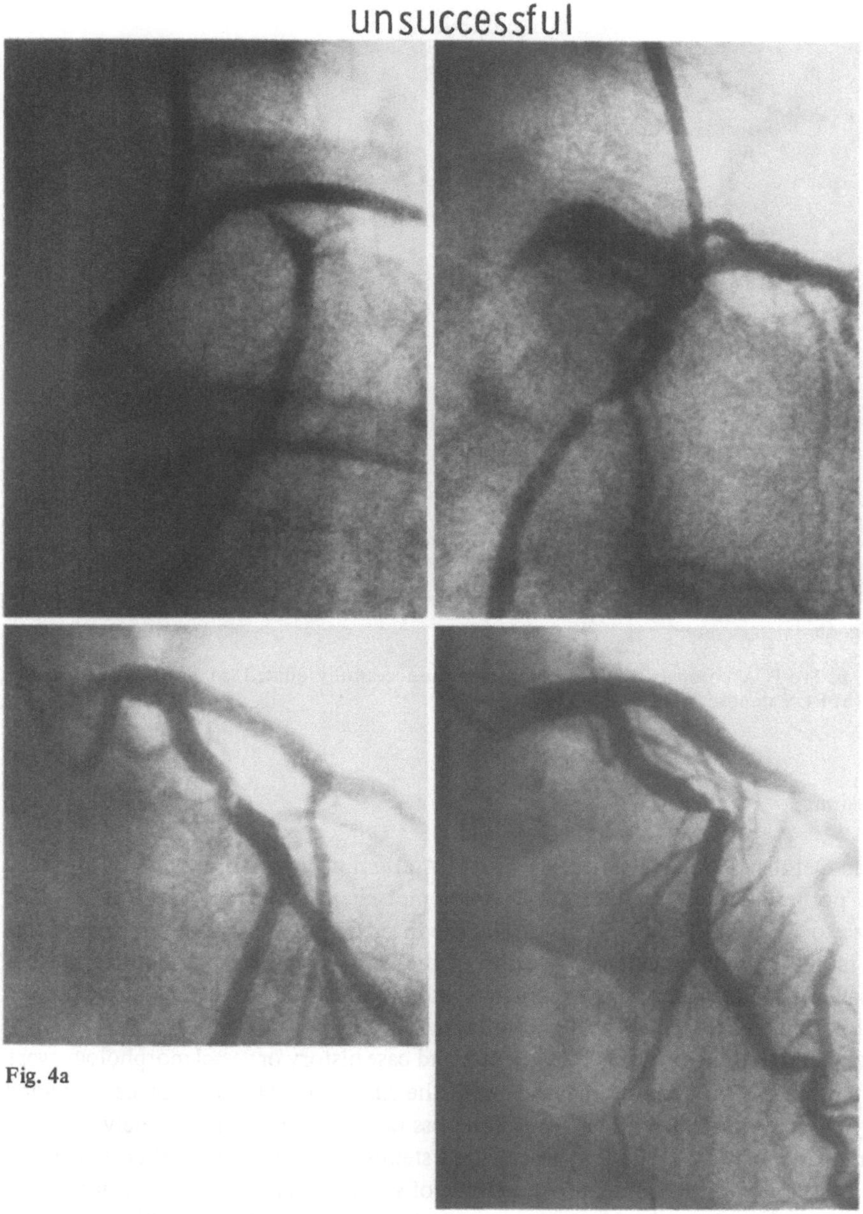

Fig. 4a

The relationship between TCA success and hemodynamic findings is given in Table 4. Successfully as well as unsuccessfully treated patients displayed a comparable mean gradient across the stenosis. Differences in the peripheral pressure curve showing constant pressure following balloon deflation or a renewed decline in pressure after an initial increase (possibly "elastic-type" stenosis) also failed to predict primary and long-term TCA success.

successful

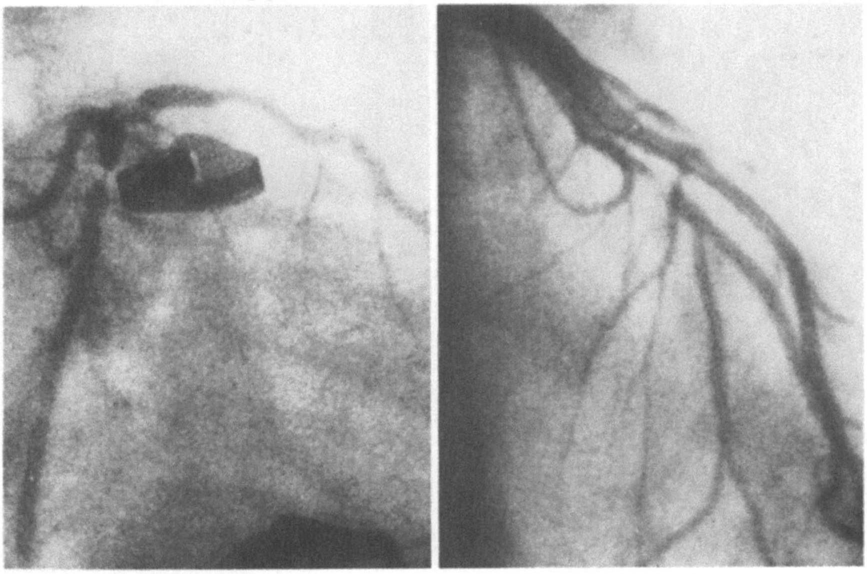

Fig. 4b

Fig. 4a, b. Pre-TCA coronary angiograms in four unsuccessfully dilated (**a**) and two successfully dilated (**b**) RCX stenoses

Conclusions

Between October 1977 and May 1981 152 TCA attempts were carried out.

The primary success rate for all TCA attempts increased from 52% for the first 50 cases to 71% for the last 50 cases. The rise in success rate is attributed to improvements in the guiding catheters, evolution of the balloon catheter (guide-wire, pliable tip, smaller diameter) increasing experience, and modification, of the technique (longer dilatation time, more frequent balloon inflations).

Strong correlations between TCA success and case history or vessel morphology were not established. This suggests that currently the success of TCA cannot be predicted reliably. A somewhat lower than average success rate is achieved in extremely tortuous segments of the RCA and RCX, in calcified stenoses, and in older patients. Even in such cases, however, the fundamental chance of success is sufficient to warrant a TCA attempt and should not lead to automatic exclusion of such patients. When patients with a short history of angina suggestive of a fresh, nonorganized coronary lesion is compared to patients with a longer history suggestive of old, organized lesions, a tendency toward better short-term results (87% vs. 78%) but poorer long-term results (52% vs. 75% at 3 months and 45% vs. 63% at 12 months) can be derived in the patient group with a short history of angina.

Changes of Coronary Obstructions in the Months Following Transluminal Coronary Angioplasty

H.-J. Engel*, M. Kaltenbach, W. Rafflenbeul, G. Kober, D. Scherer, R. Simon, P.R. Lichtlen

* Zentralkrankenhaus „Links der Weser", 2800 Bremen 61, FRG

This report concerns a special aspect of coronary angioplasty and contains the combined Frankfurt and Hannover experience in follow-up coronary angiography performed on average 3 months after PTCA. It is based on 71 patients, of whom 54 were studied in Frankfurt by Prof. Kaltenbach and Prof. Kober and 17 in Hannover.

Our interest in changes of coronary obstructions after balloon dilatation was stimulated by a 45-year-old male patient with a 61% proximal LAD stenosis (Fig. 1). The diameter of the lumen was not notably changed by PTCA and only morphometric measurement with a caliper revealed that the stenosis had been reduced mildly from 61% to 54% of the luminal diameter. This effect is more apparent than real, however, since the actual diameter of the lumen had remained unchanged at 1.2 mm. Since the patient remained symptomatic and the stress of ECG continued to be abnormal, he received an internal mammary graft to the LAD. After 2 months, the mammary graft was found to be practically occluded, but the stenosis was hardly visible any more: morphometrically it amounted to 33% of the luminal diameter, and the diameter of the lumen had increased to 2.1 mm. Since the proximal LAD stenosis had been present also on the previous angiograms performed by the referring hospital prior to dilatation, and since 0.8 mg nitroglycerin and 20 mg nifedipine had been administered prior to dilatation, the possibility of spasm is excluded for practical purposes.

Figure 2 demonstrates the angiograms of a 51-year-old male with an isolated 57% stenosis of the RCA. Balloon dilatation succeeded in reducing the stenosis to 43%, and the diameter of the lumen increased from 1.1 to 1.8 mm. The patient became asymptomatic for 4 weeks but then developed rapidly worsening new chest pain interpreted as representing unstable angina. Stress testing was felt to be contraindicated and emergency surgery was scheduled because of suspected restenosis. Angiography, however, revealed further regression of the stenosis to 29% and further increase of the diameter of the lumen to 2.5 mm. The stress test was negative at this time, and the patient was placed on nifedipine. A second restudy performed 15 months after PTCA showed a practically normal RCA.

Figure 3 shows the angiograms of our first dilatation patient in whom PTCA succeeded in reducing the stenosis from 60% to 34% and increasing the luminal diameter from 1.1 to 2.0 mm. Three months later the stenosis had become practically invisible, and the diameter had increased further to 2.5 mm.

In the patient with a 55% stenosis of the RCA shown in Fig. 4, dilatation resulted in a small linear contrast defect in the area of the stenosis suggestive of an intimal lesion

Transluminal Coronary Angioplasty and
Intracoronary Thrombolysis. Ed. by Kaltenbach et al.

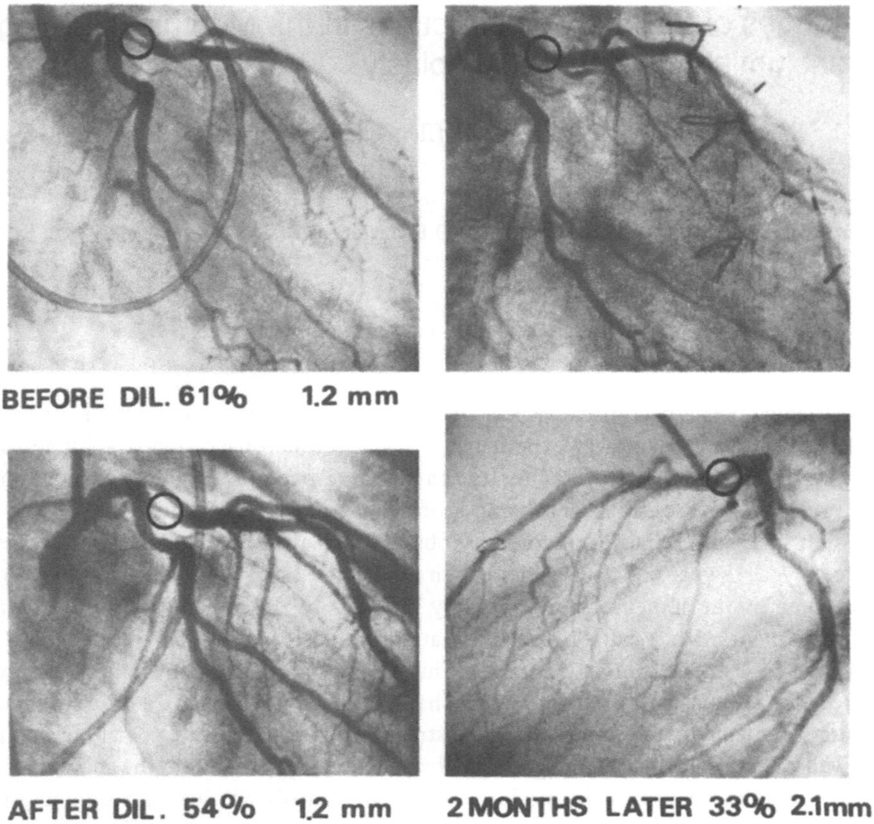

Fig. 1. Stenosis of the LAD before PTCA (*top left*) and immediately following PTCA (*bottom left*), and at control angiography 2 months later (*right*). Bottom right, LAO projection; *left* and *top right*, RAO projections

resembling a mild dissection, but reduced the stenosis to 33%. At repeat angiography 3 months later the vessel wall had become smooth and still wider. The residual stenosis was measured at 23% of the luminal diameter.

Further regression of a proximal LAD stenosis within 4 months after dilatation is also suggested by the angiograms of the 48-year-old patient shown in Fig. 5. The diameter of the lumen increased minimally from 1.7 to 1.8 mm after dilatation, but follow-up angiography showed some further improvement with a diameter of 2.2 mm.

Figures 1–5 represent examples taken from the total of 71 patients in whom control angiography after PTCA had been performed in Frankfurt and Hannover so far. Figure 6 contains a graphic summary of the effect of PTCA on coronary obstructions. The results refer to the projection in which the stenosis was seen to be most severe and were obtained by agreement of three experienced angiographers. The patients are attributed to one of three groups: those in whom a deterioration of over 10% luminal diameter was observed at repeat angiography (e.g., a 50% stenosis deteriorating to 65%), those with no change greater than 10%, and those in whom at restudy further spontaneous improvement more than 10% had occurred. On the average of all patients, dila-

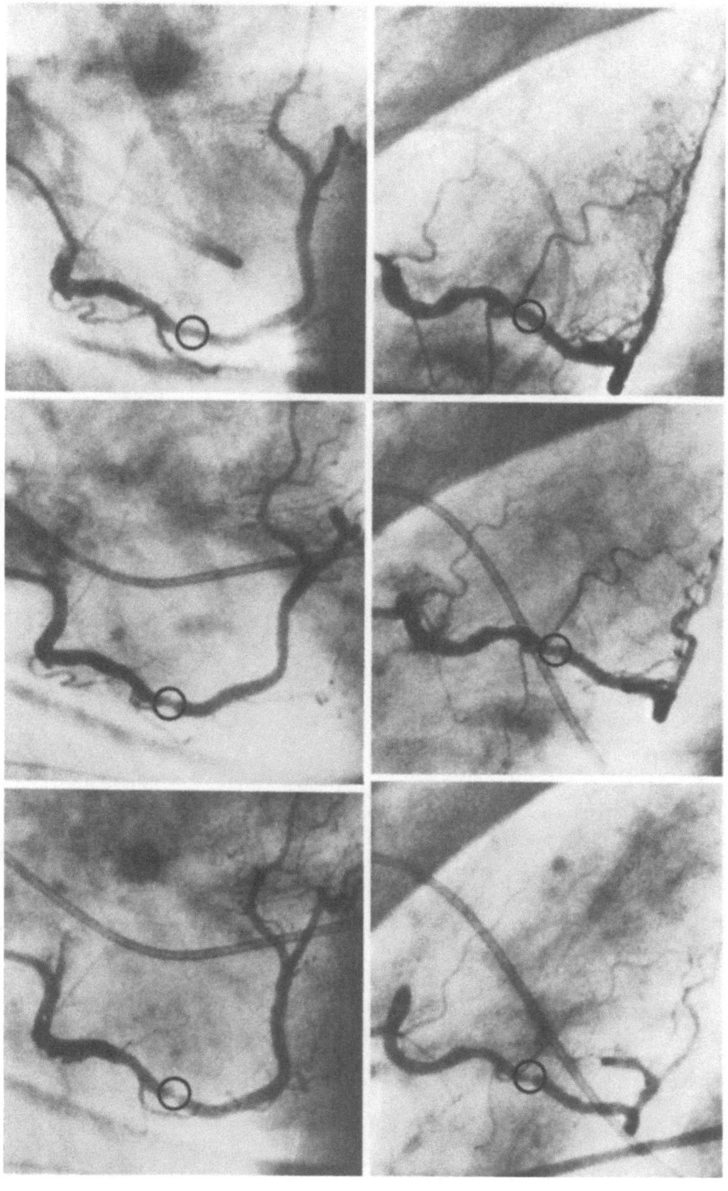

Fig. 2. Stenosis of the RCA before, immediately after, and 3 months after PTCA. *Top*, LAO projections; *bottom*, RAO projections

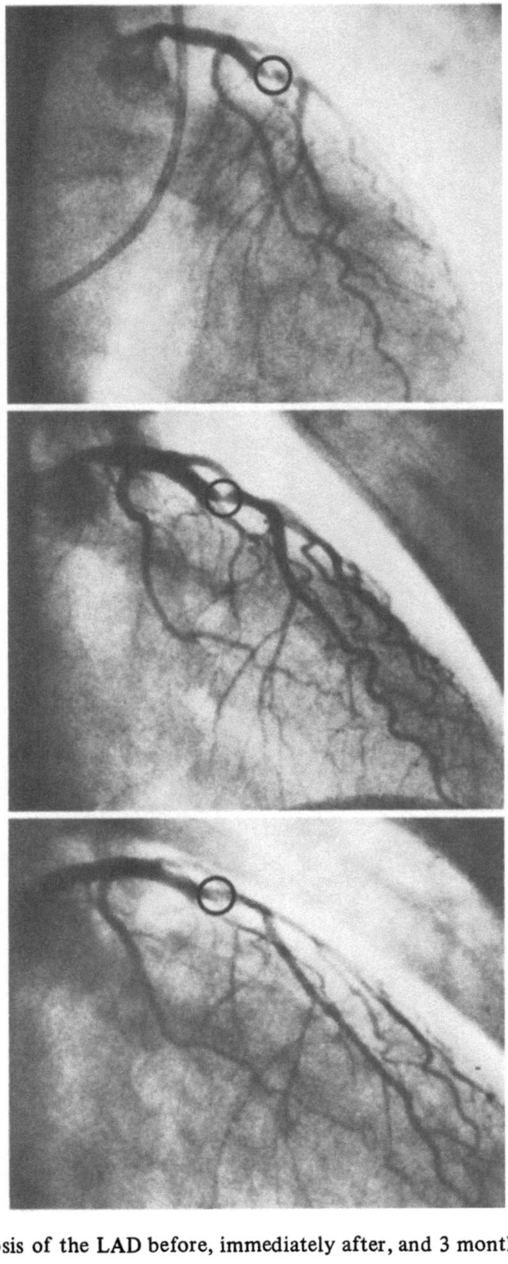

BEFORE DIL.
STENOSIS 60%
DIAMETER 1.1 mm

AFTER DIL.
STENOSIS 34%
DIAMETER 2.0 mm

3 MONTHS LATER
STENOSIS 11%
DIAMETER 2.5 mm

Fig. 3. Stenosis of the LAD before, immediately after, and 3 months after PTCA, RAO projection

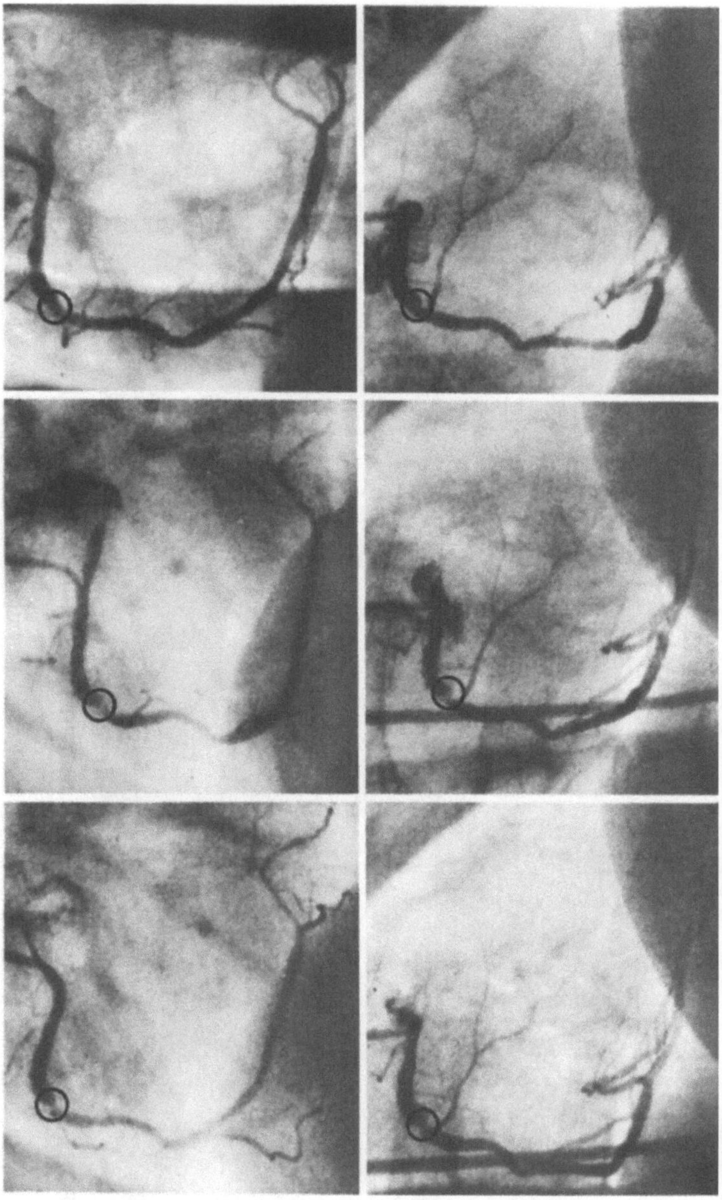

BEFORE DIL. 55% 1.3mm AFTER DIL. 33% 1.9mm 3 MONTHS LATER: 23% 2.1mm

Fig. 4. Stenosis of the RCA before, immediately after, and 3 months after PTCA. *Top,* LAO projections; *bottom,* RAO projections

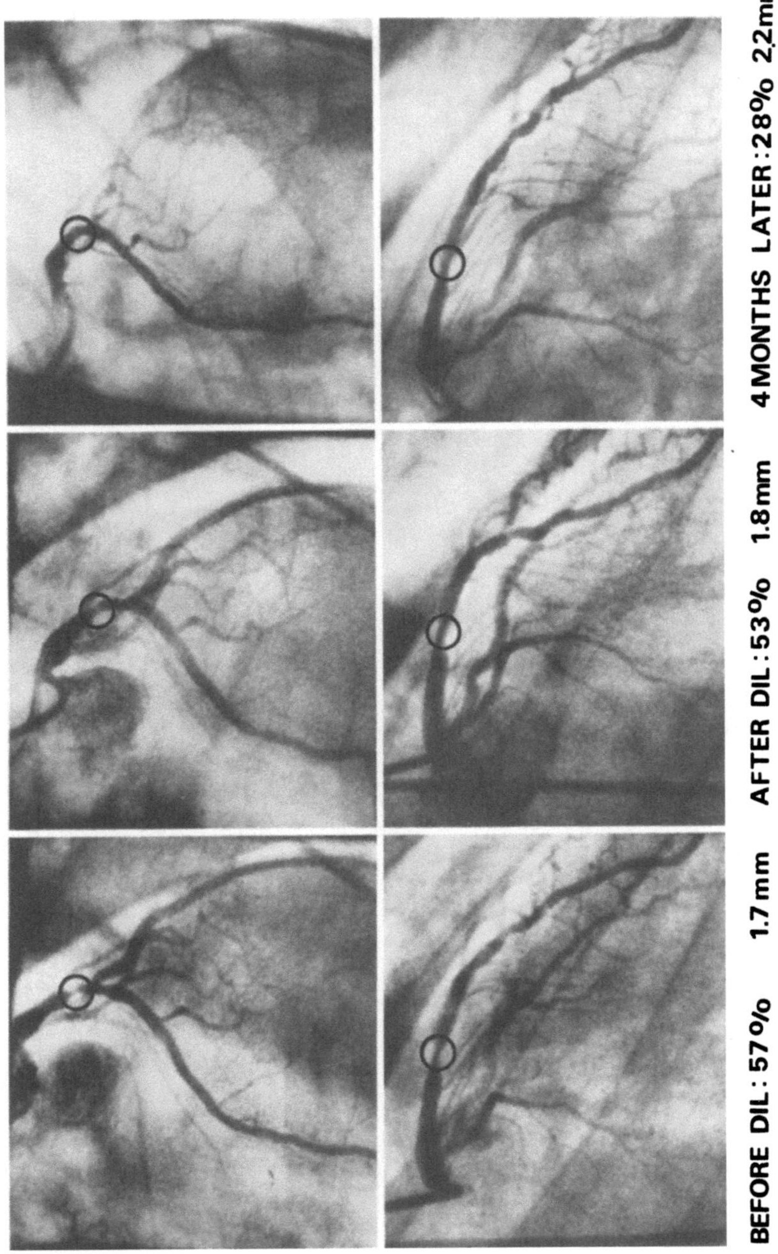

Fig. 5. Stenosis of the LAD before, immediately after, and 4 months after dilatation. *Top*, LAO projections; *bottom*, RAO projections

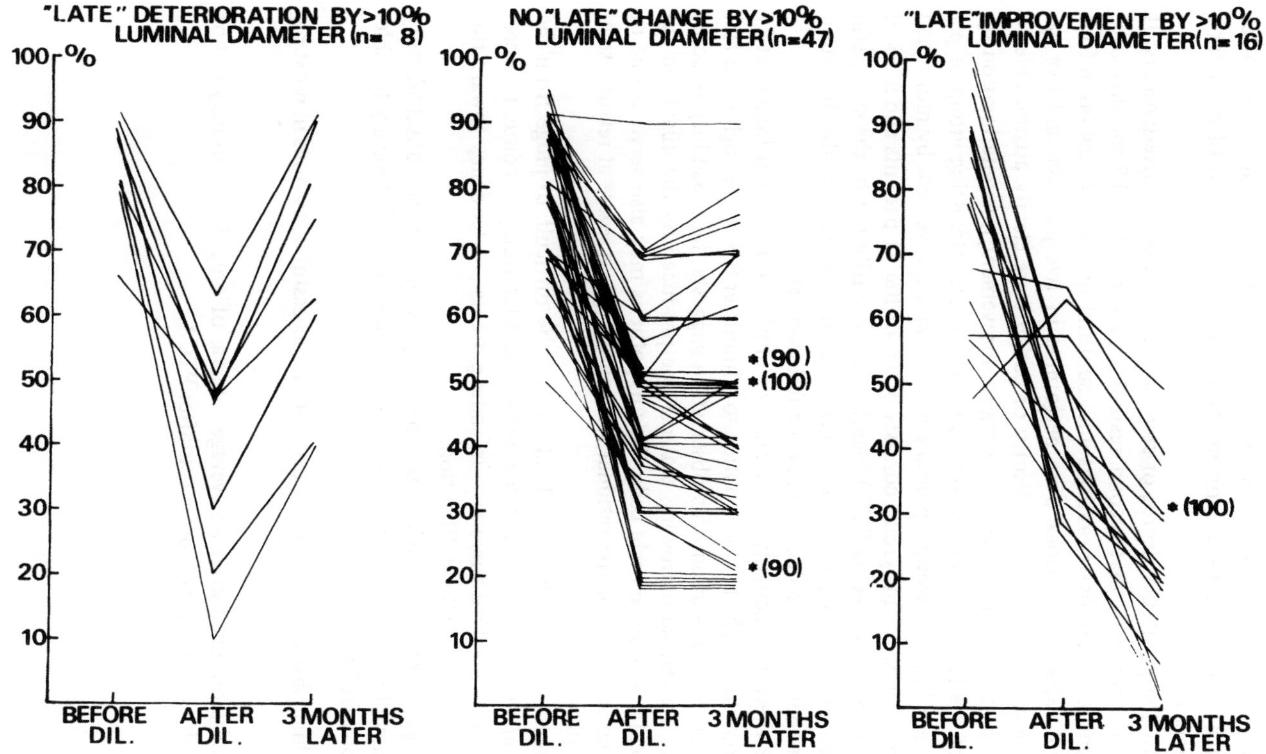

Fig. 6. Immediate and "late" effect of PTCA on coronary obstructions. Patients are divided into three groups according to the result of the restudy: deterioration *(left)*, no change (*center*), and further improvement *(right)*. The *asterisks* refer to late deteriorations observed at second restudies after 4–15 months following PTCA, with *figures in parentheses* schowing the percentage of occlusion

tation reduced the stenosis from 80.0% to 44.0% ($P < 0.005$), and at restudy after 3 months there was a further mild improvement to 40.9% which was of borderline statistical significance ($P \sim 0.05$).

Reoccurrence of the pre-PTCA degree of stenosis was observed in five patients. It must be emphasized, however, that second restudies performed 4–15 months after PTCA revealed significant late deteriorations with subtotal or total occlusions in four patients. Successful second dilatations were performed in two patients, and five patients underwent bypass grafting. The majority of patients are clearly attributable to the group containing those cases in whom neither improvement nor deterioration by more than 10% of the luminal diameter occurred. The most interesting group of patients in our view are those in whom spontaneous further improvement by more than 10% could be demonstrated. This group consists of 16 of the 71 patients and marked spontaneous improvement following PTCA significantly contributed to the successful result in all of them. In fact in 2 cases the stenosis was unchanged after the dilatation procedure but was found to have decreased at the follow-up study.

In one patient there was actually an increase of luminal obstruction immediately following dilatation. Although it is our routine to administer 0.8 mg nitroglycerin and 20 mg nifedipine prior to dilatation, this observation suggests the possibility of some residual element of functional narrowing that may be produced by the dilatation stimulus to the vascular smooth muscle cells. This hypothesis may also serve as one of various possible explanations for the residual stenosis being less severe at restudy than immediately after dilatation.

In summary, the success of ballon dilatation may be difficult to judge from the angiographic appearance of the vessel at the end of the dilatation procedure. Irrespective of the mechanisms involved there is – in some patients – a tendency toward further improvement following balloon dilatation.

We therefore suggest that the decision on bypass surgery of primarily unsatisfactory cases should be delayed until reevaluation 2–3 months after PTCA if clinically feasible.

It must be emphasized that:

Considerable residual obstructions remain even after successful dilatations in most patients.

The presented results obtained after an average interval of only 3 months may not be representative for the real long-term prognosis after PTCA.

Computerized Quantitative Coronary Angiography Applied to Percutaneous Transluminal Coronary Angioplasty: Advantages and Limitations

P.W. Serruys, F. Booman, G.J. Troost, J.H.C. Reiber, J.J. Gerbrands*, M. v.d. Brand, F. Cherrier**, P.G. Hugenholtz

Thorax Center, Erasmus University, Rotterdam, The Netherlands
* Information Theory Group, Delft University of Technology, The Netherlands
** C.H.R. de Nancy, Hôpital de Brabois, France

Introduction

Percutaneous transluminal coronary angioplasty (PTCA) is a relatively new procedure [7], by means of which one tries to restore normal coronary blood flow to an underperfused area.

What constitutes a physiologically significant obstruction to blood flow in the human coronary system is still unsettled [6, 10], but diverse experimental studies have shown that the critical point, for an adequate resting blood flow, is reached when cross-sectional area has been reduced to approximately 10% of the preexisting lumen [8]. Quantitation of percentage lumen narrowing observed by angiography is limited to comparing the luminal diameters at two different points of the vessel. Because we cannot see the arterial wall itself, we do not always appreciate the changes occurring in it that produce the variations of luminal dimensions we consider as a focal narrowing. The so-called normal caliber of a coronary vessel in its prestenotic and poststenotic segment is in fact a subtle combination of stenotic and ectatic areas, and this creates a problem in the quantification of the degree of luminal narrowing.

Moreover, assessment of the percentage of reduction of a lesion from a single projection can only be achieved by assuming circular cross sections, an assumption that will certainly not be true in general. The resulting error may be reduced by incorporating two orthogonal projections and computing elliptical cross sections. However, with the frequent eccentric lesions even this last approach provides poor results, as can be shown by the following example. Figure 1 portrays and depicts the complex problems stemming from a slit-like stenosis having a crescent shape. In cases such as this, even three or more views will not "provide a faithful portrayal of their severity" [4].

A lateral "view" of the crescent would suggest a 10% reduction in lumen diameter; a left oblique would be consistent with a 25% narrowing and an anteroposterior would imply a 60% stenosis. Even a technique of quantitating area stenosis from two orthogonal measurements and computing area based on an elliptical model would fail to describe accurately the severity of this lesion. However, some clue to the presence of this grossly asymmetrical lesion will exist, because the density of contrast medium is markedly reduced in that area, even though the caliber seems normal. Unexplained diminution of the opacity of a contrast-filled lumen (density changes) should alert the angiographer to the severity of the luminal narrowing.

Transluminal Coronary Angioplasty and
Intracoronary Thrombolysis. Ed. by Kaltenbach et al.

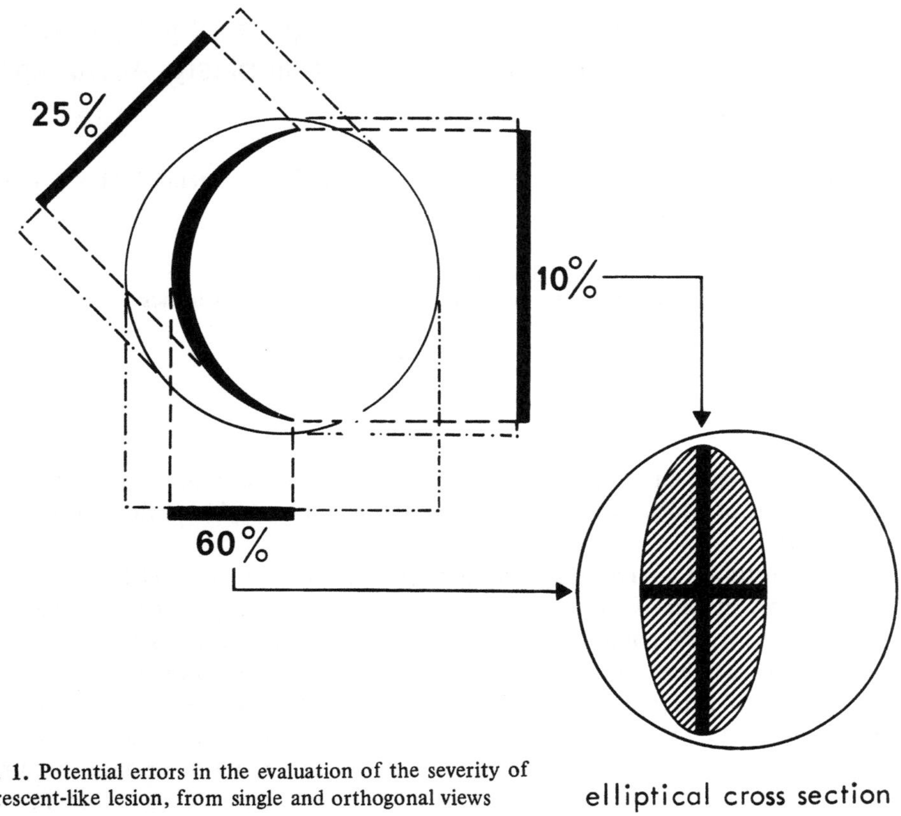

Fig. 1. Potential errors in the evaluation of the severity of a crescent-like lesion, from single and orthogonal views

From the above, it is clear that an objective and reproducible technique of quantitating cross-sectional area stenosis and normal luminal area in absolute terms and in relative percentage changes is seriously needed, in order to evaluate the efficacy of transluminal coronary angioplasty.

Over the last few years we have developed and implemented a computer-based Coronary Angiography Analysis System (CAAS), that allows the accurate assessment of percentage diameter narrowing of coronary lesions by means of automated contour detection principles [2, 3, 5, 9]. Further developments over the last year have been directed towards the quantitative analysis of the density changes in coronary vessels due to luminal narrowing. The question then arises of whether we can derive a relationship between the thickness of the irradiated object and the density level in the angiographic image. If this is feasible, the percentage area stenosis of the analyzed lesion can be computed (Fig. 2) from a single projection. As a next step, it should be possible to obtain a three-dimensional reconstruction of the arterial segment by combining the contour and density information of an analyzed lesion in two orthogonal projections.

In this paper, we describe briefly the methodology we have developed to analyze a coronary obstructive lesion quantitatively.

Cineangiograms of 28 patients who underwent PTCA were analyzed with the Coronary Angiography Analysis System and the results before and after dilatation are pre-

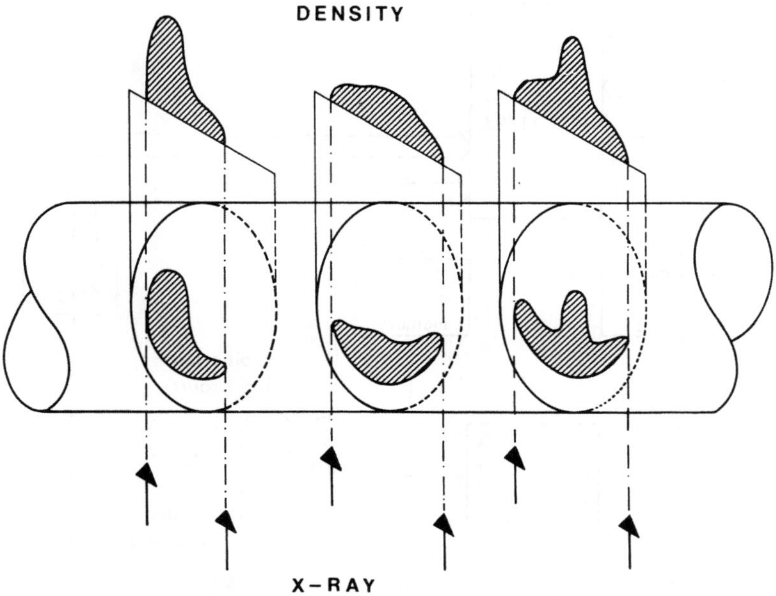

Fig. 2. Schematic illustration of the relationship between the irradiated object thickness and the density in the angiographic image

sented. In the first study group (cinefilms supplied by Prof. F. Cherrier) the severity of the obstructive lesion was evaluated in absolute terms as well as in percentage diameter reduction, derived from the automatically detected contours. In the second study group (Thorax Center) the severity of the lesion was expressed in percentage area stenosis derived from the densitometric measurements.

Quantitative Analysis of Coronary Obstructions

The quantitative analysis of selected coronary segments was carried out with the Coronary Angiography Analysis System, a block diagram of which is shown in Figure 3. The central processor is a PDP 11/34 minicomputer with a 32 K word memory. A 35-mm frame of a coronary cineangiogram is mounted on a Tagarno projector and converted into video format with a high-resolution video camera. Regions of interest are digitized with the video analog-to-digital (A/D) converter and stored in the memory of the minicomputer for subsequent processing. Detected contours, graphics, and patient data can be superimposed on the original video image with a refresh memory and displayed on the video monitor. The user communicates with the system by means of a keyboard and a writing tablet.

To obtain the computer-detected contours of a selected coronary segment, the user must indicate a number of center positions with the writing tablet, such that straight line segments connecting consecutive pairs of these points are within the artery (Fig. 4a). These line segments form the tentative centerlines for the arterial segment. Immediately after the user has indicated the last point of the tentative centerline, the contour de-

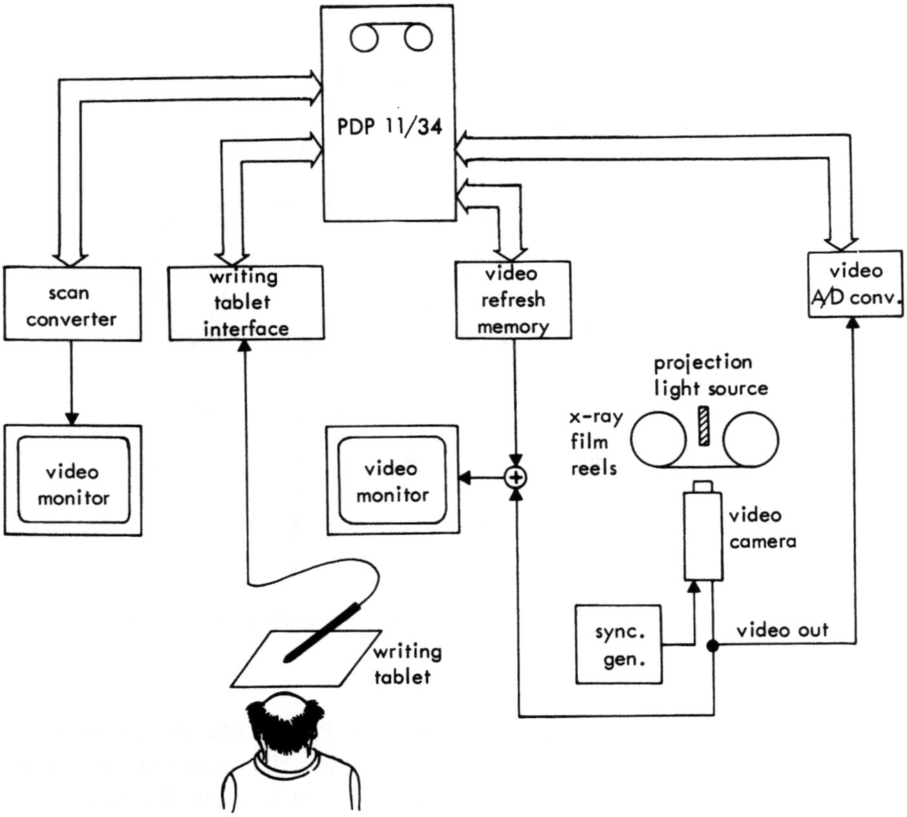

Fig. 3. The Coronary Angiography Analysis System

tection mechanism proceeds automatically, starting at the first position of the centerline. The centerline determines the positions of regions of interest, encompassing the arterial segment, to be digitized. The size of these regions equals 64 x 64 picture elements (pixels) (Fig. 4b). Figure 5 is an example of a selected cineframe of a left anterior descending artery in right inferior oblique projection, before PTCA. The outer borders of a digitization matrix encompassing the coronary obstruction are superimposed on the original image.

To better understand the principles of the automated detection of the contours and of the density measurements in the coronary artery the two-dimensional brightness function of this region of interest is displayed as a three-dimensional structure with the brightness level plotted along the z-axis (Fig. 6). The x- and y-axes correspond with the horizontal and vertical video scan directions. The coronary artery can be recognized as a mountain ridge, with a decrease in the height of the mountain at the location of the obstruction. In principle, the thickness of the contrast filled artery is proportional to the logarithm of the brightness level above the background (Lambert-Beer's law).

On each scan line perpendicular to the corresponding centerline segment, two contour positions are determined from the changes in brightness values. For this purpose

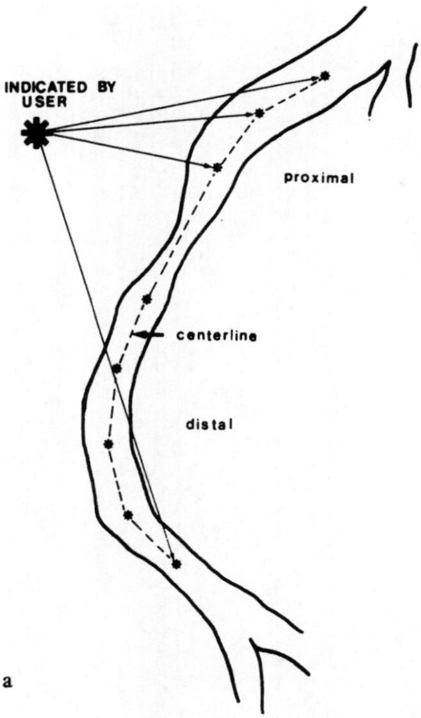

a

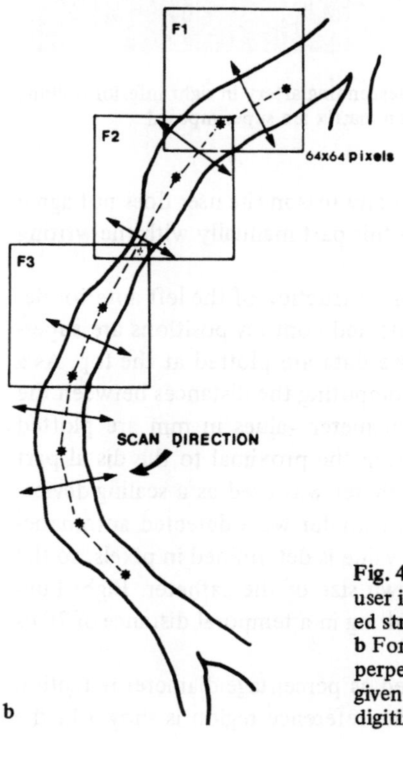

b

Fig. 4a. To analyze a selected coronary arterial segment the user indicates a number of center positions. The interpolated straight line segments function as the tentative centerline. **b** For the schematic drawing of **4a** the scan directions perpendicular to the corresponding centerline segments are given as well as the positions of the 64 X 64 matrices to be digitized

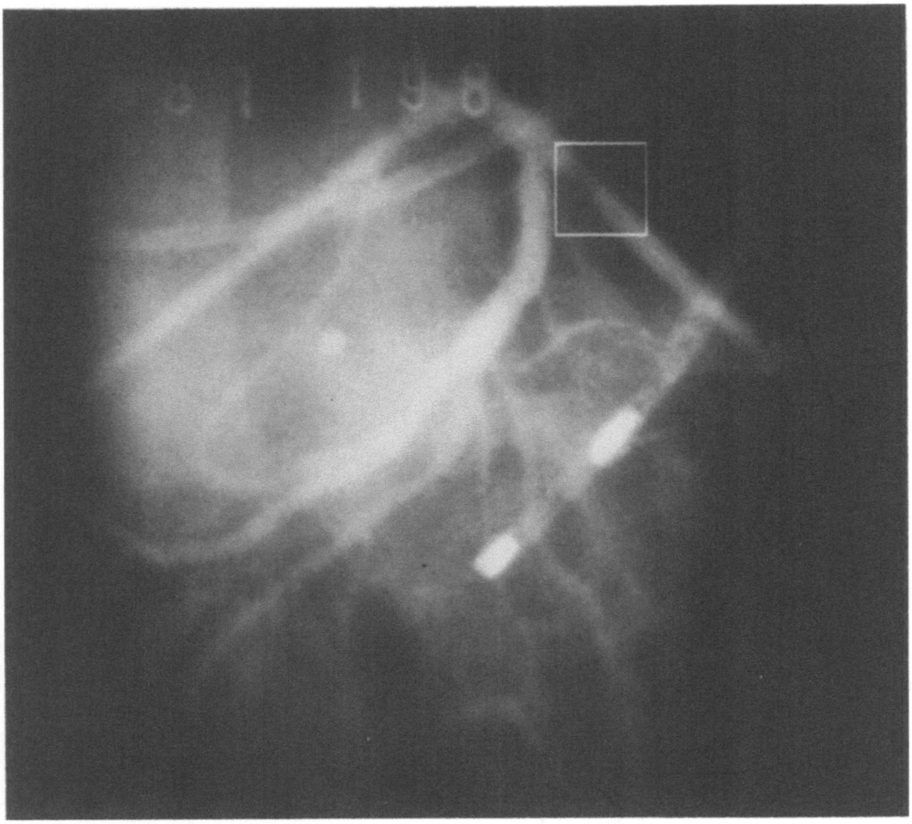

Fig. 5. Example of a selected cineframe of a left anterior descending artery in right inferior oblique projection, before PTCA. The outer borders of a digitization matrix are superimposed

an averaging derivative function is employed. If for any reason the user does not agree with part of the detected contour, he may correct this part manually with the writing tablet.

Figure 7 shows the output of the system for an obstruction of the left anterior descending artery in lateral projection. Here, the detected contour positions are superimposed on the original video image. Administrative data are plotted at the top. As a first step the diameter function is determined by computing the distances between the left and right contour positions. The calibrated diameter values in mm are plotted along the ordinate and the centerline positions from the proximal to the distal part along the abscissa. In this case, the intracardiac catheter was used as a scaling device. To this end, the contours of part of the projected catheter were detected automatically in the way described above. A mean diameter value is determined in pixels, so the calibration factor can be computed from the known size of the catheter. Eight hundred pixels are distinguished on each video line resulting in a temporal distance of 70 ns between neighboring pixels.

The severity of the obstruction can be expressed as percentage diameter reduction with respect to a user-defined reference region. The reference region is shown in the

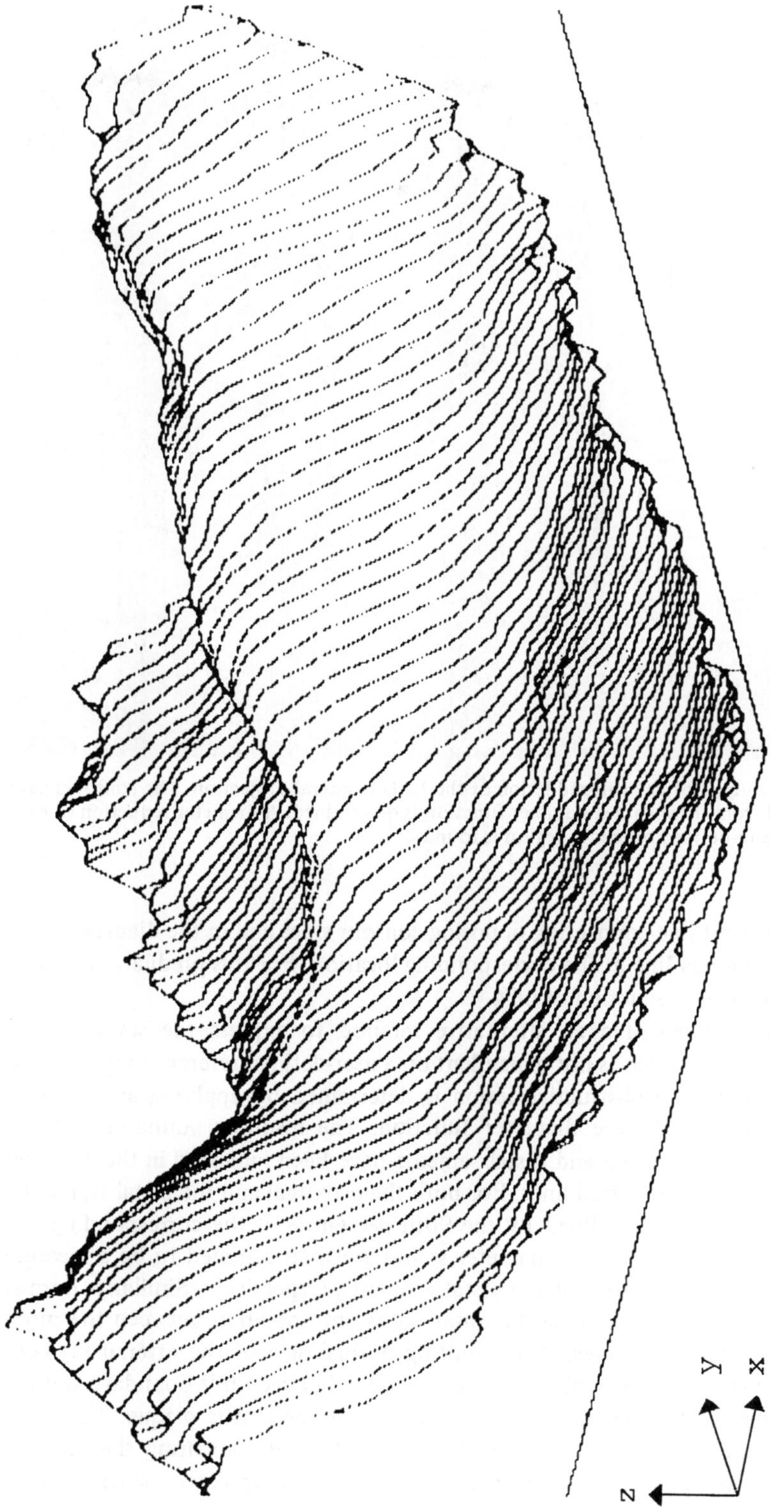

Fig. 6. Three-dimensional representation of the brightness function of the matrix of Fig. 5

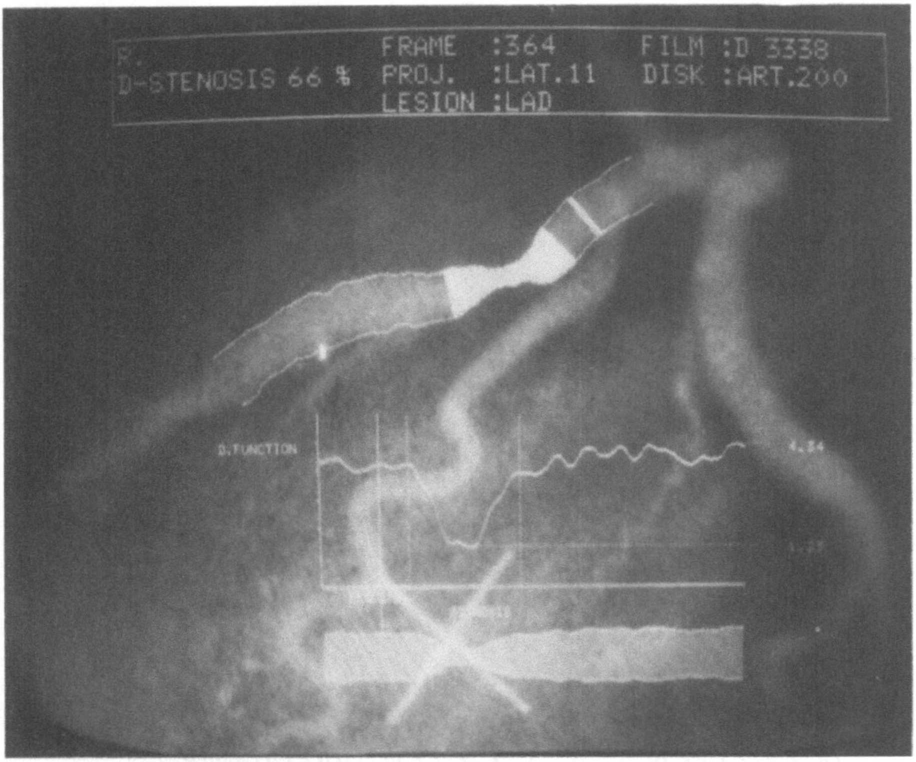

Fig. 7. Computer output of an analyzed lesion of the LAD in lateral projection. The contours have been detected and from these data a diameter function is determined. A diameter reduction of 66% with respect to a user-defined reference region is found

artery by the straight line connecting opposing contour sides and in the diameter function by the continuous line at the corresponding location. For this predilatation situation we find a diameter reduction of 66%.

We have also implemented an alternative method to express the severity of a coronary obstruction, which is not dependent on a user-defined reference region. First of all, the extent of the obstructive lesion is determined by applying an averaging first-derivative function to the diameter function. The resulting boundaries of the obstruction with the proximal and distal sements have been indicated in the diameter function in Fig. 7 with the dotted lines. For both the proximal and the distal segment a reference diameter value is defined by the 90th percentile of the corresponding diameter values. These two reference diameter values are then assumed to be a measure for the normal size of the proximal and distal segments, respectively. Similarly, normal sizes over the obstructive lesion can be obtained by interpolation between the proximal and distal reference values. The resulting normal size of the arterial segment of Fig. 7 is shown in Fig. 8, with the difference area between this boundary and the detected contours marked, being a measure for the atherosclerotic plaque. The interpolated percentage diameter stenosis is then computed by comparing the minimal diameter value at the obstruction with the corresponding interpolated diameter value.

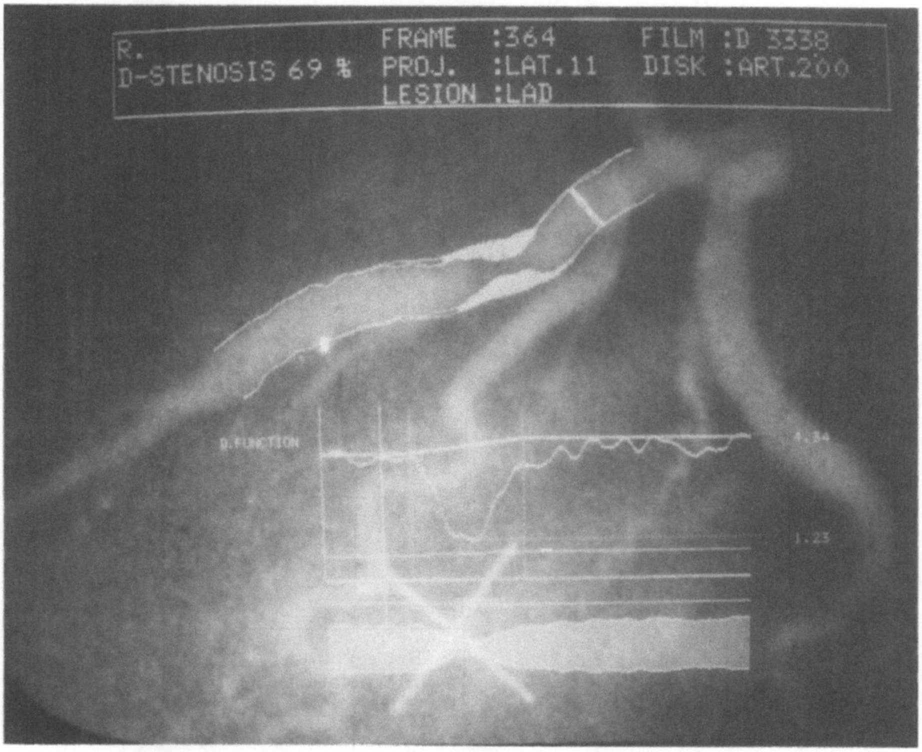

Fig. 8. For the lesion of Fig. 7 the normal size of the artery has been estimated from the normal proximal and distal diameter values (90th percentile). The marked area is a measure for the atherosclerotic plaque. An interpolated diameter stenosis of 69% results

For Fig. 8 an interpolated diameter stenosis of 69% results. Further evaluations of this method are necessary to determine its diagnostic value.

However, it has been explained that percentage diameter reduction measured in a single projection is of limited diagnostic value. Computation of the cross-sectional area reduction from the percentage diameter narrowing in the single view requires the assumption of circular cross sections, an assumption which hardly ever holds. To circumvent these limitations we have developed a densitometric procedure to determine the changes in cross-sectional areas of a coronary segment by using the density information within the artery. This requires the calibration of the brightness levels in terms of the amount of X-ray absorption (Lambert-Beer's Law). To this end, ten calibrated frames of homogeneous density levels are digitized at the start of the analysis procedure. These density levels correspond with the different light intensities at the output of the X-ray image intensifier with various amounts of absorption. Each frame is divided into 432 subimages of size 28 × 28 pixels. For each density frame the average brightness level in each of the subimages is computed. This results in a total of 432 local transfer functions; intermediate function values are obtained by interpolation. In this way the nonlinear and nonhomogeneous effects of the film processing and the film video-projection system are taken into account.

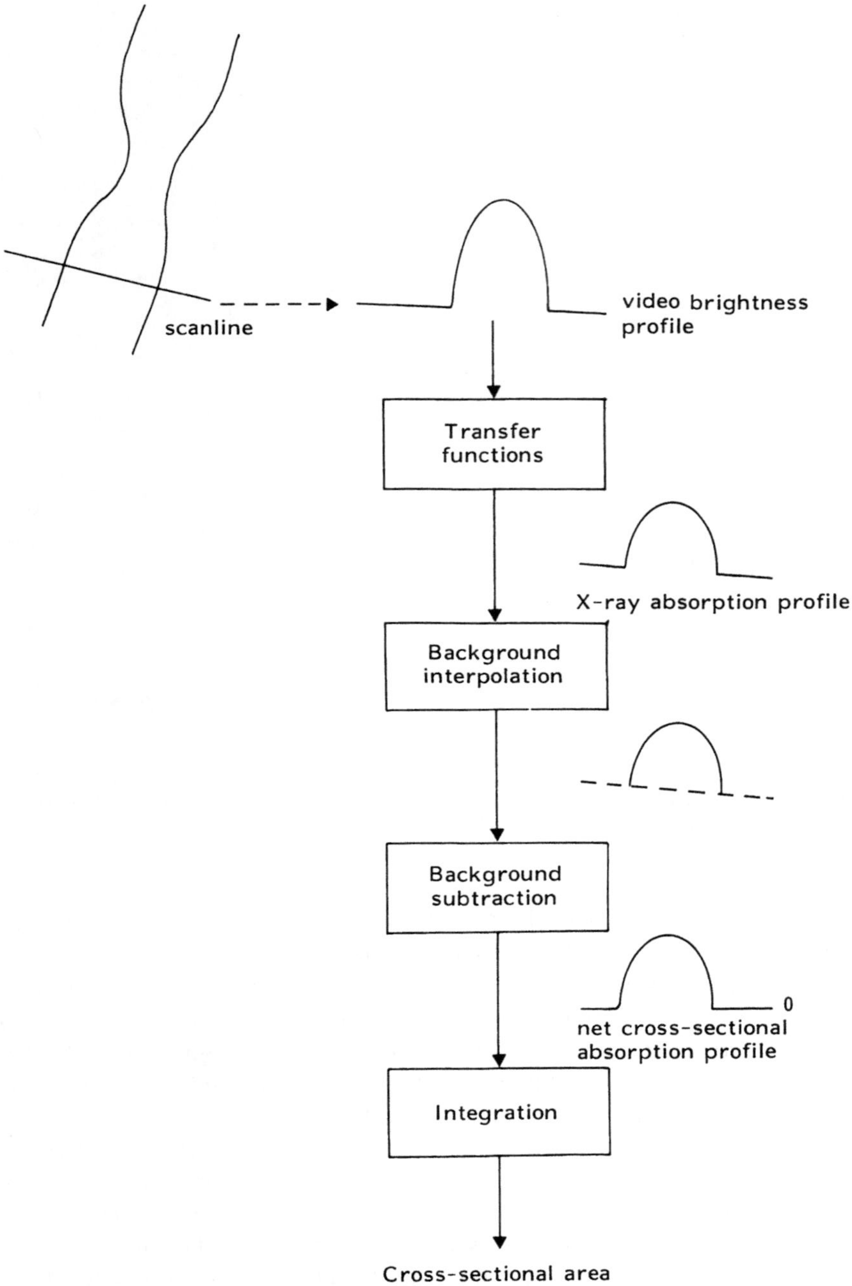

Fig. 9. Schematic drawing for determining the cross-sectional area data from the densitometric information within the artery

The procedure for determining cross-sectional areas can be explained with the schematic drawing of Fig. 9. When detecting the contour positions of a selected arterial segment in the way described above, the video brightness profile along a scan line can now be transformed into an X-ray absorption function my means of the transfer functions. Next, for each scan line the background below the arterial segment is estimated by a linear interpolation between measured background levels at both sides of the artery. By subtracting the interpolated background function from the X-ray absorption function between the contour positions, a net cross-sectional absorption function is determined. Integration of this function provides a measure for the cross-sectional area at this particular scan line. By repeating this procedure for each of the scan lines of the arterial segment, an area function A (i) is computed. It is clear that a homogeneous mixing of the contrast agent with the blood must be assumed for the measurements to be correct.

Figure 10 shows the clinical case of Fig. 5 with the computed diameter function and area function. The severity of the obstruction can now be expressed as a true percentage area reduction, by comparing the minimal area value at the obstruction with the mean area value at the selected reference position. For this particular obstruction we found an area obstruction of 86%. In this case a diameter reduction of 51% was computed from the diameter function. Assuming a model with circular cross sections

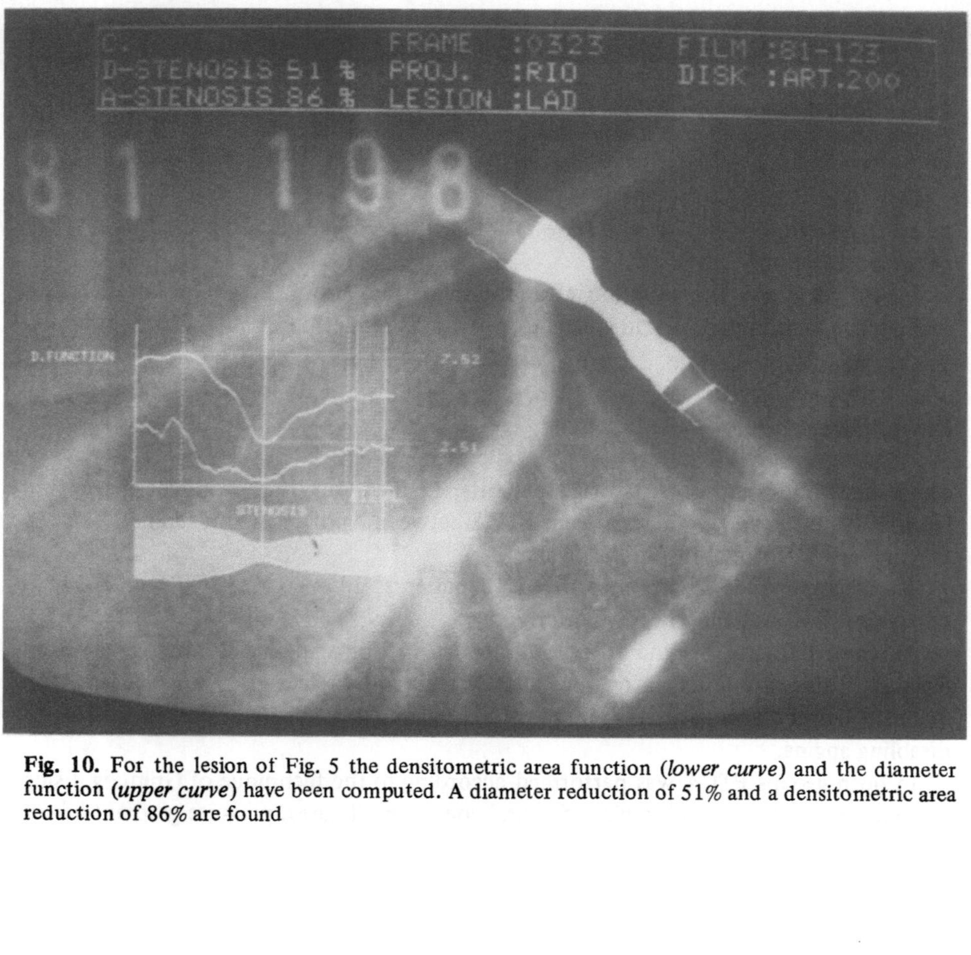

Fig. 10. For the lesion of Fig. 5 the densitometric area function (*lower curve*) and the diameter function (*upper curve*) have been computed. A diameter reduction of 51% and a densitometric area reduction of 86% are found

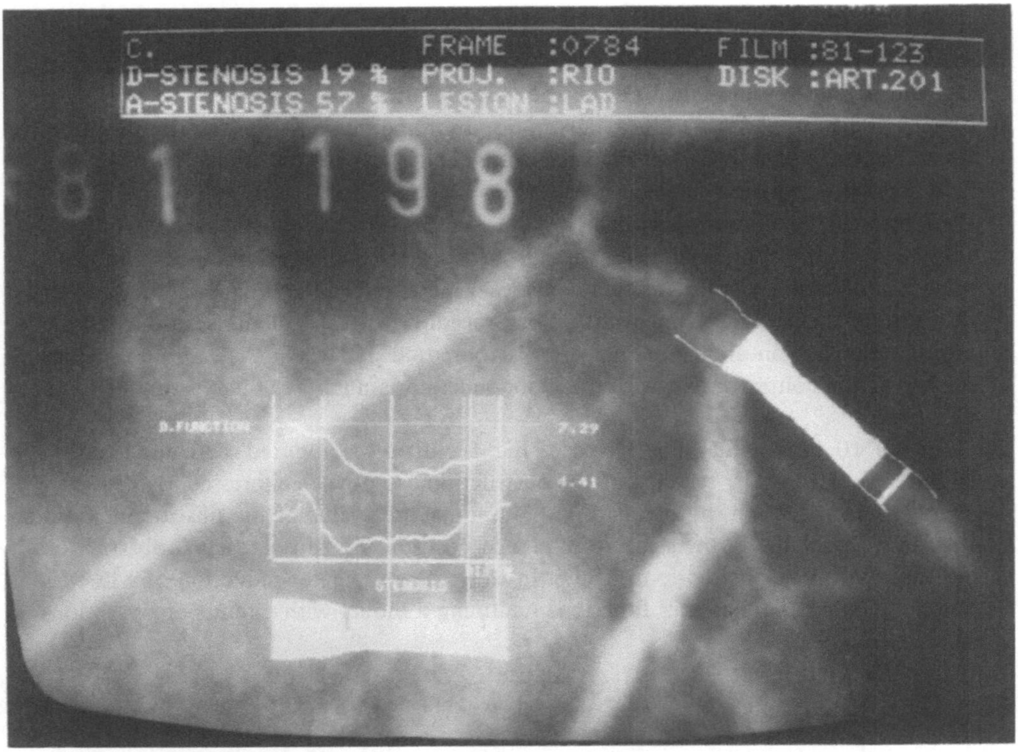

Fig. 11. Postdilatation measurements for the lesion of Fig. 5. A diameter reduction of 19% and a densitometric area reduction of 57% are found

an area reduction of 76% would have resulted, thus underestimating the true severity of the obstruction.

Figure 11 shows the situation after the dilatation. From the computer analysis a diameter reduction of 19% and a densitometric area reduction of 57% were found.

Patient Material

The first study group consists of 15 patients, 12 men and three women (age ranging from 29 to 62 years), who underwent PTCA between April 1980 and January 1981 at the University Hospital of Brabois, Nancy.

The second study group consists of 13 patients, 11 men and two women, who underwent PTCA at the Thorax Center.

All these patients met the criteria of a short history of pain (less than 1 year), an isolated obstructive lesion in one coronary vessel, and an accessible stenosis less than 1 cm in length. The patients were also likely candidates for operation as a result of disabling angina.

In both groups PTCA was performed according to the technique of Grüntzig, using the equipment of Schneider, via a femoral route. In all cases, pressure gradient across the obstructive lesion was recorded before and after dilatation. The dilatation catheters were either 20–30 or 20–37 catheters. The inflation pressure ranged from 4 to 7 atm, while the duration of the inflation was usually 15–25 s.

Attempts at dilating the stenotic lesion were repeated as long as the gradient across the lesion persisted (four to ten times). Prior to the procedure all patients received aspirin and a calcium antagonist; beta-blockers were not discontinued. During the procedure heparin, low-molecular-weight dextran, and nitroglycerin were administered intravenously. In some patients (Thorax Center) direct intracoronary injection of nifedipine and nitroglycerin was performed before the dilatation and when ST-T changes and chest pain occurred during PTCA. To visualize the effect of the procedure, coronary angiography was performed immediately before and after transluminal angioplasty. Lateral, anteroposterior, oblique, and hemiaxial views were usually obtained.

Results

In the first study group the quantitative analysis was limited to computation of the diameter values, derived from the detected contours. The severity of the obstructive lesion was expressed in relative percentage narrowing and in absolute values (mm).

For statistical analysis of the data, the projection in which the severity of the lesion was found to be greatest was selected for each patient. The postdilatation measurements were performed in the same projection selected for predilatation measurements. The results for the 15 lesions of the first study group are summarized in Table 1. On average, the reference diameter remains unchanged after PTCA. The obstruction diameter increases from 1.0 ± 0.3 mm to 2.2 ± 0.5 mm ($P < 0.001$). The diameter of stenosis, determined with respect to the user-defined reference diameter, decreases from 71% ± 6% to 37% ± 11% ($P < 0.001$). The percentage area stenosis, which is computed from the percentage diameter stenosis (assuming circular cross sections), decreases from 91% ± 4% to 60% ± 4% ($P < 0.001$).

The results of the percentage diameter stenosis determined according to the interpolated technique do not differ from the percentage diameter stenosis, calculated with respect to the user-defined reference regions.

Table 1. Effect of PTCA on 15 obstructive lesions in the first study group. Quantitative measurements derived from detected contours

Measurements	Before PTCA	After PTCA	*P*
Reference diameter (mm)	3.4 ± 0.8	3.6 ± 0.9	NS
Obstruction diameter (mm)	1.0 ± 0.3	2.2 ± 0.5	< 0.001
Diameter stenosis (%)	71 ± 6	37 ± 11	< 0.001
Area stenosis (%)	91 ± 4	60 ± 4	< 0.001
Interpolated diameter stenosis (%)	72 ± 7	41 ± 13	< 0.001

All values are expressed as mean ± standard deviation. Student's paired t test was used to determine probability

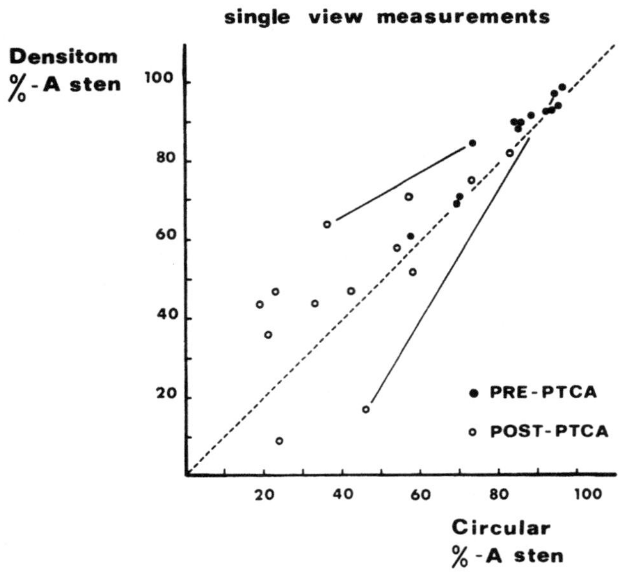

Fig. 12. Comparison of the densitometric percentage area stenosis with the circular percentage area stenosis for 13 patients

In the second study group, the densitometric percentage area stenosis was used to assess the changes in cross-sectional area after PTCA and compared to the circular percentage area stenosis from the diameter measurement. All these data were obtained from single projections. The comparative data are shown in Fig. 12. Before PTCA, there exists a good agreement between the densitometric percentage area stenosis and the circular percentage area stenosis. After PTCA, important discrepancies between these two types of measurements are observed. It is suggested that these discrepancies in results after PTCA can be accounted for by asymmetric morphological changes in luminal cross section which cannot be assessed accurately from diameter measurements in a monoplane view.

Discussion

As demonstrated elegantly by Block et al. [1] in rabbit arteries with experimentally induced atherosclerotic lesions, transluminal angioplasty may provoke splitting of the intimal surface of the atherosclerotic lesion. In their experience, the splits frequently extend to the internal elastic membrane, and angiography performed after transluminal angioplasty in these rabbits frequently shows an irregular column of contrast in the region of angioplasty. As suggested by the authors, the irregularities of their angiographic pictures must almost certainly represent contrast material within the splits of the atherosclerotic plaque produced by the angioplasty procedure. Recently, human autopsy material of coronary arteries that had undergone angioplasty was analyzed and showed changes identical to those seen in animal models.

These authors therefore conclude that "the close correlation between the changes seen in experimentally induced atherosclerosis after experimental angioplasty and in human coronary arteries after transluminal coronary angioplasty indicates that the mechanism of successful angioplasty in most cases is splitting of the atheromatous plaque which causes (erratic) enlargement of the vascular lumen." In keeping with this statement, our angiographic study suggests that changes in the luminal area of an artery, produced by the mechanical disruption of its internal wall cannot be assessed accurately from the detected contours of the vessel on a monoplane angiographic view.

In other words, the diagnostic value of this type of measurement is limited by the fact that the angioplastic changes are eccentric in nature. To obviate this limitation, the use of densitometry to compute cross-sectional areas from single views is advocated.

References

1. Block PC (1982) Correlation of the effects of transluminal angioplasty in experimentally induced rabbit atherosclerosis with pathological changes in human coronary heart disease.
2. Booman F, Reiber JHC, Gerbrands JJ, Slager CJ, Schuurbiers JCH, Meester GT (1979) Quantitative analysis of coronary occlusions from coronary cineangiograms. Comput Cardiol Proceedings 1979, p 177
3. Cherrier F, Booman F, Serruys PW, Cuilliere M, Danchin N, Reiber JHC (1981) L'angiographie coronaire quantitative. Application à l'évaluation des angioplasties transluminales coronaires. Arch Mal Coeur 12: 1377
4. Gensini GG (1975) Coronary angiography. Futura, New York
5. Gerbrands JJ, Reiber JHC, Booman F (1980) Computer processing and classification of coronary occlusions. In: Gelsema ES, Kanal LN (eds) Pattern recognition in practice. North-Holland, Amsterdam Oxford New York, pp 223
6. Gould KL (1980) Dynamic coronary stenosis. Am J Cardiol 45:286
7. Grüntzig AR (1978) Transluminal dilatation of coronary artery stenosis. Lancet 1:263
8. Mates RE, Gupta RL, Bell AC, Klocke FJ (1978) Fluid dynamics of coronary artery stenosis. Circ Res 42:152
9. Serruys PW, Steward R, Booman F, Michels R, Reiber JHC, Hugenholtz PG (1980) Can unstable angina pectoris be due to increased coronary vasomotor tone? Eur Heart J 1:71
10. Winbury MM, Howe BB (1979) Stenosis: regional myocardial ischemia and reserve. In: Winbury MM, Akibo Y (eds) Ischemic myocardium and antianginal drugs. Raven Press, New York, p 55

Techniques

Cinefluoroscopic and Video Imaging in Percutaneous Transluminal Coronary Angioplasty

J.R. Margolis

South Miami Hospital, South Miami, Florida, USA

Routine coronary angiography is best performed with high-resolution video imaging systems. Such systems provide optimal patient safety, and assure that a complete study has been performed. Unfortunately, many laboratories which produce excellent cine films have less than optimal video systems.

The unique requirements of percutaneous transluminal coronary angioplasty (PTCA) demand even more sophisticated video imaging. Because of the subselective nature of PTCA, the need for unusually accurate assessment of obstructive lesions, and the need to visualize small coronary artery branches and the tiny balloon catheter, high-resolution high-magnification imaging is required. Most existing systems obtain high magnification by electronically altering the electron beam in the image intensifier. This alteration in the electron beam attenuates the amount of light transmitted. Because of this attenuation, electronic magnification requires increased kVp for a given mAs. The increased kVp increases radiation dose. Since most PTCA work is done with patients in mid- or quiet respiration, and frequently in an angulated view, higher than ordinary kVp is needed. At high levels of electronic magnification, e.g., in the 4 in. mode of a trimode image intensifier (I.I.) the high kVp required may hamper resolution to such an extent that this mode cannot be used. The long fluoroscopy times frequently required for PTCA make it desirable to use the lowest possible fluoroscopy dose. Since electronically magnified imaging systems require higher radiation doses, an alternative form of image magnification is desirable.

At South Miami Hospital a system is presently in use that appears to meet all the diverse needs of PTCA. This system uses a standard 9 in./6 in. cesium iodide I.I., 80-line grid, newvicon TV chain, and electronic video image enhancer. Fluoroscopy dose is variable from 50 to 150 μR/s. In the 9 in. mode 50–90 μR/s provides excellent video images. In the 6 in. mode 90–150 μR/s is usually required. For normal-sized patients, even using angulated views, 90 μR/s is adequate for PTCA work. The cine dose of this system, as measured after the grid, is 28 μR/frame in 9 in. mode and 46 μR/frame in the 6 in. mode. Moderately high quality cineangiographic imaging of coronary arteries can be accomplished with a dose as low as 18 μR/frame in the 9 in. mode, but resolution of small coronary artery branches is impaired at this dose level.

The South Miami Hospital system employs two biplane C-arms, each of which is capable of obtaining all angulated views. Both C-arms are controlled electronically, and move independently. Because of this independence, virtually any combination of RAO and LAO and any combination of craniocaudal angulations are obtainable. This is par-

Transluminal Coronary Angioplasty and
Intracoronary Thrombolysis. Ed. by Kaltenbach et al.

ticularly useful in PTCA work, where the area of interest can be visualized simultaneously in the best view in two planes. For both C-arms, image tube to X-ray tube distances are fixed as short as possible. Collimation is rectangular via automatic collimators, which are coupled both to I.I. mode and zoom lens focal length (see below). The X-ray table consists of vinyl fabric stretched on a stainless steel frame. Two fiber "windows" have been inserted into the steel frame on either side at the level of the heart. These windows are relatively radiolucent, and allow imaging through or across the edges of the table. The vinyl table top has zero filtration.

The unique features of this system are two sets of zoom lenses, which are electronically coupled in such a way that video and cine images are exactly matched. Nearly continuous adjustment of focal length between 70 and 150 mm is available in two planes. Separate adjustment of magnification for each plane is easily done, and LED digital displays of focal length setting are provided. As a safety feature the cine lens acts as a master while the video lens serves as a slave, i.e., the focal length presented on the digital display will always be that of the cine lens. The video lens is adjusted by electronic circuitry to match the cine lens. This ensures that the image seen on the video monitor is identical to that which will appear on film. Malfunction in the system, which is rare, will be reflected by the image seen on the video screen. During the period of over 4 years that this system has been operative at South Miami Hospital, there has been no instance where the image produced on the film differed from that seen on the video monitor.

Figure 1 shows the zoom lens system. An electronic sensor identifies the position of the cine lens. This information is transmitted to a logic circuit (processor), which in turn transmits the information to the digital display and controls a motor connected to the video lens. A bidirectional momentary switch mounted on the digital display panel directs the processor to change the position of the cine lens to the desired focal length. With a change in position of the cine lens the slave video lens follows. A position sensor on the video lens is connected to an automatic collimator, which changes X-ray beam collimation in a manner appropriate for the image field required. Advantages of this zoom lens system can be summarized thus:

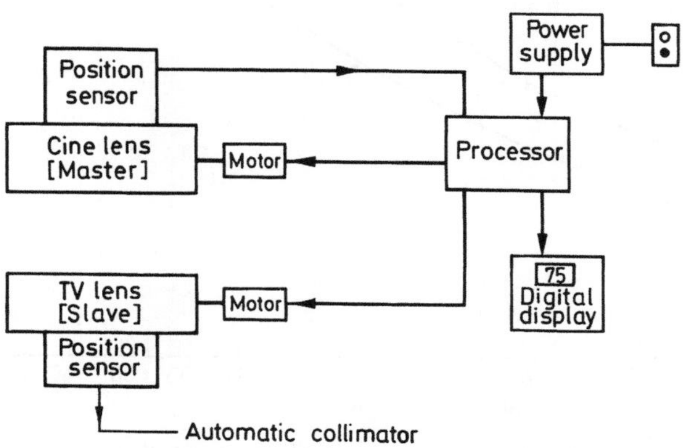

Fig. 1. The zoom lens system

Optical magnification superior to electronic magnification:
- Better resolution
- Less distortion
- Lower radiation dose
- Lower kV

Higher magnification for PTCA
Wider field for ventriculography
Variable Magnification for:
- Different patients
- Different heart sizes
- Visualization of collaterals
- Visualization of individual stenoses

In actual tests on cardiovascular phantoms and on patients optical magnification has been proven to be superior to electronic magnification in terms of resolution, distortion, and radiation dose. Even medium-priced zoom lenses have resolution capabilities which are far superior to the best image intensifiers. With optical magnification only the central portion of the I.I. is used, thereby minimizing distortion.

Optical magnification of the image from an I.I. requires no increase in radiation dose. Electronic magnification from the 9 in. mode to the 6 in. mode requires about 15% more kVp for given mA and pulse width. In the South Miami Hospital system, measured radiation dose in the 6 in. mode is 1.67 times higher than that in the 9 in. mode. A 4 in. mode would require an additional increment in radiation dose.

Figure 2 illustrates the relationship between required kVp and I.I. mode for various size patients, comparing the 9 in. and the 6 in. modes. For this demonstration a plastic

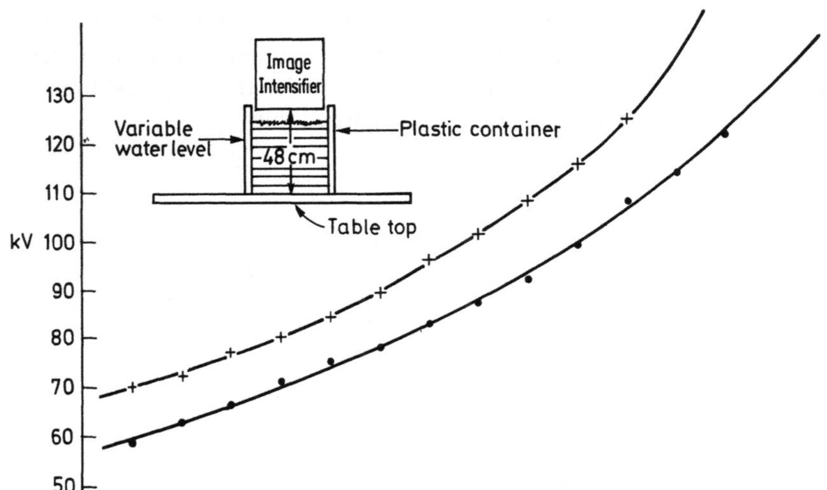

Fig. 2. Relationship between kV and simulated body thickness, in 6″ (+-+) and 9″ (.-.) modes, with X-ray tube current at 400 mA and a pulse width of 7.5 ms

container filled with water was placed on top of the X-ray table. The I.I. was kept at a fixed distance of 48 cm from the table top. The water level in the container varied from 14 to 38 cm. These distances are equivalent to patient thicknesses encountered in routine angiography and PTCA using various RAO, LAO, and angulated views. X-ray tube current was fixed at 400 mA. Pulse width was 7.5 ms. kV was adjusted electronically for optimal density using a standard auto-kV system incorporating a photo pickup. At all body thicknesses, as simulated by the water level, required kV was higher in the 6 in. mode than in the 9 in. mode. As body thickness increased the distance between the two curves widened in an exponential manner. For very large thicknesses (greater than 34 cm) kV requirements exceeded the capability of the system in the 6 in. mode but not in the 9 in. mode.

For coronary angiography optimal imaging is obtained in the range of 65–80 kVp. Using the 9 in. mode this optimal range can be used for standard size patients in almost all views, and for large patients in many views (Fig. 2). In the 6 in. mode kVp in the optimal range was used only at water levels corresponding to small patients with standard views.

Image quality deteriorates at kVp higher than 90. In the 6 in. mode water levels corresponding to moderate-size patients in angulated views and large patients in all views required kVp well in excess of 90 (Fig. 2). In the 9 in. mode kVp in excess of 90 were required only for water levels corresponding to the thicknesses of large patients with angulated views.

The ability to vary magnification with a zoom lens adds flexibility to any image intensification system. Even magnified I.I. modes (6 in. and 4 in.) can be made more magnified with the high focal length settings on the zoom lens system. This is particularly desirable for PTCA work. The low focal length zoom lens settings can be used to provide a wider field for ventriculography. This is especially helpful in dealing with abnormally large ventricles, and in assessing valvular regurgitation. In the 9 in. mode with a 70-mm focal length setting field size is adequate to encompass ventricles up to 450 ml, and still assess mitral regurgitation without panning. In the 6 in. mode with a 70-mm setting field size is adequate to encompass ventricles up to 250 ml.

Ability to vary magnification in a continuous way allows one to adjust for different patient sizes and different heart sizes. In filming larger patients magnification which occurs by virtue of a greater distance between the I.I. and the heart can be compensated for by appropriately decreasing focal length. This allows the cardiac surgeon to more accurately assess the true size of vessels which he will encounter. With large hearts excessive panning may be required to visualize the entire coronary arterial tree. This can be compensated for by appropriately decreasing focal length.

For the visualization of collateral circulation it is frequently desirable to include the entire heart within the image field. When this is done by switching from a 6 in. mode to a 9 in. mode, the coronary arteries are usually too small for adequate interpretation. Adjusting focal length to exactly incorporate the heart, and nothing more, obviates this problem.

Individual stenoses that are of marginal hemodynamic significance may be better evaluated by obtaining highly magnified views. In PTCA work, it is desirable to obtain such magnified views before and after the procedure, in order to accurately assess results.

The following examples give equivalent field sizes of optical and electronic magnification. Assuming that the standard cine lens has a focal length of 100 mm: a 6 in. intensifier with a 70-mm focal length lens has a field equivalent to that of an 8½ in. I.I.; a 6 in. I.I. with a 150-mm focal length lens has a field equivalent to that of a 4 in. I.I.; a 9 in. intensifier with a 70-mm focal length lens has a field equivalent to that of a 12½ in. I.I.; and a 9 in. intensifier with a 150-mm lens has a field equivalent to that of a 6 in. I.I.

At South Miami Hospital we routinely use the 9 in. mode with 85-mm focal length settings for ventriculography. For large ventricles, congenital heart disease, and patients with significant valvular regurgitation we use the 9 in. mode with a 70-mm setting. Routine coronary arteriography is done in the 9 in. mode with the 150-mm setting (equivalent to a 6 in. I.I. with a standard lens). For larger patients, the 9 in. mode with 143- or 137-mm focal length settings is used for routine coronary angiography. We use the 6 in. mode with focal length settings varying from 120 to 150 mm for PTCA work. When PTCA is performed on large patients, we use the 9 in. mode and 150-mm focal length setting in order to obtain the improved video image afforded by lower kVp requirements. When routine coronary angiography is performed on a patient who is a potential candidate for PTCA, highly magnified views of the lesion in question are routinely obtained.

The zoom lens system described above has been functional at South Miami Hospital since February, 1977. During this period there have been no major breakdowns, nor has it been necessary to discontinue a procedure because of malfunction of the system. At no time has information been lost due to system malfunction. The other components of the South Miami system have been functional since November, 1979. They have proved to be as useful for routine work as for PTCA.

Summary

Unusually high-resolution high-magnification imaging systems are required for PTCA. It is desirable that such systems perform at relatively low radiation doses and low kV. At South Miami Hospital a system is presently in use that appears to meet all of the diverse needs of PTCA. Unique features of this system include biplane C-arms capable of obtaining all angulated views, and matched zoom lenses for TV and cine chains. Optical magnification through zoom lenses has been proven to be superior to electronic magnification in terms of resolution, distortion, and radiation dose. The systems have been extremely reliable over several years, when used both for routine angiography and for PTCA.

Biplane Isocentric Coronary Angiography in Diagnosis and Interventional Therapy

T. Bonzel, H. Löllgen, K. Wink, H. Just

Medizinische Universitätsklinik, Abteilung Innere Medizin III, Kardiologie, 7800 Freiburg, FRG

Since the introduction of coronary angiography in 1959 and 1960 by Sones and Gensini continuous efforts have been made to improve the diagnostic accuracy of this technique. Advances were mostly accomplished in the technical field, especially regarding image quality, but also in the versatility of the systems, e.g., by establishing new angulated views. According to Judkins [1] "the issue in coronary angiography is information versus risk". Today, with interventional coronary therapy this issue regains special importance. In our experience biplane coronary angiography is one way to improve the relationship "information versus risk".

The study presents 10 months experience of biplane isocentric coronary angiography (BIC) with a double C-arm cineangiographic system. The system allows angulation of each of two independent C-arms laterally, caudally, and cranially for RAO, LAO, and hemiaxial views. Both C-arms can be rotated around a common center which is called the isocenter. This permits successive biplane coronary angiograms in various conventional and hemiaxial projections without moving the patient or the floating table. Since May 1980 more than 300 routine biplane coronary studies have been performed with a mean of three left coronary (LCA) and two right coronary (RCA) injections resulting in six LCA views and four RCA views. Most common biplane angulations were: 20° RAO + 70° LAO, 45° RAO + 45° LAO, and 45° RAO with 30° caudal + 45° LAO with 30° cranial hemiaxial angulation for LCA; and 45° RAO + 45° LAO and 45° RAO with 30° caudal + 45° LAO with 30° caudal hemiaxial angulation for RCA. For coronary interventional therapy, projections were chosen with special regard to the morphology of the diseased segment and good visualization of coronary branching, e.g., for dilatation of proximal LAD stenosis BIC angulations were usually 30° RAO + 45° LAO with 30° cranial. With increasing experience examination and fluoroscopy time could be reduced significantly by BIC compared to single-plane coronary angiography. In cineangiographic evaluation and in cardiological-cardiosurgical conferences simultaneous double projections proved to be useful for immediate recognition of anatomy and for grading of coronary stenosis (Figs. 1, 2).

Discussion

We could prove that BIC is feasible in routine coronary investigation, when cranial and caudal angulations of both systems are possible. For the experienced investigator fluoro-

Transluminal Coronary Angioplasty and
Intracoronary Thrombolysis. Ed. by Kaltenbach et al.

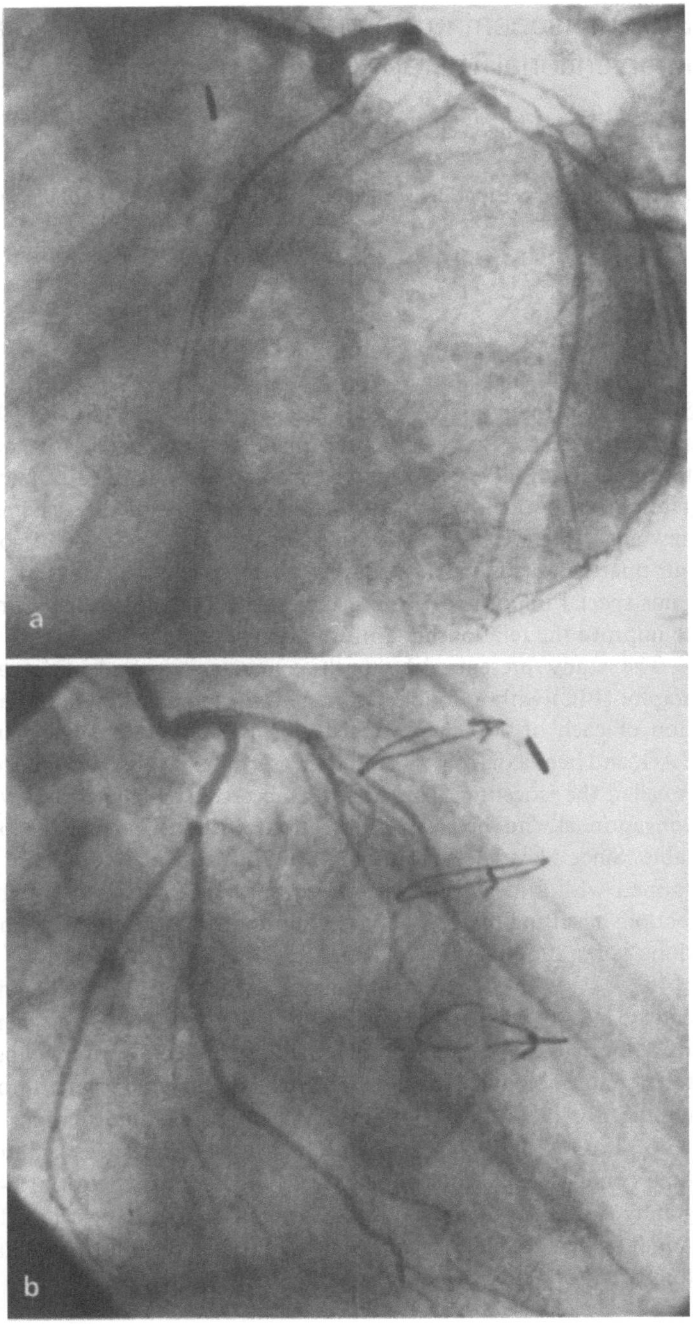

Fig. 1a, b

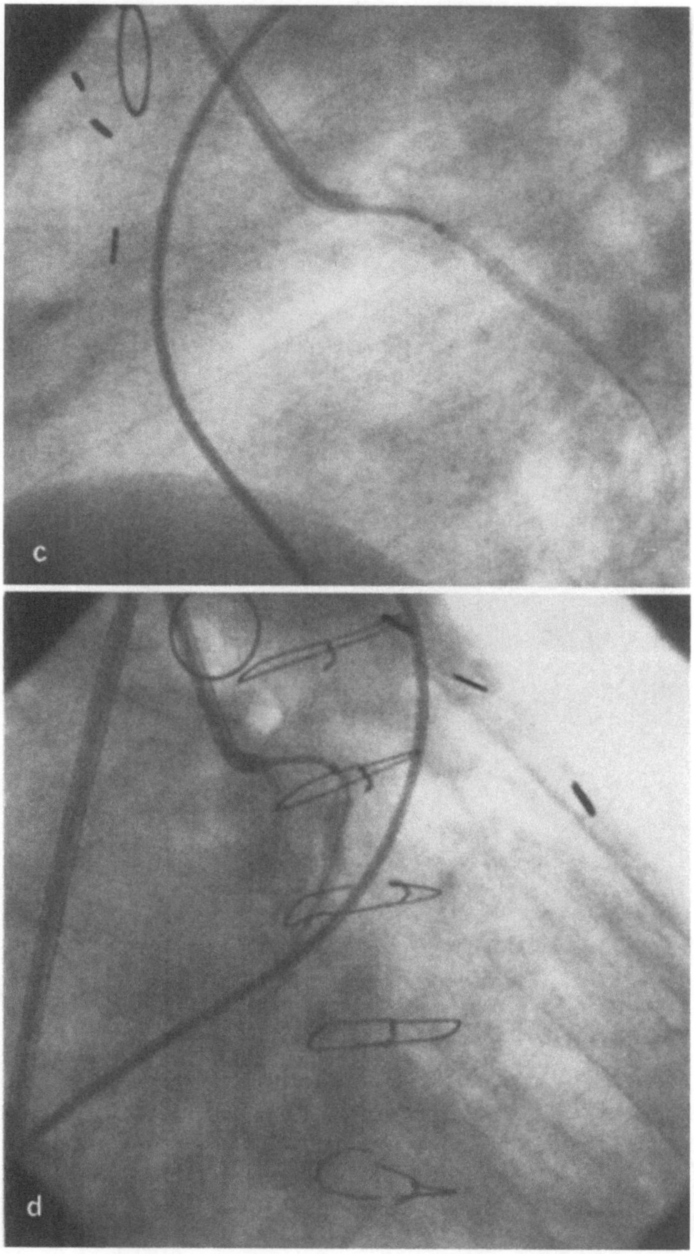

Fig. 1c, d

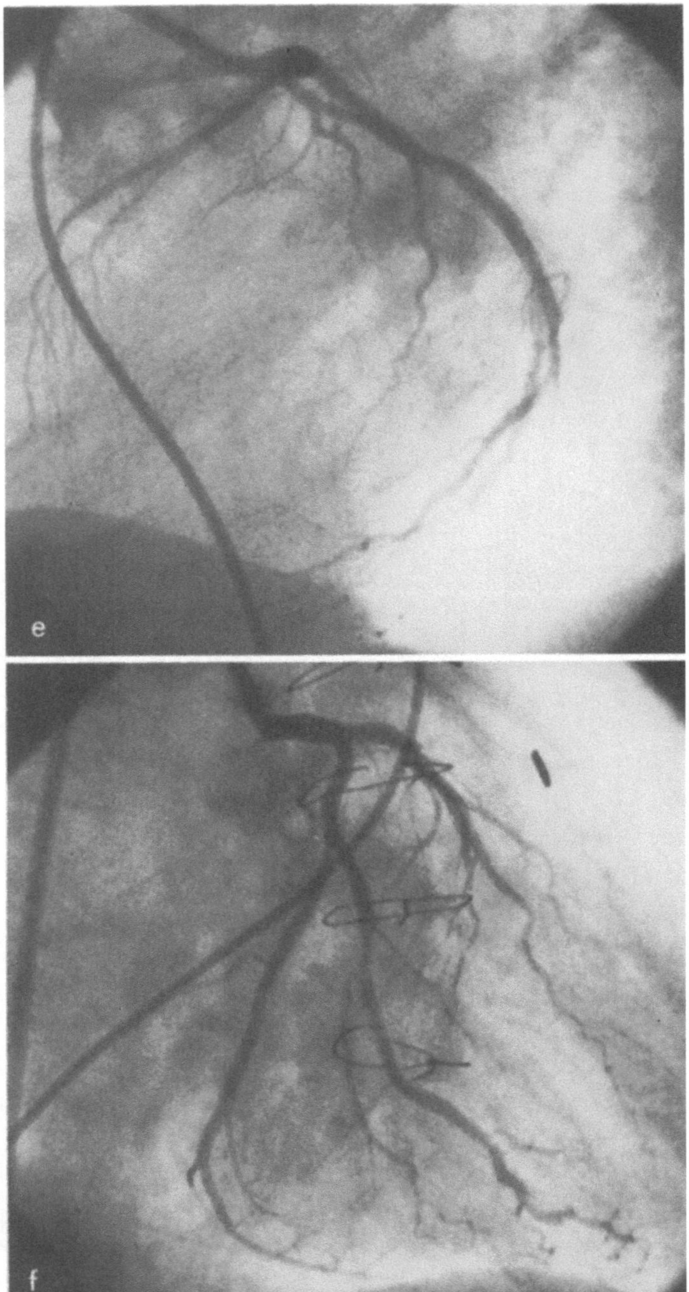

Fig. 1e, f

Fig. 1a–f. Biplane views of a severe lesion of the circumflex artery and of the successful dilatation of this stenosis in a patient with a patent LAD bypass graft and total LAD occlusion as well as recent onset of angina with mild exercise and occasionally at rest. **a** Cx lesion in LAO view; **b** RAO view; **c** balloon inflation in LAO view; **d** RAO view; **e, f** biplane views of Cx after successful dilatation

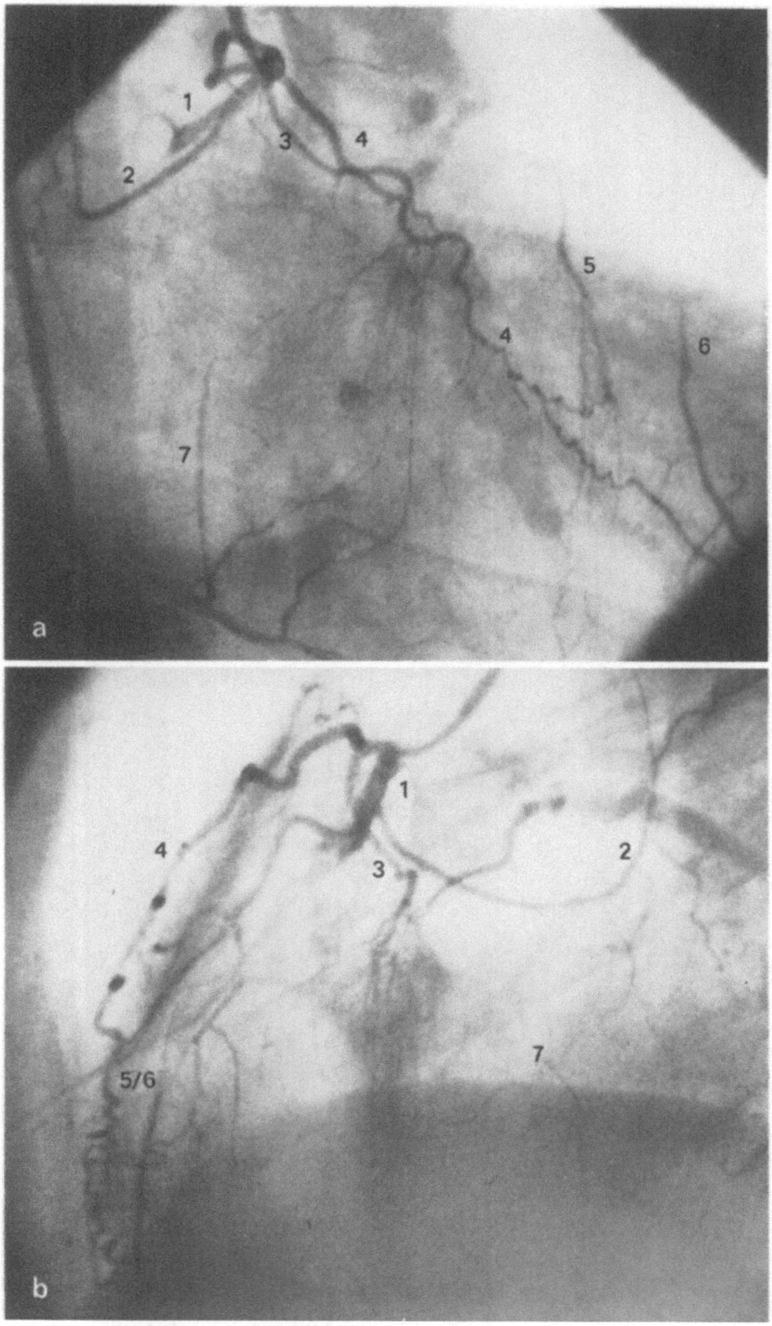

Fig. 2a, b

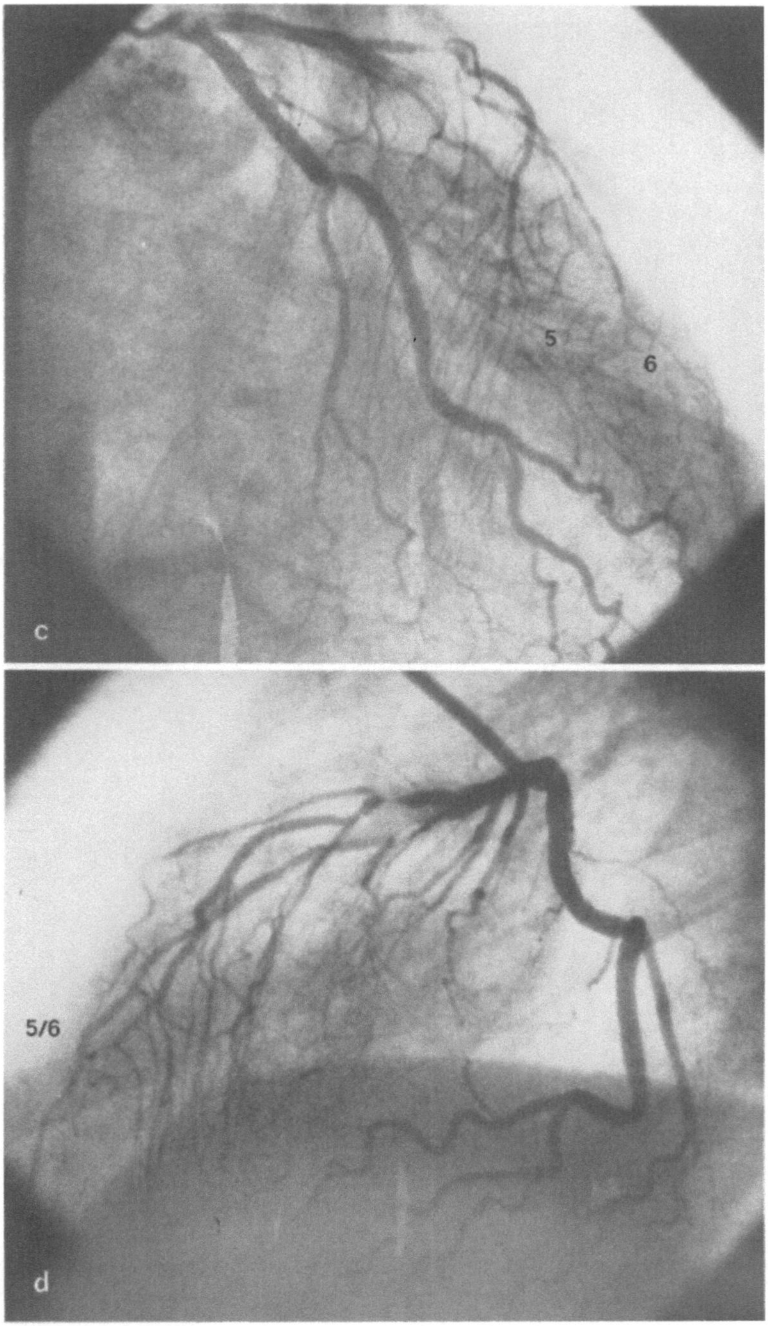

Fig. 2c, d

Fig. 2a–d. Biplane views of a diseased coronary system with additional congenital abnormalities: complete occlusion of the RCA, first septal perforator coming from the RCA, double LAD with tight stenosis, and competitive flow by collaterals from the conus branch. Filling of the distal RCA by collaterals. **a** RAO; **b** LAO; **c** RAO; **d** LAO. *1*, RCA occluded; *2*, atrial (sinus node) branch; *3*, first septal perforator; *4*, conus branch giving epicardial collaterals to double LAD branches *5* and *6*; *7*, AV node artery. Recognition of anatomical situation is facilitated by simultaneous biplane views scopy time and investigation time can be reduced and immediate information is improved. Intubation time of the tip of the catheter in the coronary ostium is also reduced, decreasing the risk of intima lesions as described by Lichtlen for the Judkins technique [2]. Advantages are obvious in coronary dilatation and in intracoronary thrombolysis. In coronary dilatation the pathway of the dilatation catheter within the stenotic vessel can be followed by biplane fluoroscopy and deviations into coronary side branches are easily recognised. The results of dilatation can be estimated with one injection in two planes. In intracoronary thrombosis detailed information on the occluded or stenotic coronary segment and on the progress of thrombolysis are immediately available by BIC with the injection of only a few ml of dye.

In our opinion patient management is an often underestimated part of the issue "information versus risk." In teaching conferences and in cardiosurgical conferences understanding of the coronary anatomy and of the morphology is facilitated remarkably with synchronized biplane projection, especially in patients with complex anatomical and pathological abnormalities.

In summary the advantages of BIC are:

1. Improved information on coronary anatomy and morphology with less contrast medium by reducing the number of injections
2. Reduced risk for high risk patients
3. Reduction of radiation and investigation time
4. Increased safety in coronary interventional therapy
5. Easier evaluation and therapeutic management

Complications did not occur and using the Judkins technique important disadvantages of BIC were not observed. If judged according to Judkins criterion, BIC positively changes the relationship "information versus risk."

References

1. Judkins MP, Gander MP (1974) Preventions of complications of coronary arteriography. Circulation 49:599–602
2. Lichtlen PR (1979) Koronarangiographie. Perimed, Erlangen (Beiträge zur Kardiologie, Band 11, pp 154–155)

Percutaneous Transluminal Coronary Angioplasty: Comparison of Brachial and Femoral Artery Methods

G. Dorros, S.H. Stertzer, R.K. Myler, M. Kaltenbach, D.A. Spring

Medical College of Wisconsin, 811 East Wisconsin Avenue, Suite 930, Milwaukee, Wisconsin 53202, U.S.A.

In 1977, Gruntzig [2] achieved the first successful coronary angioplasty with the guiding catheter introduced into the femoral artery via the Seldinger technique. In 1978 three centers, New York, Milwaukee, and Frankfurt, began developing coronary angioplasty guiding catheters which were introduced into the brachial artery. The major difference between the techniques was that the femoral method utilized preshaped guiding catheters, while the brachial method utilized a multipurpose guiding catheter which could intubate either coronary ostium. The present brachial and femoral guiding catheter systems are capable of consistently intubating either coronary ostium.

This communication reports the data of four centers that have been involved with coronary angioplasty since 1978. One center exclusively uses the brachial method, one the femoral method, and two both techniques. The results of these centers were pooled and statistically analyzed to determine the relationship between the utilized technique and the accomplishment of successful coronary angioplasty. In addition, a comparison was made between the individual vessels which had an attempted coronary angioplasty.

There were 646 coronary angioplasties (Table 1) attempted in 587 patients between November 1977 and April 1981. The stenosis was crossed in 475 cases (74%), with a primary success achieved in 422 cases (89%). A restenosis occurred in 51 instances (12%).

There were 302 angioplasties attempted using the brachial artery method (Table 2) with the stenosis crossed in 228 cases (75%) and a primary success achieved in 198 in-

Table 1. Overall results of PTCA by vessel attempted

Vessel	Attempts	Stenosis crossed	Stenosis not crossed	Primary success	Primary failure	Restenosis
LAD	396	315	81	286	29	33
LCX	34	22	12	22	0	2
RCA	168	100	68	83	17	9
SVG	23	14	9	11	3	4
LMCA	25	24	1	20	4	3
Total	646	475	171	422	53	51

Transluminal Coronary Angioplasty and Intracoronary Thrombolysis. Ed. by Kaltenbach et al.

Table 2. Results of PTCA by method used

Method	Vessel	Attempts	Stenosis crossed	Stenosis not crossed	Primary success	Primary failure	Restenosis
Brachial	LAD	159	130	29	114	16	5
	RCA	93	60	33	51	9	7
	LCX	20	15	5	15	0	2
	SVG	17	11	6	8	3	2
	LMCA	13	12	1	10	2	1
	Subtotal	302	228	74	198	30	27
Femoral	LAD	237	185	52	172	13	18
	RCA	75	40	35	32	8	2
	LCX	14	7	7	7	0	0
	SVG	6	3	3	3	0	2
	LMCA	12	12	0	10	2	2
	Subtotal	344	247	97	224	23	24
	Total	646	475	171	422	53	51

stances (87%). A restenosis occurred in 27 cases (14%). There were 344 femoral angioplasties (53%) with the stenoses crossed in 247 cases (72%) and a primary success achieved in 224 instances (91%). A restenosis occurred in 24 cases (11%). There was no statistically significant difference between the techniques in crossing the stenosis, achieving a primary success, or occurrence of a restenosis.

There were 396 left anterior descending stenoses attempted (Table 3) with the stenosis crossed in 315 cases (80%) and a primary success achieved in 286 cases (91%). A restenosis occurred in 33 cases (12%). When the brachial method (Table 4) was used

Table 3. Overall results of LAD and RCA

Vessel	Attempts	Stenosis crossed	Primary success	Restenosis
LAD	396 (80%)	315 (80%)	286 (91%)	33 (12%)
RCA	168 (26%)	100 (60%)	83 (83%)	9 (11%)

Table 4. Comparison of brachial and femoral techniques for LAD and RCA stenoses

Method	Vessel	Attempts	Stenosis crossed	Primary success	Restenosis
Brachial	LAD	159	130 (82%)	114 (88%)	15 (13%)
Femoral	LAD	237	185 (78%)	172 (93%)	18 (10%)
Brachial	RCA	93	60 (65%)	51 (85%)	7 (14%)
Femoral	RCA	75	40 (53%)	32 (80%)	2 (6%)

the stenosis was crossed in 130 of 159 attempts (82%) with a primary success achieved in 114 cases (88%). A restenosis occurred in 15 instances (13%). When the femoral technique was utilized the stenosis was crossed in 185 of 237 attempts (78%) with a primary success in 172 instances (93%). A restenosis occurred in 18 cases (10%). There was no statistically significant difference between the brachial and femoral techniques in the ability to cross the stenosis, achieve a primary success, or occurrence of a restenosis.

There were 168 right coronary stenoses attempted (Table 3) with the stenoses crossed in 100 cases (60%) and a primary success achieved in 83 cases (83%). A restenosis occurred in 9 cases (11%). When the brachial method (Table 4) was used the stenosis was crossed in 60 of 93 cases (65%) with a primary success achieved in 51 instances (85%). A restenosis occurred in seven instances (13%). When the femoral technique was utilized the stenosis was crossed in 40 of 75 attempts (53%), and a prinary success was achieved in 32 instances (80%). A restenosis occurred in two cases (6%). There was no statistically significant difference between techniques in ability to cross the stenosis, achieve a primary success, or occurrence of restenosis.

When the individual vessels were compared, the results demonstrated that a left anterior descending artery stenosis is statistically significantly more likely to be crossed than a stenosis in any other vessel, the right coronary artery ($P < 0.001$). If the left anterior descending artery stenosis is crossed, then this stenosis is statistically significantly more likely ($P < 0.05$) to be successfully dilated than a right coronary than a right coronary artery stenosis. There is also a statistically significant difference ($P < 0.05$) between the left anterior descending artery and left circumflex artery, left main coronary artery, and saphenous vein graft in crossing the stenosis, but not in dilatation of the stenosis.

There is no statistically significant difference in the occurrence of a restenosis in any native arterial segment successfully dilated, regardless of the technique used, while a restenosis in a saphenous vein graft successfully dilated was statistically more likely ($P < 0.05$) to recur than a stenosis successfully dilated in the native arterial segment (Table 1).

Summary

There is no statistically significant difference between the brachial artery and femoral artery methods in successfully crossing a stenosis (regardless of the arterial segment attempted), in achieving a primary success once the segment was crossed, or in the occurrence of a restenosis.

A left anterior descending artery stenosis is statistically more likely to be crossed and successfully dilated than a right coronary artery stenosis. The incidence of restenosis is the same in all native arterial segments dilated, while a saphenous vein graft stenosis is more likely to recur ($P < 0.05$).

These results indicate that coronary angioplasty can be effectively achieved by either the brachial or femoral artery methods. Thus, angiographers should utilize the technique with which they are most familiar.

References

1. Dorros G, Stertzer SH, Bruno MS, Kaltenbach M, Myler RK, Spring DA (to be published) The brachial artery method to (percutaneous) transluminal coronary angioplasty
2. Gruntzig AR, Senning A et al. (1979) Nonoperative dilatation of coronary-artery stenosis: percutaneous transluminal coronary angioplasty. N Engl J Med 301:61

Complications

The Role of the Percutaneous Intra-aortic Balloon in Emergency Situations Following Percutaneous Transluminal Coronary Angioplasty

J.R. Margolis

South Miami Hospital, South Miami, Florida, USA

Abrupt coronary artery occlusion is the single most important complication of percutaneous transluminal coronary angioplasty (PTCA). Even with meticulous technique and even in well-selected patients this complication can be expected to occur approximately 5% of the time. Abrupt occlusion is an acceptable complication, if patients can have subsequent coronary artery bypass surgery with neither compromise of the quality of surgery nor perioperative myocardial infarction. In the last five instances of coronary artery occlusion complicating PTCA we have exchanged the PTCA guiding catheter and sheath for a percutaneous intra-aortic balloon, using standard techniques. This maneuver rendered the patient so stable that it was possible to proceed with an unhurried bypass procedure, which was identical in all instances to the procedure that would have been performed in an elective setting. There were no instances of perioperative myocardial infarction.

Patients ranged in age from 40 to 55 years. There were four men and one woman. Three patients had attempted dilatation of left anterior descending stenoses, two patients had attempted right coronary artery dilatations (Table 1). All attempted stenoses were 80% or greater, as measured in the worst view. Two patients had subtotal occlusions before PTCA. Only one of five patients had angiographic evidence for collaterals. Three of the four patients without evident collaterals had correspondingly low distal pressures. In three patients, abrupt occlusion occurred during a period of 10–30

Table 1. Patient data

Patient	Vessel attempted	Stenosis (%)	Collaterals	Distal pressure (mmHg)	Peak CK-MB[a] (IU)
1	LAD	95	No	80/40 (64)	49
2	RCA	85	No	25/15 (20)	26
3	RCA	80	No	18/14 (16)	43
4	LAD	85	No	20/10 (15)	42
5	LAD	99	Yes	49/24 (36)	39

LAD, left anterior descending; RCA, right coronary artery.

[a] Peak CK-MB measured during 36 h after attempted PTCA and subsequent coronary artery bypass surgery (normal values < 50 IU).

Transluminal Coronary Angioplasty and Intracoronary Thrombolysis. Ed. by Kaltenbach et al.

min following apparently successful dilatation. Two patients had occlusion during passage of the dilatation catheter across the stenosis.

At the time of abrupt occlusion all patients had typical coronary pain, elevated pulmonary artery and pulmonary capillary wedge pressures, and electrocardiographic changes of epicardial injury. One patient also had hypotension, bradycardia, and ventricular premature beats. Pain, electrocardiographic changes, and elevated pulmonary artery pressures persisted despite administration of additional intravenous and intracoronary nitroglycerin and narcotics.

Percutaneous transluminal coronary angioplasty was performed according to standard techniques. All procedures were done with an operating room and cardiac surgery team on standby. Blood had been previously typed and crossmatched. A full surgical preparation had been done. An intra-aortic balloon pump, intra-aortic balloon catheters, and introducing sheaths were physically present in the catheterization laboratory. Immediately prior to attempted PTCA all patients had percutaneous insertion of a radial artery line and Swan-Ganz catheter. All patients were premedicated with diazepam, atropine, heparin, nifedipine, and intravenous nitroglycerin. Rheomacrodex and nitroglycerin infusions were continued throughout the angioplasty procedure. All procedures were performed via a percutaneous transfemoral approach through a standard USCI sheath.

When patients experienced chest pain and electrocardiographic changes, the presence of abrupt occlusion was confirmed angiographically. All patients were then given additional intravenous and intracoronary nitroglycerin and buccal nifedipine. Angiography was repeated following the administration of these medications.

Once a decision was made to transfer the patient to the operating room, the sheath in the femoral artery was exchanged over a 0.038 in. Teflon-coated guide wire for a 12F "Percor" sheath (especially fabricated for insertion of the percutaneous intra-aortic balloon). A 40-cc Percor intra-aortic balloon catheter was evacuated, moistened, and wrapped in the usual way, inserted through the sheath, and positioned fluoroscopically in the thoracic aorta. Hemostasis between the sheath and balloon catheter was obtained with #2 silk ties. Following demonstration of satisfactory balloon counterpulsation the sheath and balloon catheter were sutured in place.

In all instances, balloon counterpulsation was accomplished in less than 5 min, which includes time required for exchange of the sheaths, preparation of the balloon catheter, and preparation and venting of the pumping system. A few additional minutes were required to suture the balloon catheter in place and to cover the insertion site in a sterile manner.

Within 1 min of initiation of intra-aortic balloon counterpulsation chest pain abated, electrocardiographic changes returned to baseline, and pulmonary artery pressure became normal. All five patients remained pain-free, free of ischemic electrocardiographic abnormalities, and hemodynamically stable throughout the period of transfer to the operating room, preparation for surgery, induction of anesthesia, and initiation of cardiopulmonary bypass.

All hearts appeared to the eyes of the operating surgeon to be contracting normally. In no instance was the myocardium discolored. All three patients who had left anterior descending occlusion received internal mammary artery grafts, as is the custom in this institution for elective bypass to the LAD. Stability afforded by the intra-aortic balloon allowed the additional time necessary to harvest the internal mammary artery.

On the basis of serial CK-MB determinations (Table 1), serial electrocardiograms, and postoperative gated wall motion studies there was no evidence for perioperative myocardial infarction in any patient. There were no complications related to insertion or removal of the intra-aortic balloon. All patients had uncomplicated postoperative courses, and were entirely free of cardiovascular symptoms at the time of last follow-up.

Insertion of an intra-aortic balloon delays transfer from the cardiovascular laboratory to the operating room, and subsequent initiation of the surgical procedure. A retrospective analysis was made to determine the extent of this delay. Carefully kept protocols from the cardiovascular laboratory and operating room provided accurate data for analysis. The group of five patients who had intra-aortic balloon insertion was compared to a group of four patients who had had emergency surgery following abrupt occlusion from PTCA prior to our using the intra-aortic balloon for this indication. A second comparison group consisted of six patients who had elective coronary artery bypass surgery immediately following unsuccessful but uncomplicated PTCA. The results of this analysis are outlined in Tables 2 and 3.

Table 2. Transfer and preparation times (minutes) for the intra-aortic balloon cohort

Patient	Transfer to operating room[a]	Preparation for surgery[b]	Total
1	30	40	70
2	31	60	91
3	32	35	67
4	39	55	94
5	34	45	79

[a] Time from decision to transfer to arrival in operating room, including time for intra-aortic balloon insertion.
[b] Time from arrival in operating room to beginning of surgery.

Table 3. Comparison of mean transfer and preparation times (minutes) in the three cohorts

Cohort	Transfer to operating room[a]	Preparation for surgery[b]	Total
Elective	33	44	66
(n = 6)	(11–51)	(33–65)	(51–88)
Emergency			
No IAB	24	38	62
(n = 4)	(23–26)	(20–50)	(43–76)
IAB	33	47	80
(n = 5)	(30–39)	(35–60)	(67–90)

Figures in parentheses indicate range; IAB, intra-aortic balloon.
[a] Time from decision to transfer to arrival in operating room, including time for intra-aortic balloon insertion.
[b] Time from arrival in operating room to beginning of surgery.

For the five patients who had intra-aortic balloon counterpulsation, mean time for insertion of the balloon catheter and transfer to the operating room was 33 min, with a range of 30–39 min. The 33-min mean time was identical to that for the elective group, but was 9 min longer than the mean transfer time for the group of patients who had emergency surgery without prior intra-aortic balloon insertion. This 9-min delay can be accounted for by the 3–5 min required for preparation and insertion of the intra-aortic balloon, 2–4 min to affix and drape the balloon catheter, and 1–3 min additional transport time mandated by the bulky nature of the balloon console.

Time from arrival in the operating room to skin incision varied widely in all three groups. Mean time was shortest in the emergency group, who did not have prior intra-aortic balloon insertion. It was longest in the intra-aortic balloon group, but the differences between the three groups were small. The intra-aortic balloon may have delayed initiation of surgery because of the need to position the bulky console, additional electrode wires, and the external portion of the balloon catheter.

Total time accumulated from time of decision to transfer the patient to the time of skin incision was essentially identical for the intra-aortic balloon and elective groups. However, surgery began 18 min earlier in the emergency group (Table 3). Although this significant time difference is at least partially accounted for by the various factors listed above, the extremely stable nature of the intra-aortic balloon patients may have provided a milieu of less urgency for personnel involved in transfer and preparation for surgery. Similar transfer and preparation times for the elective and intra-aortic balloon groups suggest that this way was the case.

Discussion

Following abrupt occlusion of a major epicardial coronary artery, in the absence of good collateral circulation a myocardial infarction is likely unless immediate recanalization is accomplished. The amount of permanent myocardial damage is a function of the time between occlusion and reinstitution of adequate blood supply, but the extent of myocardial damage is also dependent upon myocardial oxygen demand during the ischemic period. Hearts protected by hypothermia and cardioplegia and vented beating hearts on cardiopulmonary bypass can tolerate long ischemic periods without significant myocardial damage. In the five patients described above, initiation of intra-aortic balloon counterpulsation erased all clinical evidence of myocardial ischemia in a prompt and dramatic way.

There are three possible mechanisms to explain the protection offered these patients by the intra-aortic balloon: reversal of spasm in the occluded artery, augmentation of collateral blood flow, and reduction of myocardial oxygen demand. Since all five arteries remained occluded despite the administration of intravenous and intracoronary nitroglycerin and buccal nifedipine, it is unlikely that intra-aortic balloon counterpulsation reversed spasm in any of these patients, and certainly not in all five. Increased aortic pressure during diastole with its concomitant augmentation of coronary artery filling may have improved collateral flow. Collateral flow may have been further augmented by reduction in left ventricular diastolic pressure. Reduction of myocardial oxygen demand is the most likely explanation for the salutory affects of balloon counterpulsation in these patients with abrupt occlusion of only a single vessel. Since all patients were at rest, sedated, and under treatment with continuous nitroglycerin infusion and nifedipine, the additional unloading affect of balloon counterpulsation may have reduced myocardial oxygen demand to a near basal level.

Most patients with abrupt occlusion following PTCA can be operated on safely without intra-aortic balloon counterpulsation (there were no perioperative myocardial infarctions in the four patients who had emergency surgery without balloon support). However, despite prompt operative intervention transmural myocardial infarctions of significant size have been reported to follow complicated PTCA. As PTCA is attempted more frequently in patients with multivessel disease or in those who have had prior coronary artery bypass surgery, the incidence of myocardial infarction following abrupt coronary artery occlusion can be expected to increase. Use of intra-aortic balloons in such patients may limit myocardial necrosis.

Insertion of intra-aortic balloons in these five patients appears to have delayed the start of surgery by an average of 18 min. Only a small portion of this time can be attributed to the insertion procedure itself. Some additional delay is inherent in the logistics of transferring a patient with intra-aortic balloon in place. A major portion of the delay is probably attributable to the marked stability of these patients following initiation of balloon counterpulsation. Although some delay may have been occasioned by a false sense of security, the stable circumstances may also have permitted more careful patient positioning, skin preparation, etc.

If emergency surgery following complicated PTCA results in a less complete operation than that which would have been performed on an elective basis, a patient has been harmed by the attempted PTCA. Stability offered by intra-aortic balloon counterpulsation allows time for an unhurried and complete operation. Use of the internal mammary artery in the three patients in this series with LAD occlusion lends support to this concept.

Patients undergoing streptokinase infusion for spontaneous coronary thrombosis are in some ways analogous to patients who have abrupt occlusion following PTCA. In both groups it is expected that blood flow to the affected area will be restored within a few hours of coronary artery occlusion, and that myocardial infarction will be either prevented or limited. Experience with the five patients described above suggests that insertion of a percutaneous intra-aortic balloon prior to streptokinase infusion may protect myocardium during the time required to reestablish flow. Since such patients usually have severe residual stenoses after clot lysis, continued balloon counterpulsation may hasten repayment of oxygen debt, especially to the subendocardium.

On the basis of a limited experience, use of intra-aortic balloon counterpulsation following complicated PTCA appears to be a useful adjunct to emergency coronary artery bypass surgery. Intra-aortic balloon insertion probably delays the start of surgery by no more than 5–10 min. This short delay is more than compensated for by the extremely stable condition of these patients during transfer to the operating room, induction of anesthesia, and initiation of cardiopulmonary bypass.

Summary

Five patients with coronary artery occlusion complicating PTCA had percutaneous insertion of an intra-aortic balloon prior to transfer to the operating room for emergency coronary artery bypass surgery. Balloon insertion was accomplished by simply exchanging the PTCA guiding catheter and sheath over a guide wire for a larger sheath suitable for intra-aortic balloon insertion. Concomitant with coronary artery occlusion, all five patients experienced angina, ischemic electrocardiographic changes, and elevations of pulmonary artery pressure. Chest pain, ECG changes, and hemodynamic abnormalities were promptly reversed upon initiation of intra-aortic balloon counterpulsation. All patients were brought to the operating room in stable condition, and remained stable throughout induction of anesthesia and initiation of cardiopulmonary bypass. All hearts appeared to the eyes of the operating surgeon to be contracting normally. Stability afforded by the intra-aortic balloon allowed time to harvest the internal mammary artery for the three patients with left anterior descending occlusions. No patient had evidence for perioperative myocardial infarction. There were no complications related to insertion or removal of the intra-aortic balloon. Insertion of the intra-aortic balloon appears to delay initiation of surgery by no more than 5–10 min. The experience with these five patients suggests that intra-aortic balloon counterpulsation following complicated PTCA may be a useful adjunct to emergency coronary artery bypass surgery.

Emergency Reopening of Right Coronary Occlusion After Angioplasty Using Guide Wire and Thrombolysis

U. Sigwart, A. Essinger, M. Grbic, U. Gleichmann*, H. Sadeghi

Centre Hospitalier Universitaire Vaudois, Lausanne, Switzerland

* Gollwitzer-Meier-Institut, Bad Oeynhausen, FRG

This communication describes a case in which an acute coronary artery occlusion after right coronary artery angioplasty was successfully reopened with the help of a large guide wire and local intracoronary streptokinase infusion.

Case Report

A 55-year-old patient was admitted for coronary angioplasty. Eight weeks prior to admission, the patient had been hospitalized for acute anteroseptal myocardial infarction. Four weeks prior to admission, cardiac catheterization revealed a subtotal proximal stenosis of the left anterior descending coronary artery and two significant stenoses of the right coronary artery. A localized akinesia of the anterior wall was also present. The patient had intermittently been hypertensive and left renal artery stenosis was suspected on the basis of a previous nonselective angiogram.

The indication for aggressive treatment of the coronary artery stenoses was based upon the patient's symptomatology, the prognostic significance of the three remaining lesions, and the patient's personal strong desire to undergo transluminal angioplasty even in the face of an elevated risk.

On admission, the patient was in no distress and well compensated. Blood pressure was 130/80 mmHg with a heart rate of 72. There was a discreet third heart sound but otherwise no clinical evidence of left ventricular dysfunction. The electrocardiogram was compatible with a localized anterior septal scar. The chest X-ray failed to reveal cardiomegaly or pulmonary congestion. Blood chemistry and urine analysis were within normal limits.

Following routine premedication with aspirin (1 g) for 2 days and continuation of the nitrate therapy, a complete left and right heart catheterization using standard technique was performed. A selective right renal artery injection showed marked kinking of the origin of the vessel with a moderately important stenotic lesion. This stenosis was not considered accessible for transluminal dilatation. Left ventriculography and coronary angiography revealed precisely the same findings as already demonstrated: localized left ventricular anterior akinesia, a subtotal proximal stenosis of the left anterior coronary artery after the first septal branch (Fig. 1a) and two significant lesions of the proximal right coronary artery (Fig. 2a), the distal part of which was si-

Transluminal Coronary Angioplasty and
Intracoronary Thrombolysis. Ed. by Kaltenbach et al.

tuated between two right ventricular branches. There was no collateral visualization of the distal left anterior descending coronary artery.

After injection of 10 000 units heparin, the subtotal stenosis of the left anterior coronary artery was dilated at a pressure of 6.5 bars. The result was satisfactory in respect to anatomical and hemodynamic aspects (Fig. 1b). The right coronary artery ostium was easily intubated; a first dilatation was performed on the proximal right coronary artery stenosis situated distally from a large atrial branch. The balloon also passed the second stenosis without major difficulties; the balloon dilatations, however, failed to reveal any significant increase in luminal diameter. Control injections (Fig. 2b) showed the stenosis still to be present, without evidence of either dissection or thrombosis. The catheters were removed without antagonizing the heparin action by protamine sulfate.

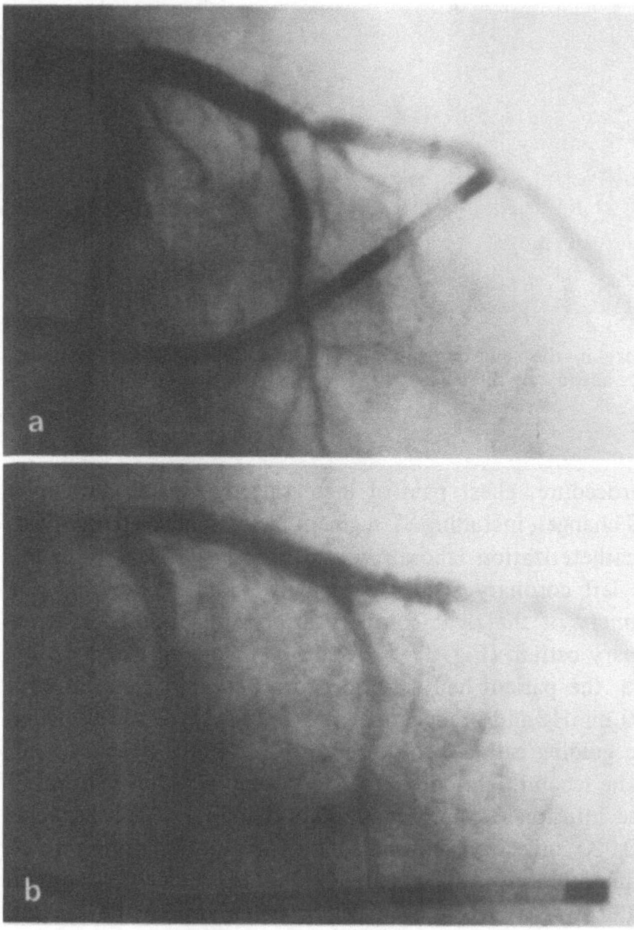

Fig. 1a, b. Subtotal proximal stenosis of the left anterior descending coronary artery. **a** before coronary angioplasty; **b** after coronary angioplasty

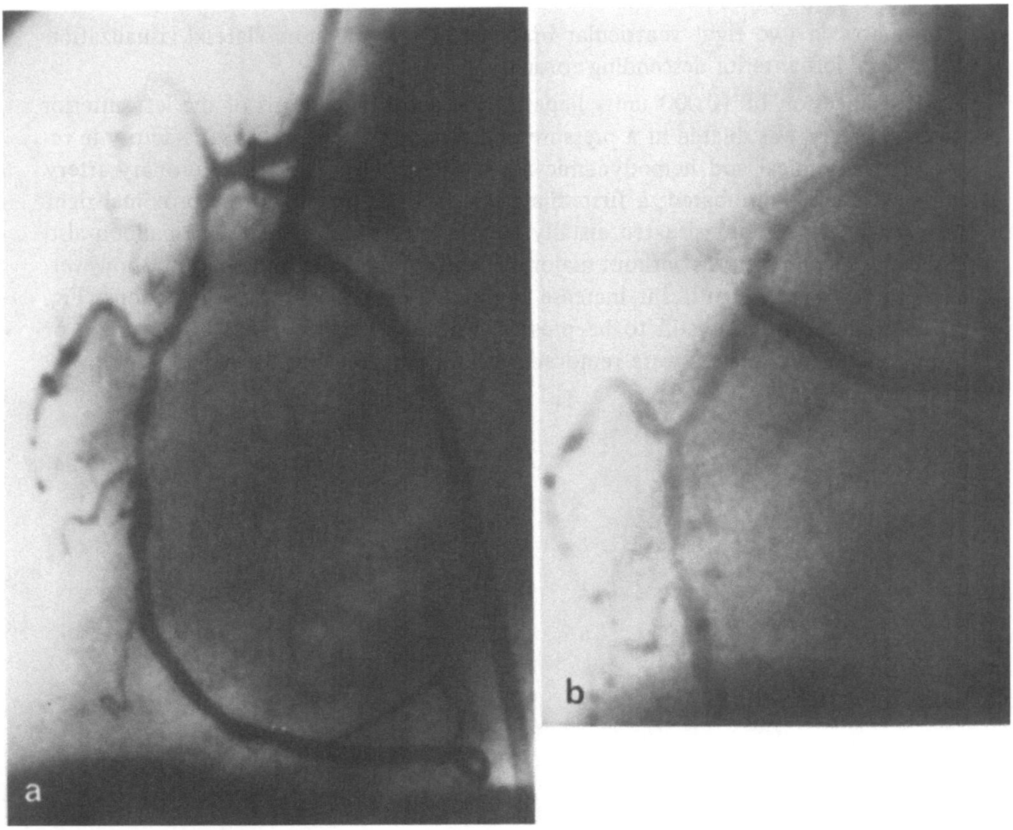

Fig. 2a, b. Right coronary artery in the same patient. **a** two consecutive significant stenoses; **b** the second stenosis could not be adequately dilated

Three hours after the procedure, chest pain of increasing magnitude developed associated with inferior ECG changes, including ST segment elevation. The patient was immediately taken to the catheterization laboratory and a control coronary angiography was performed. The left coronary artery was widely patent, opacifying in a retrograde manner the periphery of the right coronary artery. Injection of contrast medium into the right coronary ostium (Fig. 3a) showed a complete occlusion of this vessel. During the procedure, the patient had developed profound hypotension with systolic blood pressure of 40 mmHg and bradycardia. A 5 F guide wire was immediately introduced through the guiding catheter into the coronary artery and easily advanced up to the region of the second right coronary artery stenosis. After removal of the guide wire, streptokinase infusion (Streptokinase Kabi, Globopharm, Küssnacht, Switzerland) was begun. 150 000 units were infused over a 5-min period during which the patient regained an adequate blood pressure and a normal heart rate. Control angiography revelaed the right coronary artery again to be patent up to the second, nondilatable, coronary artery stenosis. Furthermore, the large right ventricular branch of the right coronary artery also showed an adequate flow.

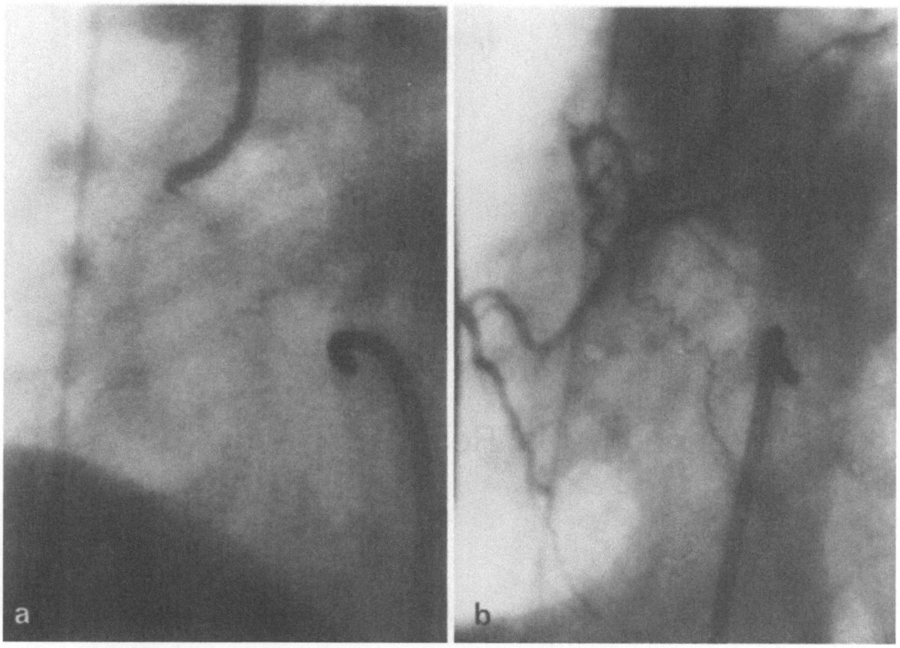

Fig. 3. a A complete occlusion of the right coronary artery in the same patient; b reopening with guide wire and streptokinase

Despite the prompt recovery after reopening of the proximal right coronary artery, it was decided to perform bypass surgery in view of the importance of the distal segment of the right coronary artery. A balloon counterpulsation was instituted and the patient was transferred in stable condition to the operating room. A double bypass procedure was performed. In postsurgical recovery was uneventful and the patient was discharged 1 week after the operation. To date (10 months later) he is free of symptoms.

Conclusion

The case presented here stresses the importance of patient monitoring after dilatation procedures, particularly as no perfect result had been obtained after angioplasty. The monitoring should include 12-lead ECG tracings at regular intervals and competent surveillance. Since reintervention may be a life-saving procedure, the necessary material for recanalization should be readily available and at hand. Streptokinase for coronary thrombolysis appears to be a most helpful adjunct in the treatment of postdilatation complications.

Experimental Results

Morphology and Pathogenesis of Coronary Artery Stenosis, Relevant to Intraluminal Dilatation

W.F.M. Fulton

University of Glasgow, Department of Materia Medica, Stobhill General Hospital, Glasgow, G21 3UW, Scotland

Introduction

The introduction of techniques for intraluminal dilatation of coronary artery stenosis gives new importance to the nature of the disease in the arterial wall responsible for the stenotic lesions. Accordingly the evidence arising from a clinicopathological study of the coronary arteries has been examined with this point in view. The paper presented to the conference was mainly a pictorial demonstration of some of the features of stenotic lesions, rather than an analysis of observations.

Material and Methods

Ninety-two hearts (82 with fatal coronary artery disease) have been examined post mortem by techniques which included stereoarteriography in three stages and mounted 2-mm serial transverse sections of major coronary arteries and branches [2]. The injection medium was bismuth oxychloride in gelatine, introduced into each cannulated coronary orifice at 80 mmHg pressure. Stereoradiographs were taken of the intact heart (I), the heart after partial dissection (II), and the coronary arteries after excision en bloc (III). Arteriograms I and II were exposed on Kodak Industrex C film and arteriograms III on Industrex M film. After formol saline fixation, decalcification and embedding in gelatine the excised arteries were sectioned from end to end at 2-mm intervals. The stereoarteriograms were used as an aid to obtaining true transverse sections where possible. The sections were mounted semi-permanently in glycerine agar. Selected 2-mm blocks were submitted for histopathology. Frozen sections were examined by normal and polarized light, unstained and stained with Sudan IV for fat. Paraffin sections were stained with haematoxylin and eosin, MSB stain for fibrin and collagen, and stained for iron by the Prussian blue method.

Prepared as above and examined by incident and transmitted light in a dissecting microscope with a magnification of × 6–× 40 these 2-mm thick transverse sections were remarkably informative in regard to microanatomy. Comparison with selected histopathological sections allowed considerable confidence in morphological interpretation of the unstained thick sections. The thick sections had certain advantages:

a) Completeness of sections, no loss of information in processing
b) Serial observations from fairly healthy to severely diseased lesions and throughout the length of the obstruction
c) Greater numbers of observations than would otherwise be feasible.

Over 300 excised arteries yielded some 10 000 2-mm thick transverse sections.

Transluminal Coronary Angioplasty and Intracoronary Thrombolysis. Ed. by Kaltenbach et al.

Observations on Morphology of Stenoses

Stenotic lesions were studied in two circumstances:

a) Those that underlay fatal acute thrombotic occlusion
b) Those that were free from recent thrombus at the time of death

The latter are the subject of this paper. There was no essential difference between the two in regard to the basic underlying intimal disease. Rupture of the intimal lining with haemorrhage into the diseased artery wall, however, was not surprisingly a more frequent feature of the stenoses complicated by thrombosis. Nevertheless haemorrhage into the artery wall was also found, with less frequency, in arterial lesions without thrombosis.

Obstructive lesions, which were 1 mm or less in diameter or one-quarter or less of previous lumen (media-to-media) diameter were classed as severe stenoses. Lesions between these dimensions and 1.5 mm in lumen diameter, or one-third of media-to-media diameter, were classed as moderate stenoses. Obstructive lesions with multiple channels or hairline lumen were classed as canalized thrombotic occlusions and are not described in this paper. This does not mean to say that single channels in severe stenosis were not, at least sometimes, the product of the same process.

The correlated evidence of magnified (× 8) stereoarteriography and of serial and selected transverse sections allowed microanatomical reconstruction of the stenotic lesions throughout their length (see Fig. 1, 2, 4).

Colour Changes

In the unstained sections the colour changes dependent on altered blood pigment were eloquent evidence of at least one component in the genesis of these lesions. Such colour changes were not represented in tissues processed for paraffin sections and stained by any of the conventional methods.

These colour changes could be traced in sections from different lesions, and from the same lesions at different levels, from the dark red-brown of recent haemoglobin-containing thrombus or haemorrhage through all tints of brown, brown-orange, yellow, sometimes brick red, to pale yellow. When examined in frozen sections, atherosclerotic plaques showing this pigmentation contained varying amounts of neutral fat and cholesterol crystals, much as in the generality of pale atheromatous lesions. The pigment seemed, however, to be a feature of the background amorphous debris in which the lipid material was embedded. In general, the paler the atheromatous lesion the greater the proportion of lipid in its composition, but many exceptions occurred. On following serial 2-mm sections from unobstructed lumen to severe stenosis, characteristically relatively pale atherosclerosis gave way, sometimes abruptly, to deeply pigmented lesions (Fig. 2). The structure and material composing such lesions was similar to that found at the ends of old thrombotic occlusions [1, 2, 3, 4].

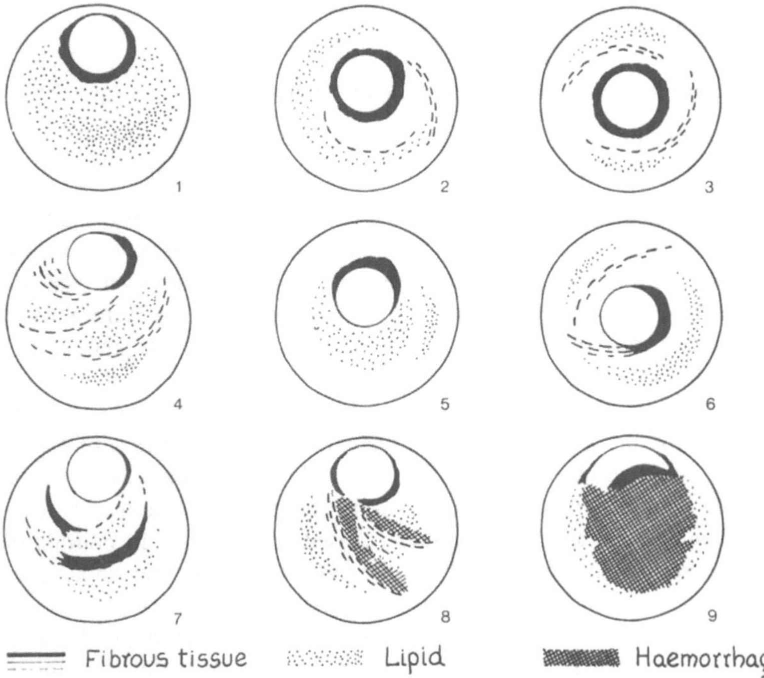

Fig. 1. Some microanatomical features of severe coronary stenosis. Note positions of lumen, varying thicknesses of fibrous wall of lumen, various distributions of fibrous layers and lipid in underlying atherosclerotic lesions. Haemorrhage occurring spontaneously dissects the structure of the plaque. Similar dissection is likely to follow mechanical dilatation. *1* Eccentric lumen, bordered by normal wall on outer aspect and by thick fibrous layer and soft atheroma on inner aspect. *2* Intermediate lumen position, fibrous wall uniformly thick. *3* Lumen central. *4* Eccentric lumen, wall uneven thickness, atheroma a compound of crescentic layers. *5*, *6* Much as 2, *3* but lumen lining thin in part. *7* Thin wall to lumen, thick fibrous layers deeply placed. *8* Haemorrhage dissecting fibrous layers (as in *4*). *9* Massive haemorrhage into atheroma (as in *1*) with compression of lumen.

Composition

Characteristically, lesions causing severe stenosis had complex structure and/or pigmentation as described above. Exceptions occurred but were relatively infrequent. The manner in which such lesions appear to have been derived from recurrent layers of thrombus or episodes of intimal haemorrhage have been described [2, 3]. This interpretation gives the only explanation acceptable to me for the multiple crescentic layers composing the atherosclerotic lesion, the tendency for rupture at interfaces between these layers, the asymmetrical distribution of disease within the artery, the pigmentary evidence of degenerated haemoglobin and some other features such as iron deposition and intimal blood channels. In some lesions it seemed probable that the lumen had never been completely closed by thrombus or haemorrhage. In others the most likely interpretation was temporary acute occlusion with early new channel formation. The latter seemed particularly likely in those instances where the lumen was in contact at one side with nearly normal arterial wall, and where old myocardial damage was evident in the relevant territory.

Position of Lumen

The lumen in severe stenosis was placed in individual sections at any point between true centre and extreme periphery (Fig. 1). Thus it might be *central* surrounded by a layer of fibrous tissue and this in turn by a zone of soft lipid-laden debris. The thickness of the periluminal fibrous tissue might be uniformly thin (a new microns only), substantially thick (0.5 mm or more), or thick and extremely thin at different points on its circumference. The surrounding soft amorphous lipid-containing

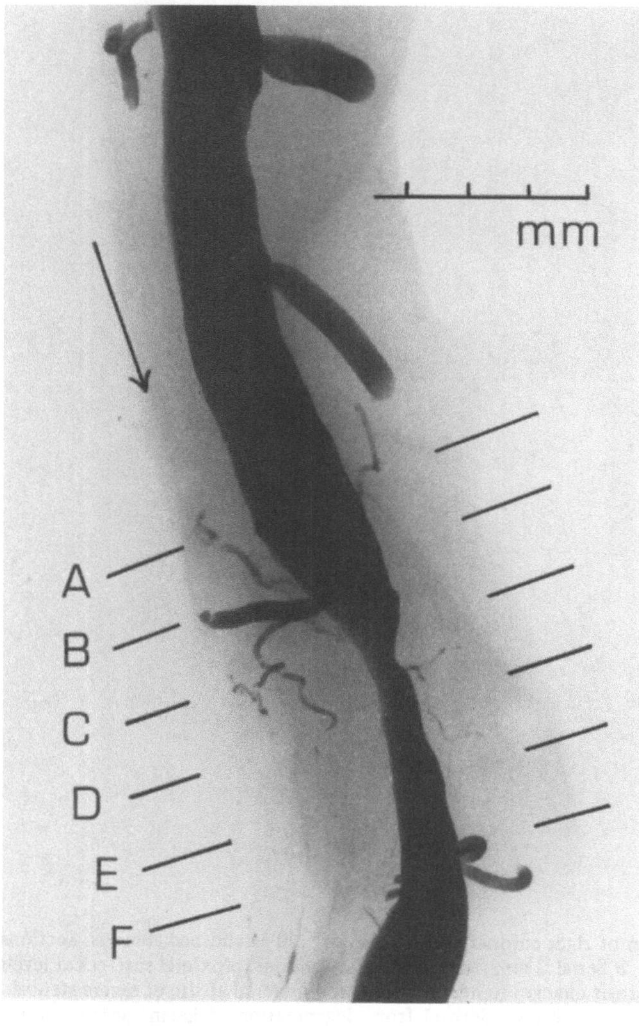

Fig. 2a

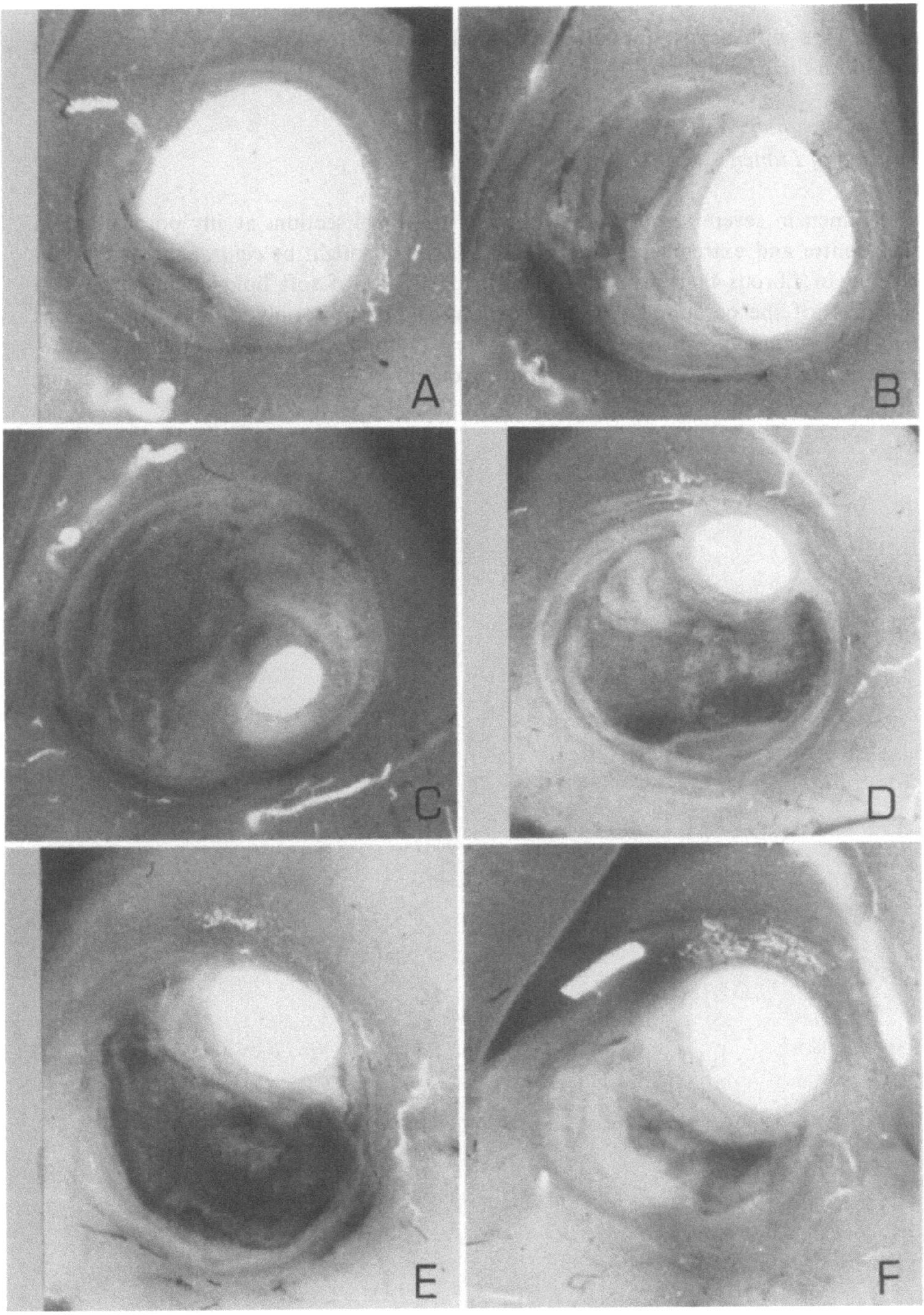

Fig. 2b

Fig. 2. a Portion of arteriogram of right coronary artery showing old established stenosis. Sections in **b** are taken at levels shown. **b** Serial 2-mm thick transverse sections, proximal surfaces at levels in **a**. Relatively pale atherosclerosis changes to deeply pigmented material at site of severe stenosis. The pigmentation was a deep orange-brown derived from degeneration of haemoglobin. Lumen eccentric. Formalin fixation, no staining

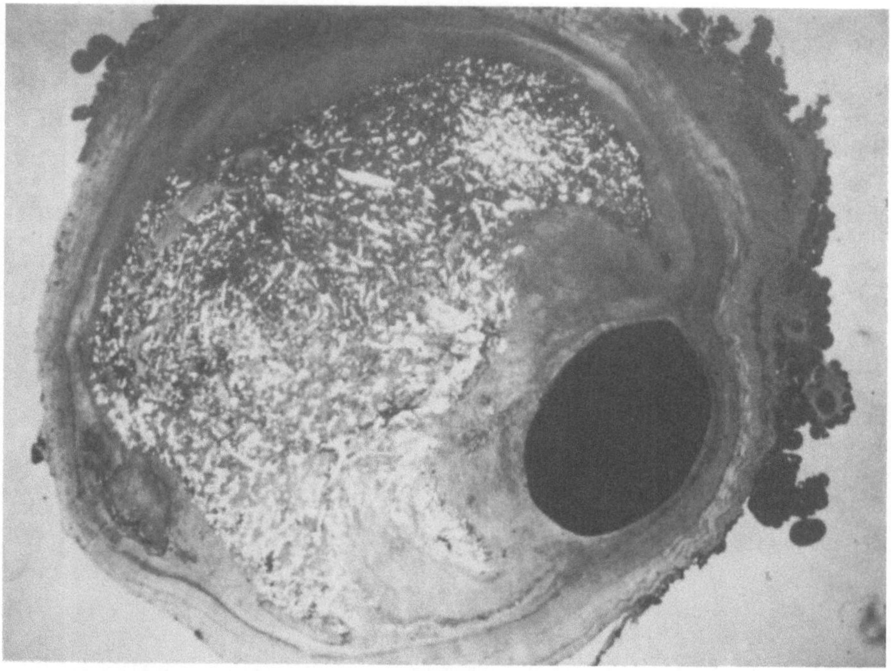

Fig. 3. Frozen section of section *C* in Fig. 2b. Polarized light shows heavy deposition of cholesterol in structureless, soft material. The lumen is supported by a thin, nearly normal wall on its outer aspect and by a thick fibrous wall against the atheroma.

material might be divided into compartments by fibrous layers (Fig. 4), and at its periphery might have portions as hard as bone from calcification.

In other lesions the lumen was placed at the extreme *periphery*, bordered for nearly half its circumference by virtually normal arterial wall (Fig. 3). At this site the wall contained a normal-looking muscle coat of normal thickness. Its morphological character suggested a potential for contraction on the one hand and stretching to the limit of the outer layers by internally applied pressure on the other, and for retraction after dilatation. At the opposite side of the lumen in such lesions lay a large atheroma. The media overlying it was often thinned, stretched and probably weakened. Again the atheroma might be a single soft structure composed mainly of debris containing cholesterol and neutral fat (Fig. 3), or it might have a more complex structure with fibrous bands breaking it into a compound of crescentic layers (Figs. 5, 6). The lining of the lumen in contact with the atheroma varied greatly in thickness.

It is, however, important to realise that the majority of lesions did not quite conform to these descriptions. *Intermediate positions* of the lumen were represented, from off-centre to nearly peripheral, the lumen being separated from the medial coat by a layer of some thickness. While such lesions of this category may well have medial coats capable of compressing the lumen, the thickness and fibrous nature of the material completely surrounding the lumen on all sides might well resist stretching, and dilatation by intraluminal forces be effected only by its rupture.

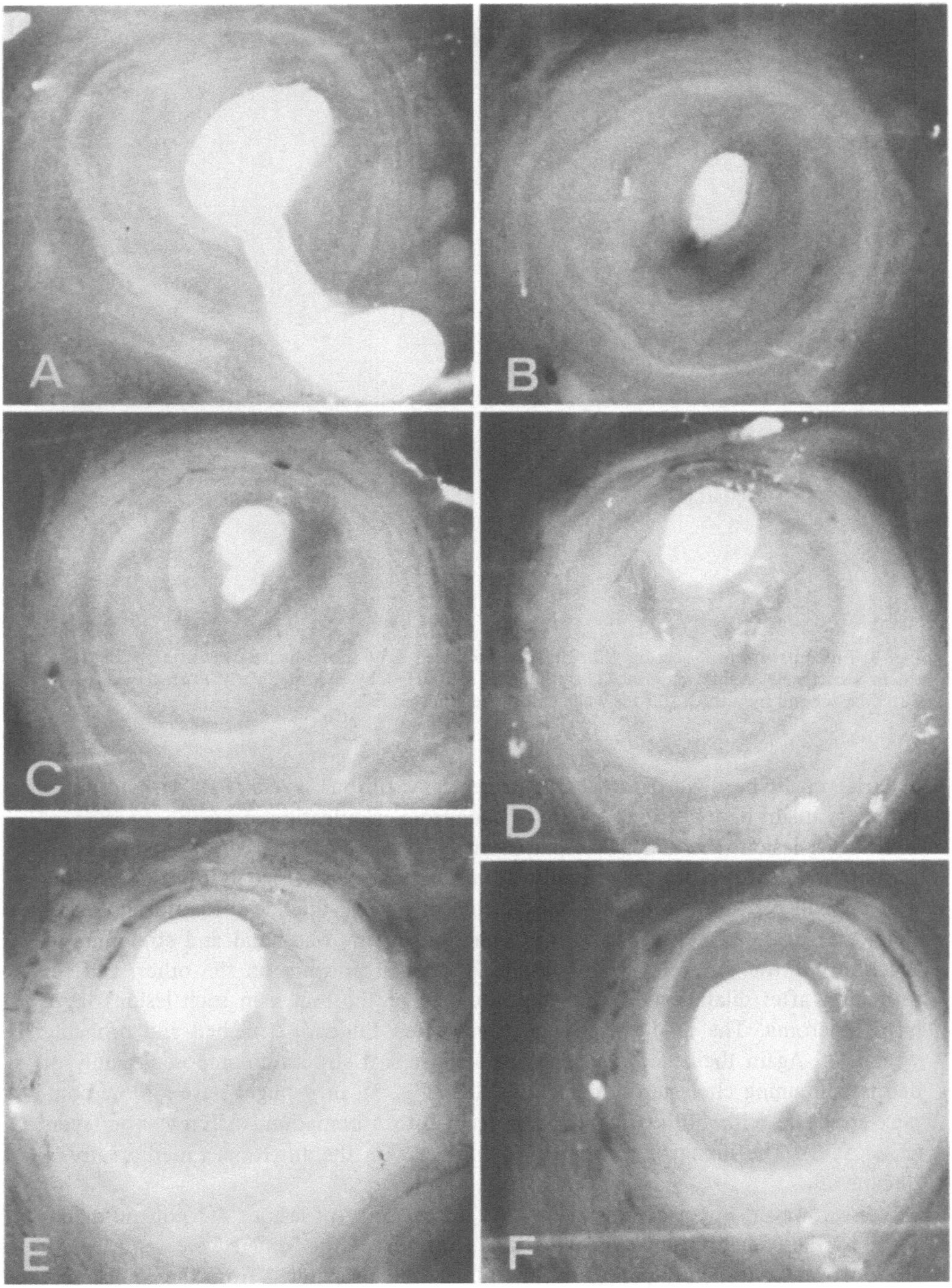

Fig. 4. Serial sections through a stenotic lesion which had a similar arteriogram to Fig. 2a. It can be seen that the lumen is central in proximal part (*A*, *B*) and becomes eccentric (*C, D, E*) and again central (*F*).

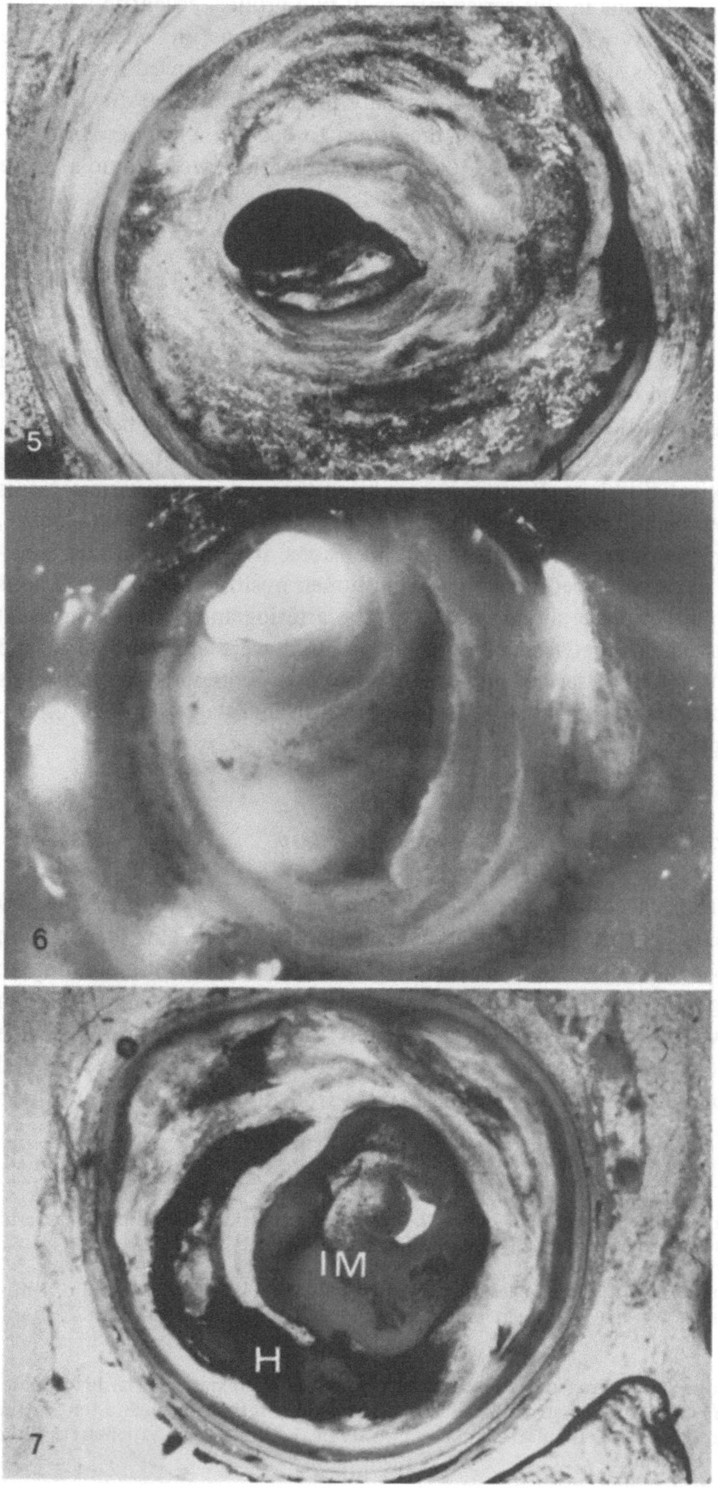

Figs. 5–7

Classification of the lesions in this series into only two groups, eccentric and concentric, would be arbitrary. Moreover, when the entire lesions are examined the position is not so simple as single sections might suggest. When followed from end to end, a stenosed lumen may firstly be found centrally placed and further down the lesion emerge, as it were, to the periphery of the artery to become a fully eccentric lesion. Alternatively the converse may take place; all combinations were found in more extensive lesions (Fig. 4).

Prediction from the Arteriogram

It might be supposed that the angiographic character of a stenosis would allow a valid opinion on the peripheral or central position of the lumen. Indeed, perhaps particularly with very short lesions, the arteriograms and transverse sections could be in accord. But more often the arteriographic appearances were unreliable, particularly in the longer and more complicated lesions. Bearing in mind that the post-mortem arteriograms were of a far higher technical quality than obtainable so far in clinical angiography, and that in addition they were viewed in three dimensions, it would seem that considerable reservation must be placed on opinions on lumen position in stenotic lesions based on arteriographic evidence alone. Moreover, the arteriograms ("lumenograms") did not reliably distinguish between stenotic lesions that were apparently old and "stable" and lesions of more recent origin, still manifestly composed of thrombus and presumably more friable, or composed of later transitional stages between thrombus and atherosclerosis.

The State of the Vessel Wall Apart From the Stenotic Lesion

A catheter passed along a coronary artery will commonly traverse a lumen lined by atherosclerotic disease. For the most part, where the lumen was greater than 50% in diameter or thereby the atherosclerotic material appeared stable with a lining to the lumen that might be expected to sustain gentle manipulation without break in its continuity. However, not infrequently the underlying lesions, even in quite wide channels, were friable, with the subendothelial layer extremely thin or defective and the atheroma composed of autolytic material derived from thrombus or haemorrhage

Fig. 5. Frozen section from 2-mm section *B* in Fig. 4. Multiple concentric rings of fibrous material with lipid deposition near periphery (partially polarized light). Unstained

Fig. 6. A typical complex atherosclerotic lesion composed of several layers of material of different consistency. These layers may represent previous episodes of thrombus deposition. Unstained, incident light

Fig. 7. Haemorrhagic dissection. Frozen section, partially polarized illumination. The black material is haemorrhage (*H*) exploring the structure of the atheromatous intima through a rent in the luminal lining. Dark grey material is injection medium (*IM*) in the lumen partly penetrating the haemorrhagic material. Unstained of apparently fairly recent date. Indeed, under the comparatively mild stresses of gently reintroduced diastolic pressure (80 mmHg) into the collapsed coronary artery post mortem, breaks in the lining of such lesions and their exploration by injection medium occurred at some point in the epicardial arteries in the majority of hearts [in addition to those in which the injection medium followed a track commenced by haemorrhage in life (Fig. 7)].

Comment

The bearing that these morphological characters may have on the outcome of intraluminal distension is speculative. I have not had the opportunity of studying cases following this procedure. Nevertheless a study of structure may permit more than a wild guess at the possibilities. It would not be necessary to have witnessed the event to predict the likely outcome for an egg, a tube of toothpaste or a tomato sandwich if trodden on heavily, provided that the structures had been carefully studied. Accordingly, it may be deduced from the composition of stenotic lesions that under mechanical dilatation certain structures may stretch, others may resist stretching or may rupture and softer material will be displaced. It would seem inevitable that in some instances the soft lipid-laden debris will be squeezed through a ruptured intimal lining into the arterial lumen, to travel downstream and to impact. It is also inevitable that blood platelets and fibrinogen will be brought into contact with freshly broken surfaces of collagen and with other thrombogenic material. Such rifts in the endothelial lining promote thrombus and arterial occlusion when they occur spontaneously. It would seem likely, therefore, that the same will sometimes occur when the injury is induced mechanically and that haemorrhage will enter the intima and explore its weakened structure. Haemorrhagic dissection of the intima may be extensive and may compress and so obstruct the lumen.

The extent to which adverse structural effects can be limited by selection of cases and complications limited by peri- and post-procedure management, is not the subject of this communication. The purpose is to draw attention to the basis in the disease underlying severe stenosis which makes such precautions desirable.

Acknowledgements. The current research programme is supported by a grant from the Scottish Home and Health Department. Acknowledgement is made of the cooperation of the clinical and nursing staff of the Coronary Care Unit and the departments of Pathology and Radiodiagnosis, Stobhill General Hospital, Glasgow.

References

1. Duguid JB (1946) Thrombosis as a factor in the pathogenesis of coronary atherosclerosis. J Pathol Bacteriol 58:207
2. Fulton WFM (1965) The coronary arteries: arteriography, microanatomy and pathogenesis of obliterative coronary artery disease. Chas Thomas, Springfield
3. Fulton WFM (1978) Coronary thrombotic occlusion in myocardial infarction and thrombus in the pathogenesis of atherosclerosis. In: Carson LA et al. (eds) International conference on atherosclerosis. Raven Press, New York, pp 75–89
4. Morgan AD (1956) The pathogenesis of coronary occlusion. Blackwell, Oxford

Morphology and Pathogenesis of the Aortocoronary Bypass Stenosis

M. Stolte*, A. Heidbrink, M. Schmuziger

Pathological Institute of the University of Erlangen-Nuremberg and the Rehabilitation Center Bad Krozingen

The aims of coronary surgery – the abolition of angina pectoris, the improvement of effort tolerance, and the extension of life expectancy – are attained by coronary revascularization [8, 9, 10, 14, 16], but in some cases primary or secondary stenoses or occlusions of the aortocoronary bypass vein (ACBV) can lead to postoperative recurrent angina pectoris or myocardial infarction [1, 3, 6, 12, 13, 15, 18, 19]. Reoperation and the creation of a new aortocoronary bypass can improve the symptomatology and prevent the infarction. In order to be able to eliminate bypass strictures without the need for surgery, using percutaneous transluminal angioplasty, the pathogenesis of these stenoses and their differing morphology must be known.

Material and Methods

We have subjected 152 ACBVs to histological examination. Of these veins, 125 were obtained as autopsy specimens from 82 patients and 27 were removed from 20 patients 1 1/2 and 6 years after primary surgery. Of the ACBVs obtained at autopsy, 98 were from early-death patients and 27 from patients who had survived between 17 days and 8 years from operation.

Results and Discussion

Autopsy Material

In our early-death cases the main causes of the 39 thrombotic occlusions and 38 stenoses of the 98 bypass veins were atherosclerosis in the region of the coronary anastomosis, stenosed or small outflow tract (Fig. 1), and technical surgical problems [18]. Six of the seven bypass occlusions seen in the 27 late-death cases were due to technical reasons; in one instance, the cause of a fresh bypass thrombosis was a progression of the stenosing coronary artery sclerosis distal to the bypass anastomosis. The main

* Pathologisches Institut, Krankenhausstr. 8–10, 8520 Erlangen, FRG

Transluminal Coronary Angioplasty and
Intracoronary Thrombolysis. Ed. by Kaltenbach et al.

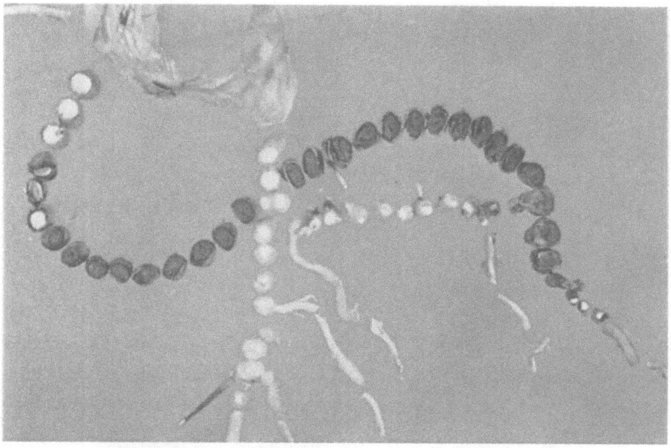

Fig. 1. Thrombosis of the aortocoronary bypass vein due to a small outflow tract

cause of the seven stenoses of these 27 bypass veins was a narrowing of the coronary anastomosis due to atherosclerosis in this location. On three occasions an old parietal thrombosis was found, and in one case the two veins were under tension; in three cases surgical technical shortcomings were the cause of the stenosis.

Reoperation Material

Based on pathological findings, the 27 bypass veins removed between 1 1/2 and 6 years after primary surgery were divided into long-segment and short-degment stenoses. In the group of long-segment stenoses, we differentiated those with and those without adaptive fibrosis of the intima:

Long-segment stenoses (n = 18)
1. Without adaptive intima fibrosis (n = 9)
2. With adaptive intima fibrosis (n = 9)

Short-segment stenoses (n = 9)
1. Organized parietal thrombosis (n = 1)
2. Atheroma in the bypass vein (n = 8)

In the nine cases without adaptive intima fibrosis, the vein is usually occluded by an organized thrombosis, and the fibrosed wall of the vessel has collapsed and is waved and ellipsoid in form (Fig. 2). The absence of adaptive fibrosis of the intima and the presence of the old organized thrombosis show that the occlusion of the bypass occurred in the early postoperative phase. Causes of these occlusions are technical problems, excessive peripheral resistance, and little blood flow.

The nine cases with high-grade concentric fibrosis of the intima show that the peripheral resistance is high, so that a very high transmural pressure has acted upon the walls of the bypass vein, with the result that this excessive intima fibrosis occured reactively (Fig. 3).

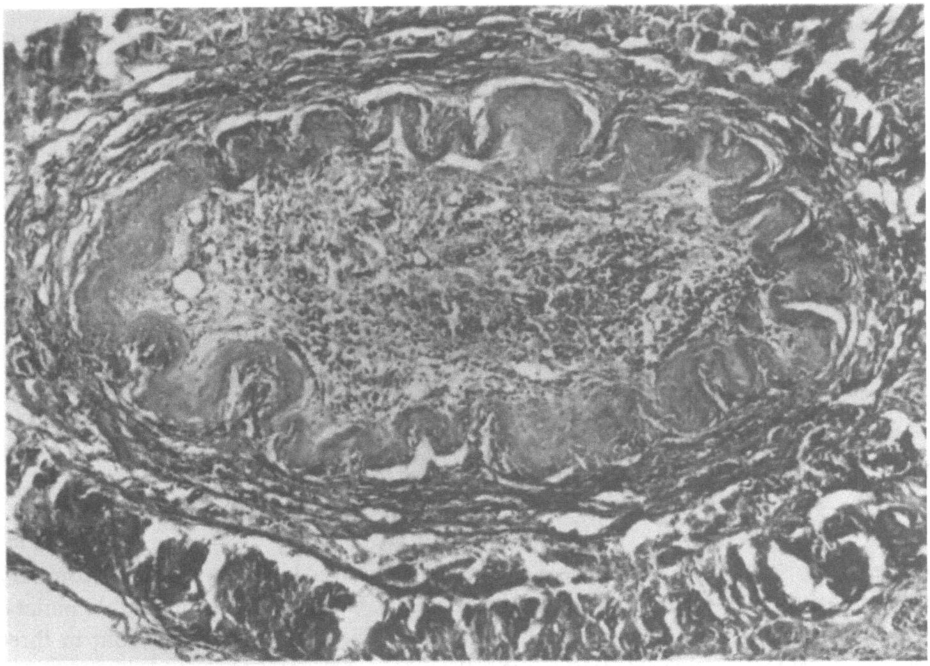

Fig. 2. Organized thrombosis of the bypass vein without adaptive intima fibrosis and "waved" wall. Masson-Goldner × 41

Our nine short-segment stenoses were diagnosed 1 1/2–6 years after the primary operation. In eight of these nine cases we found a stenosing atheroma of the bypass vein. In five of them the covering layer of the atheroma had broken away – probably at re-operation – and had given rise to a fresh occlusive thrombosis (Fig. 4). In only single case was a parietal thrombosis the cause of a short-segment stenosis. Seven of eight patients with atheromatosis of the bypass vein presented – as in other cases documented in the literature [1, 2, 3, 6, 12, 15, 20] – with hyperlipidemia. The other patient was a heavy smoker.

In Fig. 5, the pathogenesis of the bypass vein stenoses has been schematically summarized. The vein undergoes a regular transformation: the arterial pressure provokes a concentric fibrosis of the intima and the devascularization of the venous wall caused by surgical preparation leads to an ischemic fibrosis of the media [4, 5, 17, 18, 20]. Stenoses or occlusions of the bypass veins can be caused by numerous factors. In the first instance (Fig. 5), an early thrombotic occlusion can be caused by low-level blood flow or atherosclerosis in the region of the coronary anastomosis. The causes of an excessive stenosing fibrosis of the intima are: turbulence due to the formation of angles, a big difference in caliber between the bypass vein and the coronary artery [11, 20], adhesions, neighbouring inflammation [7], preexisting phlebosclerosis, and traumatic damage to the venous wall during surgical preparation.

Long-segment, concentric stenosing fibrosis is probably dependent upon the peripheral resistance, and thus on the pressure acting upon the walls of the vein. Elliptical

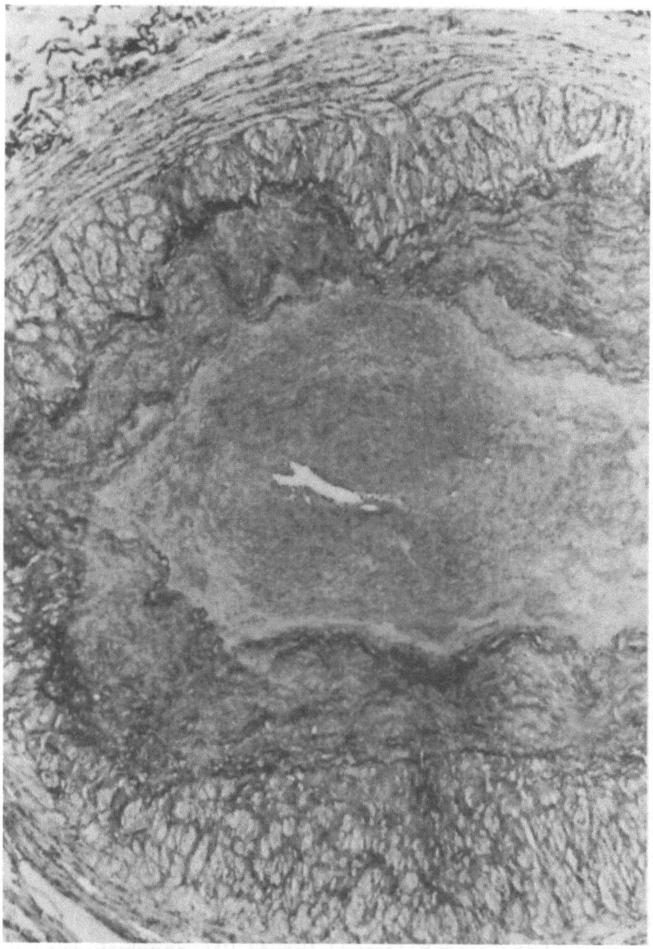

Fig. 3. Excessive fibrosis of the intima. Elastica-van Gieson × 50

deformation of the transplanted vessel with and without occlusion is an indication of primary or secondary tension, local adhesions, or early organized thrombotic occlusions.

The most frequent short-segment strictures that occur in the late postoperative phase appear to be due to atheroma. The histological structure of the atheroma suggests, from the morphological point of view, that it would be readily dilatable with the balloon catheter.

Summary

We have subjected 152 ACBVs to histological examination: 125 were autopsy specimens, 27 were removed at surgery. The stenoses or occlusions of 98 ACBVs obtained

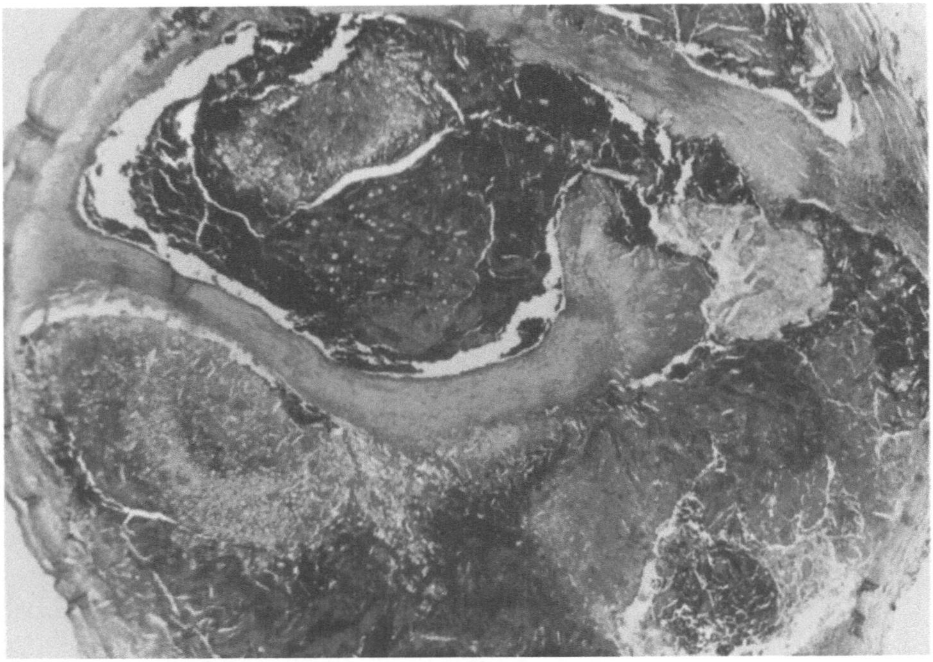

Fig. 4. Stenosing atheroma of the aortocoronary bypass vein with exulceration of the covering layer and fresh occlusive thrombosis. Masson-Goldner × 14

at autopsy from early-death patients, and 27 obtained at autopsy from late-death patients, were often due to technical surgical causes, atherosclerosis in the coronary part of the anastomosis, or outflow tract stenosis. Of 27 surgically removed bypass veins, the stenosis or occlusion affected a long segment in 18 cases and a short segment in nine cases. On the basis of the morphology of the ACBV, conclusions may be drawn as to the time of development of the stenosis and its pathogenesis:

Long-segment occlusions or stenoses without adaptive fibrosis of the intima represent thrombosis that developed shortly after surgery (due to technical problems), atherosclerosis in the region of the coronary anastomosis, or excessive peripheral resistance.

Long-segment stenoses with high-grade concentric fibrosis of the intima are the sequelae of a very high peripheral resistance and little blood flow.

Short-segment stenoses in otherwise regular ACBVs are usually atheromas.

In only a single case was an organized parietal thrombosis the cause of a short-segment stenosis; in the other eight cases, atheroma was found. These eight atheromas developed 1 1/2–6 years after the primary operation. The histological structure of these short-segment atheromas reveals that such a stenosis can be dilated with the aid of a balloon catheter.

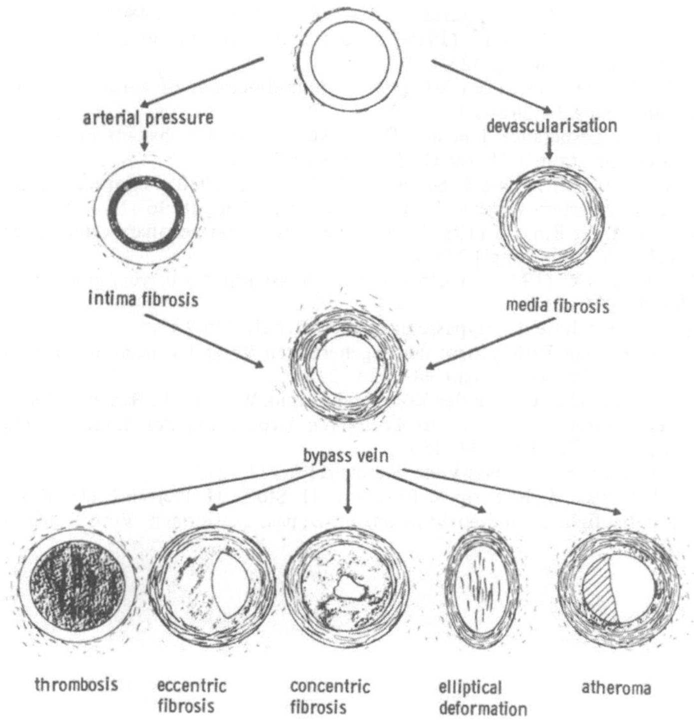

occlusion of anastomosis < flow	pre-existing phlebosclerosis surgical trauma of the vein turbulences	tension adhesions torsion	hyper-cholesterolaemia hyper-triglyceridaemia

Fig. 5. Scheme of the regular and pathological transformation of the aortocoronary bypass vein

References

1. Barboriak JJ, Pintar K, Korns M (1974) Atherosclerosis in aortocoronary vein grafts. Lancet 14:621–624
2. Barboriak JJ, Batayias GE, Pintar K, Tieu TM, Van Horn DL, Korns ME (1977) Late lesions in aortocoronary artery vein grafts. J Thorac Cardiovasc Surg 73:596–601
3. Barboriak JJ, Pintar K, Van Horn DL, Batayias GE, Korns ME (1978) Pathological findings in the aortocoronary vein grafts. Atherosclerosis 29:69–80
4. Borst, Enderlein (1909) Über Transplantation von Gefäßen und anderen Organen. Dtsch Z Chir 99:54–163
5. Brody WR, Kosek JC, Angell WW (1972) Changes in vein grafts following aortocoronary bypass induced by pressure and ischemia. J Thorac Cardiovasc Surg 64:847–853
6. Bulkley BH (1979) Pathology of coronary bypass graft surgery. Am Heart J 98:539–540
7. Bulkley BH, Hutchins GM (1978) Acute postoperative graft phlebitis. A rare cause of saphenous vein-coronary artery bypass failure. Am Heart J 95:757–760
8. Cooley DA, Wukasch DC, Bruno F et al. (1978) Direct myocardial revascularisation: Experience with 9, 364 operations. Thorax 33:411

9. Dittrich H (1977) Ergebnisse der Koronarchirurgie. Dtsch Ärztebl 10:643–648
10. Flemma RJ, Mullen DC, Lepley D, Assa J (1979) A comparative synchronous coronary surgery survival study. Ann Thorac Surg 28:423
11. Furuse A, Klopp EH, Brawley RK, Gott VL (1972) Hemodynamics of aorta-to-coronary artery bypass. Ann Thorac Surg 14:282–293
12. Grondin CM, Campeau L, Lesperance J et al. (1979) Atherosclerotic changes in coronary vein grafts six years after operation. J Thorac Cardiovasc Surg 77:24–31
13. Hacker RW, Torka M, Golling FR, Reiss J, Schmidt HJ, Stolte M (1980) Perioperative myocardial infarction in coronary artery surgery. J Thorac Cardiovasc Surg 28:96–101
14. Hacker RW, Torka M, Van der Emde J (1981) Life expectancy after coronary artery bypass surgery. J Thorac Cardiovasc Surg [Suppl] 29:37
15. Lie JT, Lawrie GM, Morris GC (1977) Aortocoronary bypass saphenous vein graft atherosclerosis. Am J Cardiol 40:906–914
16. Lichtlen P (1978) Langzeitresultate der Bypasschirurgie. Med Welt 29:423
17. Leu HJ, Brunner U (1973) Zur Pathogenese der degenerativen Veränderungen an autologen Venentransplantaten. Dtsch Med Wochenschr 98:2433–2436
18. Stolte M (1975a) Morphologische Analyse der Koronarchirurgie. Witzstrock, Baden-Baden
19. Stolte M (1975b) Verschlußursachen des aortokoronaren Bypass und der durch ihn überbrückten Stenose. Verh Dtsch Ges Pathol 59:469
20. Stolte M (1977) Die aortokoronare Bypass-Vene. Klinikarzt 6:211–218
21. Stürzenhofecker P, Schmuziger M, Rentrop P, Roskamm H, Stolte M, Pietsch K (1978) Faktoren, die die Verschlußhäufigkeit eines aortokoronaren Bypass bestimmen. Verh Dtsch Ges Kreislaufforsch 44:214

A New Guiding Catheter for Intubating Aortocoronary Bypass Grafts by the Femoral Approach

M.I.H. El Gamal, H. Bonnier, R. Michels

Catharina Hospital, Eindhoven, The Netherlands

The right Judkins-type guiding catheter is routinely used for percutaneous transluminal angioplasty of bypass grafts. In the period between October 1980 and April 1981 we attempted to dilate 14 stenosed aortocoronary bypass grafts, ten to the left anterior descending (LAD) and four to the right coronary artery (RCA). Repeated dislodgement of the tip of the Judkins-type guiding catheter while advancing the balloon dilatation catheter prevented entry into the grafts in five cases (one RCA, four LAD grafts).

In four of the five cases (one RCA, three LAD grafts), a second attempt was made with a special guiding catheter (Fig. 1). This has a smoothly curved tip 4 cm long making an angle of 80° with the shaft. The smooth curve and the superior orientation of

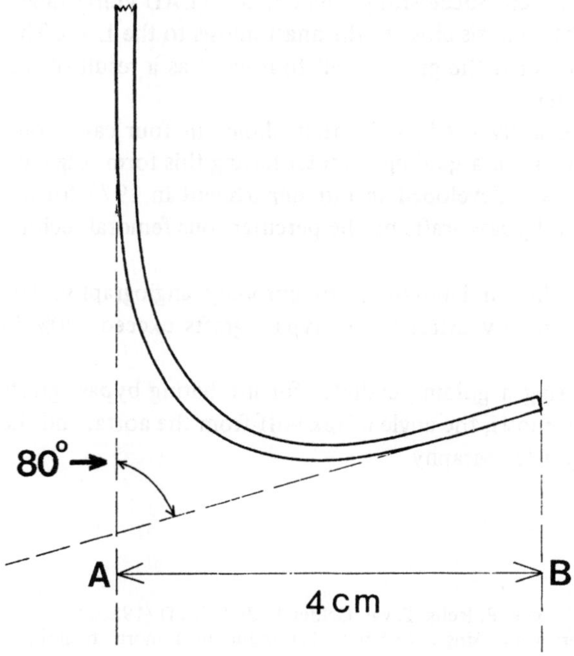

Fig. 1. Special guiding catheter. Adapted from El Gamal et al. (1980)

Transluminal Coronary Angioplasty and
Intracoronary Thrombolysis. Ed. by Kaltenbach et al.

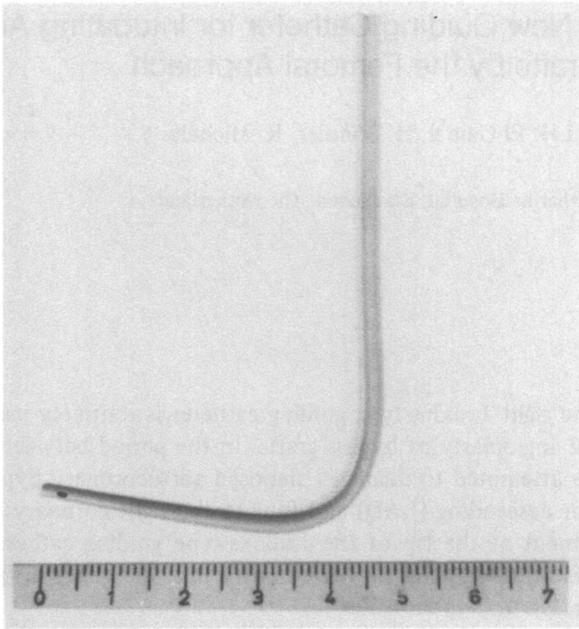

Fig. 2. Coronary catheter form which the special guiding catheter was developed

the tip offered extra stability during advancement of the dilatation catheter. Three cases (one RCA, two LAD grafts) were successfully dilated, one (LAD graft) failed because of inability to cross a tight stenosis close to the anastomosis to the LAD. The balloon dilatation catheter easily entered the grafts in all four cases as a result of the stable position of the guiding catheter.

The guiding catheter was successfully used as the first choice in four cases (one RCA, three LAD grafts). The idea to use a guiding catheter having this form originated from a coronary catheter that was developed in our department in 1977 for intubating both coronary arteries and bypass grafts by the percutaneous femoral technique [2] (Fig. 2).

This catheter is routinely used in our laboratory for coronary angiography. The success rate in intubating both coronary arteries and bypass grafts exceeds 90% in more than 2000 investigations.

Our policy at present in choosing a guiding catheter for intubating bypass grafts is determined by the site of anastomosis, the angle of take-off from the aorta, and the ease of intubation during coronary arteriography.

References

1. El Gamal M, Slegers L, Bonnier H, Borsje P, Relik T, van Gelder L, de Vries D (1980) Selective coronary arteriography with a performed single catheter: Percutaneous femoral technique. AJR 135:630–632
2. Judkins MP (1967) Selective coronary arteriography. Radiology 89:815–824

Histological Changes Following Transluminal Angioplasty of Experimentally Induced Atherosclerosis in Miniature Pigs

A.D. Schmidt-Moritz, M. Schneider, B. Kunkel, M. Kaltenbach

Department of Cardiology and Pathology, University of Frankfurt am Main, FRG

Introduction

Transluminal angioplasty (TAP) has evolved into a well-established method within the last few years, although little is known about the morphological changes induced by this technique. To clarify the mechanism we performed TAP in an animal model. We used miniature pigs because of their similar metabolism to humans, the occurrence of spontaneous atherosclerotic lesions, and characteristic intimal plaques after cholesterol diet.

Material and Methods

Ten miniature pigs weighing 12–16 kg were used as experimental animals. Balloon deendothelialization of segments of 1 cm in length of femoral and carotid arteries was performed with a 2F or 5F Fogarty catheter. The animals were fed a high-fat (15%), high-cholesterol (2%) diet over a period of 8 or 13 weeks. Transluminal angioplasty with a Grüntzig catheter was carried out in the diseased vessels at the end of the 7th or 12th week. The animals were killed 10–14 days after TAP. The arterial specimens were fixed with formalin, excised, and prepared for histological examination. Hematoxylin-eosin (HE), elastica-Domagk (E-D), and Sudan stains were performed.

Results

All animals displayed atherosclerotic lesions, mild in untreated arteries and severe in injured arteries. Proliferative changes occurred after 8 weeks. These showed characteristic subendothelial myofibroblast cushions (Fig. 1). The internal elastica was locally damaged (Fig. 2). Loss and disarray of the medial elastic fibers occurred. In some cases giant cells in the vicinity of elastic fiber fragments were observed (Fig. 3).

After 13 weeks predominantly atheromatous plaques were visible. These lesions showed lipid-containing foam cells, cholesterol crystals, and calcification (Fig. 4). Atheromatous plaques caused severe stenosis, in some cases subtotal occlusion (Fig. 5).

Ten to fourteen days after TAP the following histological characteristics were found:

Transluminal Coronary Angioplasty and
Intracoronary Thrombolysis. Ed. by Kaltenbach et al.

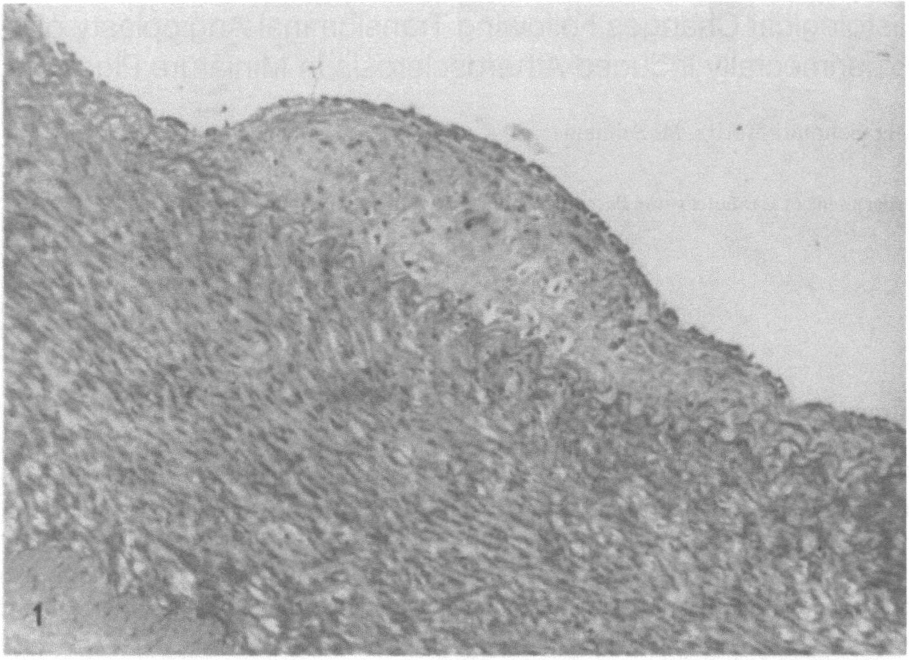

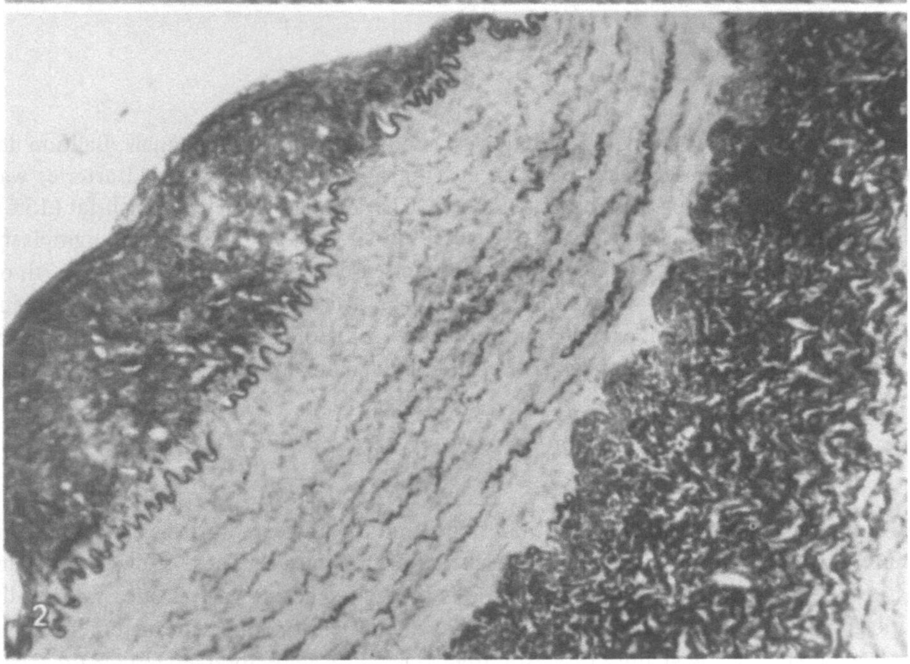

Fig. 1. After 8 weeks proliferative lesions show subendothelial myofibroblast cushions. HE × 150

Fig. 2. Disruption of medial elastic fibers in a proliferative lesion. E-D × 150

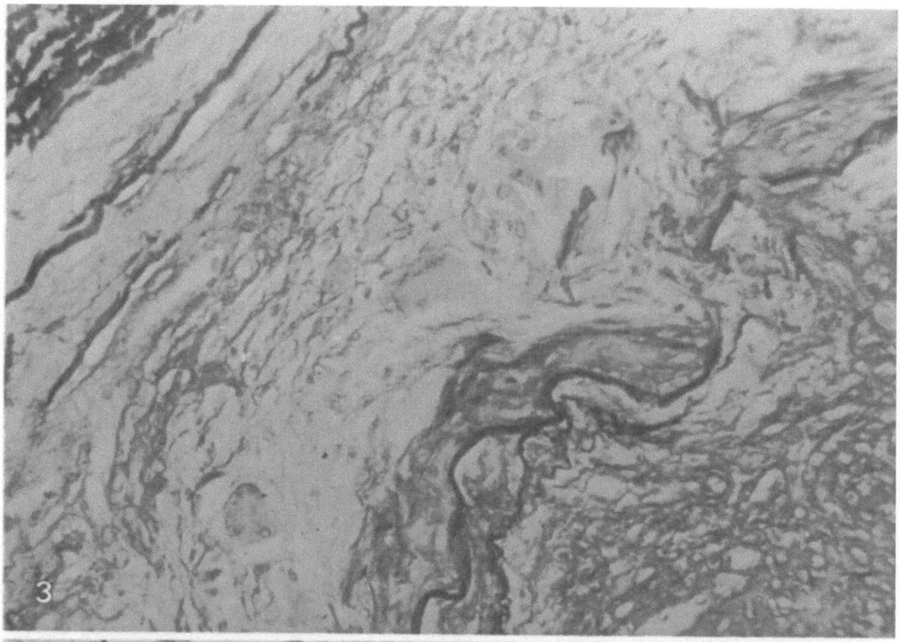

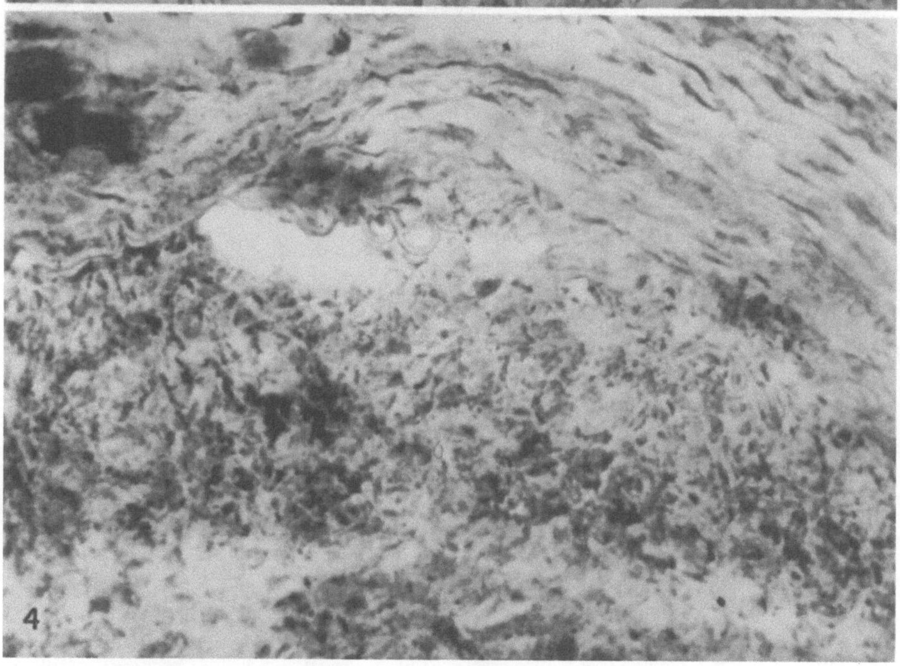

Fig. 3. Giant cells in the vicinity of elastic fiber fragments. E-D × 250

Fig. 4. Calcification (*upper right*) and diffuse lipid drops within foam cells as characteristic signs of an atheromatous lesion after 13 weeks of cholesterol diet. Sudan stain × 250

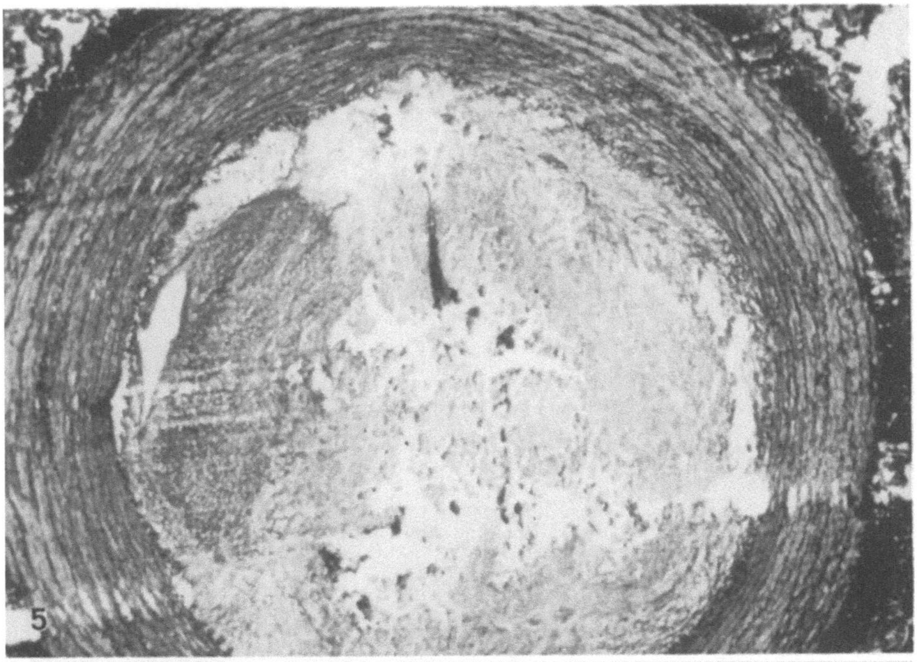

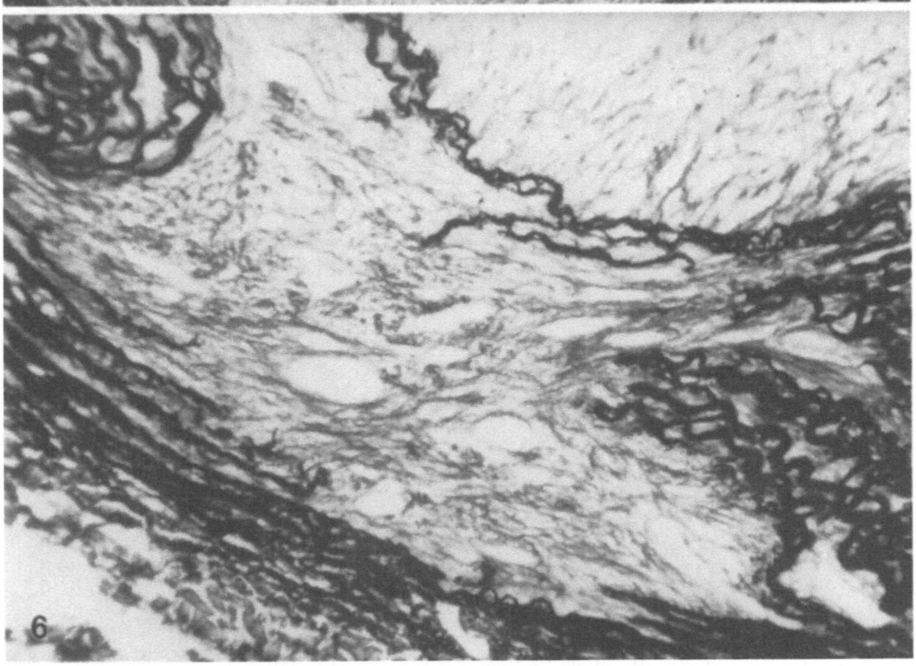

Fig. 5. Subtotal stenosis caused by an atheromatous plaque. E-D × 40

Fig. 6. Dislocation of intimal atheromatous material into medial layers after transluminal angioplasty. Medical elastic fibers are heavily damaged. E-D × 250

Proliferative lesions showed mild changes of the medial elastic fibers, which were decreased in number, displayed a corkscrew configuration, and were in disarray. Atheromatous lesions showed more serious changes. Intimal tears occurred which extended partly into medial layers. Intimal atheromatous material was displaced into the media. Elastic fibers were heavily damaged (Fig. 6).

Figure 7 semischematically summarizes the histological changes of the arterial wall in experimental atherosclerosis after TAP. Identical changes were found after TAP of a femoral artery in an autopsy specimen (Fig. 8).

Conclusions

These results show the feasibility of producing atherosclerotic lesions in miniature pigs within 8 weeks using balloon de-endothelialization combined with a high-fat, high-cholesterol diet.

The following structural changes were observed 10 to 14 days after TAP:

1. Overstretching of the medial elastic fibers
2. Intimal and medial tears
3. Dislocation of intimal atheromatous material between disrupted medial elastic fibers

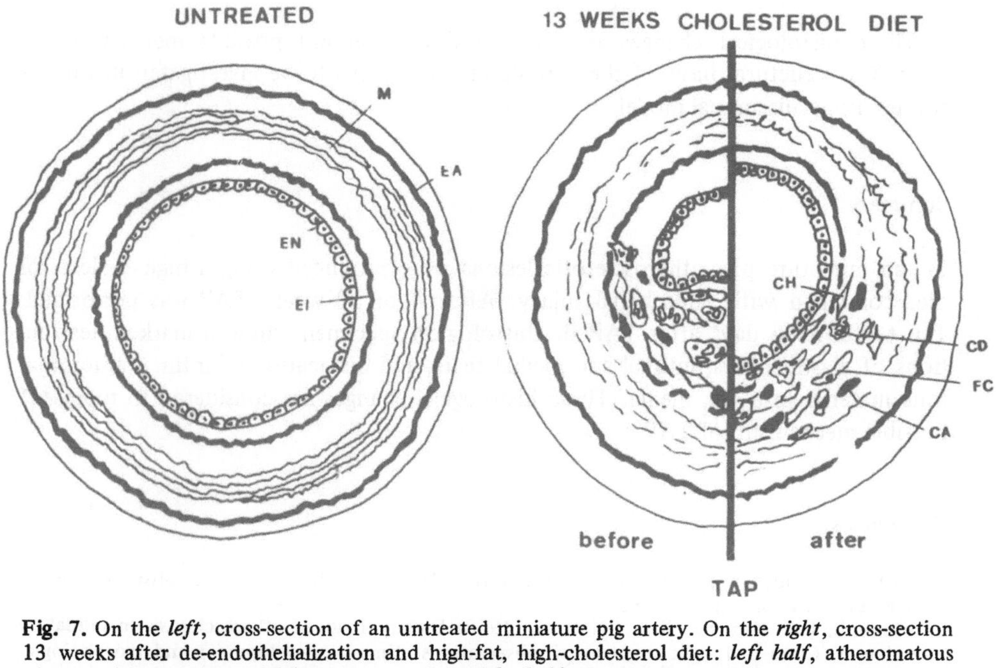

Fig. 7. On the *left*, cross-section of an untreated miniature pig artery. On the *right*, cross-section 13 weeks after de-endothelialization and high-fat, high-cholesterol diet: *left half*, atheromatous plaque with severe arterial lumen narrowing; *right half*, characteristic histological changes after TAP. CA, calcification; CD, cell detritus; FC, foam cell; EI, elastica interna; EA, elastica adventitia; EN, endothelium; M, media

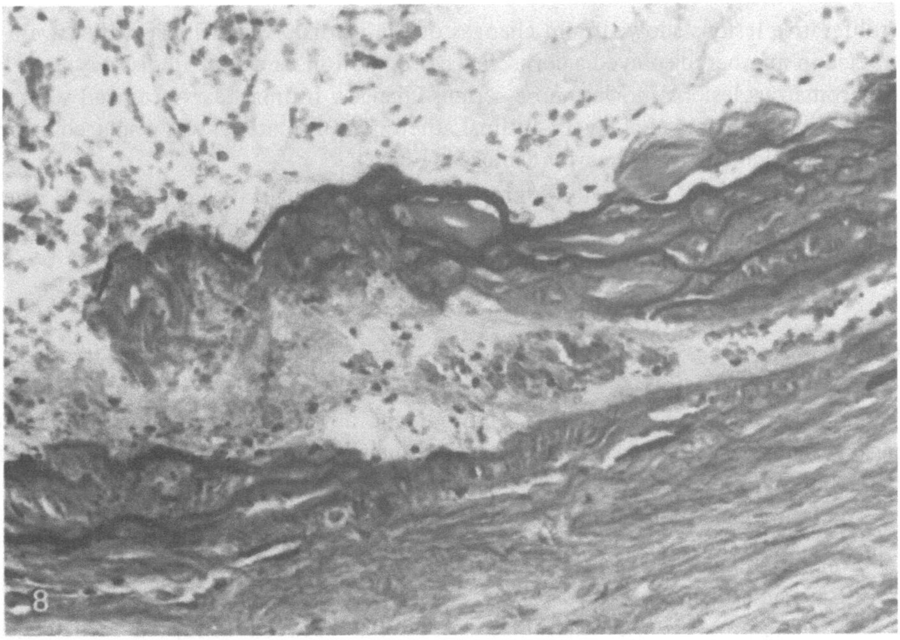

Fig. 8. Disruption of medial elastic fibers and dislocation of intimal atheromatous material into the media in an autopsy specimen of femoral artery. E-D × 250

These histological changes are considered to represent possible mechanisms of TAP. The structural basis of the chronic effect remains to be investigated in further studies using this animal model.

Summary

In ten miniature pigs atherosclerotic lesions were produced using a high-cholesterol diet combined with endothelial injury. After 8 or 12 weeks TAP was performed. Ten to fourteen days after TAP the histological specimens showed marked destructions of elastic fibers, intimal and medial tears, and dislocation of intimal atheromatous material into the media. These histological changes are considered to represent possible mechanisms of TAP.

References

1. Castaneda-Zuniga WR, Formanek A, Tadavarthy M et al. (1980) The mechanism of balloon angioplasty. Radiology 135:565
2. Florentin RA, Nam SC, Kim DN et al. (1968) Dietary induced atherosclerosis in miniature swine. I. Cross and light microscopy observations: time of development and morphologic-characteristics of lesions. Exp Mol Pathol 8:263
3. Lee KT, Lee WM (1977) Advanced coronary atherosclerosis in swine produced by combination of balloon-catheter injury and cholesterol feeding. Adv Exp Med Biol 82:597

4. Lee G, Ikeda RM, Joye JA, Bogren HG, De Maria AN, Mason DT (1980) Evaluation of transluminal angioplasty of chronic coronary artery stenosis. Value and limitations assessed in fresh cadaver hearts. Circulation 61:77
5. Moore S (1979) Endothelial injury and atherosclerosis. Exp Mol Pathol 31:182
6. Wissler RW, Vesselinowitch D (1978) Evaluation of animal models for the study of the pathogenesis of atherosclerosis. In: Hauss WH et al. (eds) International symposium: State of prevention and therapy in human atherosclerosis and in animal models, Westdeutscher, Opladen, pp 113

Correlation of the Effects of Transluminal Angioplasty in Experimentally Induced Rabbit Atherosclerosis with Pathological Changes in Human Coronary Artery

P.C. Block

Massachusetts General Hospital, Boston, Massachusetts, USA

Atherosclerosis-like lesions can be induced in rabbits by feeding them a 2% cholesterol diet. Debridement of the endothelium of the aorta and iliac arteries using a Fogarty balloon catheter accelerates the formation of atherosclerosis-like lesions in the areas of endothelial injury. Six to eight weeks after balloon debridement, atherosclerotic lesions are produced which have a high concentration of foam cells, may be calcified, and frequently cause stenosis of the arterial lumen, both of the aorta and (more prominently) of the iliac arteries. Transluminal angioplasty of such stenotic lesions in rabbits produces desquamation of endothelium and shearing of superficial portions of endothelial plaques in areas of aortic atherosclerosis (where the size of the inflated dilating balloon and the size of the aorta are almost equal). In rabbit arteries where the size of the inflated angioplasty balloon catheter and the stenotic arterial segment are more unequal (such as the iliac artery), splitting of the intimal surface of the atherosclerotic lesion almost always occurs. The splits frequently extend to the internal elastic membrane. Angiography performed after transluminal angioplasty in rabbits frequently shows an irregular column of contrast in the region of angioplasty. Such an angiographic picture is occasionally also seen in humans after angioplasty. The irregularity of the column of contrast almost certainly represents contrast material within the splits of the atherosclerotic plaque produced by the angioplasty procedure. Sequential studies done after angioplasty in rabbits show that re-endothelialization of the intimal and medial splits occurs within 3 days after angioplasty. Subsequent fibrosis and healing appear to cause retraction of the splits and further enlargement of the lumen over the first 2 weeks after angioplasty.

All animal models of atherosclerosis suffer from dissimilarities from human atherosclerosis. Consequently conclusions concerning the mechanism of transluminal angioplasty drawn from animal models, or for that matter from autopsied human material or normal arteries, have all been subject to criticism. However, human autopsy material of coronary arteries that had undergone angioplasty are now available and show changes identical to those seen in animal models.

Two patients who had died 6 h and approximately 90 h after transluminal angioplasty respectively had pathological study of their coronary arteries performed. Both patients had emergency coronary artery bypass graft procedures performed – the first for an acute dissection caused by angiographic dye after a successful angioplasty, the second because of ongoing pain 36 hours after a successful angioplasty. Pathological study of the areas of transluminal coronary angioplasty showed splitting of the athero-

Transluminal Coronary Angioplasty and
Intracoronary Thrombolysis. Ed. by Kaltenbach et al.

matous plaque in both patients. The splits extended through the atherosclerotic plaque to the internal elastic membrane. The changes seen after angioplasty in human coronary arteries were identical to those seen in experimentally induced atherosclerotic lesions in rabbits that had undergone angioplasty of the aorta and iliac arteries.

The close correlation between the changes seen in experimentally induced atherosclerosis after experimental angioplasty and in human coronary arteries after transluminal coronary angioplasty indicates that the mechanism of successful angioplasty in most cases is splitting of the atheromatous plaque which causes enlargement of the vascular lumen. Some shearing of endothelium probably also occurs.

Acute and Chronic Effects of Transluminal Angioplasty in Three Models of Experimental Atherosclerosis

T.J. Ryan, D.P. Faxon, V.J. Weber, C. Haudenschild, S.B. Gottsman, W.A. McGovern

Evans Memorial Department of Clinical Research and Department of Medicine, Section of Cardiology, University Hospital, and The Mallory Institute of Pathology, Boston University School of Medicine, USA

The development and clinical utilization of transluminal angioplasty has provided the clinician with an additional therapeutic tool in the treatment of obstructing atherosclerotic vascular disease. Data accumulating on immediate and short-term results of angioplasty have shown it to fulfil much of its early promise, but the mechanisms of action, the long-term consequences, and the possibility of lasting amelioration of obstructing atherosclerosis with this technique are questions that remain to be elucidated and experimental data are scant. The purpose of this experimental animal study was to determine the factors responsible for reduction of luminal narrowing following transluminal angioplasty and to evaluate the long-term consequences of this technique by both angiography and histopathologic examination.

Methods

Three morphologically distinct types of atherosclerotic lesion were produced in 42 3.0 kg New Zealand rabbits by combining two techniques of vascular injury with variations of cholesterol feeding. The Baumgartner technique of balloon de-endothelialization in combination with a high-cholesterol diet was used to produce predominantly concentric, soft foam lesions in 20 rabbits who formed group I. An indwelling catheter technique devised by Moore was used to produce more eccentric, fibrocellular hard lesions in combination with high-cholesterol feeding in 12 rabbits (group IIA) or with a normal-cholesterol diet in ten rabbits (group IIB). The resultant lesions formed in the left iliac artery were categorized as foam, mixed, or fibrous lesions and their distribution among the entire animal population is presented in Table 1.

Table 1. Histopathology of experimental models

Model	Lesions		
	Foam	Mixed	Fibrous
Group I (n = 20)	16	4	0
Group IIA (n = 12)	1	9	2
Group IIB (n = 10)	0	2	8

Transluminal Coronary Angioplasty and
Intracoronary Thrombolysis. Ed. by Kaltenbach et al.

After a period of 8–10 weeks in which atherosclerosis was allowed to develop, all the animals underwent angiography followed by transluminal angioplasty. Half of the animals were then killed and histologic examination carried out within 24 h. The other half were maintained on their initial diet for periods of 2 and 4 weeks at which time they underwent repeat angiography and were killed and histologically examined.

Results

The majority of animals showed angiographic lesions of at least 30% narrowing of the lumen diameter. The Baumgartner technique (group I animals) was the most effective regimen for the production of severe stenoses with eight of 19 animals showing a greater than 50% stenosis.

Acute Phase Findings

Angiography. By angiographic assessment, transluminal angioplasty was effective in reducing stenosis (defined as ⩾ 20% change) in 75% of the animals, irrespective of experimental groups. Thus, successful dilatation occurred through a spectrum of lesions. The greatest effect of angioplasty was in the most stenotic lesions. Percent stenosis was estimated in each animal by using a proximal, nondilated, but diseased segment in the left iliac artery as the control.

Acute Histopathologic Changes

In the 17 animals killed within 24 h of angioplasty, microscopic examination revealed two basic histopathologic changes depending on the morphology of the underlying lesion.

Group I. The immediate consequence of balloon dilatation of the soft foam lesions in this group was the development of significant neo-intimal fractures. This finding occurred in animals having the most successful reduction in lesion following angioplasty, while the animals with minimal or no angiographic change showed no consistent histopathologic findings (Table 2). Characteristically, the concentric, soft foam cell lesion showed a dramatic rupture through several layers of neo-intima with associated acute inflammatory changes also noted. The entire thickness of the neo-intima was ruptured with splitting and fragmentation of the internal elastic lamina. On occasion, this fracture was associated with dissection, distortion, and thinning of the original media.

Group II. The immediate consequences of angioplasty in these animals with eccentric, hard fibrocellular lesions were thinning and necrosis of the normal vessel wall without evidence of neo-intimal fracture (Table 3). The noninvolved portion of the vessel wall consistently showed thinning, loss of nuclei in the media, and the appearance of being stretched. The absence of smooth muscle cell nuclei was associated with the presence of necrotic material distributed throughout the media.

Table 2. Immediate results of angioplasty in group I

Animal	Dilatation (%)	Fracture	Dissection	Thinning
1	65	++++	–	–
2	53	++	++	+
3	50	++++	–	–
4	10	+	–	–
5	0	–	–	–
6	0	–	–	–

Table 3. Immediate results of angioplasty in groups IIA and IIB

Animal	Dilatation (%)	Fracture	Dissection	Thinning
1	100	–	++	+
2	58	–	–	++
3	45	–	–	+
4	43	–	–	+
5	40	–	–	+++
6	35	–	–	+
7	22	–	–	+
8	19	–	–	++
9	19	–	–	+
10	0	–	–	–
11	0	–	–	–

Long-term Findings

Angiography. Seven of the group I animals underwent repeat angiography and were killed 2 weeks following their angioplasty. Five animals did not exhibit any change in the degree of stenosis of the dilated segment, one animal demonstrated an increase in stenosis and one a decrease. Six group I animals were followed 4 weeks before having repeat angiography and being killed and four of these animals exhibited an increase in the stenosis of the dilated segment.

Six group II animals were followed 4 weeks before having repeat angiography and being killed. Four animals demonstrated no change, one a decrease, and one and increase in the stenosis of the dilated segment.

Of the six animals from both groups who showed an increase in the stenosis of the dilated segment, it was noted that the animals with the most effective angioplasty frequently demonstrated the most progression of stenosis.

Chronic Histopathologic Changes

The three animals exhibiting a decrease in the stenosis at chronic follow-up did not demonstrate specific histopathologic characteristics. However, pathologic examination of dilated segments that showed angiographic progression revealed a variety of morphological patterns that included: (1) multilamination, (2) thrombosis with various stages of recanalization, and (3) deposition of connective tissue within the original neo-intimal tear. In some cases, there was a striking picture of fibrocellular tissue reminiscent of the original neo-intimal tear with spaces filled in by loose connective tissue rich in lipid that created a further occlusive process with new fibrocellular cap. New vascular spaces penetrating from the original media could also be seen.

Discussion

Although there are various limitations to any one experimental model of atherosclerosis, this study demonstrated that the New Zealand rabbit can be utilized to produce a spectrum of morphological lesions that lend themselves to the study of balloon dilatation. When both concentric, soft foam lesions and eccentrically located, fibrous hard lesions of greater than 30% stenosis are subjected to angioplasty, successful dilatation occurs in three-quarters of the animals. Histologic examination carried out immediately following angioplasty shows intimal fracture and rupture of the neo-intimal tissue of soft lesions extending down to and including the internal elastic lamina. When eccentric, fibrocellular lesions are subjected to balloon dilatation, there appears to be no disruption of the lesion itself, but rather stretching and thinning of the adjacent normal vessel wall takes place. This appears to cause necrosis of smooth muscle cells of the media.

When one looks at the longer-range consequences of angioplasty in this rabbit model, there appears to be angiographic progression of disease in the initially dilated segment in approximately one-third of the animals. Animals showing the greatest improvement immediately following angioplasty seem to demonstrate the more accelerated progression of disease. Histologic examination of these dilated segments that have shown angiographic progression reveals the deposition of layers of loose or thick fibrocellular tissue alternating with lipid-laden cells in a multilaminated fashion. Remnants of the original neo-intimal tear of the foam cell lesion are visible with spaces filled in by loose connective tissue rich in lipid. These findings suggest that it is a continuation of the initial repair process that leads to further occlusion.

It is also to be noted that in 15% of the animals studied long term, there was further regression of the original stenosis following angioplasty. Although no specific histologic picture emerged in these few animals, it is clear that further study is needed to fully understand the mechanisms responsible for the success or failure of transluminal angioplasty. It seems likely that factors that influence the repair process of vascular tissue will be a fruitful area for such research.

Summary

We therefore conclude that: 1) both endothelial denudation and indwelling catheter with and without high-cholesterol diet provide suitable rabbit models for the study of transluminal angioplasty; 2) effective angioplasty is possible in each model; 3) dramatic intimal rupture, medial damage, and inflammation may result in some lesions while marked destruction of the normal vessel wall may occur in others; 4) proliferating neo-intimal processes occurring even after successful angioplasty may lead to potentiation of luminal narrowing; and 5) the frequent presence of occlusive thrombi 2 or 4 weeks after angioplasty suggests that alteration of coagulation may be important in maintaining luminal patency after this procedure.

Effect of 5 kg/cm^2 Pressure on Atherosclerotic Vessel Wall Segments

M. Kaltenbach, J. Beyer, H. Klepzig, L. Schmidts, K. Hübner

Department of Cardiology and Pathology, University Hospital, Theodor-Stern-Kai 7, 6000 Frankfurt a.M., FRG

Dotter and Judkins as well as Grüntzig ascribed the reopening of atherosclerotic obstructions achieved by transluminal angioplasty partially to a compression of atheromatous material [4, 6]. As a simplified model for the effect of angioplasty the compression of snow was taken. Several experiments performed in animals [1, 2, 9] and human postmortem coronary arteries [1, 3, 5, 7, 8] predominantly revealed changes described as desquamation of endothelial cells, splitting of vessel wall layers, and breaks of elastic fibrils. Compression of fluid-containing tissue appears not possible, since fluid is incompressible. This experimental study was performed to reveal the influence of 5 atm pressure on the morphology and the weight of postmortem atherosclerotic vessel wall segments.

Methods

Fresh human postmortem aortoiliac arteries were removed and segments with and without atherosclerotic changes excised. A total of 88 segments were investigated. Changes in morphological structures (n = 40) as well as in fluid content (n = 48) were analyzed.

Balloon compression of the tissue with a pressure of 5 atm was simulated by application of 5 kg weight on a segment area of 1 cm^2 (Fig. 1). This pressure was applied twice for a period of 5 s, i.e., for a total of 10 s. Significance of differences was calculated by means of Student's t test.

Results

Histologic changes showed a significant dependence on the degree of fibrosis of the atherosclerotic plaque (Table 1). In plaques with mild fibrosis (group 1) reduction in thickness was noted in ten of 18 cases (Fig. 2). Horizontal fissures and ruptures in the vessel wall were rarely seen (three of 18 cases). A rupture in a plaque was never observed.

In contrast, plaques with a high degree of fibrosis (group 2) never showed a reduction in thickness (Fig. 3), whereas predominantly horizontal fissures (in 11 of 22 cases) and ruptures in the vessel wall (in six of 22 cases) were seen (Fig. 4). In three of

Transluminal Coronary Angioplasty and Intracoronary Thrombolysis. Ed. by Kaltenbach et al.

Table 1. Microscopic changes following 5 kg/cm² pressure

Changes	Mild fibrosis (n = 18)	High-degree fibrosis (n = 22)
Reduction in thickness	10	0
Horizontal fissures	3	11
Rupture in vessel wall	3	6
Rupture in plaque	0	3
No change	1	4

22 cases ruptures within the plaque appeared. No changes were observed in one case in group 1 and four cases in group 2.

The fluid content (Table 2), evaluated by comparing the weight before and after pressure application, showed in group 1 a reduction of 17%, significantly greater than in group 2 (10.9%) and in segments which were considered normal (group 3) and served as control.

Conclusion

It is concluded that one acute effect of angioplasty may be a reduction in volume of atherosclerotic obstructions achieved by fluid expression from atherosclerotic tissue. Marked volume reduction and fluid expression can experimentally be achieved by the

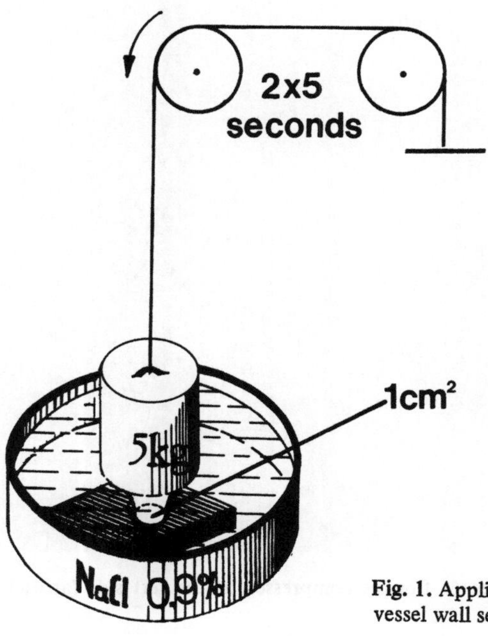

Fig. 1. Application of 5 kg/cm² pressure on atherosclerotic vessel wall segments

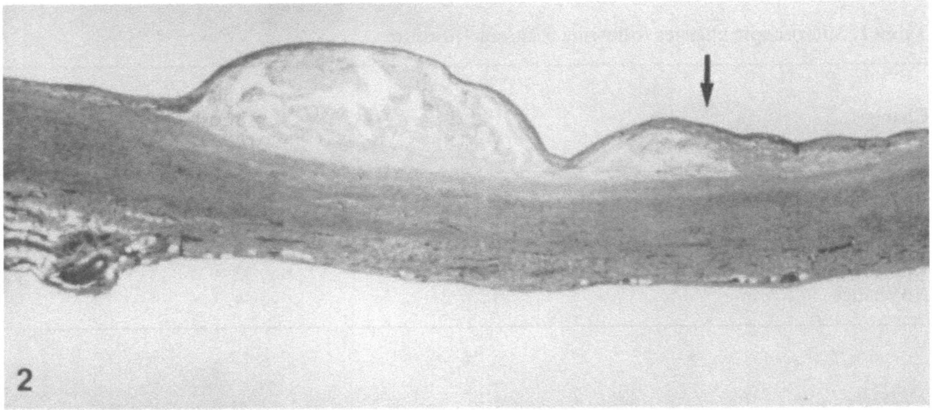

Fig. 2. Atherosclerotic plaque with mild fibrosis compressed at the right side. Reduction in thickness at the right (arrow)

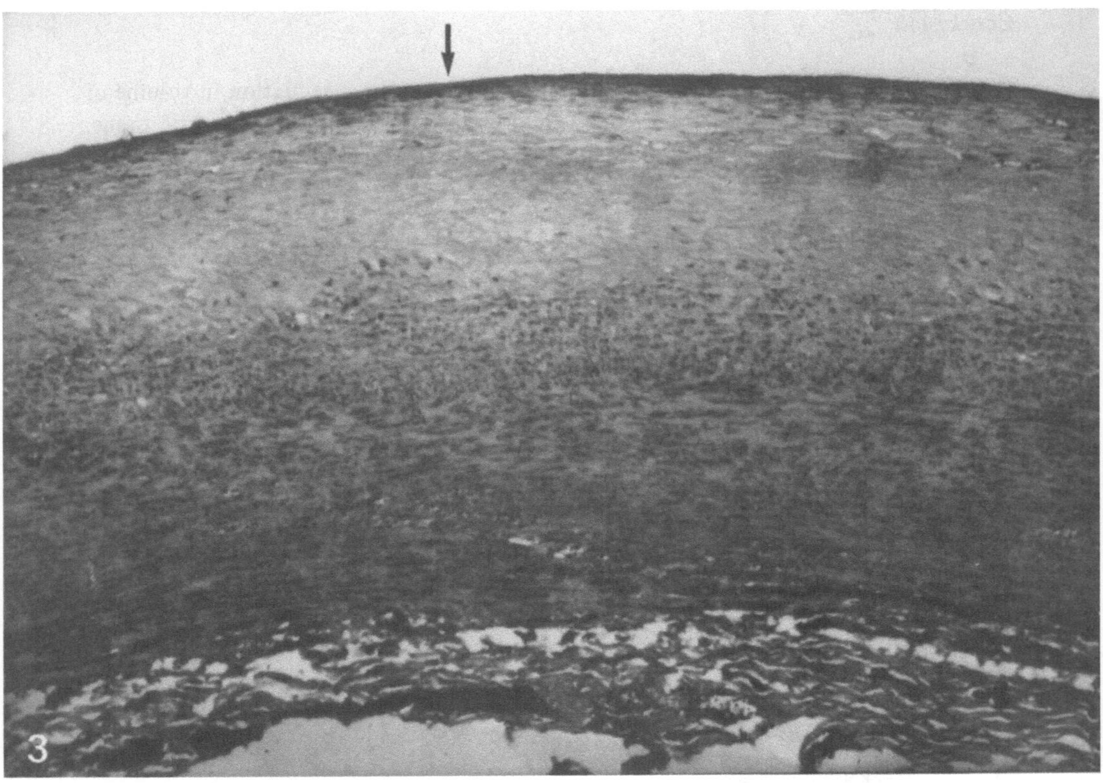

Fig. 3. Atherosclerotic plaque with high degree of fibrosis compressed at the left side (arrow). No reduction in thickness

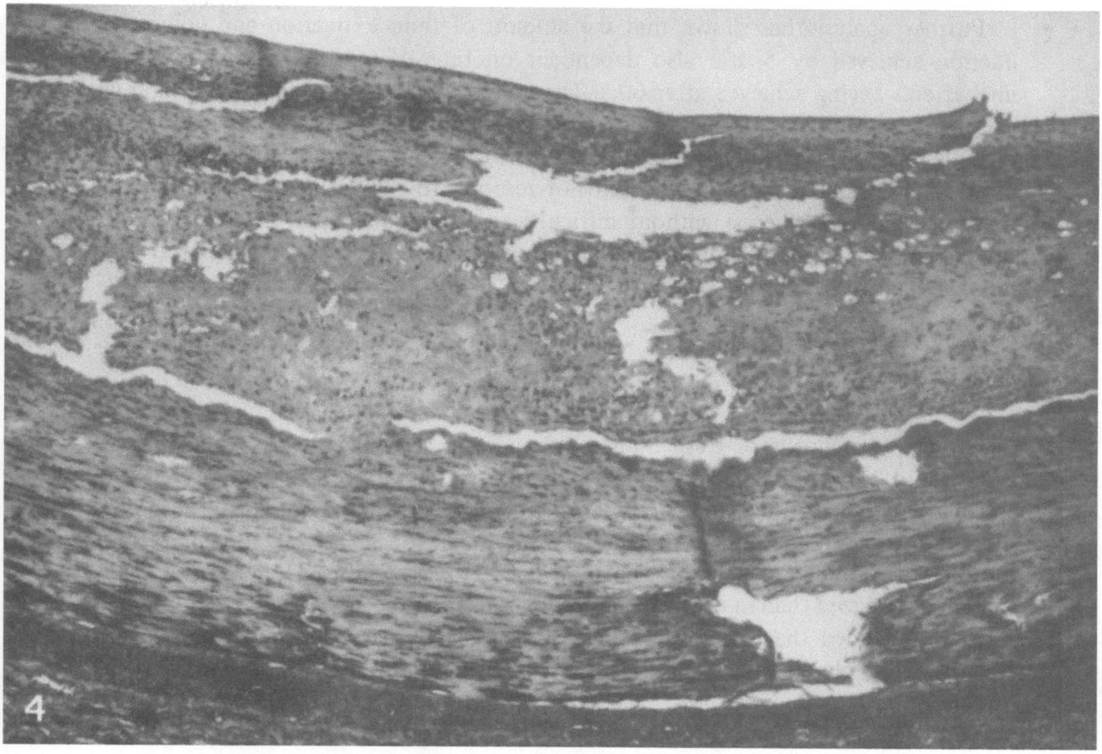

Fig. 4. Atherosclerotic plaque with high degree of fibrosis. Horizontal fissures and ruptures in the vessel wall

application of 5 kg/cm^2 over a period of only 10 s. It was more easily achieved in nonorganized than in organized atherosclerotic plaques.

Also in these experiments the well-known alterations such as endothelial desquamation, horizontal splitting, and vertical ruptures within different layers of the arterial wall as well as within the atheromatous tissue were observed. The experiments, however, demonstrate that particularly in nonorganized atheromatous tissue, i.e., in plaques with only a mild degree of connective tissue, a considerable volume reduction can be achieved by fluid expression alone, without other mechanisms involved.

Table 2. Changes in weight following 5 kg/cm^2 pressure

Fibrosis	No. of segments	Reduction in weight (mean ± SD)	P
Mild (group 1)	20	17,0% ± 3,15%	< 0.05
High-degree (group 2)	19	10,9% ± 1,93%	< 0.05
Normal vessel (group 3)	9	12,4% ± 1,19%	< 0.05

Decrease in weight in group 1 was significantly greater than in groups 2 and 3 ($P < 0.05$)

Further analysis has shown that the amount of fluid extraction and volume reduction achieved by 5 atm also dependent on time of pressure application, maximal effects beeing achieved after 60 s. The concept was transferred to clinical application of transluminal coronary angioplasty and dilatation was performed as long as possible. We have carefully extended the time of pressure inflation of the balloon to more than 1 min in patients who did not respond to shorter periods and tolerated longer periods of ischemia without difficulties. It was found that the result of dilatation can be markedly improved, i.e. the number of stenoses considered as "not dilatable" decreased from 17% to 6%.

Summary

Eighty-eight specimens of fresh human postmortem aortoiliac artery segments were investigated concerning morphological structure and fluid content before and after application of 5 kg weight on 1 cm^2 area. Fifty percent of the nonorganized lesions showed marked reduction in thickness, while in organized lesions no reduction in thickness was observed. Reduction in fluid content was significantly more pronounced in nonorganized than in organized atheromatous tissue.

It is concluded that the acute effect of angioplasty, particularly in nonorganized atherosclerotic plaques, may be at least partially achieved by fluid expression.

References

1. Baugham KL, Pasternak RC, Fallon JT, Block PC (1980) Coronary transluminal angioplasty in autopsied human hearts [Abstr]. Circulation 58 [Suppl]:80
2. Block PC, Baugham KL, Pasternak RC, Fallon JT (1980) Transluminal angioplasty: correlation of morphologic and angiographic findings in an experimental model. Circulation 61:778
3. Castaneda-Zuniga WR, Formanek A, Tadacarthy M et al. (1980) The mechanism of balloon angioplasty. Radiology 135:565
4. Dotter CT, Judkins MP (1964) Transluminal treatment of arteriosclerotic obstruction. Description of a technique and preliminary report of its application. Circulation 30:654
5. Freudenberg H, Wefing H, Lichtlen PR (1978) Risks of transluminal coronary angioplasty. A postmortal study. Circulation 58 [Suppl]:80
6. Grüntzig AR, Schneider JA (1978) Die Perkutane Dilatation chronischer Koronarstenosen – Experiment und Morphologie. Schweiz Med Wochenschr 107:1588
7. Lee G, Ikeda R, Joye JA, Bogren HG, Maria AN, Mason DT (1980a) Evaluation of transluminal angioplasty of chronic coronary artery stenosis. Circulation 61:77
8. Lee G, Ikeda R, Mason DT et al. (1980b) Effective dilatation of human coronary artery obstruction due to atherosclerosis utilizing a balloon tip catheter. Circulation 58 [Suppl]:80
9. Pasternak RC, Baugham KL, Fallon JT, Block PC (1980) Scanning electromicroscopy after coronary transluminal angioplasty of normal canine coronary arteries. Am J Cardiol 45:591

Overview

M. Kaltenbach

Department of Cardiology and Pathology, University Hospital, Theodor-Stern-Kai 7, 6000 Frankfurt a.M., FRG

After more than 4 years experience with coronary angioplasty and over 10 years experience with peripheral angioplasty, there is unequivocal agreement that localized atherosclerotic obstructions can be widened and that in the majority of patients the process of obstruction in the approached lesion can be stopped.

The findings presented by Williams et al. and Kober et al. show that the acute success of the procedure can to some extent be predicted: a short noncalcified stenosis with a concentric appearance and smooth wall contours, in a patient with a short history of anginal pain, can be dilated with a likelihood of success of more than 70%. On the other hand calcified stenoses, stenoses with eccentric appearance and irregular contours, and stenoses in patients with a long-standing history of angina pectoris have been approached with the procedure, and good results have been achieved in a considerable number of patients. The acute success rate, however, is lower in this second group.

Thus the individual probability of success can only be predicted to a certain degree. Even more difficult to predict is the chronic outcome after successful TCA. It is well established that in the weeks following the procedure the dilated lesion can develop a smoother angiographic appearance and a further widened diameter while in other patients slow or rapid reoccurence of stenosis is apparent. Almost all recidivations documented so far in our series have occured within the first 3 months after the procedure.

Despite better acute success, the likelihood of recurrence appears higher in patients with a short history of angina pectoris. From this observation it can be speculated that the long-term result of angioplasty is related to the natural history of the approached atherosclerotic plaque, i.e., to the moment in the natural course of the disease at which angioplasty is performed. The fresh, unorganized plaque may be easily dilated but reveal a strong tendency toward restenosis due to rapid proliferation. The old, already organized lesion in a patient with a long-standing history is more difficult to dilate but may have less tendency toward reocclusion due to the fibrotic character of the atherosclerotic process in its final stage.

In the contribution of Engel et al., from repeated angiograms it is shown that both progression and regression of stenoses after successful TCA can be seen. Among the possible explanations for regression, long-standing coronary spasm has to be considered. Quantification of coronary narrowing as used by Engel et al., and in a different method by Serruys et al., appears of particular importance in this context.

Transluminal Coronary Angioplasty and
Intracoronary Thrombolysis. Ed. by Kaltenbach et al.

From various contributions it can be seen that angioplasty is still a rapidly developing technique, and the tools of tomorrow will certainly be different from those of today. However, the balloon with a low-compliance hull appears a major step forward, and to date no consistently different approach has been designed.

From the NIH registry (Kent, Mock et al.) it is apparent that the complications rate of angioplasty is essentially related to personal experience. The contribution of Margolis shows encouraging results with the use of intra-aortic balloon pumping in complicated cases. There seems, however, still to be discussion about the indication for this procedure. The difficulty lies in deciding in which type of complication balloon pumping is mandatory before surgery. Apparently, in patients developing cardiac shock after TCA this procedure may be the only way of reestablishing a condition in which surgery can be performed with reasonably good results.

The problem of intracoronary thrombosis after "controlled injury" to the endothelium is approached in a case report from Sigwart. In this instance successful intracoronary lysis reestablished flow and apparently prevented infarction. In Chapter 1 this problem has been discussed in connection with the use of antithrombotic medications throughout the angioplastic procedure (Kaltenbach et al.).

Through our understanding of possible mechanisms involved in the process of angioplasty, it is apparent that experimental work is mandatory in order to gain better information about the possible influence of different events. Fulton gives a fascinating demonstration of the possible mechanisms involved as seen from postmortal specimens. Stolte reports on the pathoanatomy of aortocoronary bypass lesions which in the first part of this book are discussed in regard to the results of TCA. Schmidt-Moritz, Block, and Ryan share their observations in experimental atherosclerosis in pigs and rabbits. In the process of acute widening of a critical coronary stenosis, different mechanisms such as stretching of the media, intimal dissection, and desquamation of atherosclerotic material may be involved. The question of whether atherosclerotic lesions can be dimished in volume simply by compression via fluid expression is approached in an experimental study on atherosclerotic tissue specimens, which shows that fluid expression can be a mechanism for volume diminution of atherosclerotic obstructions. It appears to be more easily achieved in nonorganized than in organized plaques.

New Applications of Transluminal Angioplasty

Coronary Angiography in Combination with Opacification of Other Arteries and Simultaneous Transbrachial Dilatation of Peripheral and Abdominal Arteries

K. Bachmann, G. Raab, W. Niederer

Medizinische Poliklinik, University Erlangen-Nürnberg, Östliche Stadtmauerstr. 29, 8520 Erlangen, FRG

The high incidence of peripheral artery occlusive disease in coronary heart disease, and vice versa, is well documented in both autopsy and clinical studies [1, 5, 8, 9, 10, 11, 12, 13, 16, 17, 20, 21, 22, 23, 27, 28, 30, 31, 34, 37, 38, 39, 41, 42, 43]. The risk in operative treatment in one region of vascular complication in another, such as stroke or myocardial infarction, has been emphasized by surgeons. In order to reduce mortality and morbidity in cardiovascular surgery from cerebral, coronary, and peripheral ischemic events, they recommended the extension of preoperative angiographic evaluation [2, 6, 7, 28, 29, 33, 35, 40]. The diagnostic and prognostic aspects of a "Topographic multimorbidity" may not be overlooked. Severe peripheral artery disease is common not only in symptomatic but also in asymptomatic coronary patients. Therefore both the coronary patient and the patient with peripheral occlusive arterial disease should be suspected of having generalized atherosclerosis.

To identify the "candidate at risk" we started in 1971 to combine selective coronary angiography and left ventricular angiography with opacification of the abdominal aorta, iliac artery, femoral artery, and extracerebral arteries [3, 4, 32, 36]. In patients with arterial hypertension the total angiography includes selective angiography of the renal arteries. One year later, in 1972, the same policy was introduced as "total body angiography" in the department of Favaloro in Buenos Aires [15, 18, 24]. Total cineangiography seems to be a rational diagnostic approach which may be recommended when the following requirements are fulfilled:

1. The extension of selective coronary angiography to total angiography must be without additional risk to the patient with regard to the invasive procedure, contrast material, and X-ray exposure.
2. Total angiography must be more sensitive than noninvasive procedures in detecting peripheral arterial occlusive disease.
3. Total cineangiography may lead to therapeutic consequences not afforted by noninvasive procedures. The high rate of "false negative" diagnoses is significant, and masked arterial occlusive disease and the inability of clinical methods to detect early stages of cerebral, abdominal, and peripheral atherosclerosis are additional strong arguments for total cineangiography in coronary patients.

Transluminal Coronary Angioplasty and Intracoronary Thrombolysis. Ed. by Kaltenbach et al.

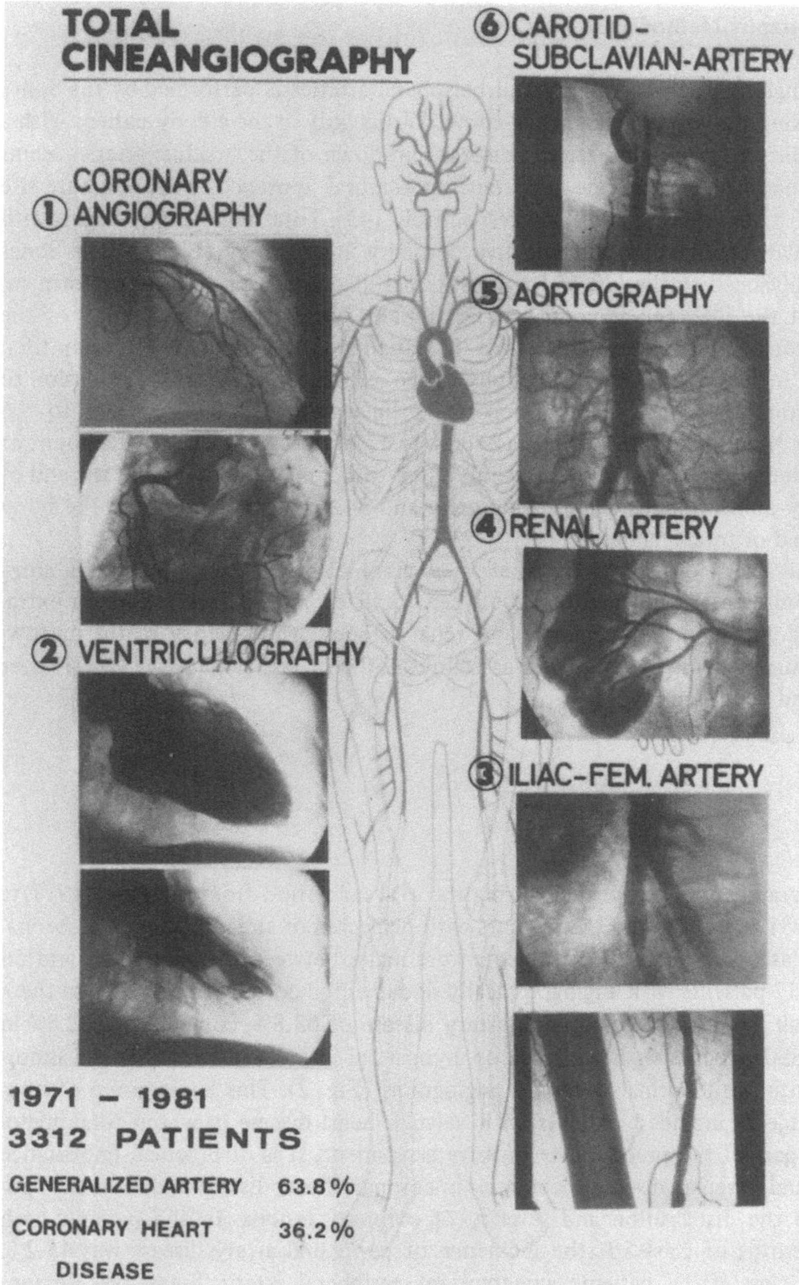

Fig. 1. Total angiography in patients with coronary heart disease begins with coronary angiography including left ventricular angiography (1, 2). Then the catheter is advanced to the iliac artery for filling of the iliac and femoral artery (3). The procedure ends with opacification of the abdominal aorta (5) and the supra-aortic arteries (6). In patients with arterial hypertension total angiography is extended to the renal arteries (4)

Total Angiography Method

Combined angiography of coronary and peripheral arteries is performed by the Sones technique using the right transbrachial route. Particularly in the elderly patient with a high probability of peripheral arterial disease, cut-down of the brachial arteries seems to be less complicated than the percutaneous femoral approach, with puncture site complication rates of 2.2% and 7.9% respectively [45]. Total angiography begins with left ventricular angiography and selective coronary angiography (Fig. 1). The Sones catheter is advanced to the left and right external iliac artery in order to perform angiography of the iliac and femoral arteries. Finally we perform angiography of the abdominal aorta and extracerebral vessels. In patients with arterial hypertension total angiography includes selective angiography of the renal arteries. With this extension to selective coronary angiography the fluoroscopic time is increased from 2.8 to 8.6 min and the X-ray dosage from 610 rads/cm^2 to 1530 rads/cm^2. The total amount of contrast material injected averages 104 ml, equal to 1.3 ml/kg body wt., at the end of the coronary and left ventricular angiography and 242 ml, equaling 3.1 ml /kg body wt., at the end of total angiography.

Peripheral artery disease is classified angiographically in the same way as coronary artery disease. We differentiate between localized and diffuse lesions in extracerebral, abdominal, pelvic, femoral, and renal arteries. The severity of the narrowing of the lumen diameter is graded as follows: 50% or less (I), 51%–75% (II) over 75% (III), and occlusion (IV).

Results

Total angiography was performed during the 10-year period from February 1971 to February 1981 in a total of 3312 patients with suspected or already diagnosed coronary heart disease. The majority of subjects were males between the ages of 41 and 56 years. In 2432 patients with angiographically documented coronary heart disease there was an overall incidence of peripheral artery disease of 63.8%, compared to 12.8% in a group of 880 patients with a history of myocardial infarction, chest pain, or abnormal ECG buth with normal coronary angiograms (Fig. 2). This latter group of noncoronary subjects included patients with valvular heart disease in whom total angiography was part of the preoperative invasive assessment. It is of practical importance that peripheral vascular disease is common in coronary heart disease and correlates positively with the distribution and severity of coronary lesions. In 467 patients with coronary stenosis of class I/II the incidence of peripheral artery disease was 45.2%. In 1965, in class III/IV patients, concomitant peripheral artery disease was demonstrated angiographically in 68.2%, 16.5% having a more than 75% stenosis or occlusion in at least one peripheral artery. These patients must therefore be considered as potential candidates for operative management of peripheral artery disease.

Moreover, the extent of coronary artery disease indicates the likelihood of "Topographic multimorbidity". In coronary patients with one-vessel disease extracoronary manifestation of atherosclerosis grade I/II is documented angiographically in 20.0%

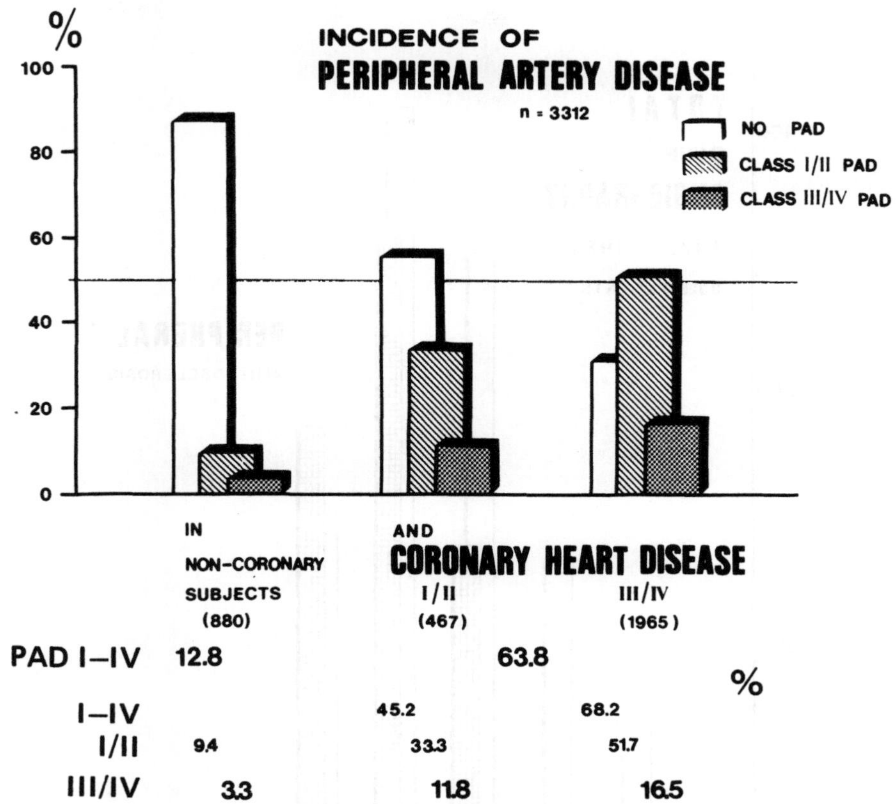

Fig. 2. Incidence and severity of peripheral artery disease (PAD) in 2432 patients with angiographically documented coronary heart disease, compared to 880 subjects in whom coronary heart disease was excluded by coronary angiography

and grade III/IV in 7.5% of the subjects. However, in four-vessel disease the rate of concomitant peripheral vascular disease increases to 56.0% and 21.8% respectively.

As far as the topography of noncoronary vascular disease is concerned, location of lesions in the superficial femoral artery dominates with 58.2%, while the incidence of coronary heart disease and atherosclerosis of extracerebral arteries has an incidence of 16.2% only.

Furthermore, there is an age-related increase in angiographically documented extracerebral, abdominal, and peripheral atherosclerosis with an incidence of 15% between 31 and 35 years and 72% between 61 and 65 years (Fig. 3). The occurrence of atherosclerosis in the subgroup of hemodynamically effective lesions with a greater than 75% reduction in vessel diameter or occlusion (grade III/IV), increases from 8% to 21%.

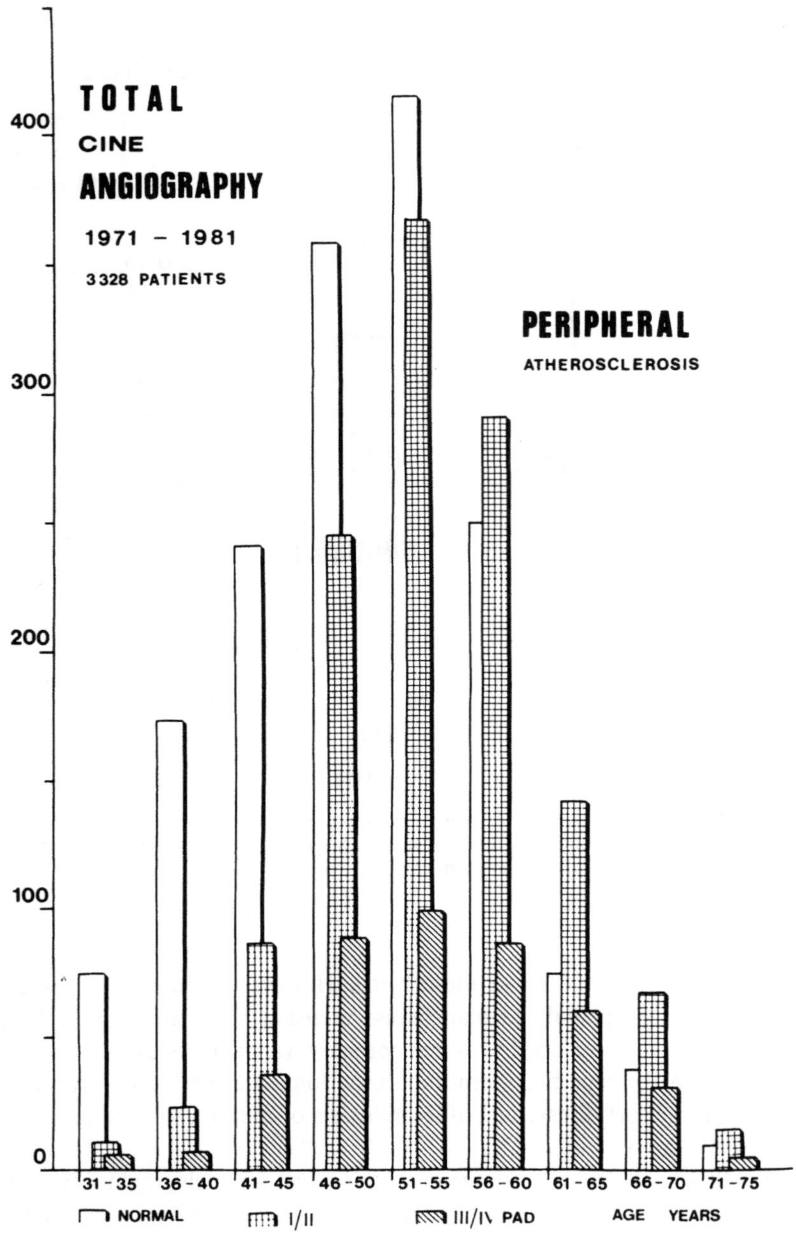

Fig. 3. Age-related distribution of peripheral atherosclerosis demonstrated angiographically in 3328 patients with suspected or diagnosed coronary heart disease

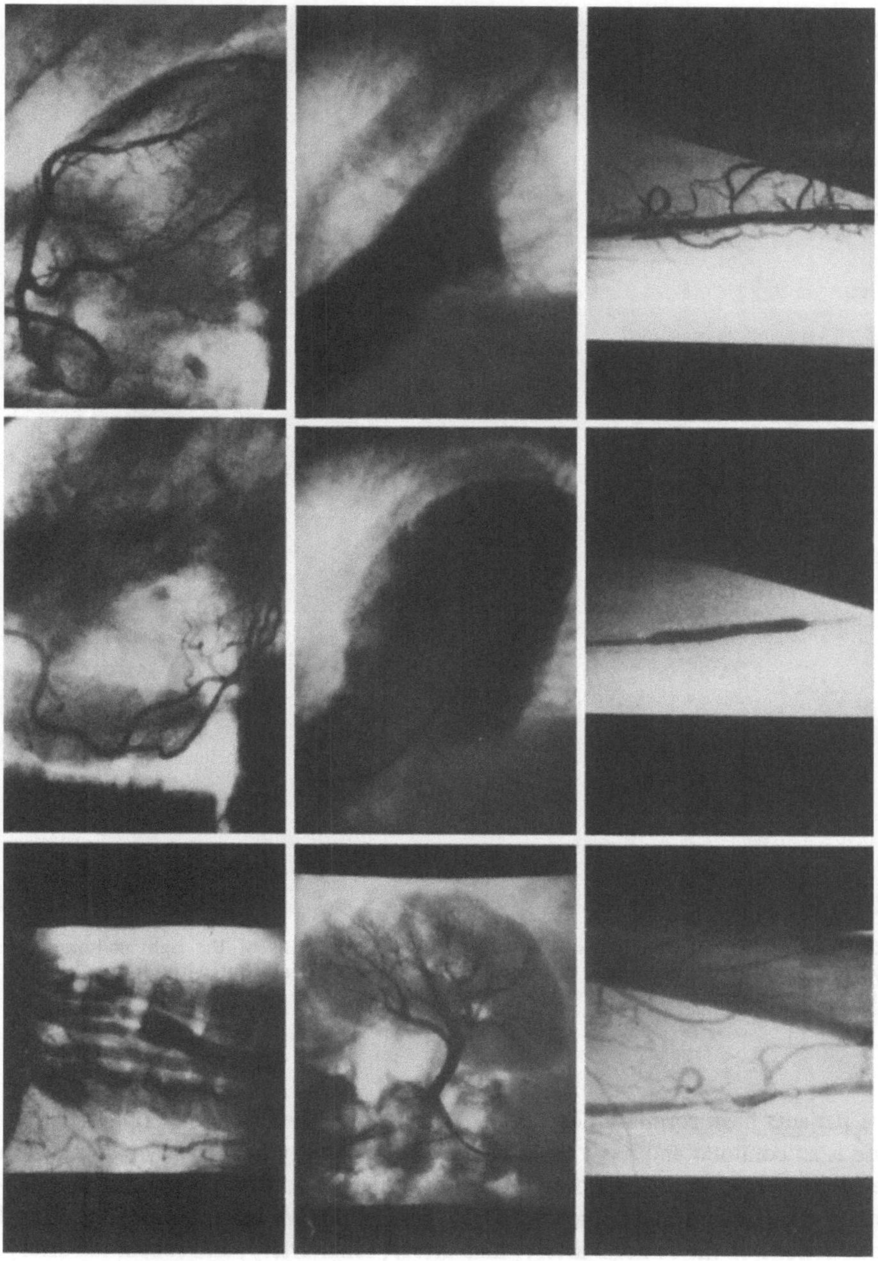

Fig. 4. Transbrachial transluminal dilatation of severe stenotic lesions of the left femoral artery in a 51-year-old woman with exercise-induced chest pain and arterial hypertension

Transbrachial Transluminal Dilatation

Summing up the results of total angiography, it appears that in two-thirds of the cases coronary heart disease is part of a generalized atherosclerosis and only one-third

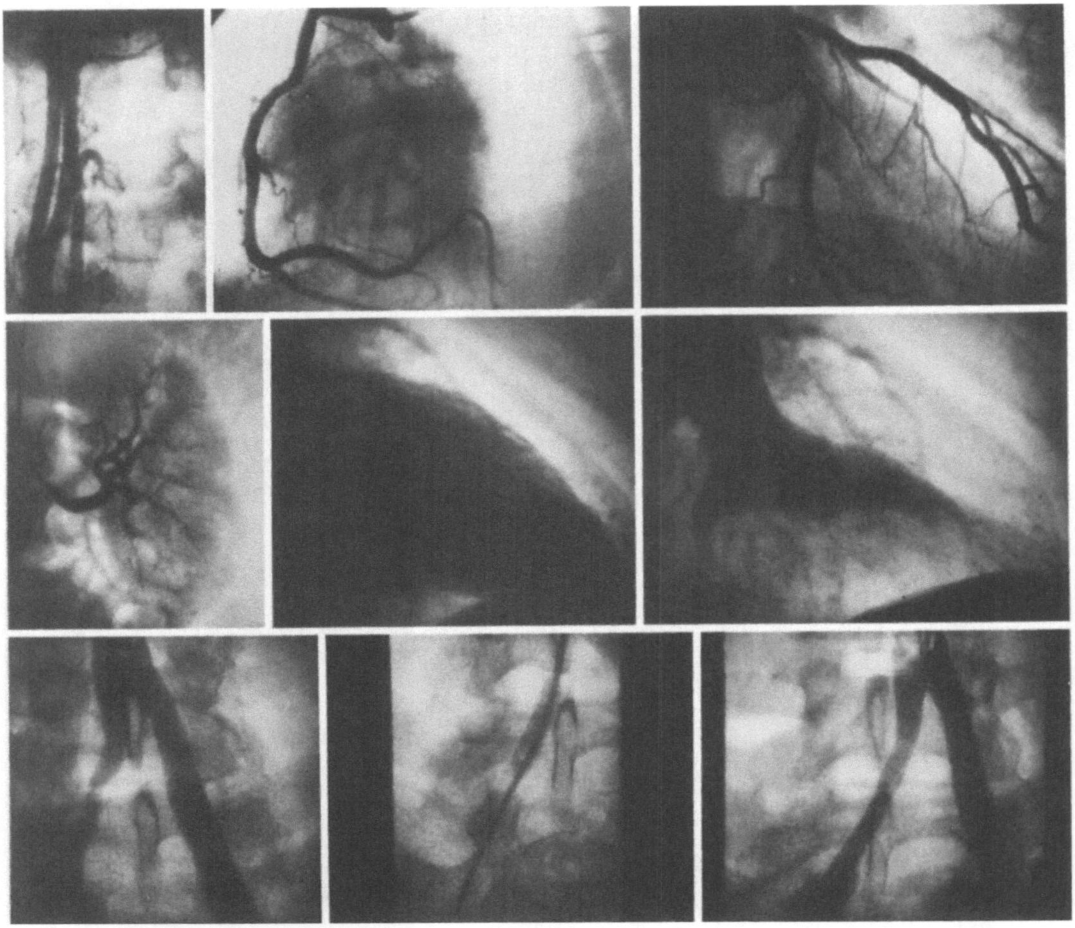

Fig. 5. Transbrachial transluminal dilatation of high-grade stenosis of the right common iliac artery in a 37-year old man with suspected coronary heart disease but without symptoms of occlusive arterial disease

of the patients have coronary heart disease exclusively. The fact that peripheral artery disease is so common and has a more than 50% probability in coronary patients with three-vessel disease or patients over the age of 60 led us to develop transluminal dilatation by the transbrachial approach (BTD) (Figs. 4, 5). We have successfully dilated stenotic lesions of the femoral artery, iliac artery, renal artery, and subclavian artery, and we have performed BTD with the special Grüntzig dilatation catheter, 7F-9F with a length of 150–160 cm, in 13 patients with a total of 18 arterial stenoses. Dilatation was successful in seven of eight femoral arteries, in five of seven iliac arteries, in both of two renal arteries and in one left subclavian artery. This brings the overall primary success rate up to 83.3%. There were three patients in whom the stenosis of the common iliac artery (two cases) or the left superficial femoral artery (one case) was so severe that the balloon segment of the dilatation catheter could not be passed through.

One the other hand, in a 54-year-old woman three high-grade segmental stenoses, one in the left subclavian artery and two in the superficial right and left femoral artery were dilated successfully during the same invasive procedure. All BTDs remained without complication. Thus the transbrachial approach has the following advantages over percutaneous transfemoral dilatation (PTD) introduced by Dotter [14] and improved by Grüntzig [19]:

1. It is not a separate procedure but immediately follows the combined angiography of coronary and peripheral arteries. It uses the same approach both for diagnosis and therapy.
2. It necessitates no interruption of anticoagulant therapy. Dilatation of peripheral arteries is possible even in patients in whom anticoagulation is a must, such as those with heart valve prostheses. Moreover, BTD facilitates anticoagulation instead of the recommended platelet-inhibition drug therapy [44].
3. It has a significantly lower local and overall complication rate than PTD. Furthermore, the local complication rate is reduced to the accepted minimum for the Sones technique.
4. Sequential dilatation of multiple peripheral vessels is easily achieved in combination with the diagnostic procedure.
5. BTD introduces the dilatation catheter via the brachial artery – a site of lower intraluminal risk than the femoral artery.

Summary

At present total angiography can be recommended for:

1. Coronary patients with three- and four-vessel disease or those over the age of 60 years in whom the probability of concomitant peripheral artery disease exceeds 50%.
2. Patients with symptoms of coronary or peripheral artery disease only, probably requiring operative treatment.
3. Patients with arterial hypertension, in order to evaluate potential renal vascular disease.

Total angiography offers at the time of diagnosis the possibility of subsequent therapeutic dilatation of critically stenosed abdominal, peripheral, and renal arteries using the same transbrachial approach as the Sones catheter. Transbrachial intraluminal dilatation seems to be superior to the percutaneous transfemoral method because of its high primary success rate and lower complication rate.

References

1. Allen EV, Willius FA (1929) Disease of coronary arteries associated with thrombo-angitis obliterans of extremities. Ann Intern Med 3:35
2. Anderson RP, Bonschek LJ, Wood J, Chapman R, Starr A (1974) Surgical management of coexisting coronary artery and valvular heart disease. Am J Surg 128:383

3. Bachmann K (1976) Total cineangiography. In: Coronary Angiography and Angina pectoris. Symp Europ Sos Cardiol et PR Lichtlen. G Thieme, Stuttgart
4. Bachmann K, Raab G, Niederer W (1980) Total cineangiography in patients with coronary heart disease. 22 Ann Meet Amer Coll Angiol Vienna
5. Barmeyer J, Buchwalsky R, Blümchen G et al. (1976) Der Verlauf der Arteriosklerose an den Koronar- und Beinarterien. Dtsch Med Wochenschr 101:443
6. Berndt TB, Hancock EW, Shumway NE, Harrison DC (1974) Aortic valve replacement with an without coronary artery bypass surgery. Circulation 50:967–971
7. Bernhard VM, Johnson WD, Peterson JJ (1972) Carotid artery stenosis: association with surgery for coronary artery disease. Arch Surg 105:837
8. Blümchen G, Kiefer H, Reindell H (1971) Periphere Arterien – Koronararterien. Aktuelle Probleme in der Angiologie, 14. Huber, Bern
9. Böhme H (1976) Koronare Herzkrankheit und periphere arterielle Verschlußkrankheit. Muench Med Wochenschr 118:187
10. Bollinger A, Lichtlen P, Kaindl F, Mannheimer E (1922) Koinzidenzuntersuchungen bezüglich peripherer Arteriopathie und Koronarsklerose. Wien Z Inn Med 53:455
11. Bonati F, Dettori AG: Frequenza delle lesioni coronariche in pazienti affetti da arteriopatie periferiche.
12. Contorni L, Visconti W (1958) Compromissione coronarica in corso di arteriopatia cronica obliterante periferica. G Ital Chir 14:424
13. Crepaldi G, Fellin R, Briani G, Baggio G, Manzato E, Veronese R (1977) Prevalence of coronary artery disease and peripheral artery disease in patients with different types of primary hyperlipidemia. Atherosclerosis 26:593
14. Dotter CT, Judkins MP (1964) Transluminal treatment of arteriosclerotic obstruction. Description of a technique and a preliminary report of its application. Circulation 30:654
15. Favaloro RG (1979) Direct myocardial revascularisation: a ten year journey. Am J Cardiol 43:109
16. Friedman SA, Pandya M, Greif E (1973) Peripheral arterial occlusion in patients with acute coronary heart disease. Am Heart J 86:415
17. Gordon T, Kannel WB (1972) Predisposition to atherosclerosis in the head, heart and legs. The Framingham study. JAMA 221:661
18. Grinfeld LR, De la Fuente LM, Shinji K et al. (1974) Total body angiography in patients with diffuse atherosclerosis [Abstr]. Am J Cardiol 33:141
19. Grüntzig A, Hopff H (1974) Perkutane Rekanalisation chronischer arterieller Verschlüsse mit einem neuen Dilatationskatheter. Dtsch Med Wochenschr 99:2502
20. Heitz J (1924) Claudication intermittente et angine de poitrine. Arch Mal Coeur 17:673
21. Jipp P, Sedlmeyer J, Scheumann J, Brunn HD, Mueller-Wiefel H, Borm D (1971) Koronarielle Zirkulationsstörungen bei arteriosklerotischem Verschluß von Extremitätenarterien. Z Kreislaufforsch 60:851
22. Kübler W, Schütz E, Gries FA et al. (1974) Periphere arterielle Verschlußkrankheit, angiographisch nachweisbare Koronarsklerose und Konstellation von Risikofaktoren bei Patienten mit pectanginösen Beschwerden. Dtsch Med Wochenschr 99:2201
23. Linhart J, Hejl Z, Geizerova H, Santrucek M (1974) Intermittent claudication and angina pectoris in two age groups of male population of Prague-2. Cas Lek Cesk 113:918
24. Londero HF, De la Fuente LM (1977) Transbrachial selective arteriography of the neck vessels. Our experience in 258 cases. Cathet Cardiovasc Diagn 3:425
25. Lukasik E, Liszewska-Pfejfer D (1977) Obliterative arteriosclerosis of extremitees in patients with coronary heart disease. Cor Vasa p 138
26. Matthes D, Opherk K, Mörl H (1978) Nachweis einer peripheren obliterierenden Arteriosklerose bei Patienten mit koronarer Herzerkrankung und eingeschränkter Koronarreserve. Vasa 7.138
27. McDonald L (1953) Ischemic heart disease and peripheral occlusive arterial disease. Br Heart J 15:101
28. Mörl H (1978) Früherkennung arteriosklerotischer Gefäßerkrankungen. Internist (Berlin) 19.636
29. Okies JE, McManus O, Starr A (1977) Myocardial revascularisation and carotid endarterectomy. a combined approach. Ann Thorac Surg 23:560
31. Philips DF (1980) Coronary arteriography in patients with peripheral vascular disease. Cleve Clin Q 47:206
30. Pandya M, Greif E (1973) Peripheràl arterial occlusion in patients with acute coronary heart disease. Am Heart J 86:415

31. Philips DF (1980) Coronary arteriography in patients with peripheral vascular disease. Cleve Clin Q 47:206
32. Raab G, Bachmann K, Niederer W (to be published) Risiko, Aussage und Indikation der totalen Angiographie (TA). Z Kardiol
33. Ranson HC, Imparato AM, Clauss RH, Reed GE, Hass WK (1969) Factors in the mortality and morbidity associated with surgical treatment of cerebrovascular insufficiency. Circulation 39, 40 [Suppl]:I–269
34. Rossier PH, Maier C, Thurlimann E (1947) Sclerose coronaire et endoangeite oblitèrante. Acta Cardiol (Brux) 2:201
35. Rubio PA, Guinn GA (1975) Myocardial infarction following carotid endarterectomy. Cardiovasc Dis 2:402
36. Schebelle K, Bachmann K, Niederer W, Petenyi M, Rupp K (1975) Vergleichende koronare und periphere Angiopathie bei 250 Patienten. Z Kardiol 41:121
37. Schettler G, Nüssel E (1974) Neuere Resultate aus der epidemiologischen Herzinfarktforschung in Heidelberg. Dtsch Med Wochenschr 41:2003
38. Schoop W (1973) Koinzidenz von koronaren und peripheren Durchblutungsstörungen, experimentelle und klinische Befunde. In: Gottstein U (ed) Koronarinsuffizienz – periphere Durchblutungsstörungen. Huber, Bern Stuttgart Wien, pp
39. Selvaag O (1956) Coronary (ischemic) heart disease in patients with arteriosclerosis obliterans. Acta Med Scand [Suppl] 319:59
40. Shore RT, Johnson WD (1974) Combined surgical treatment for coronary artery surgery complicated by extracranial carotid disease. Chest 66:336
41. Silvestre A, Desaneto A, Johnson JM, Desser KB, Benchimol A (1979) Abnormal electrocardiographic responses to exercise in patients refered for non-invasive evaluation of occlusive peripheral arterial disease. Am J Cardiol 43:713
42. Tillgren C (1965) Obliterative arterial disease in the lower limbs. III. Prognostic influence of concomitant coronary heart disease. Acta Med Scand 178:121
43. Tomatis LA, Fierens EE, Verbrügge GP (1972) Evaluation of surgical risk in peripheral vascular disease by coronary arteriography: a series of 100 cases. Surgery 71:429
44. Zeitler E (1978a) Drug treatment before and after percutaneous transluminal recanalisation (PTR). In: Zeitler E, Grüntzig A, Schoop W (eds) Percutaneous vascular recanalisation. Springer, Berlin Heidelberg New York, pp 73–77
45. Zeitler E (1978b) Complications in and after PTR. In: Zeitler E, Grüntzig A, Schoop W (eds) Percutaneous vascular recanalisation. Springer, Berlin Heidelberg New York, pp 120–125

Transluminal Angioplasty for Vertebral Basilar Artery Stenosis

H.C. Smith, T.M. Sundt, D.G. Piepgras, R.E. Vlietstra, A.W. Stanson, J.K. Campbell

Mayo Clinic and Foundation, Cardiovascular Division, Rochester, Minnesota 55901, USA

In recent years, the development and application of a balloon catheter technique for dilating arterial stenoses (transluminal angioplasty) has generated considerable interest. This technique has been successfully employed to reduce symptomatic stenoses in the coronary [7], renal [8, 9], and iliofemoral [2, 8] arteries. Relief of symptomatic stenoses in other arterial systems is currently under consideration or initial trials. This report describes our initial experience with balloon catheter dilatation of intracranial vertebral or basilar artery stenoses in four patients with severe brains stem, cerebellar, or posterior cerebral symptoms poorly responsive to medical or prior surgical therapy.

Case Reports

Case I. This 48-year-old diabetic male first experienced episodic diplopia and vertigo in early 1979. His symptoms progressed to include tinnitus, ataxia, scotomata, diminished coordination, and transient daily right hemiparesis unresponsive to intravenous heparin therapy. A severe (95%) focal stenosis of the basilar artery was demonstrated by angiography (Fig. 1). He was transferred to Mayo Clinic, and in August 1979 a right superficial temporal artery to right posterior cerebral artery graft was performed. The patient remained on warfarin and free of symptoms for 3 months. Following minor head injury he developed mild left hemiparesis, right hypoalgesia, and frequent transient cortical blindness (which were unresponsive to all medical measures, including continuous heparin infusion), and his systolic blood pressure rose to 230 mmHg. Angiography revealed a patent graft, but poor flow. In November, a saphenous vein graft from the left external carotid artery to the left posterior cerebral artery was performed. Postoperative studies demonstrated good graft flow. The patient remained asymptomatic on aspirin and dipyridamole (Persantine) for 2 months. In January 1980 he noted loss of graft pulsation, diplopia, and a right homonymous visual field defect. Despite surgical removal of clot, vein graft patency could not be maintained, and a palliative left occipital artery to left posterior cerebral artery graft was performed, with relief of diplopia.

Three months later he was transferred again to Mayo Clinic when daily episodes of cortical blindness, dysarthria, and right arm weakness occurred in hospital on full anticoagulant therapy. On May 13, under general anesthesia, the extracranial portion of the left vertebral artery was surgically exposed at the base of the skull, a 14-gauge

Transluminal Coronary Angioplasty and
Intracoronary Thrombolysis. Ed. by Kaltenbach et al.

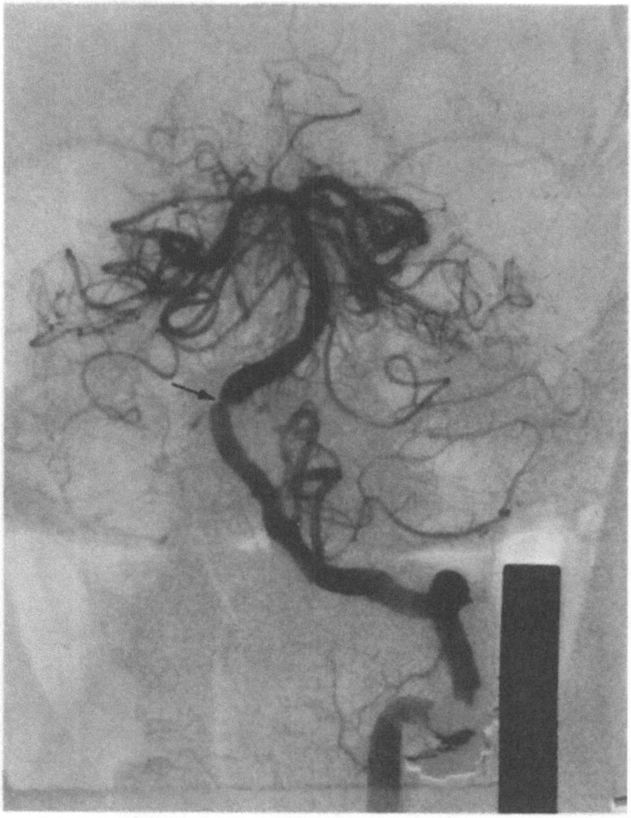

Fig. 1. Basilar artery subtraction angiogram in case 1. High-grade stenosis (*arrow*) at the origin of the basilar artery. The small occluded right vertebral artery (*below arrow*) faintly fills with dye retrogradely. The distal basilar artery and posterior cerebral arteries are normal. Note the tortuosity of the vertebral artery which must be traversed by a dilatation catheter if an alternative approach from the subclavian artery is employed. (From Mayo Clinic Proc. 55.673–680, 1980 with permission)

sheathed needle was inserted, the needle withdrawn, and a 4F Gruntzig catheter (3.0 mm balloon diameter) advanced through the sheath under portable fluoroscopic control through the basilar artery stenosis (Fig. 2). A 55 mmHg systolic pressure gradient was noted across the stenosis and there was marked delay in contrast media run-off from the artery distal to the stenosis. Several inflations of 20 s duration at 4 atm were performed. Because of persistence of the pressure gradient a 3.7 mm diameter balloon catheter was substituted and two inflations at 5 atm were performed, with reduction in the gradient to 10 mm (Table 1). After fluoroscopic demonstration of a 50% residual stenosis and rapid distal run-off of contrast media the catheter and sheath were withdrawn. Purse-string closure of the vertebral artery was required. The patient received preoperative antiplatelet therapy (dipyridamole 75 mg t.i.d.). The patient awoke promptly, with no neurologic deficit. Heparin was avoided because of the surgical aspect of the procedure. However, transient quadriplegia developed 12 h after surgery which responded to intravenous heparin and did not recur. Following angio-

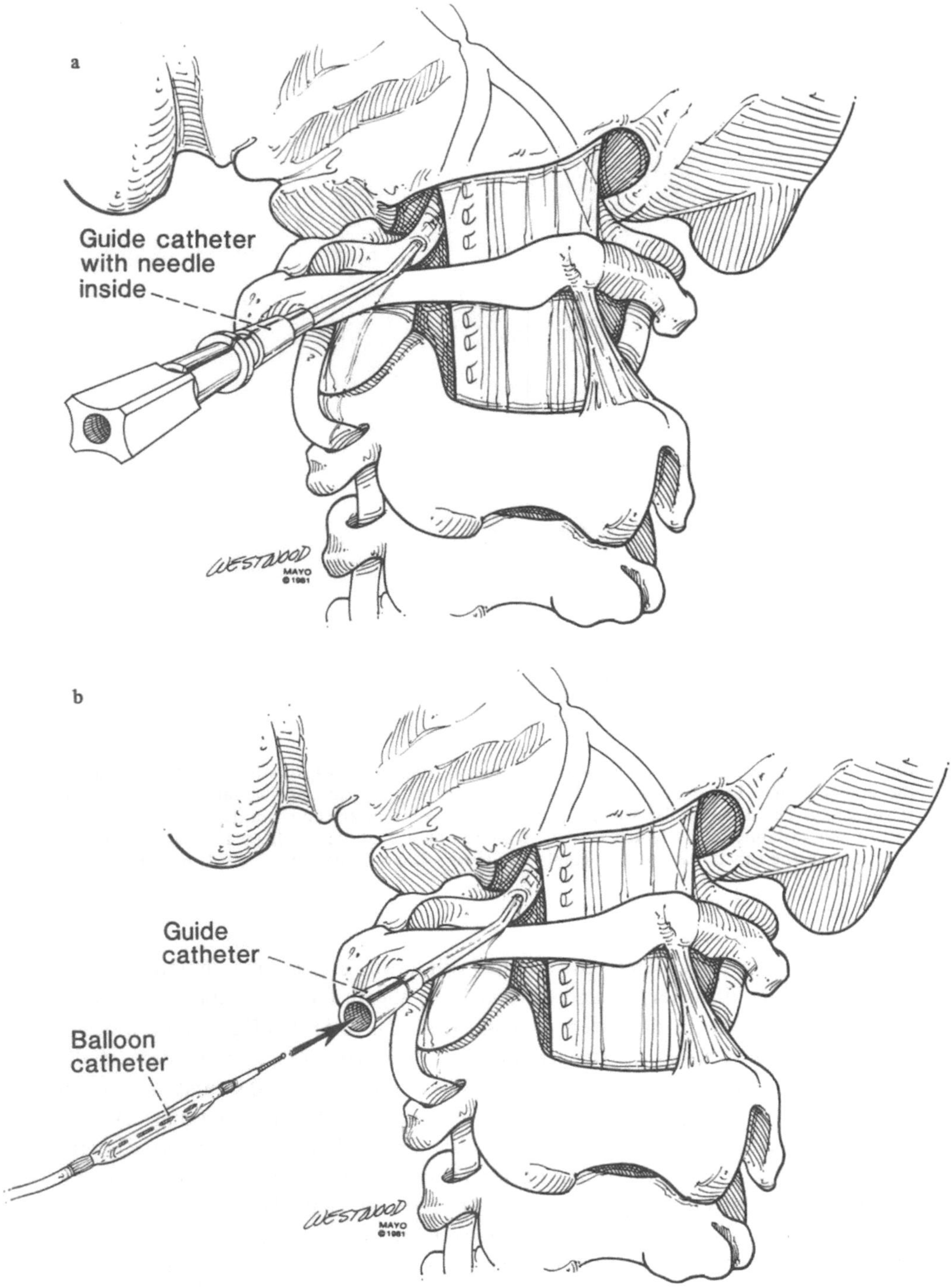

Fig. 2. a Bent 14-gauge sheathed needle inserted into exposed extracranial portion of vertebral artery. **b** Needle has been removed and dilatation catheter is passed through sheath into vertebral artery and advanced under fluoroscopic control to basilar artery

Table 1. Vertebral artery transluminal angioplasty

		Diameter of Stenosis (%)		Stenosis systolic pressure gradient (mmHg)	
Patient	Age	Before	After	Before	After
1	48	90	40	55	10
2	56	95	30	75	15
3	66	90	30	50	10
4	42	90	20	70	30
Mean values		92	30	62	17

graphic demonstration of a residual 50% stenosis on the 10th postoperative day, verapamil (80 mg q.i.d.) was stopped and the patient was discharged on Coumadin and dipyridamole.

He remained active without visual disturbances or ataxia until 11 weeks after angioplasty, when ataxia and blindness recurred. He was transferred to Mayo Clinic where

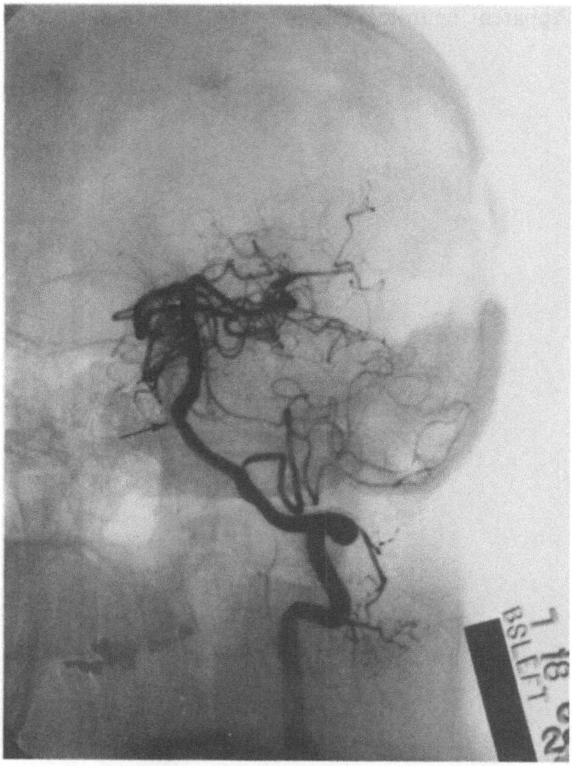

Fig. 3. Dilated area (*arrow*) of basilar artery in case 1 shows a residual 30% stenosis with apparent further regression from the 50% stenosis (not shown) noted 1 week after dilatation. Excellent opacification of all distal vessels, with no evidence of embolic occlusion. (From Mayo Clinic Proc. 55:673–680, 1980 with permission)

repeat angiography (Fig. 3) demonstrated further regression of the stenosis, no distal embolization, and rapid distal run-off. His symptoms cleared several hours after angiography. Because of suspected basilar artery spasm, verapamil 80 mg q.i.d. was started. In the follow-up period, now 24 months from angioplasty, he remains active and free of symptoms.

Case 2. This 56-year-old veterinarian first experienced vertebral-basilar transient ischemic attacks (TIAs) in March 1980, with symptoms of transient vertigo, nausea, generalized decreased coordination, and diplopia. Despite Coumadin therapy, six similar unprovoked attacks occurred over the next 5 months. In August his TIAs were worse, with additional symptoms of transient right-sided paralysis, dysarthria, drowsiness, and inability to swallow. A severe (95%) focal stenosis was demonstrated angiographically (Fig. 4).

When the patient experienced two similar severe TIAs (but with left-sided paresis) on the following two days, despite intravenous heparin, he was transferred to Mayo Clinic. Daily vertiginous spells persisted, and on September 4 a transluminal angioplastic procedure was performed on the basilar artery stenosis. The procedure details are similar to those outlined in case 1 and the angiographic and hemodynamic results are outlined in Table 1. Heparin was employed in the immediate postoperative period. The patient awoke promptly without apparent neurologic deficit. The following day nau-

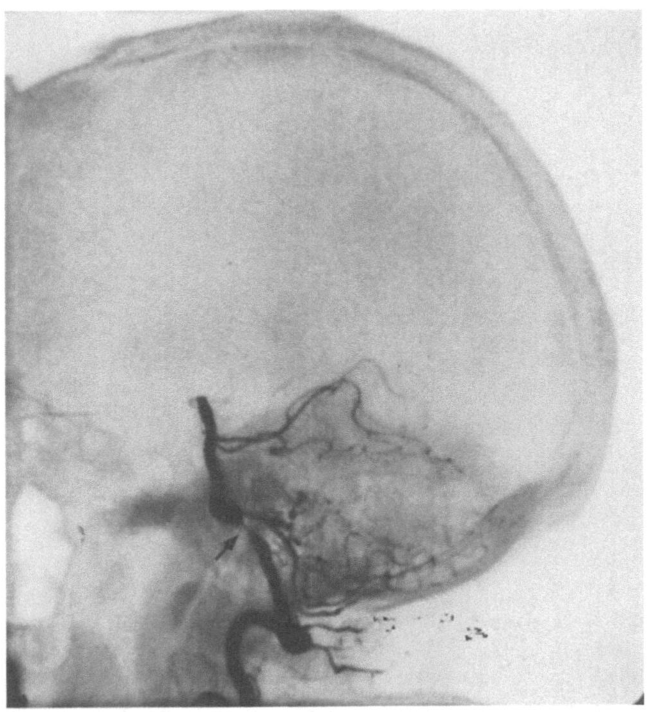

Fig. 4. Predilatation angiogram (lateral view) in case 2. High-grade (95%) stenosis (*arrow*) of basilar artery with poststenotic dilatation. Distal vessels are free of disease. (From Mayo Clinic Proc. 55:673–680, 1980 with permission)

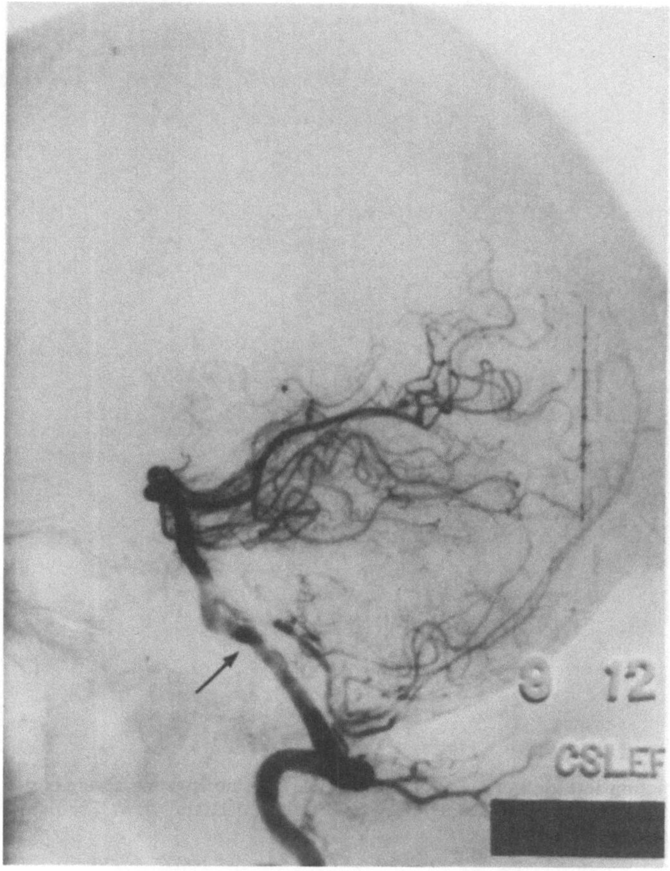

Fig. 5. Postdilatation subtraction angiogram in case 2. Basilar artery is now widely patient at site of previous stenosis (*arrow*) with more extensive filling of distal circulation. (From Mayo Clinic Proc. 55.673–680, 1980 with permission)

sea and left gaze paresis and nystagmus were noted. These improved and angiography on the 8th postoperative day (Fig. 5) revealed only minor (20%) residual stenosis and excellent distal run-off. The patient was discharged on dipyridamole, aspirin, and verapamil, and returned to veterinary practice. Subsequent neurologic examination was normal with no residual nystagmus or gaze paresis noted. He is active and free of symptoms 21 months after angioplasty.

Case 3. This 66-year-old male first experienced transient light-headedness, syncope, diplopia, and ataxia in July 1979, and sustained a brain stem infarct in September 1979. He continued to have vertebral-basilar TIAs in late 1979, and was treated with Coumadin. His symptoms progressed so that by September 1980 he had dysarthric spells while lying down, in addition to his usual symptoms, and he was transferred to Mayo Clinic for surgical consideration. He was noted to be ataxic, with a positive right Babinski reflex. Angiography demonstrated severe stenosis (approximately

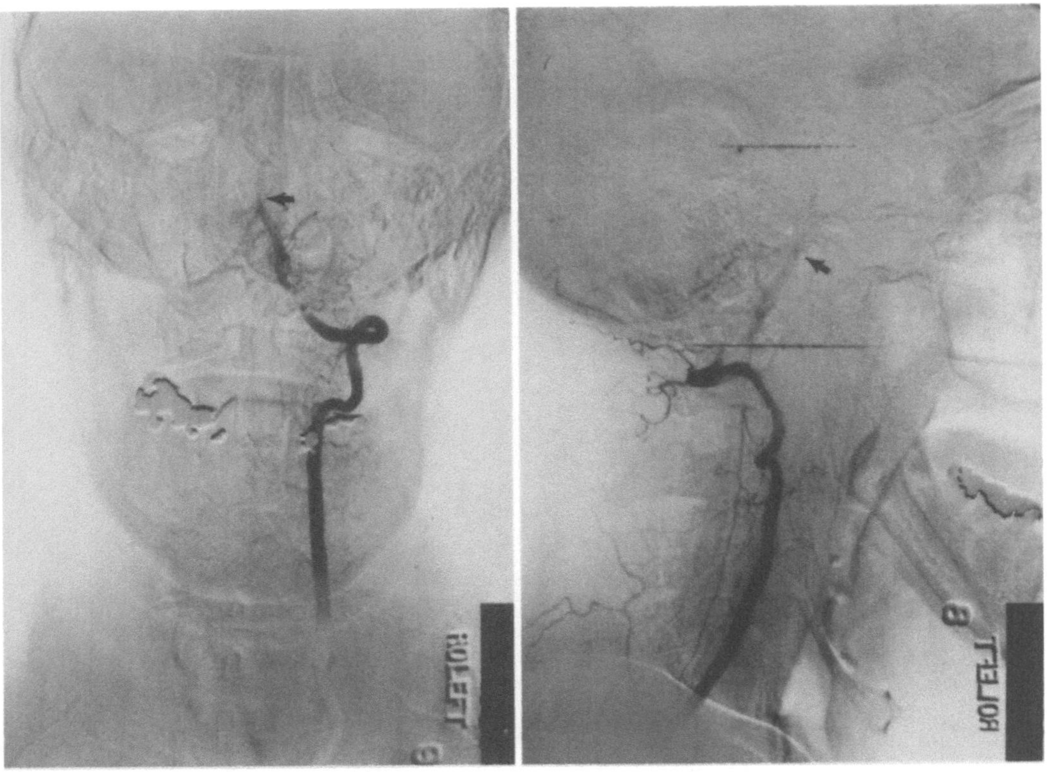

Fig. 6a, b. Predilatation subtraction left vertebral angiograms in case 3 demonstrating severe basilar artery stenosis and poor antegrade filling of distal vessels. *a* PA view; *b* lateral view. The right vertebral artery was occluded (*arrow*)

90%), of the left vertebral artery and a hypoplastic occluded right vertebral artery. Very poor antegrade opacification of the basilar artery was noted and this vessel was opacified by collaterals from the anterior spinal artery and a small posterior communicating artery from the left carotid artery (Fig. 6).

Transluminal angioplasty was performed in the usual manner (Table 1). The patient awoke promptly from the anesthesia, but the following morning his ataxia was worse and neurologic findings were consistent with a right cerebellar infarct. Angiography 8 days later demonstrated that the left vertebral artery was totally occluded at the C_2 level, probably due to thrombus. He has made a moderate recovery, but his ataxia persists.

Case 4. This 42-year-old male insulin-dependent diabetic underwent coronary artery saphenous vein bypass grafting and right carotid endarterectomy in 1975, at age 36. Further coronary artery bypass surgery was performed in 1977 and in 1979 he underwent bilateral iliofemoral artery surgery for occlusive vascular disease. He sustained a left hemisphere stroke following further surgery in late 1979 for reocclusion of his right femoral artery. Cerebral angiography demonstrated a patent right internal carotid artery. However, the left internal carotid artery was totally occluded at its origin.

The right vertebral artery was either occluded or absent. Much of the left hemisphere filled through the left vertebral artery, which had a severe stenosis just distal to the posterior inferior cerebellar artery (PICA). Because the majority of the left hemisphere was dependent upon continued blood flow through this stenosed vessel, the patient was referred to Mayo Clinic for consideration of surgery. However, all veins suitable for external carotid – posterior cerebral artery grafting had been employed for his previous cardiac and vascular bypass graft procedures and the posterior cerebral arteries were themselves atherosclerotic. Thus, although the vertebral artery angiographic anatomy was not optimal for angioplasty (long tubular plaque and minor diffuse disease), other therapeutic options were not available. Angioplasty was performed in a manner similar to the preceding cases. There was difficulty advancing the catheter beyond proximal irregularities to the high-grade stenoses, but apparently successful dilatation was achieved (Table 1). Because of persistent and considerable bleeding from multiple small areas in the surgical wound, the heparin given immediately after dilatation was reversed by protamine and fresh platelets were given. When the patient did not awaken promptly from anesthesia, angiography was performed (Fig. 7). This demonstrated dilatation of the basilar artery stenosis (residual 20% ste-

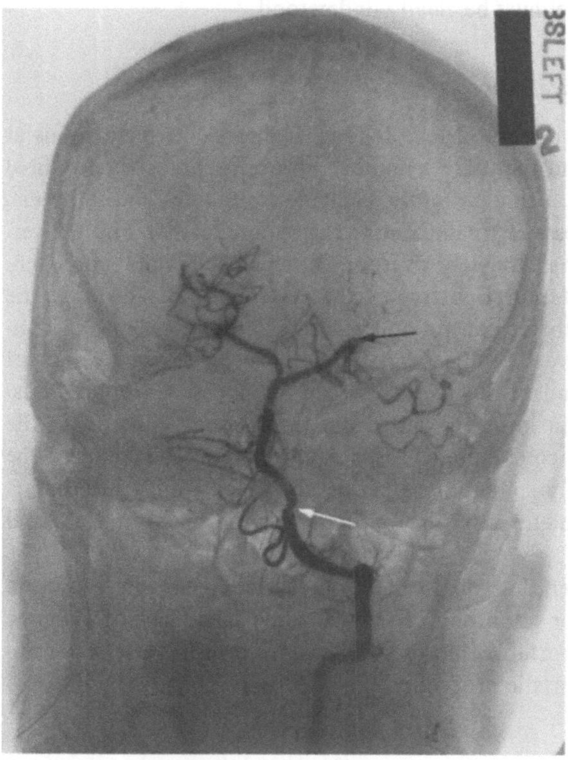

Fig. 7. Postdilatation angiogram in case 4. In contrast to the predilatation angiogram (not shown), the high-grade stenosis was reduced to residual 20% stenosis (*white arrow*). However, there was apparent distal embolic occlusion of left posterior cerebral artery (*black arrow*). Other views demonstrated embolic occlusion of the right superior cerebellar artery

nosis) and rapid movement of contrast media through the dilated segment. However, there was a small intimal flap in the dilated area and apparent distal embolic occlusion of the left posterior cerebral artery, the right superior cerebellar artery, and the left anterior inferior cerebellar artery. The patient did not regain consciousness and expired the following day.

Discussion

Vertebral basilar ischemic symptoms are usually caused by intracranial stenoses, because extracranial vertebral artery stenoses are often protected by an extensive collateral system [3, 4, 6]. For patients with ischemic symptoms not responsive to anticoagulants, if the vertebral artery stenosis is proximal to the PICA an external cartod (occipital branch) to PICA graft may be employed [10]. For those with stenosis of the basilar artery or vertebral artery distal to the PICA there are few surgical options. The basilar artery is largely inaccessible, and to date basilar artery bypass grafts have had disappointing results.

While transluminal dilatation of the vertebral or basilar artery may be of significant clinical benefit in these circumstances, the unique technical requirements and hazards of this particular procedure must be clearly understood.

Necessity and Hazards of the Surgical Approach

The extracranial portion of the vertebral artery is long and particularly tortuous at the level of the C_1–C_2 arches, and there are a number of arterial branches proximal to the origin of the basilar artery. Using currently available techniques and catheters, there is a low probability of successfully manipulating the balloon catheter up the vertebral artery and through a basilar artery stenosis from a brachial or femoral approach. While surgical exposure of the extradural portion of the vertebral artery distal to the C_1–C_2 arches provides better catheter control and placement, there are several limitations to this approach. Excessive bleeding from the surgical incision may restrict the use of antiplatelet or anticoagulant therapy. This occurred in case 4 despite immaculate hemostasis prior to heparin infusion, and distal thromboembolism from the dilated arterial segment may have contributed to this patient's demise. Trauma to the extracranial vertebral artery at the puncture site can also occur, and this trauma possibly contributed to the complete occlusion of the vertebral artery at this level in our third patient.

Finally, most neurosurgical operating room suites do not have fixed high-resolution radiographic systems, and the poor resolution of the video image and lack of dynamic image storage capability of most portable fluoroscopic systems provides less than optimal visualization during the angioplastic procedure.

Distal Embolization

While distal embolization is reported to occur in 3%–5% of patients undergoing iliofemoral angioplasty, it is rarely reported as a complication of coronary angioplasty.

This low incidence probably reflects our inhability, to detect microembolism, which in the coronary circulation may have little clinical significance. The vertebral basilar system has a limited tolerance for microembolism, and brain stem infarction can occur from occlusion of the small penetrating arteries that arise from the vertebral and basilar arteries [5]. The occurrence of macroembolism, as in our fourth patient, may have severe or fatal results. This low tolerance for microembolism may be the most significant determinant of the ultimate clinical utility of transluminal angioplasty of atheromatous lesions in the vertebral basilar artery system.

Adjunctive Medical Therapy

Because transluminal angioplasty is a recent development, the evaluation of various medications employed before, during, or after this procedure has been limited. While no clinical randomized trials have been reported, the likelihood that collagen exposed by the dilatation procedure will serve as a nidus for platelet deposition and thrombus formation prompts most centers performing coronary angioplasty to prescribe an antiplatelet or anticoagulant regimen or both. In our first and fourth patients, heparin and antiplatelet agents were either withheld or reversed. In both patients, clinical or angiographic findings suggested intra-arterial thrombus formation or embolism, which in the first patient promptly resolved with heparin therapy.

Because of a demonstrated propensity for coronary artery spasm after angioplasty, the calcium antagonists verapamil and nifedipine are now employed by most centers performing coronary angioplasty to reduce or prevent arterial spasm. Allen et al. have shown that the basilar artery, like the coronary artery, relies upon an extracellular source of activator calcium [1], and they have further demonstrated in a dog model that cerebral artery spasm can be blocked by calcium antagonists.

The occurrence of transient blindness and ataxia in our first patient 11 weeks after angioplasty was not associated with any angiographic evidence of restenosis, intra-arterial thrombus, or embolism. Its disappearance shortly after angiography (radiographic medium has predominant vasodilator effects) and its failure to recur in the 10 subsequent months on verapamil therapy strongly suggests transient basilar artery spasm.

Clinical Indications

The angiographic criteria for vertebral basilar transluminal angioplasty are likely to be similar to those employed for coronary angioplasty; an arterial stenosis that is preferably single, severe, discrete, and noncalcified, with downstream vessels relatively free of disease.

There are, however, several major clinical differences between coronary and basilar artery angioplasty. The latter is currently a surgical procedure, and the inability in some cases to employ antiplatelet or anticoagulants can, as noted in our initial experience, impose several limitations on this procedure and reduce the likelihood for success.

The second major difference is that coronary angioplasty is considered as an alternative to the standard surgical approach. Failure to obtain a satisfactory result or complications of coronary angioplasty are not associated with a high morbidity or mortality because the surgical option can be promptly exercised and the myocardial ischemia relieved. In contrast, for patients with basilar or distal vertebral artery stenosis there may be no reasonable surgical alternative. Failure to dilate a basilar artery stenosis or the development of a complication can have severe consequences, such as a severe stroke or death.

The feasibility of 1 year's complete relief from severe vertebral basilar ischemic symptoms by transluminal angioplasty has been demonstrated by this initial experience. The severe potential risks of this procedure have also been demonstrated. On the basis of this initial experience, it would presently seem prudent to reserve this procedure for those patients with severe vertebral-basilar system ischemia that is unresponsive to prior conventional anticoagulant and surgical therapy.

References

1. Allen GS, Banghart SB (1979) Cerebral arterial spasm. 9. In vitro effects of nifedipine on serotonin-, phenylephrine-, and potassium-induced contractions of canine basilar and femoral arteries. Neurosurgery 4:37–42
2. Alpert JR, Ring EJ, Freiman DB et al. (1980) Treatment of stenosis of the iliac artery by balloon catheter dilation. Surg Gynecol Obstet 150:481–485
3. Castaigne P, Lhermitte F, Gautier JC et al. (1973) Arterial occlusions in the vertebro-basilar system. a study of 44 patients with post-mortem data. Brain 96:133–154
4. Fisher CM (1970) Occlusion of the vertebral arteries: causing transient basilar symptoms. Arch Neurol 22:13–19
5. Fisher CM, Caplan LR (1971) Basilar artery branch occlusion: a cause of pontine infarction. Neurology (Minneap) 21:900–905
6. Fisher CM, Gore I, Okabe N, White PD (1965) Atherosclerosis of the carotid and vertebral arteries: extracranial and intracranial. J Neuropathol Exp Neurol 24:455–476
7. Gruntzig A (1978) Transluminal dilatation fo coronary-artery stenosis. Letter to the editor. Lancet 1:263
8. Katzen BT, Chang J, Knox WG (1979) Percutaneous transluminal angioplasty with the Gruntzig balloon catheter: a review of 70 cases. Arch Surg 114:1389–1399
9. Kuhlmann U, Vetter W, Furrer J, Lutolf U, Siegenthaler W, Gruntzig A (1980) Renovascular hypertension: treatment by percutaneous transluminal dilatation. Ann Intern Med 92:1–6
10. Sundt TM Jr, Whisnant JP, Piepgras DG, Campbell JK, Holman CB (1978) Intracranial bypass grafts for vertebral-basilar ischemia. Mayo Clin Proc 53:12–18

Catheter Dilatation in Subclavian Steal Syndrome

K. Mathias

Abteilung für Röntgendiagnostik, Universität, 7800 Freiburg, FRG

Patients with significant narrowing of the innominate or proximal subclavian artery may develop reversal of blood flow in the vertebral artery of the affected side, diverting blood from the cerebral circulation into the arm arteries, especially during exercise. This entity was first recognized by Harrison in 1829 and definitely attributed to a subclavian steal by Smyth in 1866 [3]. The symptoms (Table 1) may be intensified by cerebrovascular disease in other vessels. In the past vascular surgery was the only means of treatment for this circulatory impairment.

Since 1978 we have applied catheter dilatation to patients with subclavian steal syndrome [13, 14, 15]. Additional indications for angioplasty of supra-aortic arteries are fibromuscular dysplasia of the internal carotid and vertebral arteries and atherosclerotic stenosis in bilateral vertebral artery disease [11].

Materials and Methods

Based on favorable experience with angioplasty in peripheral vessel disease in more than 750 patients, and after animal experiments with carotid artery stenosis, we began dilatation treatment of the supra-aortic arteries in March 1978. Up to October 1981 catheter dilatation was attempted in 21 patients (13 males and eight females) with subclavian steal syndrome (Table 2). The patients had a mean age of 53 years with a range of 15–73 years.

The diagnostic work-up includes Doppler ultrasound studies and selective arteriograms of the aortic arch vessels. The treatment plan is laid down after discussing the

Table 1. Symptoms of subclavian steal syndrome in 21 patients

Cerebral symptoms	*n*	Brachial symptoms	*n*
Vertigo	4	Abnormal fatigue	20
Diplopia	1	Pain at rest	1
Temporary blindness	1	Cold sensations	16
Temporary blurred vision	2	Numbness	5
Drop attacks	1	Emboli	1
Mental signs	2		
Headache	4		

Transluminal Coronary Angioplasty and
Intracoronary Thrombolysis. Ed. by Kaltenbach et al.

Table 2. Results of angioplasty in subclavian steal syndrome in 21 patients

Results	n	%
Primary success rate	19	88
Patency rate (15 months)	17	81
Clinically cured	15	72

different modalities of management with the neurologist, angiologist, and vascular surgeon. The patients are informed about the technique of catheter dilatation and alternative procedures and their respective risks, and have to give their written consent for the intervention. The patients have the procedure performed while awake and under light sedation. Most dilatations are carried out by a transfemoral approach but the transaxillary route is preferred in patients with occlusion of the left subclavian artery and with right subclavian or innominate artery obstruction.

Using the transfemoral approach a 7- or 9F dilatation catheter (Schneider, Zürich; Cook Europe) is introduced over a 260-cm long exchange guide wire, selectively placed through a sidewinder catheter into the left subclavian or innominate artery. While advancing the catheter in the subclavian artery, entrance into the vertebral artery is avoided to prevent adverse effects on the vertebrobasilar circulation. The dilatation catheter is 100 cm long and its inflated balloon has a maximum diameter of 8–9 mm.

Blood pressure is measured before and after the passage of the stenosis. After positioning of the dilatation segment of the catheter in the stenotic portion, the balloon is inflated with dilute contrast material for 5–20 s under a pressure of 5–8 atm. The pressure is not increased further if the patient complains of tension caused by stretching of sensitive nerve fibers in the adventitia. The balloon is deflated, and another pressure recording obtained to decide whether the hemodynamic situation has improved or a second dilatation is necessary. After successful angioplasty the collapsed balloon catheter is withdrawn and a postdilatation angiogram performed.

The puncture of a pulseless axillary artery may prove difficult, but can be achieved by Doppler ultrasound guided puncture or search punctures with a thin anesthetic needle. The recently available polyethylene catheters are superior to polyvinylchloride catheters because higher pressures, which are necessary in hard sclerotic lesions, can be applied. Immediately after introduction of the catheter, at the end of the procedure, and again 6 h later 5000 IU heparin is given. For at least 6 months platelet aggregation inhibitors (1 g acetylsalicylic acid, 225 mg dipyridamole) are prescribed. Before hospital discharge and thereafter every 3 months control examinations with Doppler ultrasound are carried out.

Case 1

A 49-year-old man complained of arm weakness and recurrent dizziness without history of stroke, hypertension, or heart disease. Physical examination revealed that the left radial pulse was markedly diminished. Left brachial pressure was 125/85 compared

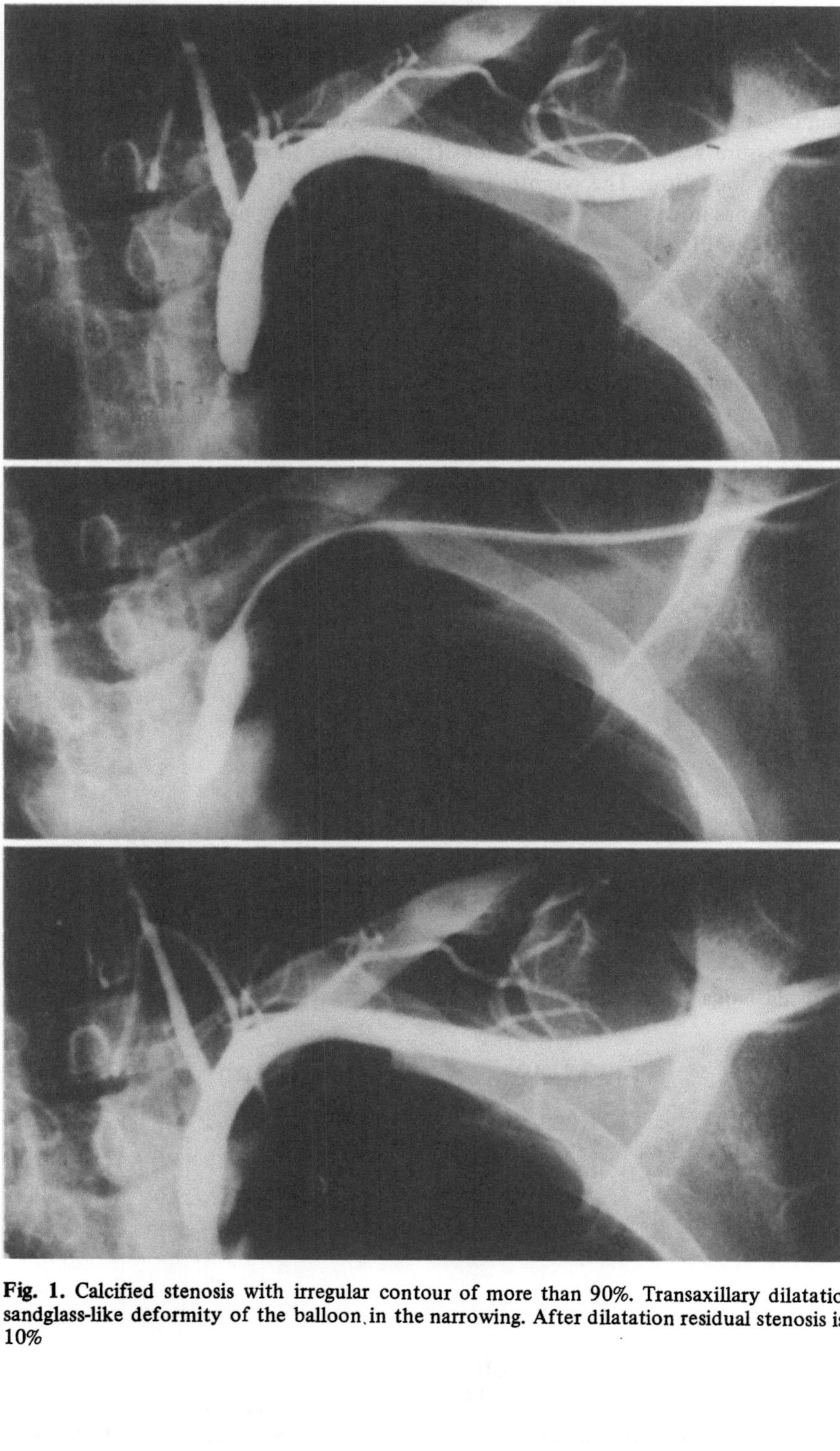

Fig. 1. Calcified stenosis with irregular contour of more than 90%. Transaxillary dilatation with sandglass-like deformity of the balloon in the narrowing. After dilatation residual stenosis is about 10%

to 185/90 mmHg on the right side. A loud harsh bruit was heard over the left supraclavicular area. Neurological examination and chemistry profile were normal, but Doppler ultrasound showed a reversed vertebral blood flow. Angiography revealed a calcified stenosis of high degree in the proximal subclavian artery (Fig. 1). After dilatation the pressure was equal on both sides (Fig. 2), and the vertebral artery showed an orthograde blood flow. The symptoms of dizziness and left arm weakness disappeared. The patient has now been free of symptoms for 12 months, as documented by control oscillography (Fig. 3).

Case 2

A 58-year-old man with claudication and coronary heart disease noticed vertigo and blurring of vision in his right eye. The right radial pulse was scarcely palpable, and a bruit was audible over the right supraclavicular fossa. Doppler ultrasound examina-

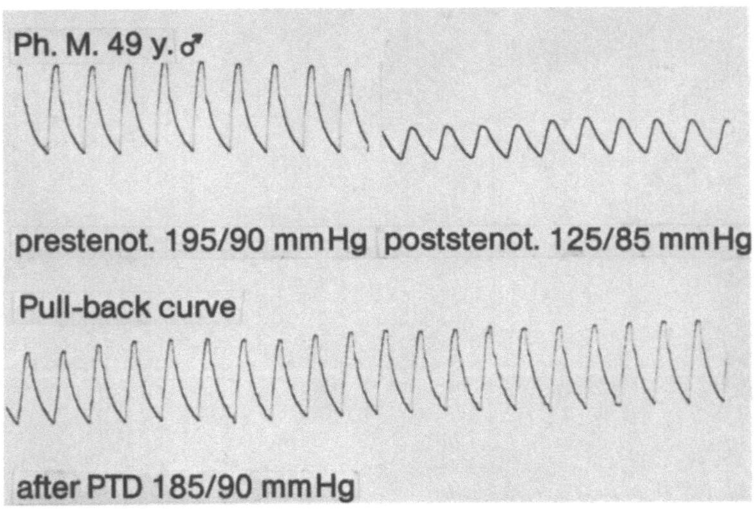

Fig. 2. After dilatation the pressure gradient is completely removed

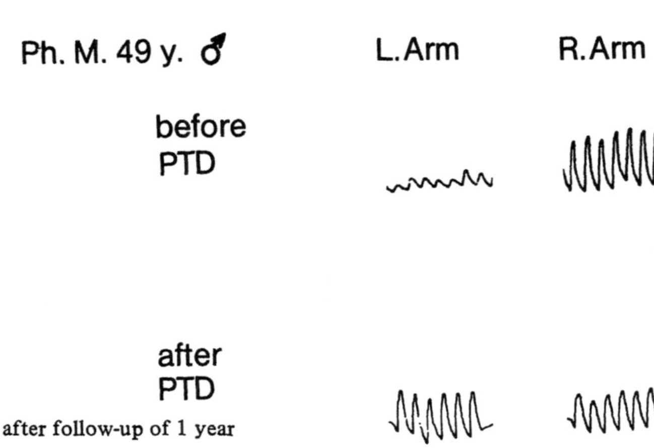

Fig. 3. Normal oscillogram after follow-up of 1 year

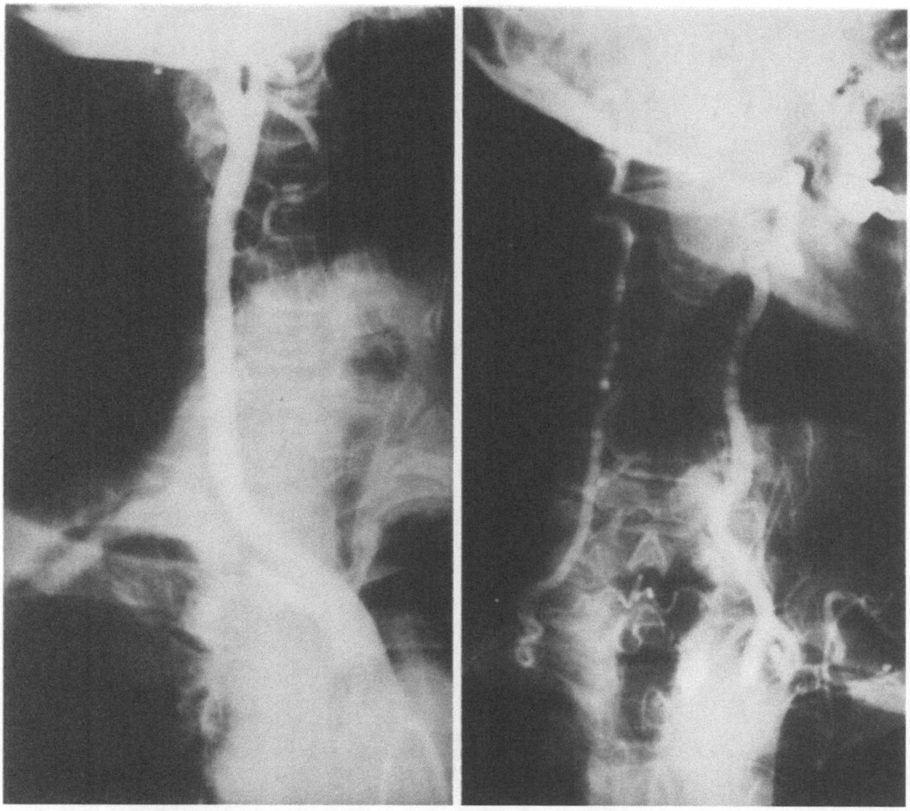

Fig. 4. Aortic arch injection: narrowing of the right subclavian artery and reversed vertebral blood flow of the affected side

tion revealed a proximal subclavian artery stenosis with reversed vertebral blood flow. These findings were confirmed by angiography (Fig. 4). The vertebral artery could not be visualized. For angioplasty a transaxillary route was chosen and a 5F diagnostic catheter advanced up to the stenosis and passed through the narrowing. Thereafter the catheter was replaced by an 7F dilatation catheter and the 90% stenosis was dilated to 6 mm. The pressure gradient of 60 mmHg was completely removed (Figs. 5, 6). The symptoms disappeared and did not recur during a follow-up period of 12 months (Fig. 7).

Results

From March 1978 to October 1981, 21 patients with subclavian artery obstructions were treated by percutaneous angioplasty. Eighteen patients suffered from a stenosis and three from a short occlusion of the subclavian artery. With exception of a hard calcification and an elastic narrowing all stenosis could be dilated, whereas two of the three occlusions could be recanalized successfully. No local complications

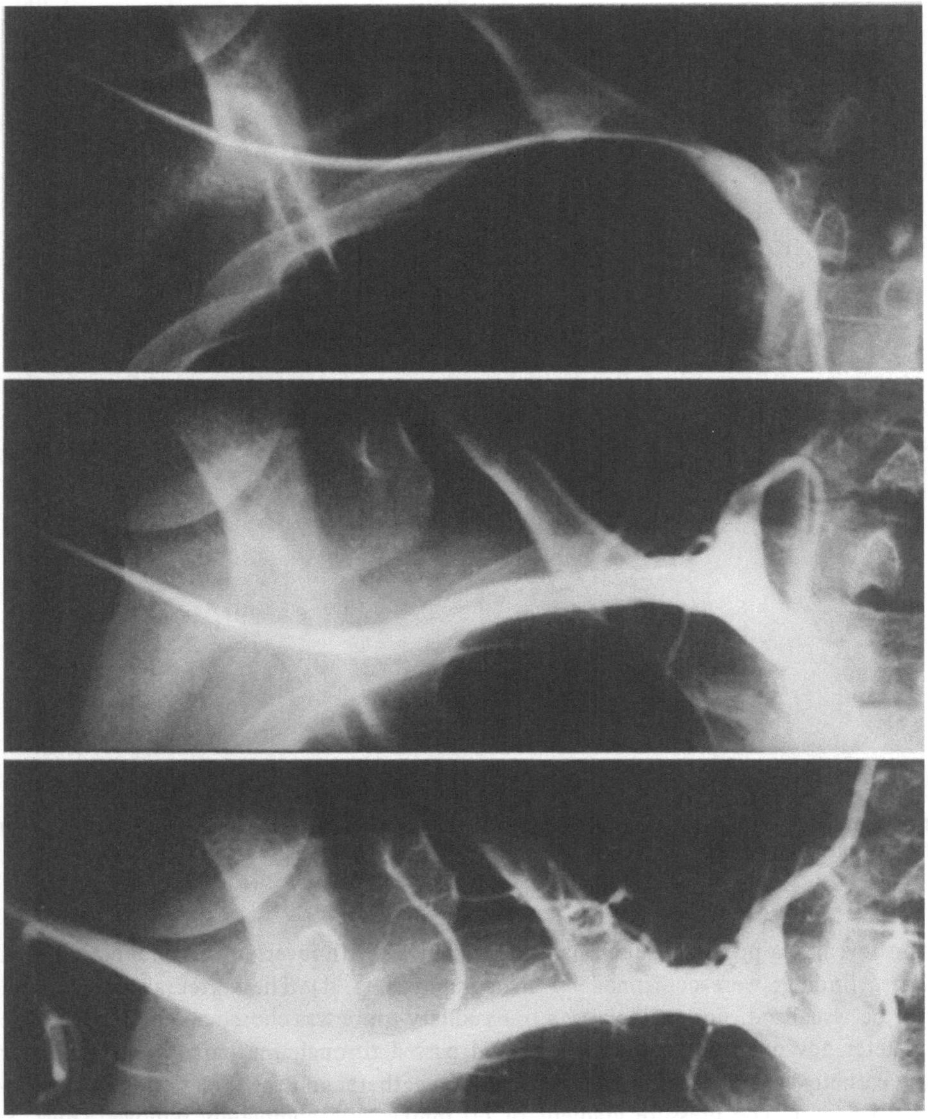

Fig. 5. Transaxillary dilatation of the subclavian artery stenosis with orthograde vertebral flow thereafter

occured during the interventions and none of the patients showed neurological signs suggesting an embolism. One patient developed a hematoma at the puncture site after transaxillary catheter dilatation which could be managed conservatively. All other patients were discharged from hospital 2–3 days after angioplasty.

The successfully treated patients have been followed up at 3-monthly intervals for between 3 and 35 months, on average 15 months. Two patients developed a recurrent stenosis 3 and 9 months after dilatation as shown by Doppler ultrasound studies and pressure recordings. No treatment has been necessary in these cases so far, as clinical signs are lacking.

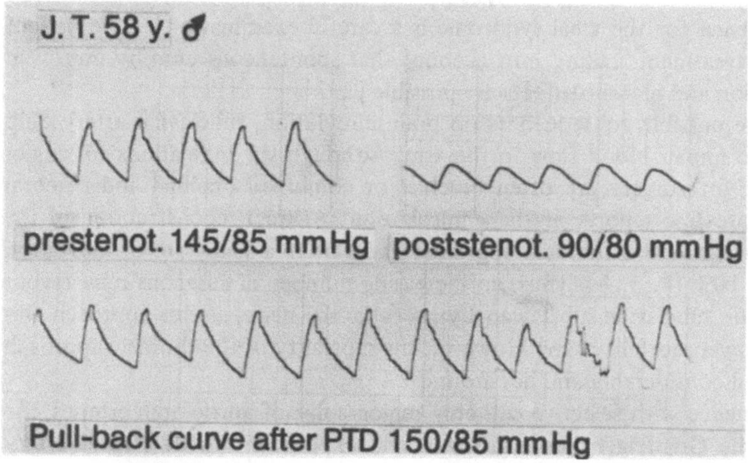

Fig. 6. Pressure recordings reveal a normal poststenotic pressure after dilatation

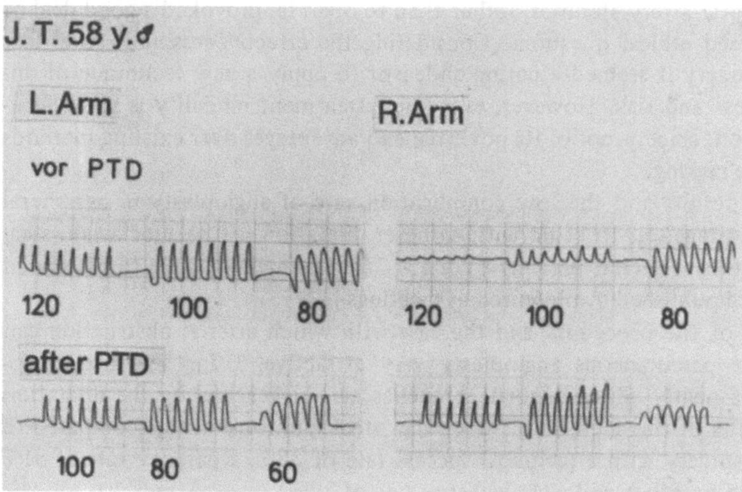

Fig. 7. Control oscillogram 1 year after dilatation confirms the good clinical effect with a normal finding on both sides

Discussion

There is still no convincing evidence that the reversed vertebral blood flow is a real steal from the brain causing a vertebrobasilar ischemia. Hemodynamic studies, both in animals [6] and in humans [10], demonstrate that the retrograde vertebral blood flow is easily compensated for by increased carotid artery flow. Regional cerebral blood flow studies failed to show any decrease of total or regional flows. The presence of an isolated subclavian steal may have consequences for the brain circulation, but the great number of asymptomatic patients with reversed vertebral flow makes it clear that are still no objective means of measuring it.

The only evidence for the steal syndrome is a careful examination of the patient before and after treatment, taking into account that spontaneous cure by improved collateral circulation and placebo effects are possible [2, 7].

Apart from the possible consequences on brain circulation, subclavian artery obliterations may also impair blood flow to the arm. Although the indications for angioplasty as well as for surgery are often brachial or combined brachial and cerebral symptoms there are few reports of the clinical results. Direct reconstruction of the obliterated artery through a thoracic approach had earlier a high rate of mortality, between 5% and 10% [4, 5, 8]. Thus, an increasing number of surgeons now favour carotid-vertebral or subclavian-subclavian bypasses in the neck, as this approach was found to have a lower mortality [16]. However, the mortality of the thoracic approach has since decreased considerably and lies around 2% [9].

Growing experience with selective catheter angiography of aortic arch arteries, the introduction of the Grüntzig balloon catheter, and experiments with carotid artery stenosis in animals have allowed trials of alternatives to vascular surgery in the treatment of supra-aortic artery obstruction [12]. The suggestion to dilate subclavian, carotid, and vertebral artery stenoses, rather than to operate, provoked a good deal of discussion and raised ethical questions. Considering the effectiveness and rather low risk of vascular surgery it seemed a daring endeavor to apply a new technique of unknown effectiveness and risk. However, every new treatment modality is viewed initially with suspicion, since proof of its potential and advantages over existing methods are supposed to be lacking.

The promising results and the low complication rate of angioplasty in peripheral vessel disease encouraged us to begin with catheter dilatation of the subclavian, steal syndrome in carefully selected patients [11, 13–15]. Meanwhile single cases treated by other groups are published or presented at meetings [1].

The simplicity of the procedure and the ease with which arterial obstruction can be removed make percutaneous angioplasty very attractive. Using selective angiographic techniques nearly all supra-aortic branches can be reached by the dilatation catheter. The results of this method in subclavian steal syndrome can be compared to those of vascular surgery with a technical success rate of 88%, a patency rate of 81% (mean follow-up 15 months), and a clinical cure rate of 72%.

It seems a fair guess that the technical success rate can be further increased with growing experience, but the long-term results, leaving calcifications and atherosclerotic material in place, will not exceed those of vascular surgery. Redilatation may become necessary in about 10% of the patients, and is justified once the low complication rate of the procedure is confirmed by a greater number of treated patients.

References

1. Bachman DM, Kim RM (1980) Transluminal dilatation for subclavian steal syndrome. Am J Roentgenol 135:995–996
2. Buchwalsky R, Genswein R, Schlosser V, Blümchen G (1977) Subclavian-Steal-Syndrom: postoperativer und spontaner Verlauf bei 27 Patienten über 3 Jahre. Thoraxchir Vask Chir 25.288–290
3. Contorni L (1973) The true story of the "subclavian steal syndrome" or "Harrison and Smyth's syndrome". J Cardiovasc Surg 14:408–411

4. Crawford ES, DeBakey ME, Morris GC, Howell J (1969) Surgical treatment of occlusion of the innominate, common carotid and subclavian arteries: a 10-year experience. Surgery 65:17–24
5. Edwards WH, Wright RS (1972) Surgical therapy in subclavian occlusive disease. Am J Surg 123:689–695
6. Eklöf B, Schwartz SI (1970) Effects of subclavian steal and compromised cephalic blood flow on cerebral circulation. Surgery 68:431–438
7. Fields WS, Lemak NA (1972) Joint study of extracranial arterial occlusion. VII. Subclavian steal – a review of 168 cases. JAMA 222:1139–1143
8. Hafner CD (1976) Subclavian steal syndrome. A 12-year experience. Arch Surg 111:1074–1082
9. Liljeqvist L, Ekeström S, Nordhus O (1979) Intrathoracic approach for subclavian and innominate artery reconstruction. Scand J Thorac Cardiovasc Surg 13:309–314
10. Magaard F, Eklund B (1975) Oscillography and digital pulse plethysmography in occlusive disease of the subclavian artery and brachiocephalic trunk. Scand J Thorac Cardiovasc Surg 9:250–261
11. Mathias K (1981) Perkutane transluminale Katheterbehandlung supraaortaler Arterienobstruktionen. Angio 3:47–50
12. Mathias K, Mittermayer C, Ensinger H, Neff W (1980) Perkutane Katheterdilatation von Karotisstenosen. Tierexperimentelle Untersuchungen. Fortschr Geb Röntgenstr 133:258–261
13. Mathias K, Gospos C, Thron A, Ahmadi A, Mittermayer C (1980) Percutaneous transluminal treatment of supraaortic artery obstruction. Ann Radiol 23:281–282
14. Mathias K, Schlosser V, Reinke M (1980) Katheterrekanalisation eines Subklaviarverschlusses. Fortschr Geb Röntgenstr 132:346–347
15. Mathias K, Staiger J, Thron A, Spillner G, Heiss HW, Konrad-Graf S (1980) Perkutane Katheterangioplastik der Arteria subclavia. Dtsch Med Wochenschr 105:16–18
16. Raithel D (1978) Behandlung des Subclavian-Steal-Syndrom. Dtsch Med Wochenschr 103:1126–1127

Overview

W.-D. Bussmann

Department of Cardiology, University Hospital, Theodor-Stern-Kai 7,
6000 Frankfurt a.M., FRG

Transluminal angioplasty of supra-aortic, carotid, vertebrobasilar, and abdominal arteries are new applications. Bachmann et al. proposes angiography in one session for different vessels of the body, as indicated. Dr. Mathias has performed angioplasty in supra-aortic arteries, especially in patients with subclavian steal syndrome, and also reports one case with successful dilatation of a carotid artery stenosis. Experience with this vessel is rather limited so far, and the same is true for angioplasty of the vertebrobasilar system. Smith and co-workers report four angioplasties performed during operation: in two patients the procedure was successful. The cerebral system has little tolerance for microembolism, which might be the most significant determinant of the ultimate clinical utility of angioplasty in this area.

Transluminal Coronary Angioplasty and
Intracoronary Thrombolysis. Ed. by Kaltenbach et al.

Coronary Fibrinolysis in Acute Myocardial Infarction

Percutaneous Transluminal Coronary Recanalization: Procedures, Results, and Acute Complications

W. Rutsch*, M. Schartl, D. Mathey, K. Kuck, W. Merx, R. Dörr, P. Rentrop, H. Blanke

Klinikum Charlottenburg of the Free University of Berlin,
Medical Clinic of the University of Hamburg, FRG,
Medical Clinic of the University of Aachen, FRG,
Medical Clinic of the University of Göttingen, FRG

Introduction

We should like to report results obtained in 232 patients treated at four West German University Hospitals in the period from 1978 to May 1981. Special attention will be given to the procedure used, rate of success, duration of therapy until recanalization was achieved, and complications encountered during the procedure, as well as to global and regional left ventricular function before and after myocardial reperfusion.

Material and Methods

Patients were included in the study when onset of persistent nitroglycerin-resistant angina pectoris was exactly defined. Three hours was generally considered as a limit for initiation of therapy, and CPK values had to be normal. Demonstration of ST segment elevation and/or demonstration of an akinetic segment in the 2D-echocardiogram were used as objective criteria of coronary artery occlusion.

Patients older than 70 years were excluded from the study for a number of reasons. Patients with a history of infarction in the regions served by the occluded vessel were excluded. High risk of potentially fatal hemorrhage in patients who underwent cardiovascular resuscitation with external heart massage, in patients with gastrointestinal bleeding and cerebrovascular hemorrhage was criterion for exclusion. Patients with serious noncardiac diseases were also excluded from the study.

The recanalization procedure began with an attempt at mechanical perforation of the thrombus with a soft-tipped guide wire when the position of the thrombus permitted the maneuver. This was the case in 22% of patients, and the attempt was successful in 41%. However, the procedure is not without risk, as perforation of the vessel with extravasation of contrast medium occurred in 2 of 97 patients (2%). The next step involved selective injection of 0.1 mg nitroglycerin or 0.1 mg nifedipine in order to exclude the possibility of coronary artery spasm. Results were poor, even in the 3% of patients in which a slight degree of recanalization was achieved. Regardless of the

* Abteilung Innere Medizin – Kardiologie –, Klinikum Charlottenburg der FU Berlin, Spandauer Damm 130, 1000 Berlin 19

Transluminal Coronary Angioplasty and
Intracoronary Thrombolysis. Ed. by Kaltenbach et al.

results obtained with these two maneuvers, selective infusion of streptokinase was performed in all cases. Three study centers administered 2000 units/min, while the fourth used 4000 units/min. Recanalization occurred at 36 min after initiation of streptokinase therapy, with a mean total dose of 71 000 units streptokinase. All patients received 10 000 units heparin IV, 500–1000 mg acetylsalicylic acid IV, corticosteroids (500–1000 mg prednisolone IV), and infusion of 3–6 mg nitroclycerin/h, when hemodynamic considerations allowed.

Results

Subtotal occlusion was found in 19.5% ± 14.2% of cases (range 5%–37%) despite all criteria of acute myocardial infarction. Selective administration of nitroglycerin and streptokinase did not result in significant dilatation of the stenosis. Attempted recanalization was unsuccessful in 19.0% ± 3.3% of cases with complete vascular occlusion (range 14%–22%), which may have been due to causes other than thrombosis.

The interval between onset of angina and initiation of streptokinase infusion was 211.3 ± 44.3 min in the patients who underwent successful recanalization (range 151–276 min). Recanalization occured at 35.5 ± 8.4 min in the entire study group (range 30–60 min), but there were clear differences related to location of occlusion and age of thrombus. Although there was a considerable degree of variation, successful recanalization in the LAD and the RCA was achieved after almost identical periods of streptokinase infusion, while occlusion of the left circumflex artery required a longer period (Table 1). Recanalization was achieved at 23 min when the thrombus was less than 2 h old. In comparison, recanalization was achieved at 31 min when therapy was initiated at 2–4 h after the onset of symptoms, and 43 min were required when the thrombus was more than 4 h old.

Table 1. Mean duration of thrombolysis related to the site of occlusion

Artery	Duration (min)
LAD	34
LCX	42
RCA	35

Arrhythmias were observed at the same time as successful recanalization in 25% ± 5% of cases (range 19%–32%). These disorders were not related to the location of occlusion and were generally benign. A few cases of more serious arrhythmias required therapy, but there were no fatalities.

Residual stenosis remained following successful recanalization (Table 2). Seven of 232 patients (3%) died within 6 h of the procedure. Five fatalities (2.1%) occurred before recanalization was achieved, and only two patients (0.9%) died within 6 h of successful recanalization. Causes of death were cardiogenic shock and other compli-

Table 2. Residual stenoses after complete thrombolysis

Stenosis	Proportion of total patients (%)
Below 50%	6
Between 50% and 75%	18
Between 75% and 90%	49
Subtotal	27

Table 3. Incidence of bleeding complications during the first 6 h after start of streptokinase infusion

Site	Proportion of total patients (%)
Arterial puncture	4.8
Other punctures	1.0
Gastrointestinal tract	0.3
Cerebrovascular system	0.3

cations of infarction. No patient died as a direct result of the procedure, nor was cardiac or noncardiac hemorrhage implicated as a cause of death. Hemorrhagic complications were rare. Large hematomas at the site of arterial puncture were the most common complication of this sort (Table 3).

Coronary recanalization in impending myocardial infarction is intended to reduce the final area of myocardial necrosis. Quantification of the therapeutic success is not without problems. The behavior of regional and global left ventricular function in the natural course of the disease is not fully understood in man. In addition, it is difficult to determine exactly the extent of ischemic or necrotic myocardial tissue.

In 22 of 68 patients in our study successfully undergoing coronary recanalization, functional parameters sufficient for quantitative analysis could be registered. Following reperfusion, the adjacent myocardial segment was examined in the 30° RAO monoplane ventriculogram. Quantification of regional wall motion disorder was performed by means of a continuous curve of the circumferential fiber-shortening velocity (VCF) over the entire left ventricular circumference. The regional wall motion as determined by contrast ventriculography is shown in Fig. 1.

This method principally allows a quantification of regional wall motion disorder to the extent that is possible by ventriculography. Parameters can be determined:

1. The length of the asynergic segment is measured between the crossing points of the curve with the lower standard range.
2. Since the total length of the ventricle is known in centimeters, the length of the akinetic segment can also be expressed in centimeters.
3. The comparison of the mean VCF value of the asynergic segment with the corresponding mean value of the lower standard range renders the percentage of reduction in regional wall motion of the asynergic segment in oppostion to the standard, $VCF_a\%$.

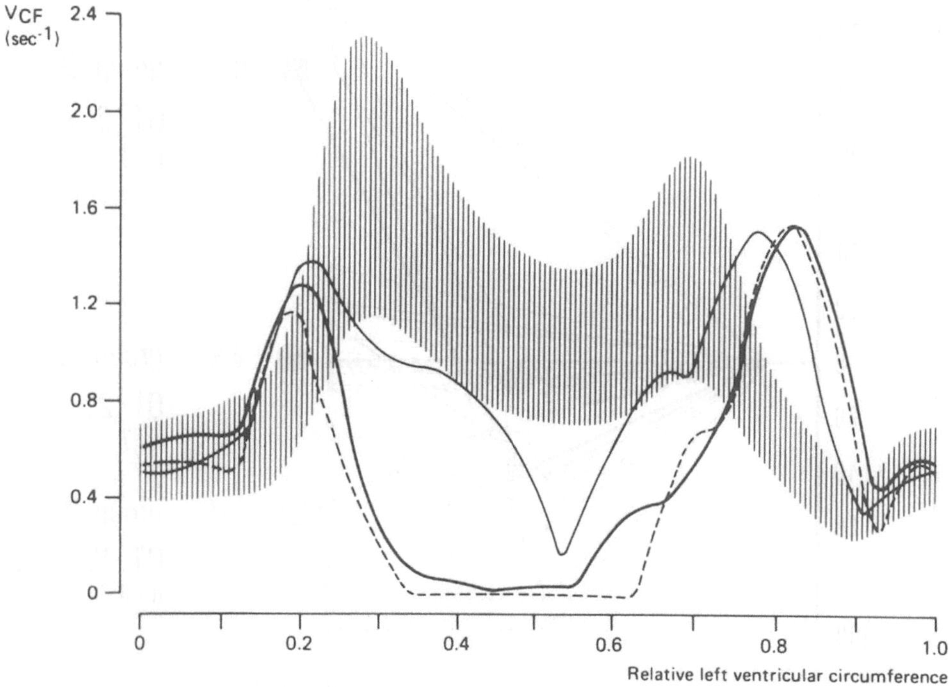

Fig. 1. Regional wall motion as determined by contrast ventriculography. The *abscissa* stands for the length of the left ventricular end-diastolic circumference, measured from the aortic valve on the left-hand side and the mitral valve on the right-hand side. The *ordinate* shows the mean VCF for a total of 300–500 points of the endocardium. The normal wall motion of ten healthy subjects is illustrated by the *shadowed area*. The *dotted line* represents the wall motion in an extensive anterior infarction and a mean VCF of zero for the anterolateral, apical, and diaphragmal segments. The *full black line* demonstrates the only slightly increased wall motion 60 min after recanalization, while the obviously much-improved wall motion 3 weeks after recanalization is shown by the *thin line*

4. The extent of wall motion disorder depends on both the length of the akinetic segment and the extent of reduction in the VCF. The product of these two parameters can therefore best describe the segmental defect. For this, the difference between the mean VCF of the lower standard range and the mean VCF of the asynergic segment is multiplied by the length of the asynergic segment: $(VCF_n - VCF_a) \times cm = VCF_a \times cm$.

These data were calculated before reperfusion as well as 60 min and 3 weeks after. The change in percentage was used to describe the actual myocardial condition. The patients were divided into three groups (Fig. 2):

Group 1, with a reduction in asynergy of 11%–100%
Group 2, with changes within the range of plus or minus 10%,
Group 3, with a more than 11% increase in asynergy.

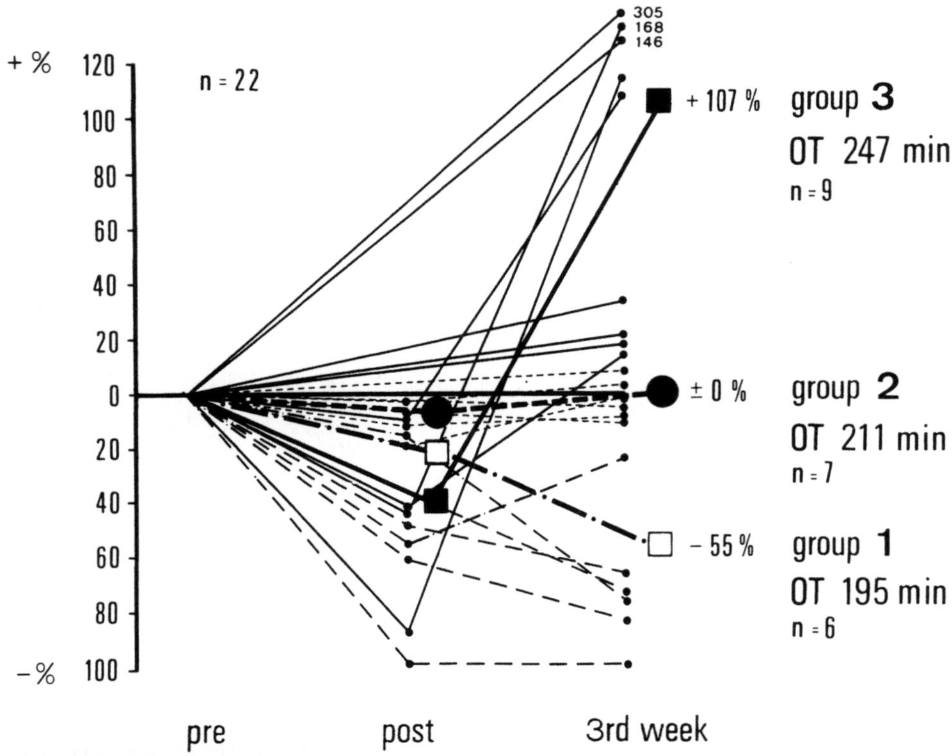

Fig. 2. Change of regional wall motion (Δ VCF_a $\times$ cm) in percent 60 min and 3 weeks following recanalization n = 22. OT, occlusion time

In all three groups the following parameters were registered at the three intervals: length of asynergy, decrease of the mean segmental VCF expressed as percentage of the norm, the product of the difference betwen mean VCF of the akinetic segment and the normal value and its length, ejection fraction, and occlusion time. Table 4 shows the mean values and standard error of the mean, the statistical significance of the differences, and the distribution of the coronary occlusion sites among the three groups. The differences in the basic values can be explained by the fact that group 2 patients nearly exclusively had anterior infarctions, group 1 showed predominance of anterior and group 3 of inferior infarctions. The length of asynergy, therefore, is greatest in group 2 and least in group 3.

The mean values of VCF_a expressed as percentage of the norm are lowest in group 2 and highest in group 3 with predominance of inferior infarction. Corresponding results were seen for the product of these two parameters and the ejection fraction.

Comparison of group 1 and group 3 three weeks after recanalization reveals statistically significant differences for the length of asynergy, for VCF_a expressed as percentage of the norm, and for the product of both. The insufficient therapeutic results in group 3, compared to group 1, are most likely due to varying total occlusion times, with 247 min in group 3 and 195 min in group 1.

Table 4

Parameter	Group									
	One ($n = 6$)			Two ($n = 7$)			Three ($n = 9$)			
	Pre	Post	Control	Pre	Post	Control	Pre	Post	Control	P
Asynergy (cm) ±	9.7	7.4	6.2	12.7	13.5	13.3	7.2	6.3	9.0[a]	0.05
	3.7	5.7	5.1	3.8	1.1	3.8	4.5	4.1	4.8	
VCF_a % ±	44	55	72[a]	23	16	25	57	75[a]	51	0.05
	30	32	27	27	8	26	22	19	22	
$VCF_a \times$ cm ±	5.3	4.2	2.4	9.4	9.9	9.4	3.1	1.8	6.4[a]	0.05
	4.1	4.0	3.0	4.1	1.6	4.1	2.7	1.8	3.9	
Ejection fraction (%) ±	55	61[a]	63[a]	47	53	38	61	69[a]	54[a]	
	8	5	9	11	8	12	7	7	14	n.s.
Occlusion time (min)	195 ± 78			211 ± 44			247 ± 41			n.s.
Artery	LAD: 4 CX: – RCA:2			LAD:6 CX:1 RCA:–			LAD:2 CX:3 RCA:4			

[a] $P < 0.05$

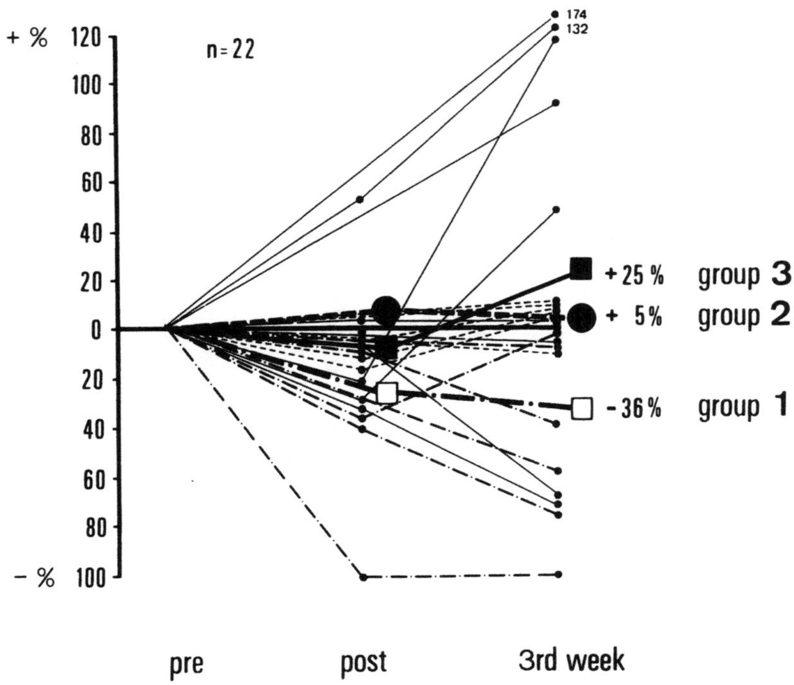

Fig. 3. Change of length of asynergy (cm) in percent 60 min and 3 weeks following recanalization (n = 22)

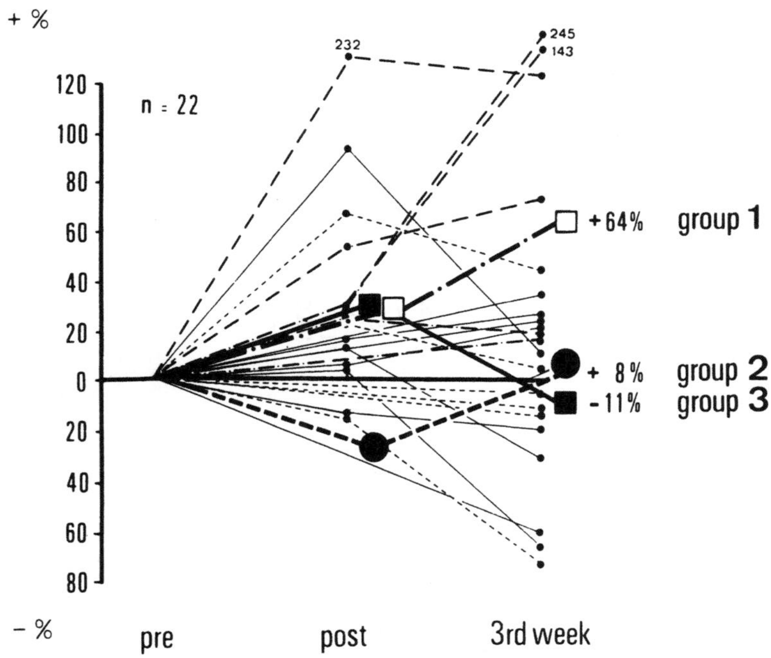

Fig. 4. Change of VCF_a values of the asynergic segment in percent (n = 22)

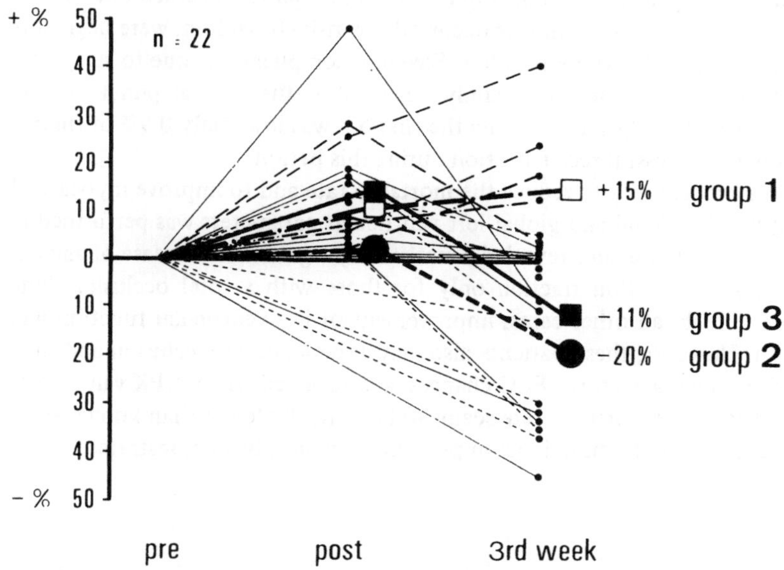

Fig. 5. Change of ejection fraction in percent 60 min and 3 weeks following recanalization (n = 22)

Figures 3–5 demonstrate the percentage changes for the single and mean values. Except in five cases the length of asynergy in the 3rd week remains unchanged or is clearly reduced – by 36% in group 1 (Fig. 3). Correspondingly, group 1 shows a 64% increased wall motion whereas the other two groups do not show any significant changes. There is a remarkable and nearly identical increase of the VCF_a in group 1 and group 3 60 min after reperfusion (Fig. 4). After the 3-week interval, only in group 1 does the ejection fraction tend to increase; it is reduced in the other two groups (Fig. 5). The varying effects of recanalization upon the depending myocardial function are best shown by analyzing the change in percentage of the asynergy determined by the product of VCF_a and the length of asynergy. While in group 3 the asynergy rises by more than 100% group 1 has a decrease of 55% (Fig. 2). Remarkably well again are the results in group 3 60 min after recanalization.

Summary

In 80% of the cases with total occlusion of a coronary artery, selective intracoronary infusion of streptokinase can achieve recanalization within a short time, depending on the location and age of the thrombus. Thrombus perforation by mechanical maneuvers or intracoronary injection of vasodilators is not sufficient and is mostly without lasting effect. Residual stenoses following complete thrombolysis were severe and in three-quarters of the cases measured more than 75% of the vessel's diameter.

Diagnostic and therapeutic procedures in a total of 232 patients turned out to have a very low risk. Reperfusion arrhythmias occurred surprisingly seldom, were negligible in most cases, and could always be handled. Bleeding complications due to streptokinase were seen in 6.4% of cases and mainly occurred at the arterial puncture site. Mortality in the overall study group during the first 6 h was low. Only 0.9% of the patients died following successful recanalization during this period.

The aim of the procedure is to reduce the mortality rate and to improve myocardial function. Analysis of regional and global left ventricular parameters was performed in a limited number of patients and revealed a statistically significant decrease of asynergy and an increase of ejection fraction only for those with a total occlusion time of less than 195 min. In all other cases, improvement of left ventricular function will be the exception. However, these patients also may experience a reocclusion and then in most cases show angina pectoris, ECG changes, and renewed rise of CPK values. For reasons as yet unclear, the mortality rate seems to be critically lower than known from conventional therapy even if a functional improvement cannot be demonstrated.

Rapid Intracoronary Thrombolysis by Subselective Administration of Thrombolytic Agents

W. Ganz

Department of Cardiology, Cedars Sinal Medical Center, Los Angeles, CA 90048, USA

The purpose of intracoronary thrombolysis in patients with evolving myocardial infarction is to reopen the occluded coronary artery and to prevent the consequences of continued myocardial ischemia. Myocardial necrosis may begin after only 20 min coronary artery occlusion. In cases of severe ischemia the process of necrosis may be completed in 3–4 h. The earliest possible restoration of flow in the occluded artery is therefore of critical importance.

In experimental studies in dogs infusion of thrombolytic agents into the immediate vicinity of an intracoronary thrombus resulted in consistent lysis within 5–10 minutes. When the agent was applied into the ostium of the occluded coronary artery, with one or more branches between the site of infusion and the clot, lysis of the clot was either delayed or unsuccessful. In accordance with these observations, it was observed in vitro that the rapidity of clot lysis increased with the concentration of the thrombolytic agent (Thrombolysin = streptokinase and plasminogen).

In clinical studies the thrombolytic agent is delivered directly to the site of occlusion. For that purpose a special 2 1/2 F catheter[1] reduced to 2F in its distal 20 cm is inserted through the lumen of a 8F angiography catheter with the tip 1–2 mm from the site of occlusion. The tip of the coronary infusion catheter is intensely radiopaque to allow its precise placement. After placement, the catheter is stretched by slight withdrawal to prevent movement of the tip into or beyond the clot as thrombolysis progresses. The catheter position is checked in at least two projections. The infusion catheter for the right coronary artery is straight. Occasionally it may be difficult to insert the infusion catheter when the tip of the angiography catheter is directed against the wall of the right coronary artery. Changing the position of the angiography catheter by slight withdrawal may eliminate the difficulty. The straight catheter may also be tried in the branches of the left coronary artery. In the case of difficulty, it is preferable to use the special catheters designed to enter either the left anterior descending (LAD) or the circumflex (CX) branch.

These catheters are shaped in three dimensions to assume the shape and orientation of the Judkins catheter and then rotate either anteriorly (for LAD) or posteriorly (for CX).

---

[1] Coronary Infusion Catheter, American Edwards Laboratories P.O. Box 11150, Santa Ana, California 92711, USA

Transluminal Coronary Angioplasty and
Intracoronary Thrombolysis. Ed. by Kaltenbach et al.

The infusion catheter is inserted into the angiography catheter through the straight arm of a side-arm (Y) adaptor (e.g. Cook). A guide tube is used to insert the catheters preshaped to enter the LAD or CX into the side-arm adaptor and the angiography catheter. Advancement of the LAD and CX catheter beyond the tip of the angiography catheter is performed slowly to allow the catheter to resume its shape as it emerges from the angiography catheter. For the same reason it is advisable to wait 15–20 s before the infusion catheter is advanced toward the LAD or CX. If the site of occlusion is more distal and the catheter shows a tendency to enter a side branch, stiffening of the catheter with 1–2 ml refrigerated saline or 5% dextrose may be helpful in preventing slippage of the catheter into side branches.

In general, penetration of the infusion catheter into the clot should be avoided, because on withdrawal the catheter may carry pieces of clot which remain unaffected by the infusion of the thrombolytic agent distally and may grow and obstruct the coronary artery.

There is sufficient space in the lumen of the angiography catheter to allow monitoring of the intracoronary pressure so that obstruction of the left main or the right coronary artery can be immediately detected. The space around the infusion catheter also allows intermittent injection of contrast medium to check for patency.

The Morphology of Coronary Thrombotic Occlusions Relevant to Thrombolytic Intervention

W.F.M. Fulton

University of Glasgow, Department of Materia Medica, Stobhill General Hospital, Glasgow, Scotland

The recently introduced percutaneous techniques of lysis and canalization of occlusive coronary thrombi have rekindled interest in the microanatomy of occlusive lesions. The clinical coronary angiogram prior to thrombolysis can give only limited information. Where occlusion is complete only the proximal face of the thrombus will be revealed, as a rule. Angiography can provide little evidence on the following features:

Severity of the stenosis that has been blocked by thrombus
Linear extent of the occlusive thrombus and its distally propagated non-occlusive extension
Composition of the thrombus
Disease of the arterial wall underlying the thrombus
State of the artery wall and lumen distal to occlusion.

However, each of these features has relevance for successful thrombolysis in the short term and for the prospects of sustained lumen patency after lysis. They can be studied only by appropriately conducted pathological examination.

The methods used in the present study have been outlined in my paper on coronary stenosis in this publication. Techniques of special importance in the study of the thrombotic occlusive lesions included the use of stereoarteriography and serial 2-mm thick mounted transverse sections throughout the length of the occlusive lesions. Correlation of the information obtained by these two methods allowed visual and graphic reconstruction of the microanatomy of the lesions. Selective histopathology gave critical information on the composition of thrombus, atheroma and intimal haemorrhagic dissection. The radiofibrinogen study [6, 8] introduced a time label in the course of thrombus formation, which allowed distinction to be made between thrombus formed close to the onset of myocardial infarction and that formed later.

Coronary Artery Stenosis Underlying Occlusive Thrombus

It is well recognised that coronary thrombosis only rarely occurs except at the site of severe atherosclerotic disease. Only by a serial section method can the point of maximum stenosis be identified. This was found to be of greater severity than I believe is generally supposed. Figure 1 indicates the lumen diameters at the point of maximum stenosis. Often the lumen was narrowed to this degree for only a few

Transluminal Coronary Angioplasty and
Intracoronary Thrombolysis. Ed. by Kaltenbach et al.

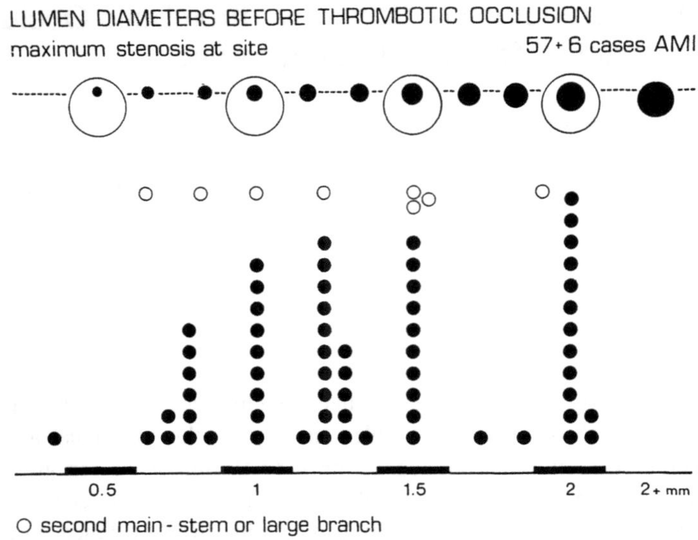

Fig. 1. Lumen diameters refer to the point of maximum stenosis as revealed by transverse sections throughout the lesion. *Solid circles* represent main-stem occlusions causally related to myocardial infarction. *Open circles* represent recent occlusive thrombus in other coronary arteries or major branches. The grouping at 1.0, 1.5 and 2.0 mm reflects observer preference for round figures (see text). In the schematic representation of stenosis a media-media diameter of 4 mm has been assumed, and 1 mm lumen diameter = 75% stenosis. Often media-media diameter was greater (5.0–5.5 mm), in which case stenosis would be relatively more severe (over 80%)

millimetres. The lumen underlying main stem occlusions was less than 1.5 mm in diameter in more than half the lesions, 1 mm or less in one-third and greater than 1.5 mm in only one-quarter. In no instance was the lumen greater than 2 mm at the narrowest point, i.e. about 50% stenosis.

Measurements of lumen diameter could be made with fair certainty in about half the lesions, the arterial wall being well defined and the contour nearly round. In other instances where the lumen was elliptical, ovoid or compressed into a less regular shape, the diameter recorded was an estimate of what it would have been had its cross-sectional area been enclosed in a circle. In about one-third of all lesions, at least at some point on the circumference of the lumen, the margins were ill defined. This made it impossible to define precisely the position of the endothelial lining on account of disruption of the plaque, usually by haemorrhagic dissection. The approximate dimensions of the lumen after death are recorded, no allowance being made for the possible size of the lumen prior to haemorrhage into the intima. These difficulties led to observer preference for approximate whole numbers, e.g. 1 mm in preference to 0.9 or 1.1 mm, hence the apparent uneven distribution in Fig. 1. Adjustment of the distribution curve can be made by grouping the lumen diameters as follows:
< 0.4, 0.4–0.6, 0.7–0.8, 0.9–1.1, 1.2–1.3, 1.4–1.7, 1.8–2.1, and < 2.1 mm lumen diameter. When this is done the totals in these groups are respectively 0, 2, 8, 11, 15, 12, 15, 0.

It is evident from the measurements of lumen diameter that successful thrombolysis alone is at best going to leave an importantly stenosed lumen in more than half the arteries and a severely stenosed lumen in about one-third.

Following complete thrombolysis angiographic display of the lumen becomes possible. It is remarkable how closely my own results correspond with those reported in this volume by Rutsch based on clinical coronary angiography after thrombolysis – all the more remarkable in view of the higher mean age of my subjects (all patients 64.4 years, males 63.6, females 65.8; range in 48 males, 38–77 years; range in 25 females, 47–77 years). It should also be noted that in my series each of the main stem occlusions (solid circles in Fig. 1) had been the cause of fatal myocardial infarction.

In addition the open circles record eight instances of fresh thrombotic occlusion of coronary main stems or branches other than the one believed to be directly responsible for the acute infarct. That second arteries can be occluded in this setting should be taken into account in deciding the extent to which the outlining of all coronary arteries at coronary angiography should be undertaken prior to thrombolysis. Some of the second lesions were definitely later than the primary occlusions but others were possibly coeval. Second thrombi have been described by Harland and Holburn [9] and Foord [3].

Length of Thrombotic Occlusions

The linear extent of complete occlusion by thrombus was measured in each of 57 lesions. The results are shown in Fig. 2. The extent to which thrombus extended proxi-

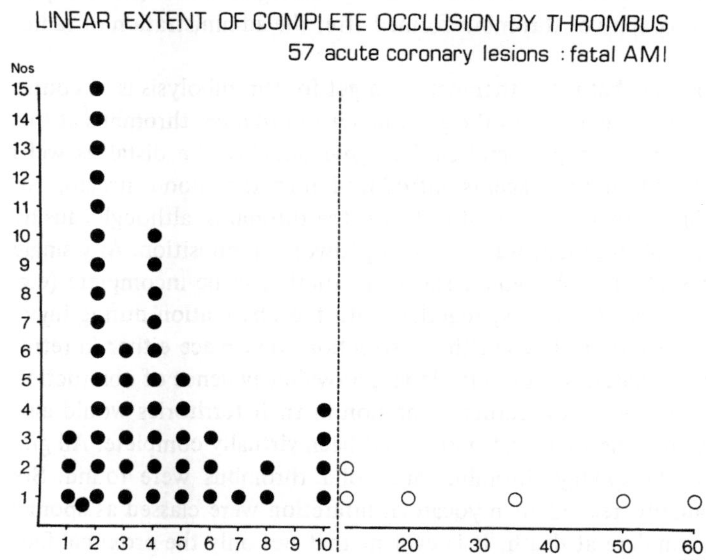

Fig. 2. Measurements of linear extent refer only to complete or virtually complete occlusion by thrombus. In most lesions non-occlusive thrombus extended proximally and/or distally, sometimes for many millimetres

mally and distally without occlusion was also measured but is not here recorded: it varied greatly. It can be seen from Fig. 2 that the extent of complete occlusion was often remarkably short. Indeed four lesions were complete for less than 2 mm and in three instances this was the entire length of the thrombus. Obstruction in 35% of lesions was complete for 2 mm or less; for 5 mm or less in 72%; for 10 mm or less in 90%. In only four lesions did complete occlusion extend for more than 12 mm, with obliteration of the lumen for 2–6 cm.

Not surprisingly the point of complete occlusion was usually at the same site as that of maximum stenosis. Also the radiofibrinogen study confirmed that at least part of the completely occlusive thrombus had been laid down early and that propagation of the thrombus continued after the administration of the radioactive label. Propagation was demonstrated in 25 of 41 cases where the radiofibrinogen was administered within 24 h and in 10 of 13 cases when it was given within 6 h of the onset. However only in eight instances, where the initial occlusive thrombus was radionegative, was the radioactive propagated thrombus completely occlusive. This observation provides strong evidence that complete occlusion may extend. A similar process may have affected lesions which were of low radioactivity throughout but with these lesions there is no evidence on the time course of secondary thrombosis.

Composition of the Thrombus

It is generally held that thrombus commences with platelet aggregation, soon builds up with platelets and fibrin, and to a greater or lesser degree incorporates red cells and white cells. My observations are in accord. Thrombi varied greatly in the relative proportion of these ingredients. With one possible exception, all occlusive thrombi contained large amounts of fibrin as revealed by histopathological stains (MSB in particular) and by autoradiography of thrombus formed after the administration of radiofibrinogen.

The portion of thrombus that is the therapeutic target for thrombolysis is of course that which causes complete occlusion. In the great majority instances thrombus at this point was "solid" and only the proximal surface (and possibly the distal as well) would be accessible to fibrinolytic agents introduced into the blood stream. An example is shown in Fig. 3. In a minority of instances the thrombus, although causing severe virtually complete obstruction, was of more openwork composition. Any single section taken through such thrombi would show obstruction to be incomplete (e.g. Fig. 4). However the stereoarteriograms, together with the observation during injection that the filling of the arteries beyond the obstruction took place either in retrograde fashion (through "collaterals") or very slowly, provided evidence of obstruction of severe grade. The presence of myocardial infarction in their territories would also be evidence acceptable to some that obstruction had been virtually complete. All gradations between obviously spongy thrombus and solid thrombus were found. Six main stem thrombi causally related to myocardial infarction were classed as spongy and three others as incomplete at death. It is evident that not only the proximal face but the full length of spongy thrombus can be percolated by thrombolytic agents introduced into the bloodstream – and at high concentration if introduced by intracoronary catheter.

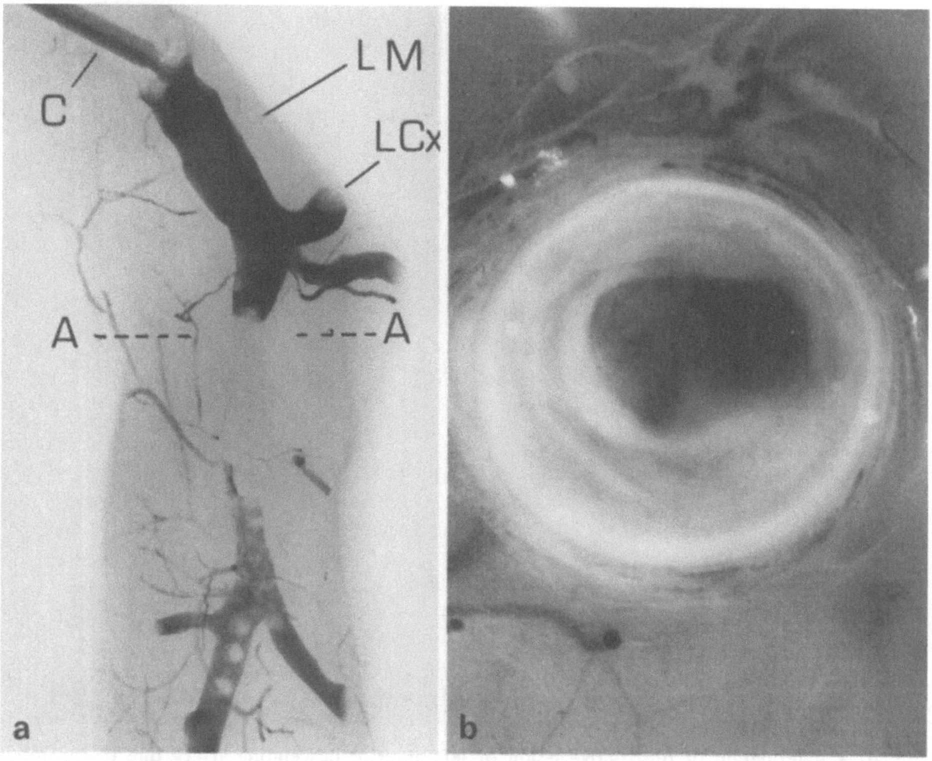

Fig. 3. a Arteriogram of complete occlusion of left anterior descending artery by solid thrombus. *C*, cannula; *LM*, left main coronary artery; *LCx*, left circumflex coronary artery. In contrast to clinical angiogram, retrograde filling through anastomoses distal to occlusion is seen in post-mortem arteriogram. **b** Section at *A-A* in Fig. 3a. Thrombus solid but not homogeneous: typical composition with greyish strands of fibrin/platelets and darker areas which incorporate more red cells

In many instances occlusion by solid thrombus was incomplete for part of its length as the result of separation of the thrombus from the arterial wall at one side. This may have resulted from shrinkage of the thrombus or from loss of tonus in the post-mortem artery [5]. Similar mechanisms in life would increase the access of thrombolytic agent to the greater length of the thrombus.

Thrombi were usually laid down in more than one episode. The time interval between such episodes is conjectural and possibly quite short as a rule; but in a few instances the first episode was clearly several weeks in duration. This may have importance in so far as older fibrin is more resistant to fibrinolytic agents.

Disease of the Artery Wall Underlying Thrombotic Occlusion

As already noted, in all lesions there was at least 50% encroachment on the lumen by atherosclerosis prior to thrombosis (Figs. 1, 3, 5). The atherosclerotic lesions were usually of a complex nature consistent with their genesis in earlier episodes of thrombus

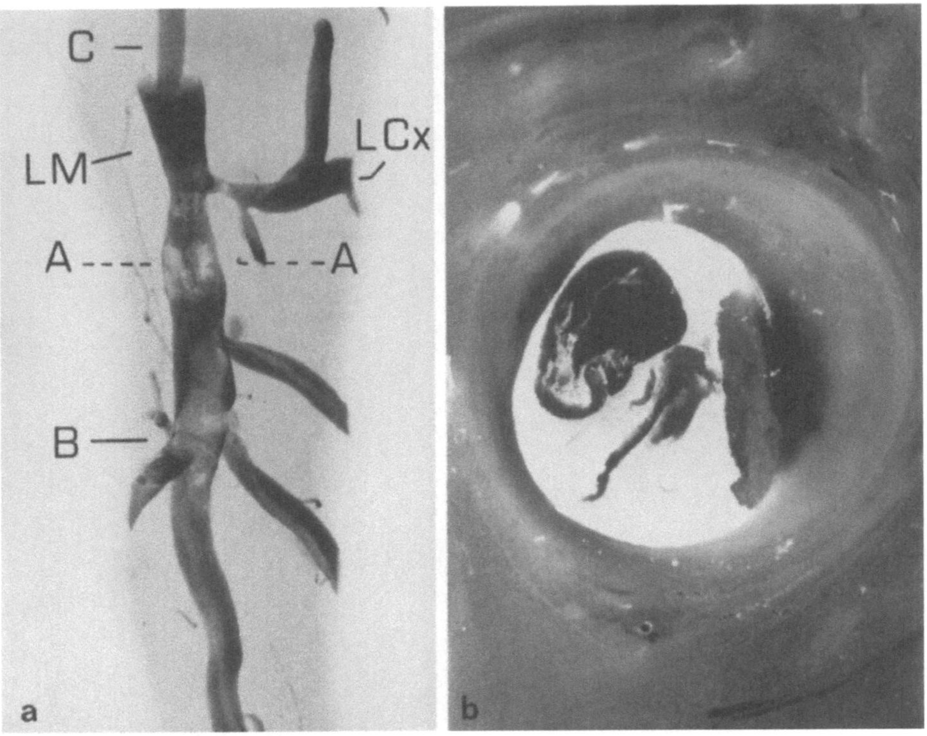

Fig. 4. a Arteriogram of obstructive lesion of left anterior descending artery due to thrombus that forms a spongework. In total the obstruction was sufficient to cause myocardial infarction and for filling during injection to be retrograde beyond the obstruction. *C* cannula; *LM*, left main coronary artery; *LCx*, left circumflex coronary artery; *B*, distal propagation with partial impaction at bifurcation.
b Section at A-A in Fig. 4a. Section through the spongy thrombus, partly pale and attached to the wall (*right*) and partly "free" in the lumen. As seen in any one section, occlusion seems far from complete but the evidence of stereoarteriography confirmed the highly obstructive nature of the total lesion

and/or intimal haemorrhage [5, 7]. The pigmented character of such lesions was described in my paper on stenosis in this volume. A minority of lesions appeared to be fairly stable but for the most part lesions complicated by thrombosis appeared to have been friable. In 47 of 63 instances a break in the luminal lining had allowed blood to burst into the diseased intima. In some 23 of 47 instances the haemorrhage was on a large scale (haemorrhagic dissection), with apparent compression of the lumen to varying degree in 20 instances (Figs. 5–7).

Tears in the intimal lining had exposed flowing blood to the material composing the underlying lesions. This was the probable cause of platelet aggregation and fibrin deposition [1, 4, 9, 11]. Mostly the overlying thrombus had sealed off the defect in the intima. In only one instance was there definite evidence that occlusion adjacent to the site of an intimal tear was composed mainly of the extruded contents of a thromboatheroma.

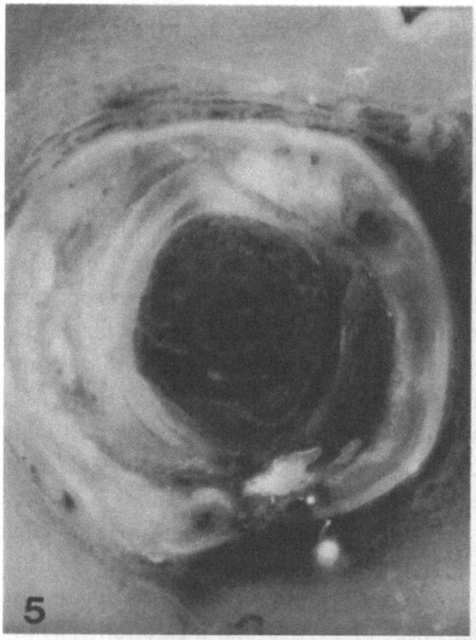

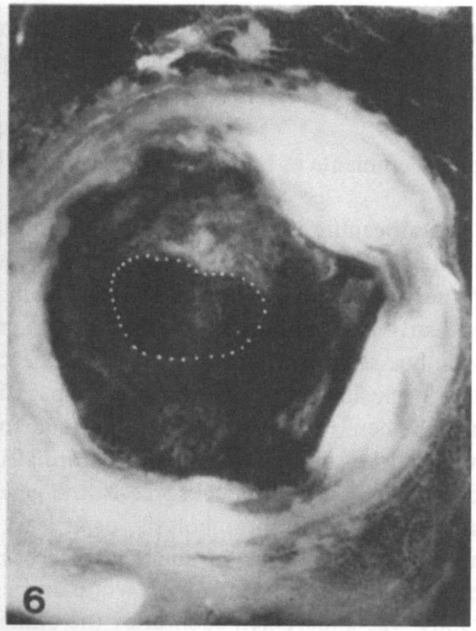

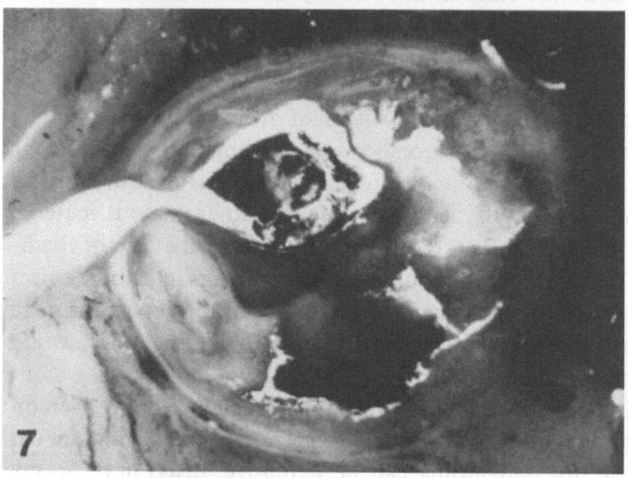

Fig. 5. Haemorrhagic dissection disrupting the intima underlying occlusive thrombus. Haemorrhage entered the intima through a tear at a higher level and is itself partially explored by pale injection medium (surface view 2 mm section)

Fig. 6. Extensive haemorrhagic dissection. The previous lumen, now occupied by thrombus, is outlined by the *white dots* (surface view 2 mm section)

Fig. 7. Diseased intima at distal extremity of a thrombotic occlusion. The lumen is occupied by white injection medium in which late, propagated thrombus is embedded. The injection medium has also explored the friable structure of the "plaque", which had manifestly been derived from an earlier thrombotic episode and which still had only a thin fibrous surface layer separating the unorganised material from the lumen (surface view 2 mm section)

Successful thrombolysis would again expose the material of the atheromatous lesions to flowing blood. Whether the thrombogenic activity of this material would be as active as in the first instance is speculative, but secondary thrombotic occlusion after thrombolysis may be due to this circumstance. Further, the contents of the atheroma now no longer blanketed by thrombus could well be extruded into the lumen to impact in small branches downstream [10]. Theoretically small infarcts could result but I have only one instance in which this appears to have occurred in the natural course of an acute occlusive coronary episode.

Some Comments in Relation to Therapeutic Fibrinolysis

If the procedure is to be successful in limiting or preventing myocardial infarction, it is evident on other grounds that thrombolysis must be undertaken early in the course of the clinical illness. It would seem from the morphological studies here reported that early intervention would also carry a greater prospect of success in so far as the thrombus seems to tend to increase in the course of time, both as extension of complete occlusion and non-occlusive propagation. It must, however, be noted that the thrombi here reported had been destined to remain completely occlusive or virtually so and to be the cause of fatal myocardial infarction. It is possible that this evidence does not apply with equal force to the generality of thrombotic occlusions in which early spontaneous thrombolysis, or at least the reopening of a channel alongside the thrombus, may occur in some instances and may possibly favour survival. In this context the observations of De Wood and colleagues [2] are relevant. Coronary angiography was undertaken soon after the clinical onset of myocardial infarction. The incidence of related complete occlusion, probably due to thrombus, was higher (89%) in those cases investigated within 3 h of onset than was found in cases between 12 and 24 h of onset (65%).

The uncovering of subendothelial structures by lysis of a thrombus occluding an intimal tear has potential for reactivation of thrombosis. Accordingly, there are strong theoretical reasons for adopting antithrombotic measures after successful thrombolysis.

As another consequence of fibrinolysis, in some instances atheromatous material is likely to be displaced into the lumen. The resultant reduction in the size of the lesion at its site of previous maximum stenosis could be a favourable result, to be offset against the possible adverse effects of small artery embolic occlusion downstream. In the presence of coronary anastomotic enlargement it is likely that such emboli would usually be sustained without major injury.

It would be natural to entertain the fear that thrombolysis might extend haemorrhagic dissection and that this might be hazardous. However, although spontaneous haemorrhagic dissection of the diseased intima can be extensive, it has never in my observations come more than perilously close to the medial coat. Rupture through the internal elastic lamina and outer coats has not been witnessed by me in the coronary arteries. Usually the process of dissection was separated from the outer coats by a fairly substantial, mainly fibrous, atherosclerotic layer, presumably formed many years earlier. It was the probably more recently formed softer structureless material lying between the outer layers and the lumen that was explored by haemorrhage. Accordingly there seems to me little probability that fibrinolysis alone will lead to rupture of the artery wall.

On the other hand instrumental disruption of the thrombus might possibly disturb the integrity of the outer layers of intimal sclerosis. Certainly a mechanical device introduced through the catheter might explore the atheromatous intima more extensively than the original haemorrhage.

These observations are not put forward to discourage these new ventures in the management of acute coronary thrombotic events but to draw attention to the possibilities for success and for complication to which a detailed study of the morphology of the lesions in question would seem to point.

Acknowledgements. The current research programme is supported by a grant from the Scottish Home and Health Department. The radiofibrinogen study was made in collaboration with Dr. D.J. Sumner, Department of Nuclear Medicine. Acknowledgement is also made to the co-operation of the clinical and nursing staff of the Coronary Care Unit and the Departments of Pathology and Radiodiagnosis, Stobhill General Hospital, Glasgow.

References

1. Constantinides P (1966) Plaque fissures in human coronary thrombosis. J Atheroscler Res 6:1–17
2. De Wood MA, Spores J, Notske R et al. (1980) Prevalence of total coronary occlusion during the early hours of transmural myocardial infarction. N Engl J Med 303:897–902
3. Foord AG (1948) Embolism and thrombosis in coronary heart disease. J Am Med Assoc 138:1009–1012
4. Friedman M, Van den Bovenkamp GT (1966) The pathogenesis of a coronary thrombus. Am J Pathol 48:19–44
5. Fulton WFM (1965) The coronary arteries: arteriography, microanatomy and pathogenesis of obliterative coronary artery disease. Chas Thomas, Springfield
6. Fulton WFM (1978a) Coronary thrombosis in myocardial infarction. In: Wilhelmson L, Hjalmarson A (eds) Acute and Long-term Medical Management of Myocardial Ischaemia, Eds. Lindgren and Soner, Mölndal, pp 59–69
7. Fulton WFM (1978b) Coronary thrombotic occlusion in myocardial infarction and the role of thrombus in the pathogenesis of atherosclerosis. In: Carlson LA et al. (eds) International Conference on Atherosclerosis. Raven Press, New York, pp 75–89
8. Fulton WFM, Sumner DJ (1979) Radiofibrinogen in a study of fatal myocardial infarction. Proc VIIth Int Conf on Thrombosis and Haemostasis [Abstr]. Thromb Haemost 42:38
9. Harland WA, Holburn AM (1966) Coronary thrombosis and myocardial infarction. Lancet 2.1158–1160
10. Jørgensen L, Chandler AB, Borchgrevink CF (1971) Acute lesions of coronary arteries in anticoagulant-treated and in untreated patients. Atherosclerosis 13:21–44
11. Sinapius D (1972) Beziehungen zwischen Koronarthrombosen und Myokardinfarkten. Dtsch Med Wochenschr 97:443–448

Fibrinogen in Successful and Unsuccessful Cases

W. Huhmann, R. Allner, H. Nieth

Med. Klinik I, Städtische Kliniken, 6400 Fulda, FRG

Angiographic findings before and during intracoronary streptokinase application in patients with acute myocardial infarctions are controversial: 23% of the patients have subtotally stenosed coronary arteries without thrombosis, 77% show thrombotic occlusions. Of these occlusions, 83% can be opened but 17% remain occluded. Moreover, in patients with infarcts of only 30 min duration thrombotic occlusion can occur during observation and in spite of streptokinase injections [1]. To find out the mechanism of these discrepancies we studied several parameters of the blood coagulation system.

Method

In 27 patients with acute myocardial infarction coronary angiography was performed immediately after hospital admission and 2000 IU/min streptokinase was administered intracoronarily. There were four groups: in 12 patients coronary arteries could be opened within 3 h of onset of chest pain (early); in seven patients opening was reached after more than 3 h (late); in four patients the arteries remained occluded (negative); and four patients had only subtotally stenosed coronary arteries (subtotal). In all of these patients fibrinogen (FG) levels were measured intravenously every 2 h for 52 h.

Moreover, plasminogen, fibrinogen, and fibrin splits were measured before treatment, every 30 min for 4 h after treatment, and 24 h after treatment. There were two groups: in five patients with intracoronary streptokinase application blood sampling was done from coronary arteries and from a peripheral vein synchronously, and in eight patients with 500 000 IU streptokinase given systemically within 30 min [2] blood sampling was done from a peripheral vein.

Results

Fibrinogen After Intracoronary Streptokinase Application

The results of fibrinogen measurements for 52 h after intracoronary streptokinase application are shown in Fig. 1. The lower part illustrates that fibrinogen in patients

Transluminal Coronary Angioplasty and
Intracoronary Thrombolysis. Ed. by Kaltenbach et al.

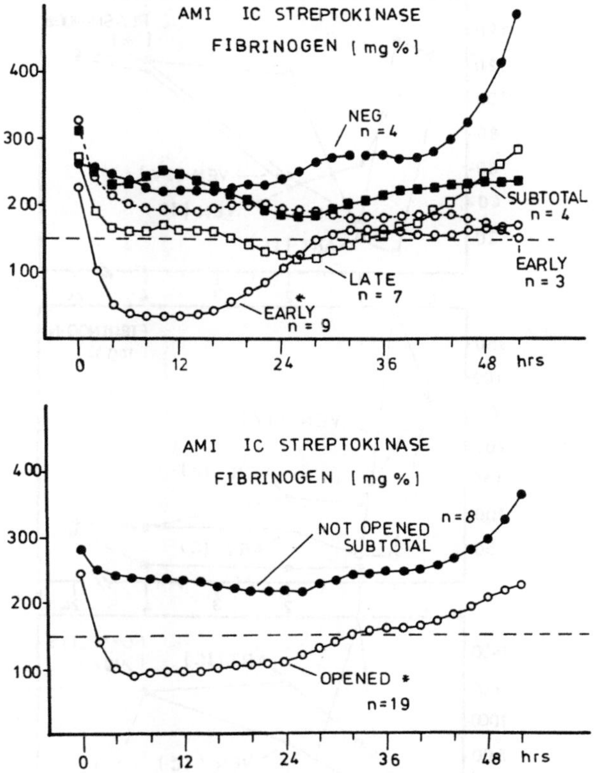

Fig. 1. Fibrinogen every 2 hours after intracoronary (*IC*) streptokinase treatment in patients with acute myocardial infarction (*AMI*). *Broken line* indicates lower normal values. *Asterisks* indicate significance ($P < 0.05$)

in whom the coronary arteries could be opened decreased significantly for more than 24 h compared to patients who could not be opened or had subtotal coronary artery stenoses.

The difference was caused by a significant decrease in the early group, whereas the late group reached only subnormal values. No change could be seen in patients where opening failed to occur or in those with subtotal occlusions. In the early group we saw three patients with infarcts of 30 min duration who developed an occlusion during our observation but could be reopened later. In these patients fibrinogen did not change.

Fibrinogen, Plasminogen, and Fibrin Splits

Figure 2 shows the results of the first 4 h of fibrinogen, plasminogen, and fibrin splits measurements in those patients in whom the arteries could be opened. During intracoronary streptokinase application fibrinogen and plasminogen decreased immediately in the coronary artery followed by venous circulation with a delay of 30 min. Plas-

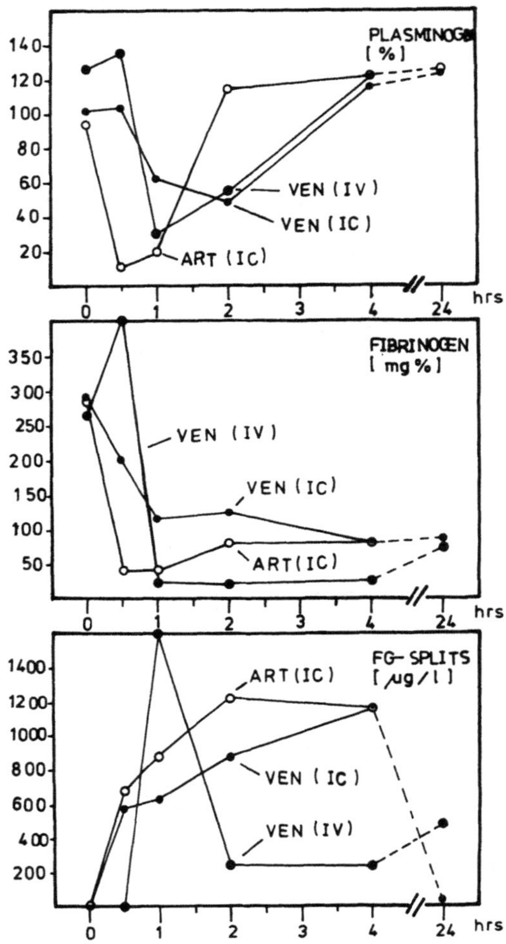

Fig. 2. Plasminogen (*PG*), fibrinogen (*FG*), and fibrin splits (FSP) in successful cases. Streptokinase was injected either intracoronarily or intravenously. Blood sampling was done from coronary artery (*ART IC*) and peripheral vein (*VEN IC*) synchronously or from the veins only (*VEN IV*)

minogen then recovered, reaching normal levels after 2–4 h . Fibrinogen, however, remained low for more than 24 h. These changes indicate that there is a systemic effect after intracoronary streptokinase application. Fibrin splits appeared at once in the coronary arteries and in the veins, reaching effective blood levels, and then remained high for more than 4 h.

After intravenous streptokinase application changes of fibrinogen, plasminogen, anf fibrin splits were similar but happened after a delay of 1 h. In patients in the intravenous streptokinase group in whom the arteries could not be opened (50%) we found significantly lower initial plasminogen values (109.7 ± 13.4% against 51.7 ± 25.7%, $P < 0.05$).

Figure 3 illustrates that creatine kinase peak activity was reached after 24 h, indicating that the arteries remained occluded [2]. This was controlled angiographically. Fi-

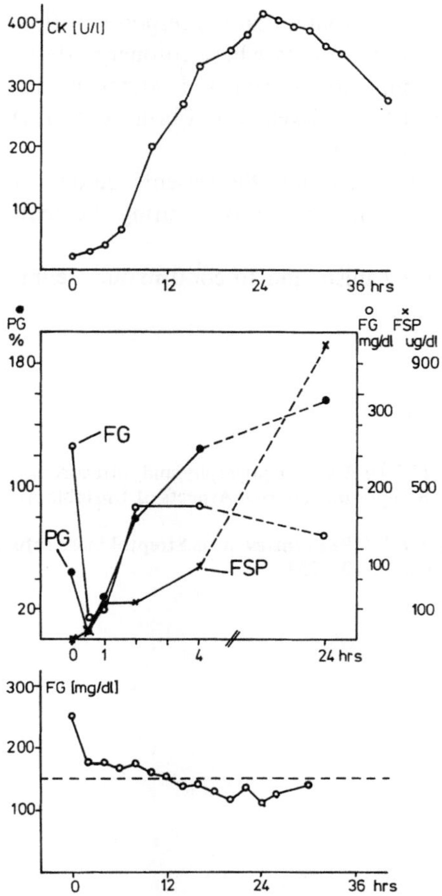

Fig. 3. Creatine kinase (*CK*), plasminogen (*PG*), fibrinogen (*FG*), and fibrin splits (*FSP*) in unsuccessful cases

brinogen in those patients was not altered very much within 48 h, showing failure to respond to treatment.

However, looking at the first 4 h plasminogen was low initially and then decreased almost to zero, but recovered to normal values after more than 2 h. Fibrinogen decreased at first but increased again, being normal during the remainder of the measurement period. Fibrin splits failed to appear initially, and first became effective after more than 4 h.

Conclusions

Different findings of coronary artery situation as well as varying response to treatment in patients with acute myocardial infarction raise the question of the mechanism of these discrepancies. In our studies of blood coagulation system during and after intracoronary or intravenous streptokinase application we found that the response of fibrinogen to treatment was entirely different in those patients where coronary arteries could be opened from those where opening could not be achieved. Moreover, unsuccessful cases started with low initial plasminogen levels and fibrin splits first appeared after a delay, reaching relatively low blood levels.

Whether these differences are due to a different situation in the patients' blood coagulation systems, to a varying response to treatment, or to shock during the acute myocardial infarction is still unknown.

More studies are necessary to find out the mechanism and to confirm our preliminary results.

Results

1. Huhmann W, Duangphung K, Krunke M, Nieth H (1980) Acute angiography and intracoronary Streptokinase in acute myocardial infarction. In: Symposium on New Aspects of Unstable Angina Pectoris, Oct 16–18 1980, Hannover
2. Schroeder R, Biamino G, Von Leitner E-R, Linderer T (1981) Intravenöse Streptokinase Infusion bei akutem Myokardinfarkt. Dtsch Med Wochenschr 106:294

Preservation of Function by Nonsurgical Coronary Artery Reperfusion

P. Rentrop, K.R. Karsch, H. Blanke, W. Rutsch, W. Merx, D. Mathey

Mount Sinai Medial Center, New York, N.Y., USA
University of Göttingen, FRG
Klinikum Charlottenburg of the Free University of Berlin
University Hospital Eppendorf, Hamburg, FRG
Dept. of Internal Medicine, University Hospital, Aachen, FRG

Reperfusion by intracoronary streptokinase infusion resulted in early and late improvement of ejection fraction and local wall motion in the majority of infarct patients treated by this method [15]. Improvement of function and preservation of R waves were more frequent and more marked than in conventionally treated patients [16]. The relationships between the functional changes and both duration of symptoms prior to hospital admission and the presence or absence of angiographically demonstrable collaterals prior to reperfusion will be analyzed in the present collaborative study.

Materials and Methods

Intracoronary streptokinase infusion (Kabikinase, Deutsche Kabi GmbH, Streptase, Behring Werke) has been applied in 209 patients in the four participating centers (Universities of Aachen, Berlin-Charlottenburg, Goettingen, and Hamburg) between June 1979 and December 1980. The diagnosis of acute myocardial infarction was based on a history of chest pain of more than 20 min duration not alleviated by nitroglycerin, ECG changes compatible with acute myocardial ischemia, and increase of CPK to pathological values upon serial determination (retrospective confirmation of the diagnosis). All patients who were suspected of having acute myocardial infarction and arrived at the hospital within 3 h (one center) or 6 h (three centers) of onset of chest pain were considered candidates for the study. To patients arriving after more than 6 h of chest pain, intervention angiography was offered only if they still had severe chest pain. Asymptomatic patients arriving more than 6 h after onset of pain were not considered candidates. Informed consent was obtained. The catheterization techniques have been described in another presentation at this symposium.

The infarct-related coronary artery was completely obstructed in 166 patients and reperfusion was achieved in 129 patients. The study group is comprised of 46 patients in whom cineventriculography was performed prior to reperfusion as well as in the chronic stage of infarction 2–4 weeks later (before any surgical intervention), and in whom patency of the recanalized vessel was found. The mean age of the patients was 56 years.

Transluminal Coronary Angioplasty and
Intracoronary Thrombolysis. Ed. by Kaltenbach et al.

In 21 patients the left anterior descending artery was recanalized, in eight patients the left circumflex artery, and in 17 patients the right coronary artery. In 23 patients collaterals to the occluded vessel were demonstrated by intervention angiography, and in the remaining 23 patients collaterals were not seen. Eight patients were admitted within 3 h of onset of chest pain (group A), 25 patients had pain for more than 3 h and less than 6 h (group B), and 13 patients had pain for more than 6 h before admission (group C). Ideally patients should be grouped according to duration of symptoms prior to reperfusion rather than prior to hospital admission. However, this information was not available in all patients. If reperfusion was achieved it occurred within approximately 30–90 minutes of hospitalization.

There was only one striking difference between the subgroups' acute coronary angiography results: collaterals to the infarcting area were visualized in only three of eight group A patients (38%) and 11 of 25 group B patients (44%), but in 9 of 13 group C patients (69%).

Volumes were calculated from monoplane RAO cineventriculograms [7]. Data presented are mean values ± standard deviations. Values of P above 0.05 were considered nonsignificant (NS).

Results

In the total study group of 46 patients ejection fraction increased significantly from 52% ± 13% prior to reperfusion to 56% ± 16% in the chronic stage of infarction ($P < 0.025$). Left ventricular end-diastolic pressure and peak systolic pressure were not significantly different during acute and chronic angiography.

In group A ejection fraction rose significantly from 51% ± 12% prior to reperfusion to 65% ± 6% at the time of chronic angiography ($P < 0.025$). Improvement of global left ventricular function occurred in seven patients in this group, and in one patient ejection fraction remained unchanged.

In group B mean ejection fraction did not change (acute, 52% ± 13%; chronic, 52% ± 16%). In six patients there was a rise of ejection fraction by at least 10%, in six patients ejection fraction was decreased at least 10% at the time of chronic angiography. It was striking that in the subgroup of ten group B patients admitted 3–4 h after onset of pain only two patients showed clear-cut improvement of ejection fraction.

In group C ejection fraction rose significantly from 51% ± 14% to 59% ± 17% ($P < 0.01$).

While there was no significant difference of ejection fraction between the subgroups prior to the intervention, the chronic ejection fraction values were significantly higher in group A than in group B ($p < 0.0125$).

There were no significant differences of pressures or heart rate between the subgroups. Left ventricular end-diastolic pressure decreased from 18 ± 6 mmHg prior to the intervention to 14 ± 6 mmHg at the time of chronic angiography in group A (NS), from 19 ± 9 mmHg to 17 ± 9 mmHg in group B (NS), and from 17 ± 8 mmHg to 16 ± 11 mmHg in group C (NS). Peak systolic pressure rose slightly from 123 ± 10 mmHg to 128 ± 23 mmHg in group A (NS), and from 124 ± 23 mmHg to 127 ±

19 mmHg in group B (NS); it decreased from 133 ± 28 mmHg to 131 ± 22 mmHg in group C (NS).

Ejection fraction rose from 51% ± 14% to 57% ± 18% in patients with collaterals, and from 54% ± 12% to 56% ± 13% in patients without angiographically demonstrable collaterals to the infarct area. Only the improvement in the group of patients with collaterals achieved statistical significance ($P < 0.025$). In group A improvement of function occurred regardless of presence or absence of collaterals. In group B no correlation between left ventricular function changes and presence or absence of collaterals could be found. In the nine group C patients with angiographically demonstrable collaterals there was a significant rise of ejection fraction from 53% ± 15% to 63% ± 15% ($P < 0.005$), whereas ejection fraction did not change in the four group C patients without collaterals (acute, 47% ± 13%; chronic, 49% ± 20%).

Discussion

The distinctive difference in functional changes after reperfusion in patients admitted to the hospital within 3 h after onset of chest pain compared to patients admitted during the 4th h after onset of symptoms is remarkable. Since reperfusion was achieved within 1 h of hospital admission as a rule, our findings suggest that the critical time for preservation of left ventricular function by reperfusion is the first 4 h after onset of ischemic symptoms.

In dogs and primates early or late improvement of local and global left ventricular function was found uniformly if reperfusion was carried out within 3 h after coronary obstruction [2, 6, 11, 12, 13, 14]. Reperfusion after 4 h occlusion was less frequently associated with return of function [13, 14]. No return of function was seen if coronary artery occlusion was released after 5 h [13, 14]. Correlative experimental studies have shown that lack of return of function after reperfusion is usually associated with the development of irreversible damage of the corresponding myocardial segment [5, 13, 14, 17].

Some experimental data suggest that reperfusion may lead to the acceleration of cell death and infarct extension [1, 9]. In the absence of a control group we cannot determine whether the marked deterioration of global function which occurred in 6 of 25 group B patients is due to reperfusion damage.

Group C was the only subgroup in which a significant correlation was found between improvement of function and presence of angiographically demonstrable collaterals. The striking angiographic finding in this group was visualization of collaterals to the infarcting area in the majority of patients. Group C, however, is not representative of patients admitted to the hospital after more than 6 h chest pain, since these patients were accepted for reperfusion only if they had continuing severe chest pain at the time of evaluation.

From experimental studies it has been known that the occlusion of a major coronary artery results in extensive loss of function and of viable myocardium if there is no collateral supply to the area perfused by the obstructed vessel [4]. Development of an adequate collateral system prior to coronary obstruction can limit or even prevent the loss of function and of myocardium [4]. In humans the natural history of left ventricular function after coronary obstruction, in the presence of collaterals, has not been studied prospectively. Retrospective angiographic [8, 10] and pathoanatomic [3] studies suggest that the loss of function and contractile tissue may be limited by "adequate" collaterals. Our data do not permit us to postulate a causative relationship between coronary artery recanalization and improvement of function in patients reperfused after more than 6 h chest pain.

References

1. Banka VS, Chadda KD, Helfant RH (1974) Limitations of myocardial revascularization in restoration of regional contraction abnormalities produced by coronary occlusion. Am J Cardiol 34:164–170
2. Blumenthal MR, Wang H, Liu LMP (1975) Experimental coronary artery occlusion and release. Am J Cardiol 36:225–233
3. Blumgart HL, Schlesinger MJ, Davis D (1940) Studies on the relation of the clinical manifestations of angina pectoris, coronary thrombosis, and myocardial infarction to the pathologic findings. Am Heart J 19:1–91
4. Blumgart HL, Zoll PM, Freedberg AS, Gilligan DP (1950) The experimental production of intercoronary arterial anastomoses and their functional significance. Circulation 1:20–27
5. Capone RJ, Most AS (1978) Myocardial hemorrhage after coronary reperfusion in pigs. Am J Cardiol 41.259–266
6. Costantini C, Corday E, Lang T et al. (1975) Revascularization after 3 hours of coronary arterial occlusion: effects on regional cardiac metabolic function and infarct size. Am J Cardiol 36:368–384
7. Dodge HT, Sandler H, Baxley WA, Hawley RR (1966) Usefulness and limitations of radiographic methods for determining left ventricular volume. Am J Cardiol 18;10–24
8. Hamby RJ, Aintablian A, Schwartz A (1976) Reappraisal of the functional significance of the coronary collateral circulation. Am J Cardiol 38:305–309
9. Lang TW, Corday E, Gold H et al. (1974) Consequences of reperfusion after coronary occlusion. Effects on hemodynamic and regional myocardial metabolic function. Am J Cardiol 33.69–81
10. Levin DC (1974) Pathways and functional significance of the coronary collateral circulation. Circulation 50:831–837
11. Maroko PR, Libby P, Ginks WR et al. (1972) Coronary artery reperfusion. I. Early effects on local myocardial function and the extent of myocardial necrosis. J Clin Invest 51:2710–2716
12. Mathur VS, Guinn GA, Burris WH (1975) Maximal revascularization (reperfusion) in intact conscious dogs after 2 to 5 hours of coronary ocfclusion. Am J Cardiol 36:252–261
13. McNamara JJ, Smith GT, Suehiro GT et al. (1974) Myocardial viability after transient ischemia in primates. J Thorac Cardiovasc Surg 68:248–256
14. Puri PS (1975) Contractile and biochemical effects of coronary reperfusion after extended periods of coronary occlusion. Am J Cardiol 36:244–251
15. Rentrop P, Blanke H, Karsch KR, Kaiser H, Koestering H, Leitz K (1981) Selective intracoronary thrombolysis in acute myocardial infarction and unstable angina pectoris. Circulation 63.307–317
16. Rentrop P, Blanke H. Karsch KR (1982) Effects of non-surgical reperfusion upon the left ventricle in man, compared with conventional treatment. Am J Cardiol 49:1–8
17. Schaper W, Frenzel H, Hort W, Winkler B (1979) Experimental coronary artery occlusion. II. Spatial and temporal evolution of infarcts in the dog heart. Basic Res Cardiol 74:233–239

Left Ventricular Function After Reopening of Occluded Coronary Arteries

W. Huhmann, K. Duangphung

Med. Klinik I, Städtische Kliniken, 6400 Fulda, FRG

Patients who survive an acute myocardial infarction have a restricted left ventricular function [5]. This is shown in Fig. 1 in a group of 42 normally treated patients who were studied hemodynamically 4 weeks after an acute myocardial infarction. Thirteen had subtotally stenosed coronary arteries and 29 had total occlusion. Mainly those with total occlusions had elevated end-diastolic pressures, high end-systolic volumes, decreased ejection fractions, and large akinetic areas.

However, spontaneous recanalization of the occluded vessel and reperfusion of the ischemic area improve left ventricular function, as can be seen in Fig. 1 where those patients with subtotal stenoses have a slightly better ventricular performance.

If reopening can be achieved within the time when myocardial muscle is still viable [1, 6] one can expect to get further improvement of ventricular function. Thus, the aim of this presentation is to show that the infarct size can be influenced in general and that there is a time within which ventricular can be significantly improved for a long period.

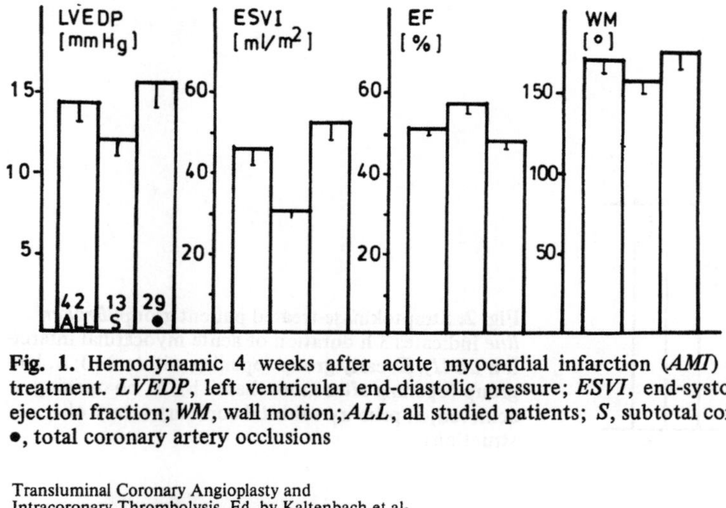

Fig. 1. Hemodynamic 4 weeks after acute myocardial infarction (*AMI*) without streptokinase treatment. *LVEDP*, left ventricular end-diastolic pressure; *ESVI*, end-systolic volume index; *EF*, ejection fraction; *WM*, wall motion; *ALL*, all studied patients; *S*, subtotal coronary artery stenoses; •, total coronary artery occlusions

Transluminal Coronary Angioplasty and
Intracoronary Thrombolysis. Ed. by Kaltenbach et al.

Method

We have treated 40 patients with acute myocardial infarction with streptokinase infusions so far. However, we only wish to present the results of those 16 patients in whom the occluded coronary artery could be reopened and who could be catheterized acutely, 4 weeks after treatment, and 3 months later.

All patients had 2000 IU streptokinase intracoronarily immediately after hospital admission and after the first hemodynamic measurements, as well as levocardiograms and coronary arteriograms.

Using Sones' technique levocardiograms were performed in 40° RAO projection injecting 20 ml Urografin 76 with a flow rate of 10 ml acutely and 40/20 ml during control angiographies. Coronary injections were done first into noninfarcted vessel and thereafter into infarcted vessel in at least two projections.

There was an early group with infarcts of 30–120 min duration from onset of chest pain to admission to hospital (Fig. 2). The arteries could be opened within 25–55 min, so that the total duration of occlusion was less than 3 h.

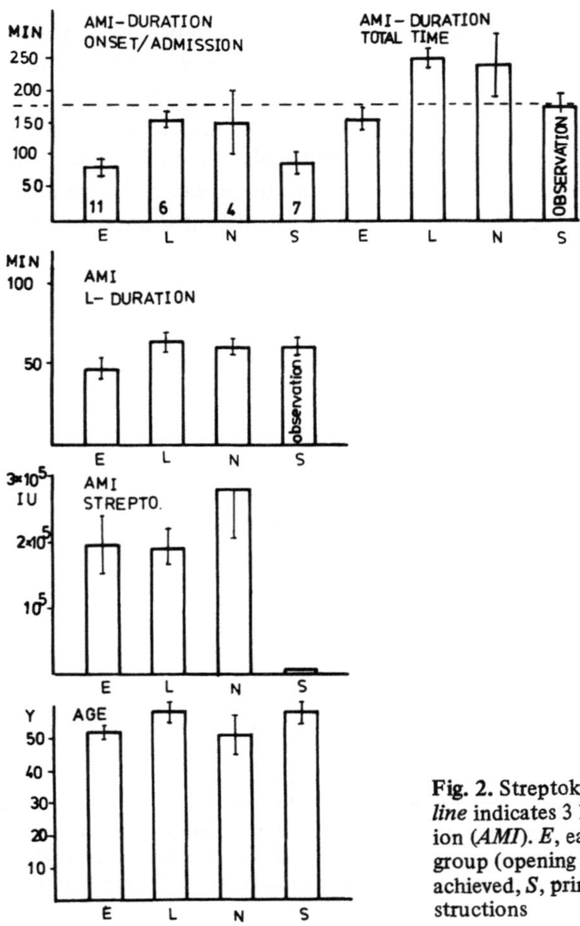

Fig. 2. Streptokinase-treated patient group. *Broken line* indicates 3 h duration of acute myocardial infarction (*AMI*). *E*, early group (opening within 3 h); *L*, late group (opening after more than 3 h); *N*, no opening achieved, *S*, primary subtotal coronary artery obstructions

We then had a late group with infarcts of 120–170 min duration. In this group opening took 45–75 min so that the total duration of the infarct was more than 3 h from onset of chest pain.

The groups with negative response to treatment and with primary subtotally stenosed arteries will not be discussed in this presentation. We wish to concentrate on the comparison between the early and late groups, who received the same total amount of streptokinase per patient.

The comparison was done statistically using the t test for two means. The figures are shown as mean values and standard error of the mean. Significances are based on $P < 0.05$.

To evaluate left ventricular function end-diastolic pressure (LVEDP), end-systolic volume index (ESVI), ejection fraction (EF), and wall motion (WM) were compared acutely and 4 weeks and 3 months after treatment.

Results

Figure 3 shows changes in LVEDP from acute values to 4 weeks and 3 months later. Acutely, early and late groups both had elevated filling pressures. Possibly due to longer infarct duration, greater impairment, and therefore larger infarct sizes the filling pressure in the late group was significantly higher than in the early group. This difference disappeared 4 weeks and 3 months later, although there were still higher pressures in the late group.

In both groups initial pressures decreased, but became normal after 4 weeks and 3 months in the early group. These changes were statistically significant. In the late

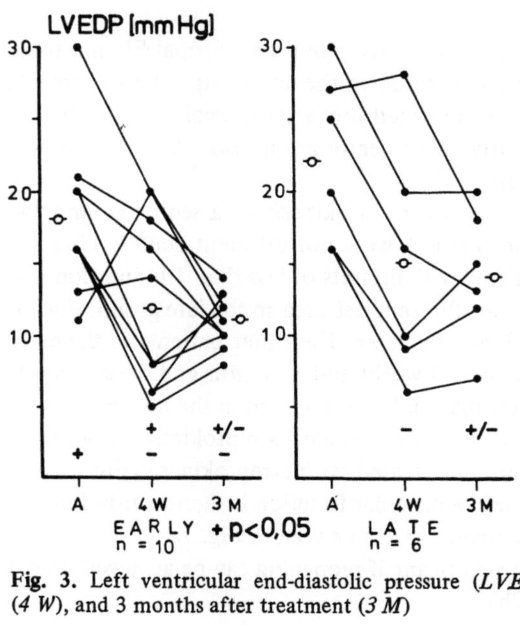

Fig. 3. Left ventricular end-diastolic pressure (*LVEDP*) acutely (*A*), 4 weeks after treatment (*4 W*), and 3 months after treatment (*3 M*)

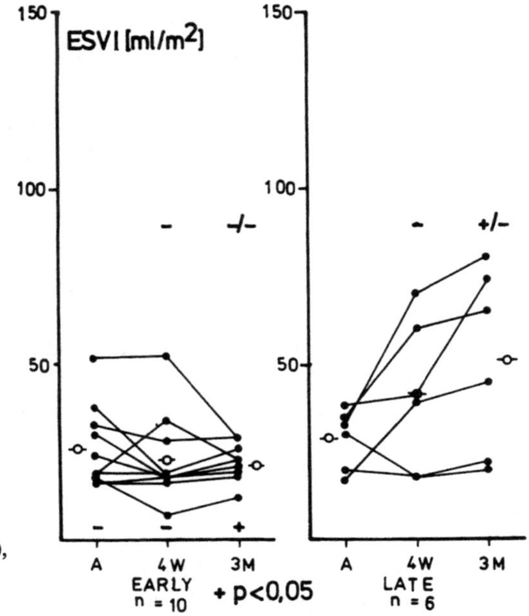

Fig. 4. End-systolic volume index (*ESVI*) acutely (*A*), 4 weeks after treatment (*4 W*), and 3 months after treatment (*3 M*)

group only the 3 months values were significantly decreased, but there were still some patients with elevated pressures.

Since filling pressures are related to cavity size they can be low if ventricles enlarge. This is shown in Fig. 4.

Initially ESVI was almost normal in both the early and late groups. Those patients of the early group who had an enlarged ventricle acutely normalized their chamber size. However, in the late group chambers got bigger and were significantly enlarged after 3 months.

During acute infarction some patients of the early group had normal EF and some had decreased EF (Fig. 5); mean EF was higher than in the late group. This difference, however, was not significant. Whereas EF remained low after 4 weeks and 3 months in the late group it increased significantly in the early group; this increase was also significantly different from the late group.

Mean values of WM, given in degrees of hypo- or akinesia of a sector around the centre of the projected left ventricular area [3], were not different acutely (Fig. 6). However, in the early group our six patients with infarcts of less than 1 h duration had hypokinetic areas which were smaller than the smallest area in the late group. Five of these patients had almost normal WM 3 months later. The other patients in the early group had only small hypokinetic zones after 4 weeks and 3 months and these changes were significant. On the other hand no change could be observed in the late group.

If we compare the findings 4 weeks after intracoronary streptokinase application with our group of 29 patients who were not treated with streptokinase (Fig. 1) and still have occluded arteries we find that left ventricular function is significantly improved after intracoronary streptokinase treatment, as can be seen in Fig. 7a.

This improvement, however, is only significant if reopening can be achieved within 3 h of commencement of infarct (Fig. 7b).

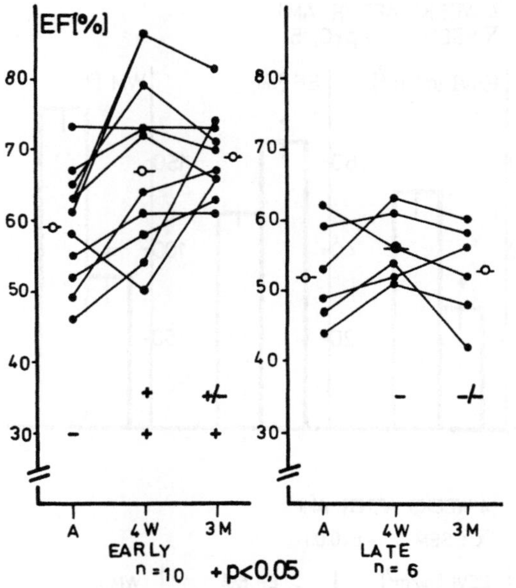

Fig. 5. Ejection fraction (*EF*) acutely (*A*), 4 weeks after treatment (*4 W*), and 3 months after treatment (*3 M*)

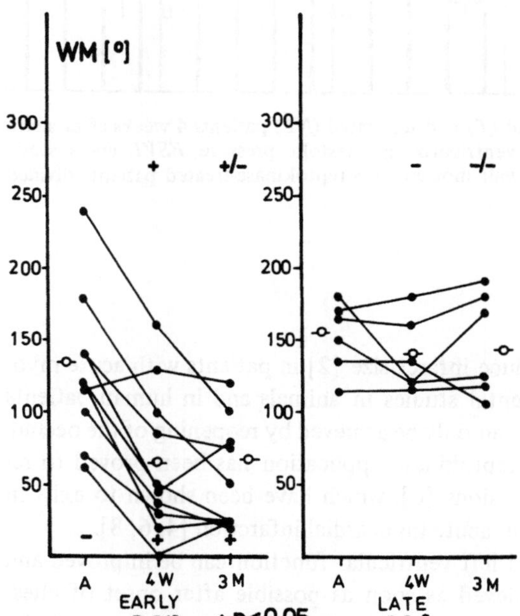

Fig. 6. Wall motion (*WM*) acutely (*A*), 4 weeks after treatment (*4 W*), and 3 months after treatment (*3 M*)

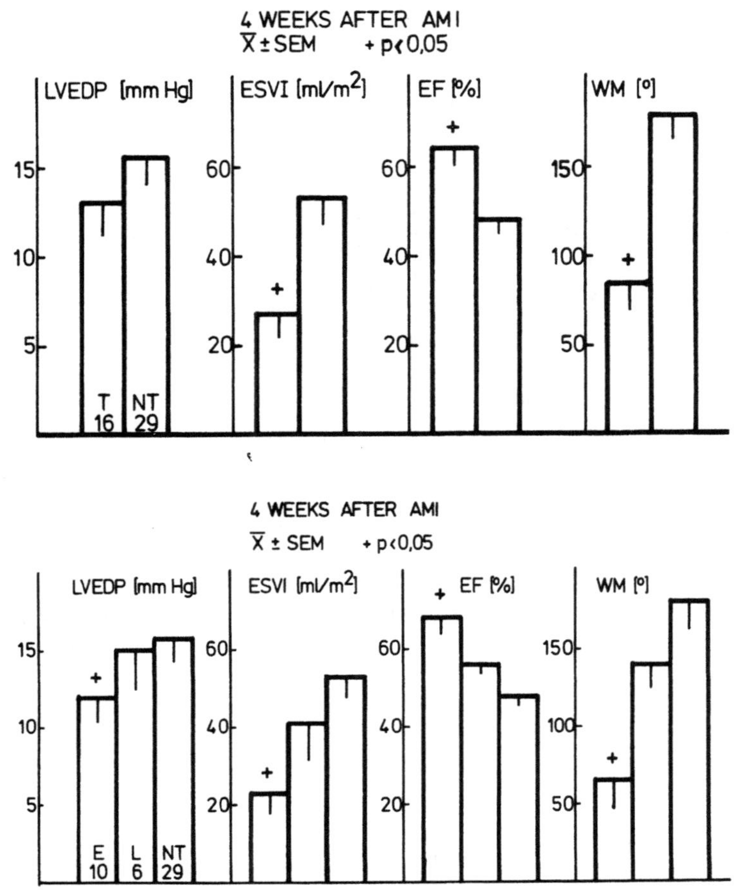

Fig. 7. a Comparison of streptokinase-treated (*T*) and untreated (*NT*) patients 4 weeks after acute myocardial infarction (*AMI*). *LVEDP*, left ventricular end-diastolic pressure; *ESVI*, end-systolic volume index; *EF*, ejection fraction; *WM*, wall motion. **b** Streptokinase-treated patients divided into the early (*E*) and late (*L*) groups

Discussion

Many attempts have been made to reduce infarct size [2] in patients with acute myocardial infarctions. However, experimental studies in animals and in human patients have demonstrated that true reduction can only be achieved by reopening of the occluded arteries [1, 6, 7]. Intracoronary streptokinase application has been proved to reopen thrombotic coronary artery occlusions [6], which have been shown to exist in almost 80% of patients suffering from an acute myocardial infarction [4, 6, 8].

In our studies we found that indeed left ventricular function can be improved and almost normalized if reopening is achieved as soon as possible after onset of chest pain. Reopening within 3 h of commencement of infarct improves left ventricular function significantly as is demonstrated here by catherization studies 4 weeks and 3 months after treatment. Reopening after more than 3 h, however, only tends to improve ventricular function; this is not significant. In some patients ventricular function even deteriorates. Whether this is due to hemorrhage remains obscure. However, accurate observations of the levocardiograms suggest that his deterioration may be produced by hemorrhage. Therefore we believe that after 3 h duration of infarct some patients do not benefit from reopening of the occluded artery. One reason may be an insufficient collateral flow and a high oxygen consumption [7]. In all our patients treated so far we have never seen collaterals in the acute angiograms. However, 4 weeks later 20% and 3 months later 50% showed collateral vessels. Other reasons include lack of improvement due to irreversible damage of myocardial cells. This coincides with experimental findings in animal studies [7].

Thus, we conclude from our studies that reopening of occluded coronary arteries in patients with acute myocardial infarctions is possible in almost 85% of thrombotic occlusions. This improves left ventricular function for at least 3 months only if reopening can be achieved within 3 h of onset of chest pain.

More studies with large numbers of patients and in particular randomized studies are necessary to confirm our initial findings.

Summary

Sixteen of 40 patients with acute myocardial infarction who were treated with 2000 IU/min streptokinase given intracoronarily in order to reopen the thrombotic occluded coronary artery could be catheterized acutely after hospital admission, and also 4 weeks and 3 months later, to study left ventricular function.

We found that in comparison to a group of 29 patients who were treated without streptokinase left ventricular function was significantly improved only if reopening could be achieved within 3 h of onset of chest pain. This improvement lasts for at least 3 months.

Reopening more than 3 h after onset of chest pain, however, only tends to improve left ventricular function as far as end-diastolic pressure, end-systolic volume index, ejection fraction, and wall motion are concerned and this tendency is significantly lower than the changes achieved by reopening within 3 h.

References

1. Baugham KL, Maroko PR, Vatner SF (1981) Effects of coronary artery reperfusion on myocardial infarct size and survival in conscious dogs. Circulation 63:317
2. Braunwald E (1976) Protection of the ischemic myocardium. W Harvey lecture
3. Huhmann W, Duangphung K (1980) Normale Wandbewegung des linken Ventrikels. Vergleich mehrerer Auswertemethoden. Z Kardiol 69:818
4. Huhmann W, Duangphung K, Krunke M, Nieth H (1980) Acute angiography and intracoronary Streptokinase in acute myocardial infarction. In: Lichtlen PR (ed) New aspects of unstable angina pectoris. Hannover, pp
5. Rentrop P, Blanke H, Karsch KR, Kreuzer H (1979) Koronarmorphologie und linksventrikuläre Pump-Funktion im akuten Infarktstadium und ihre Änderungen im chronischen Stadium. Z Kardiol 68:335

6. Rentrop P, Blanke H, Karsch KR, Kaiser H, Koestering H, Leitz K (1981) Selective intracoronary thrombolysis in acute myocardial infarction and unstable angina pectoris. Circulation 63: 307
7. Schaper W (1981) Is preservation possible? 4th Int Postgrad Course of Myocardial Infarction and Angina pectoris. Davos
8. De Wood MA, Spore J, Notske R et al. (1980) Prevalence of total coronary occlusion during the early hours of transmural myocardial infarction. N Engl J Med 303:897

Collaterals May Determine the Functional Result of Intracoronary Streptokinase Therapy After Acute Intracoronary Fibrinolysis in Acute Myocardial Infarction

H.C. Mehmel, F. Schwarz, G. Schuler, W. Mäurer, H. Tillmanns, J. Senges, W. Kübler

Medical University Clinic III, Bergheimer Str. 58, 6900 Heidelberg, FRG

The reopening of an occluded coronary artery after an acute myocardial infarction is an attractive therapeutic concept for the salvation of jeopardized myocardium. Although streptokinase infusion reopens the occluded coronary artery in the majority of cases, the functional result, as measured either by left ventricular angiography or by myocardial perfusion studies with thallium-201, is sometimes disappointing. The present study was undertaken in order to elucidate some possible factors which determine the functional result.

Methods

The angiographic data were obtained from 14 patients with acute myocardial infarction (AMI). In 12 patients the occluded coronary artery was reopened by intracoronary streptokinase infusion, which was applied according to published standards [2]. In one patient with anterior wall infarction a sluggish flow in the left anterior descending branch, and in one patient a sluggish flow in the right coronary artery, due to high-grade stenoses, were clearly improved after streptokinase infusion. Patients in whom the occluded coronary artery could not be reopened were excluded from the study. In nine of the 14 patients a thallium-201 seven-pinhole tomography was performed. The protocol was as follows:

The diagnosis of AMI was based on a typical history and on signs of acute ST elevation in the ECG. Informed consent was obtained from the patient and in every case from close relatives of the patient. Creatine kinase levels were not significantly elevated at the start of acute intracoronary streptokinase therapy. A thallium-201 perfusion study was performed, followed by monoplane left ventricular angiography in 30° RAO projection and coronary angiography. Left ventricular end-diastolic and end-systolic volumes were calculated according to standard formulas [1]. After premedication streptokinase was infused into the involved coronary artery following published recommendations [2]. Angiographic control was performed every 15 min. After reopening of the vessel, or after clear improvement of a sluggish flow due to high-grade stenosis in two patients, the streptokinase infusion was continued for another 15 min. A second left ventricular angiogram and a second seven-pinhole thallium-201 tomography concluded the acute investigation and treatment. Four weeks after the acute myocardial infarction thallium-201 tomography and left ventriculography with coronary angiography were repeated.

Transluminal Coronary Angioplasty and
Intracoronary Thrombolysis. Ed. by Kaltenbach et al.

Results

In nine patients the ejection fraction increased from 44% ± 12% (mean ± 1 SD) at the acute stage before intracoronary lysis to 58% ± 12% four weeks after the acute event ($P < 0.025$). In five patients the ejection fraction decreased from 53% ± 6% to 45% ± 7% ($P < 0.05$). In the second group no collaterals could be demonstrated in any patient. In the first group with improved ejection fraction, five of nine patients showed collaterals in the initial coronary angiogram. The situation in the two patients with high-grade stenoses was judged to be similar, because the slow flow was markedly improved after streptokinase infusion. In one patient possible collaterals were not visualized, because contrast medium was not injected into the noninvolved coronary artery. Only one patient did not show any evidence of collaterals in spite of the improvement of left ventricular function after streptokinase therapy (Fig. 1).

The time between onset of angina pectoris and reopening of the coronary artery was nearly the same for the two groups: it amounted to 4.3 ± 2.3 h in the group with improved left ventricular function and to 4.2 ± 1.0 h in the group who showed no

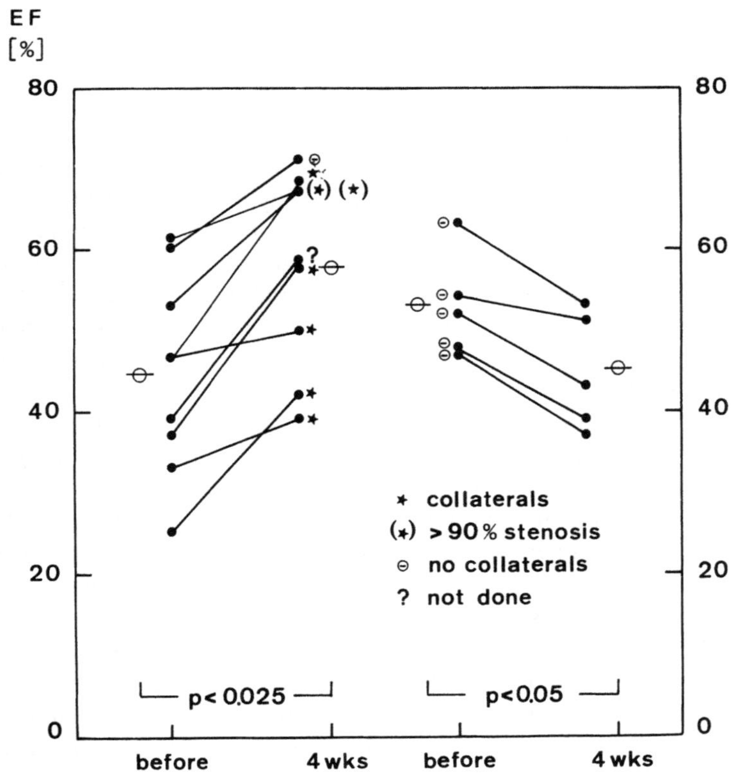

Fig. 1. Left ventricular ejection fraction before and 4 weeks after intracoronary lysis in acute myocardial infarction. In all patients the occluded coronary artery could be reopened by streptokinase infusion, in two patients a sluggish flow due to a high grade stenosis could be markedly improved

improvement in their left ventricular performance after lysis. It appears, however, remarkable that the only patient without collaterals but with improved ventricular function had the shortest interval between onset of symptoms and successful lysis: it amounted to only 1.5 h.

Although the CK and LDH kinetics are influenced by reperfusion due to lysis of a thrombus in myocardial infarction, the peak CK value may serve as a rough estimate of infarct size. In the first group of patients with improved left ventricular function the CK reached a maximum of 827 ± 480 U/liter and in the second group 1224 ± 620 U/liter. This difference is not statistically significant but it can be expected that with a greater number of patients the level of significance will be reached. It seems conceivable that the initial size of a myocardial infarction will partly determine the functional result of all subsequent therapy.

The differences in the LDH peak value are less pronounced (707 ± 313 mU/ml in the first group and 863 ± 499 mU/ml in the second group). Again it seems to be remarkable that the patient without collaterals but with improved left ventricular function after lysis exhibitis the second lowest CK and LDH maximum.

The comparison between the radionuclide and angiographic studies provides only preliminary data, because only six patients in the first group with improved left ventricular function had both complete isotope and angiographic investigation. The enhancement of myocardial perfusion appeared to be greater in the first group than in the second group when measured as reduction of disturbed perfusion in degrees of circumference of left ventricular slices. The reduction of impaired perfusion amounted to 85° ± 54° in the first group and to 41° ± 33° in the second group. The small number of patients precluded any further statistical analysis.

Conclusion

The data suggest that collaterals to the infarcted myocardium increase the tolerance of ischemia and may determine the functional result of reopening of an occluded coronary artery by intracoronary streptokinase infusion after acute myocardial infarction, although other factors, e.g., size of the infarcted myocardium, may also play a role.

References

1. Greene DG, Carlisle R, Grant C, Bunnell IL (1967) Estimation of left ventricular volume by one-plane cineangiography. Circulation 35:61
2. Rentrop P, Blanke H, Köstering H, Karsch KR (1980) Intrakoronare Streptokinase-Application bei akutem Infarkt und instabiler Angina pectoris. Dtsch Med Wochenschr 105:221

Intracoronary Fibrinolysis in Acute Myocardial Infarction. Effect on Left Ventricular Function

F. Schwarz, H.C. Mehmel, G. Schuler, K. v. Olshausen, M. Hofmann, H. Tillmanns, W. Kübler

Abteilung Innere Medizin III (Kardiologie) der Medizinischen Universitätsklinik, Bergheimer Str. 58, 6900 Heidelberg, FRG

Introduction

A variety of hemodynamic responses have been observed after intracoronary fibrinolysis in patients with acute myocardial infarction. The purpose of the present study was to analyze factors which may determine the late hemodynamic result after intracoronary fibrinolysis.

Methods

Three groups of patients with acute transmural myocardial infarction were studied. Acute transmural infarction was defined by [1] acute chest pain of more than 1/2 h duration, and [2] ST segment elevation with or without pathologic Q waves in the standard 12-lead electrocardiogram. Serum CK activity was determined every 1 h after admission to the coronary care unit. Group A contains 15 patients with successful recanalization who developed peak CK activity below 1200 U/liter within the first 3 days after infarction. Group B consists of nine patients with successful recanalization who developed peak CK activity above 1200 U/liter. Group C includes eight patients who had unsuccessful coronary artery recanalization. The left ventricular ejection fraction was determined from RAO cineangiograms before and 4 weeks after recanalization. The average time between the onset of symptoms and the beginning of catheterization was 3.6 h. Streptokinase was infused through the coronary catheter selectively into the occluded coronary artery (2000 U/min).

Results

Before reperfusion the ejection fraction was not significantly different in the three groups studied ($P > 0.05$) as shown in Fig. 1. Similarly, before reperfusion the Gensini score of obstructed coronary artery (causing infarction) excluding collaterals was not significantly different ($P > 0.05$) in the three groups (Fig. 2). This documents identical masses of jeopardized myocardium in all three groups. Four weeks after reperfusion the ejection fraction was significantly higher in group A than in both other groups (Fig. 3). Note that there was no difference of ejection fraction between groups

Transluminal Coronary Angioplasty and
Intracoronary Thrombolysis. Ed. by Kaltenbach et al.

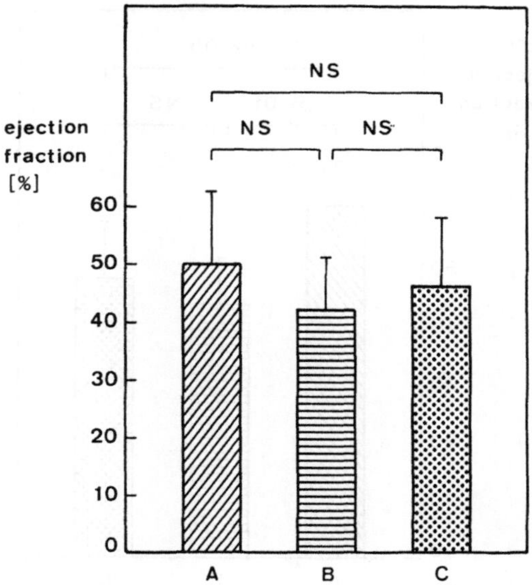

Fig. 1. The left ventricular ejection fraction before reperfusion in the three groups studied. Analysis of variance was used for statistical comparison

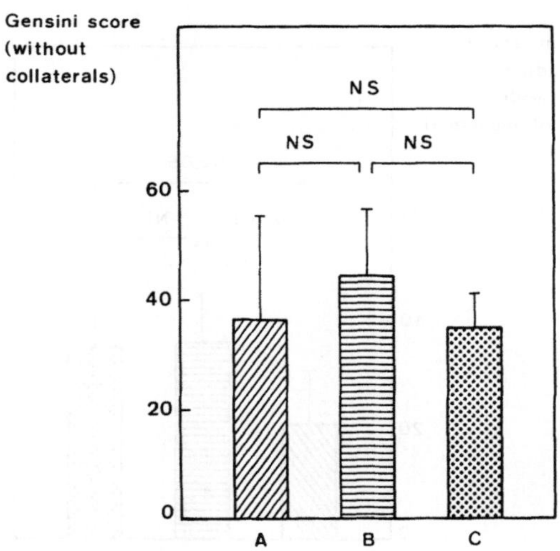

Fig. 2. The Gensini score of infarct vessel (without grading collateral supply to occluded artery) before reperfusion in the three groups

B and C. The incidence of collaterals to obstructed coronary artery was 60% in group A, 43% in group B, and 33% in group C. There was no significant difference between the three groups ($P > 0.05$). The average time between onset of symptoms and reperfusion (time of ischemia) was 4.2 h in group A and 5.1 h in group B ($P > 0.05$). In group C permanent ischemia persisted. Although differences between groups did not reach significant level, group A had a higher incidence of collaterals and a shorter time of ischemia than group B. The Gensini score was modified by including the collateral supply to obstructed coronary artery and a gradation for time of ischemia which was derived from the experimental data of Reimer and coworkers [1]. This Gensini score was significantly lower in group A than in both other groups (Fig. 4).

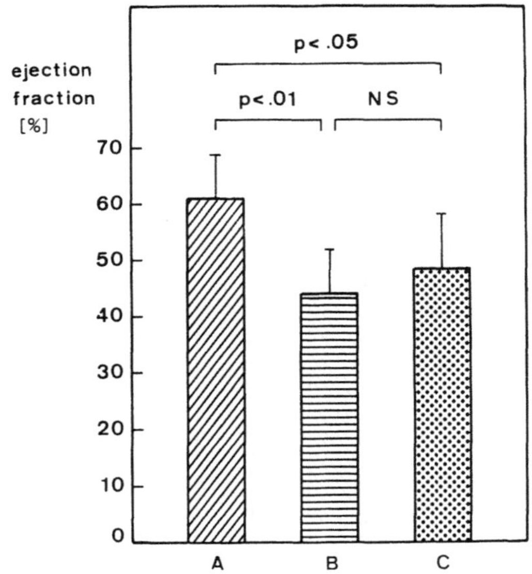

Fig. 3. The ejection fraction 4 weeks after reperfusion

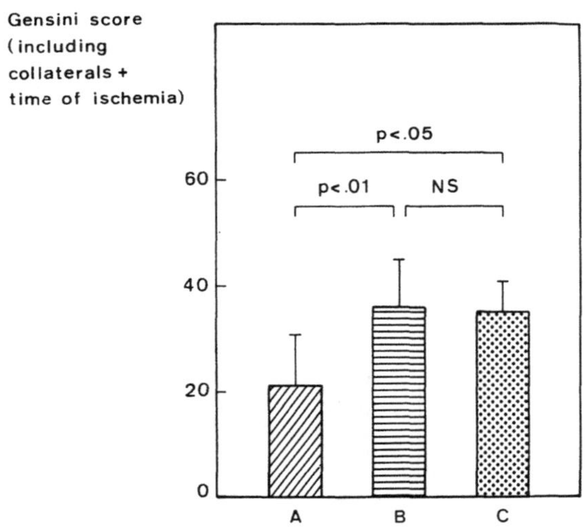

Fig. 4. The modified Gensini score including the collateral supply to obstructed coronary artery and a gradation for the time of ischemia. The grading for time of ischemia was: < 1 h ischemia, × 0.40; 1–3 h, × 0.60; 3–6 h, × 0.80; > 6 h, × 1.00. When using this system group A revealed a significantly lower Gensini score than both other groups, showing that both collaterals and time of ischemia are important determinants of the late hemodynamic result after early reperfusion in acute myocardial infarction

Conclusions

Our data show that the best hemodynamic result was obtained in group A, which represented patients with acute transmural myocardial infarctions in whom the coronary artery was reopened. Infarction was small due to the combination of collateral supply to obstructed coronary artery during coronary occlusion and a short time of ischemia before reperfusion was instituted. Group B shows patients with a reopened coronary artery. Infarction was large due to lack of collaterals and/or long duration of ischemia. Group C represents patients in whom the coronary artery was not reopened. Infarction was large due to lack of reperfusion. It has to be noted that a beneficial effect according to late hemodynamic result occurred mainly in group A whereas patients in group B had similar hemodynamic result to patients in group C. This indicates that reperfusion should be instituted within 4–5 h of onset of symptoms.

Reference

1. Reimer KA, Lowe JE, Rasmussen MM, Jennings RB (1977) The wavefront phenomenon of ischemic cell death. I. Myocardial infarct size vs. duration of coronary occlusion in dogs. Circulation 56:786

Two-dimensional Echocardiographic Findings in Patients with Evolving Myocardial Infarction Treated by Intracoronary Fibrinolysis

M. Schartl, W. Rutsch, W. Disselhoff, H. Schmutzler

Department of Cardiology, University-Hospital, Berlin-Charlottenburg

Based on the fact that thrombosis is the cause of 80% of all cases of acute myocardial infarction, we have included intracoronary application of streptokinase into our therapeutic regime [12]. The idea is to dissolve the thrombus and thus preserve myocardial tissue from necrosis.

Before intracoronary thrombolysis can be performed a quick and reliable diagnosis is required. We therefore examined whether in the early diagnosis of acute myocardial infarction two-dimensional echocardiography (2D-echo) could be helpful [8, 14]. Furthermore, we wanted to know whether 2D-echo allows a quantitative observation of the development of left ventricular function [1–4, 6, 7, 13]. Echocardiographic results were obtained with a 90-degree mechanical sector scanner (Fa. ATL).

Criteria for inclusion in our study were the following: onset of angina pectoris resistent to nitroglycerin less than 4 h previously, ST elevation in the ECG or demonstration of an asynergic segment in the 2D-echo, and CPK-level not elevated. When a patient fulfilled these criteria ventriculography and coronary angiography were performed. If an occlusion of a coronary vessel was found streptokinase was applied intracoronarily (4000 IU/min). Following a mean duration of lasis of 35 min approximately 80% of the occluded arteries were reopened.

To investigate whether 2D-echo is helpful in the early diagnosis of acute myocardial infarction two groups of patients were compared. In the first group 2D-echo was used a diagnostic tool, in the second it was not. All patients had been sent to us for intracoronary streptokinase therapy with a diagnosis of acute myocardial infarction made on the basis of chest pain and changes in the ECG. In the group in which 2D-echo was not used 26 of 30 patients had a clearly positive ECG and were proven to have an acute myocardial infarction by catheterization. In the other four cases the ECG was doubtfully positive. Catheterization revealed that in two cases an infarction had happened and in the other two it had not. This means that two patients underwent invasive diagnostic procedure needlessly.

In the group in which 2D-echo was applied 24 of 29 patients had a clearly positive ECG and an asynergy in the 2D-echo which was easy to see because of the hyperkinesia of the noninfarcted segments. The infarction was confirmed by the angiogram. In the five patients with doubtfully positive ECG, 2D-echo and angiogram showed an infarction in two cases. In the other three patients, however, 2D-echo could not demonstrate any asynergy and we therefore did not perform a catheterization. The further clinical development confirmed that there was not infarction. The comparison

Transluminal Coronary Angioplasty and
Intracoronary Thrombolysis. Ed. by Kaltenbach et al.

of these two groups demonstrates that in patients with doubtlessly positive clinical symptoms and ECG 2D-echo can confirm the diagnosis of myocardial infarction but is not necessarily required. In those patients with doubtful findings, the 2D-echo indeed can be helpful in the diagnosis or exclusion of acute myocardial infarction. Two limitations must be made. First, only in about 92% of the cases is 2D-echo sufficient in quality. Second, you cannot differentiate between acute or chronic infarction by 2D-echo: this can be done only with the help of ECG and clinical data.

Independent of the success of recanalization, in nearly all cases with myocardial infarction a regional wall motion disturbance could be observed in the follow-up study. In order to quantify this, the RAO equivalent view and the RAO monoplane angiogram were analyzed by two examiners independently using a computer program. Ejection fraction was determined using the area length method and the length of the akinetic segment was measured using a continous curve of the ventricular fiber-shortening speed [11]. Correlation between echocardiographically and ventriculographically estimated ejection fraction (Dodge, Sandler) was $r = 0.85$ before recanalization ($n = 24$), $r = 0.83$ 60 min after recanalization ($n = 21$), and $r = 0.81$ 3 weeks after recanalization ($n = 17$). The length of the akinetic segment (continuous VCF curve) correlated in a similar way ($r = 0.83$ before canalization, $r = 0.84$ 60 min after recanalization, and $r = 0.83$ 3 weeks after recanalization). Our results show that echocardiographic studies in comparison to ventriculography provide satisfactory results for a quantitative analysis of the left ventricle, although the volumes and akinetic segments are systematically underestimated.

Figure 1 demonstrated the ejection fraction in three groups determined before recanalization, 60 min after recanalization, and 3 weeks after recanalization. In the groups with unsuccessful recanalization or recanalization after more than 200 min

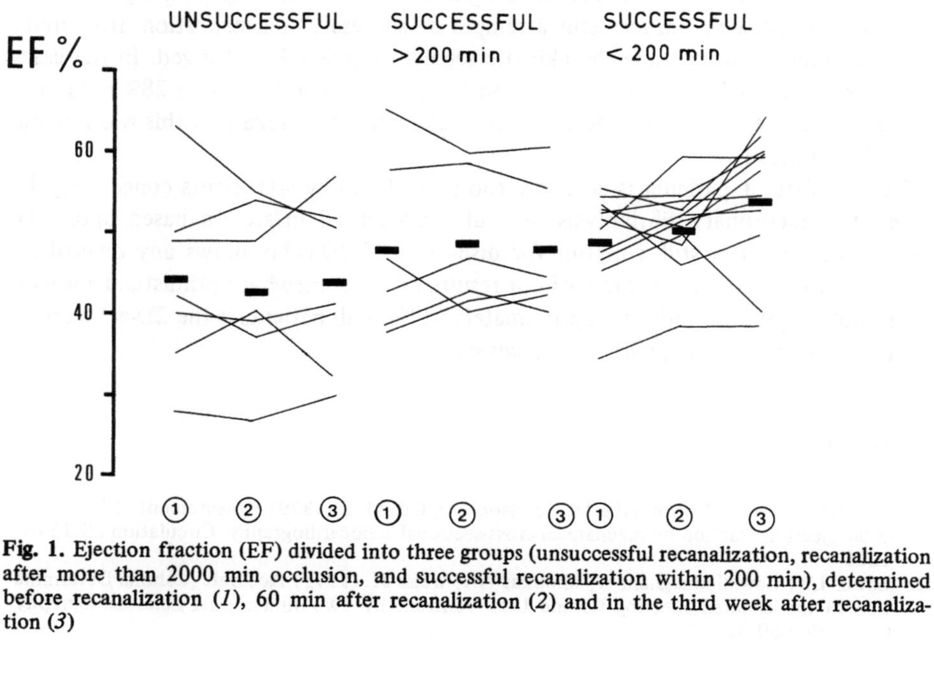

Fig. 1. Ejection fraction (EF) divided into three groups (unsuccessful recanalization, recanalization after more than 2000 min occlusion, and successful recanalization within 200 min), determined before recanalization (*1*), 60 min after recanalization (*2*) and in the third week after recanalization (*3*)

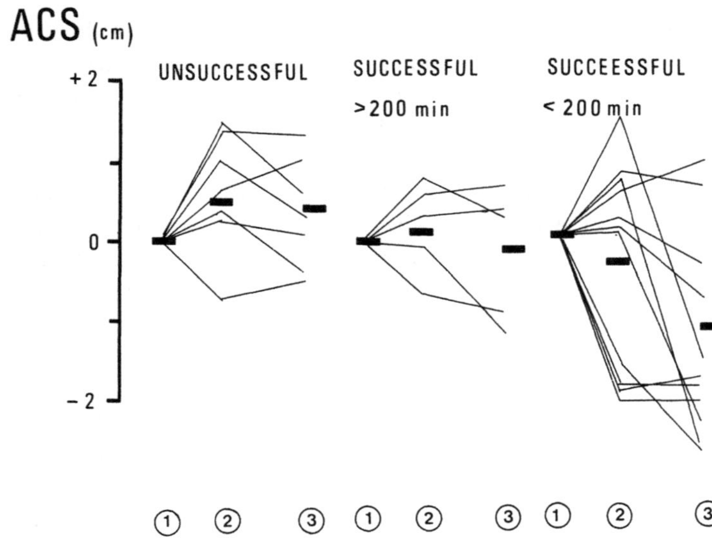

Fig. 2. The length of the akinetic segment (AKS) divided into three groups (unsuccessful recanalization, recanalization after more than 200 min occlusion, and successful recanalization within 200 minutes), determined before recanalization (*1*), 60 min after recanalization (*2*) and in the third week after recanalization (*3*)

occlusion time a change in the ejection fraction could not be observed. In the third group with successful recanalization within 200 min the ejection fraction remained unchanged at first but after 3 weeks rose from 49% to 54%, which was not statistically significant.

Figure 2 shows the results for the length of the akinetic segment. Again in the first two groups with unsuccessful attempts or successful recanalization after more than 200 min occlusion time the akinetic segment remained unchanged. In the cases of successful recanalization after occlusion lasting less than 200 min a 28% reduction of the akinetic segment could be found 3 weeks after recanalization: this was not statistically significant.

Our number of patients is certainly too small to allow statements concerning the value of intracoronary fibrinolysis in acute myocardial infarction based upon 2D-echo. Moreover, it is still a matter for discussion if 2D-echo allows any quantification at all [5, 9, 10, 15]. Because of our results we are somewhat optimistic. However, we do not forget that only in approximately 70% of all patients is the 2D-echo image sufficiently clear for the quantitative analysis.

References

1. Carr KW, Engler RL, Forsythe JR, Johnson AD, Gosink B (1979) Measurement of left ventricular ejection fraction by mechanical cross-sectional echocardiography. Circulation 59:1196–1205
2. Eaton LW, Lowell-Maugham W, Shoukas AA, Weiss JL (1979) Accurate Volume Determination in the Isolated Ejecting Canine Left Ventricle by Two-dimensional Echocardiography. Circulation 60:320–326

3. Erbel R, Schweizer P, Meyer J, Grenner H, Krebs W, Effert S (1980a) Bestimmung der Volumina und der Ejektionsfraktion des linken Ventrikels aus dem zwei-dimensionalen Echokardiogramm bei Patienten mit koronarer Herzerkrankung. Z Kardiol 69:52–61
4. Erbel R, Schweizer P, Pyhel N et al. (1980b) Quantitative Analyse regionaler Kontraktionsstörungen des linken Ventrikels im zwei-dimensionalen Echokardiogramm. Z Kardiol 69: 562–572
5. Falsetti HL, Marcus ML, Kerber RE, Skorton DJ (1981) Quantification of myocardial ischemia and infarction by left ventricular imaging. Circulation 63:747–751
6. Folland ED, Parisi AF, Moynihan PF, Jones DR, Feldman CL, Tow DE (1979) Assessment of left ventricular ejection fraction and volumes by real-time, two-dimensional echocardiography. Circulation 60:760–766
7. Grube E, Richter R, Otten H et al. (1979) Darstellung linksventrikulärer Kontraktionsanomalien mit Hilfe der zwei-dimensionalen Sektor-Echokardiographie. Dtsch Med Wochenschr 104:703–707
8. Heger JJ, Weyman AE, Wann LD, Dillon JC, Feigenbaum H (1979) Cross-sectional echocardiography in acute myocardial infarction: detection and localization of regional left ventricular asynergy. Circulation 60:531–538
9. Moynihan PF, Parisi AF, Feldman CL (1981) Quantitative detection of regional left ventricular contraction abnormalities by two-dimensional echocardiography. I. Analysis of methods. Circulation 63:752–760
10. Parisi AF, Moynihan PF, Folland ED, Feldman CL (1981) Quantitative detection of regional left ventricular contraction abnormalities by two-dimensional echocardiography. II. Accuracy in coronary artery disease. Circulation 63:761–767
11. Rutsch W, Grosse G, Krais T, Michel U, Schmutzler H (1976) Left ventricular angiography on exercise in coronary heart disease with regional disorders of left ventricular myocardium. 7th Eur Cong of Cardiology, 1976.
12. Rutsch W, Weber H, PaepRer H, Schmutzler H (1980) Maßnahmen zur Myokardperfusion beim akuten Myokardinfarkt: Transluminale, mechanische Rekanalisation und koronarselektive Thrombolyse mit Streptokinase. Z Kardiol 69:230
13. Schiller NB et al. (1979) Left ventricular volume from paired biplane two-dimensional echocardiography. Circulation 60:547–555
14. Weyman AE, Peskoe SM, Williams ES, Dillon JC, Feigenbaum H (1976) Detection of left ventricular aneurysms by cross-sectional echocardiography. Circulation 54:936–944
15. Wyatt HL et al. (1979) Cross-sectional echocardiography. I. Analysis of mathematic models for quantifying mass of the left ventricle in dogs. Circulation 60:1104–1113

Intracoronary Fibrinolysis in Acute Myocardial Infarction: Hospital Follow-up

W. Merx*, Ch. Bethge, P. Rentrop, H. Blanke, K.R. Karsch, D.G. Mathey, P. Kremer, W. Rutsch, H. Schmutzler

Dept. of Internal Medicine I of the University Hospital, Aachen
Dept. of Cardiology of the University Hospital of Göttingen
Dept. of Cardiology of the University Hospital of Hamburg
Dept. of Cardiology of the Free University of Berlin

Though it is proven that in the majority of patients with acute myocardial infarction due to complete thrombotic occlusion recanalization can be achieved by selective intracoronary infusion of streptokinase [1, 2], little is known with respect to reduction of mortality and possible late complications. With this goal in mind data on 204 patients pooled by four cardiological centers in West Germany have been evaluated.

For antithrombotic therapy, all patients surviving acute intervention and not operated on during the first day received heparin for the first days in the cardiac care unit (CCU). Heparinization was continued in 102 patients in this subacute stage, until later operation or discharge. Thirty-eight had low-dose heparin treatment in the range of 12 000–15 000 units/day, nine received doses between 15 000 and 20 000 units/day and 55 patients received daily doses exceeding 20 000 units.

With the exception of two patients who received neither heparin nor coumarin, all others (60 patients) were anticoagulated with coumarin. In 43 of them, more than half of the prothrombin time controls were in the therapeutic range, in 15 patients more than half of the prothrombin time was above the therapeutic range, and in two patients no prothrombin time values were available.

Most of the patients (119 or 58%) received, at the time of acute intervention, 1.0 g (96 patients) or 0.5 g (23 patients) acetylsalicylic acid (ASA) intravenously. Thereafter, antiplatelet therapy was continued with ASA in 39 patients: 34 patients received orally 3 × 0.5 g/day, two patients 3 × 1.0 g and three received 3 × 0.33 g in addition to 3 × 75 mg dipyridamole. Another four patients were treated with sulfinpyrazone.

While the in-hospital mortality was 24% in patients with complete thrombotic occlusion when recanalization was unsuccessful, only 7% of the patients with successful acute intervention died (Fig. 1). This significant difference is obtained in spite of the fact that within the nine deaths of the successfully treated group two noncardiac deaths – one due to peritonitis in the CCU and one due to pulmonary embolism in the general ward – are included. Thus, the cardiac mortality after recanalization was only seven of 129 patients or 5.4%. While all of these patients survived the acute intervention, in contrast six of the nine deceased patients in the group without recanalization died in cardiogenic shock when still in the heart catheter laboratory. The remaining three patients died 7 h, 16 h, and 1 day following the acute intervention.

* Abt. Innere Medizin I, Goethestraße 27/29, 5100 Aachen, FRG

Transluminal Coronary Angioplasty and Intracoronary Thrombolysis. Ed. by Kaltenbach et al.

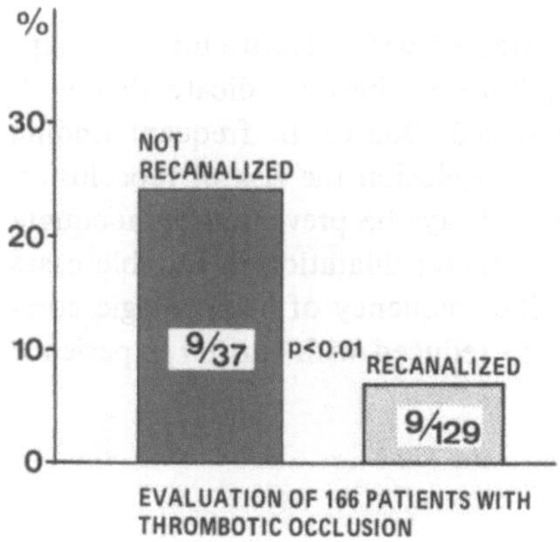

Fig. 1. Deaths among recanalized and nonrecanalized patients during hospitalization (n = 166)

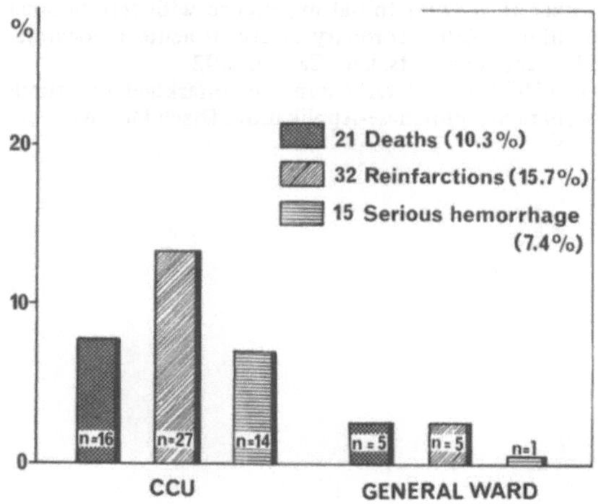

Fig. 2. Serious complications among patients in the cardiac care unit (CCU) and on the general ward (n = 204)

By far the greater part of the three serious complications – death, reinfarction, and hemorrhage – occurred in the days following the acute intervention, while patients were still in the CCU (Fig. 2). Major bleeding, defined as necessitating blood transfusion, was significantly associated with fibrinogen concentrations below 100 mg% after the infusion of streptokinase.

Of 20 patients who experienced reinfarctions according to ECG or enzyme criteria 15 were later reinvestigated. Eight showed new occlusion of the infarct vessel, in six the infarct vessel was open but distal flow was very slow, and in only one could a normal flow be seen in the infarct vessel.

Of 64 patients who were reinvestigated before discharge from hospital and who had not yet received bypass grafts or suffered from reinfarction, only five showed a reoccluded infarct vessel at coronary angiography. In none of these five, either in the CCU or in the general ward, was infarct recidivism diagnosed. Of the 59 patients with open vessels, one was recorded to have had reinfarction according to ECG criteria during his stay in the general ward. In this case, coronary angiography demonstrated a very poor flow in the infarct-related vessel. There was also "poor flow" reported in four other patients without apparent signs of reinfarction.

The results of this first large study of patients treated with selective intracoronary infusion of streptokinase as a therapy for thrombotic occlusion indicate that with successful early recanalization mortality can be reduced. Due to the frequent finding of severe stenotic lesions at the site of thrombotic occlusion the risk of reocclusion is high, especially during the first days. It cannot always be prevented by adequate anticoagulation. Early bypass surgery or balloon catheter dilatation in suitable cases is therefore the logical therapeutic consequence. The frequency of hemorrhagic complications is acceptably low and can most likely be reduced with further experience and refinement of technique.

References

1. Rentrop KP, Blanke H, Karsch KR, Kreuzer H (1979a) Initial experience with transluminal recanalization of the recently occluded infarct-related coronary artery in acute myocardial infarction. Comparison with conventionally treated patients. Clin Cardiol 2:92
2. Rentrop KP, Blanke H, Karsch KR et al. (1979b) Wiedereröffnung des Infarktgefäßes durch transluminale Rekanalisation und intrakoronare Streptokinase-Applikation. Dtsch Med Wochenschr 104:1438

Relevance of Hemorrhage After Reperfusion in Acute Myocardial Infarction

M.C. Fishbein, W. Ganz, J. Y-Rit, U. Lando, K. Kanmatsuse, J. C. Mercier

Divisions of Anatomic Pathology and Cardiology, Cedars-Sinai Medical Center, 8700 Beverly Blvd, Los Angeles, CA 90048, USA

Restoration of blood flow to ischemic myocardium would seem to be a rational way of limiting ischemic injury. Studies in dogs have shown that if reperfusion is instituted within 20 min of coronary occlusion myocardial blood flow, function, and morphology eventually return to normal [23, 24]. However, if 40 min or more elapse before flow is restored, normal perfusion may not be restored, function may not recover fully or may even worsen temporarily, and the morphological signs of myocardial injury may be more pronounced than would be expected after occlusion of the same duration not followed by reperfusion [23, 24, 26].

Whether the reperfusion merely makes already irreversibly injured myocardium look worse or whether it actually extends myocardial necrosis is controversial. As surgical bypass [9] and transluminal angioplastic techniques [20] are now applied for early reperfusion of myocardium in patients with evolving myocardial infarction, this matter is clinically relevant. This study was performed to determine whether reperfusion hemorrhage actually extends infarction or occurs in myocardium that was already irreversibly injured before reperfusion.

Methods

Six mongrel dogs were anesthetized with morphine (1.5 mg/kg), followed 45–60 min later by IV pentobarbital (30 mg/kg) supplemented by doses of 2 mg/kg pentobarbital every 30 min. The dogs were artificially ventilated 10 times/min at tidal volumes of 20 ml/kg. Heparin (100 IU/kg) was given hourly. Aortic pressure and ECG were monitored continuously. An angiographic catheter was inserted through the left carotid artery and advanced under fluoroscopic guidance into the left main coronary artery. A double-lumen 2½ F catheter with a distal lumen and a balloon (also 2½ F deflated) 2 mm from the tip was then inserted 2–3 cm into the left anterior descending coronary artery through the lumen of the angiographic catheter. The balloon was inflated with diluted Renografin until cylindrical distortion was visualized fluoroscopically; then the angiographic catheter was withdrawn into the aorta. This degree of inflation causes pressure distal to the balloon to decrease to less than 20 mmHg, indicating complete coronary occlusion (unpublished work).

The occlusion was maintained for 5½ h. Then, to label myocardial vessels with ischemic injury, 0.1 ml/kg filtered colloidal carbon suspension (Pelikan Co.) was

Transluminal Coronary Angioplasty and
Intracoronary Thrombolysis. Ed. by Kaltenbach et al.

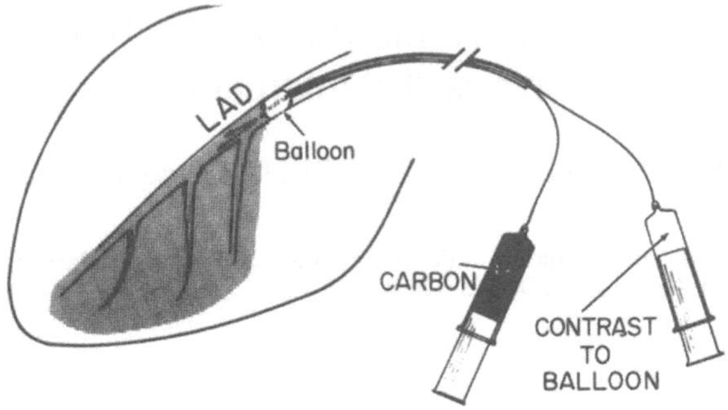

Fig. 1. Selective carbon uptake before coronary reperfusion. The diagram shows the position of the balloon-tipped catheter in the left anterior descending coronary artery. The position of the balloon was verified by fluoroscopy. After 5½ hours occlusion, carbon was injected distal to the inflated balloon to label ischemically injured vessels

injected over 5 min distal to the inflated balloon through the distal lumen of the catheter [11] (Fig. 1).

The carbon was allowed to circulate for 15 min so it could be cleared from the bloodstream and noninjured vessels by the reticuloendothelial system. The clearing of carbon from the circulation and noninjured vessels before reperfusion was confirmed initially by the absence of carbon in centrifuged blood and later by its absence in areas of nonischemic myocardium. Thus any vessel labeled with carbon was labeled before reperfusion. The balloon was then deflated to allow reperfusion of the myocardium for 30 min. Reperfusion arrhythmias (premature ventricular complexes) were not frequent or severe and were abolished by the administration of a 20-mg bolus of lidocaine. The dogs were killed and their hearts excised and cut into 1-cm thick transverse slices. Each slice was incubated in tripenyl-tetrazolium chloride (TTC), a histochemical stain for dehydrogenase activity that identifies areas of necrosis grossly [16, 31]. A planimeter was used [2, 3] to measure areas of necrosis, areas with carbon-labeled, injured vessels, and areas of hemorrhage in all gross heart slices and in giant whole-mount histologic sections of each slice. For each heart the extent of vascular injury, hemorrhage, and necrosis was measured in each slice and expressed as a percentage of the entire left ventricle. The paired t test was used to compare the percentages of necrosis and vascular injury in each heart.

The initial 5½-h period of ischemia was chosen to allow enough time for gross and microscopic recognition of the infarction [4. 15, 33] and for development of sufficient injury to result in hemorrhage after reperfusion [5, 7]. The 5-min duration of carbon injection was chosen so the injection could be performed in a short time, yet at low pressure. The 15-min period of carbon circulation was chosen to allow time for the carbon to be cleared from the blood and noninjured vessels before beginning deflation of the balloon, so that no labeling would occur after reperfusion. The 30-min reperfusion period was to allow enough time for reperfusion injury to occur [23, 24].

Thus, hemorrhage outside the area of necrosis and away from areas of carbon-labeled vessels would suggest an increase in the volume of injured tissue. If all the hemorrhage were from previously injured labeled vessels within the confines of the original area of necrosis, additional tissue destruction would not be expected.

Results

Grossly, areas of non-necrotic myocardium that stained with TTC appeared red and areas of vascular injury and hemorrhage that trapped carbon appeared black. The areas of blackening were predominantly subendocardial, with sparing of the peripheral portions of the infarct (Figs. 2 and 3).

Microscopic examination of giant whole-mount histologic sections confirmed gross findings. Microscopically, infarcts delineated by TTC showed increased eosinophilia and waviness of fibers, spaces presumed to represent interstitial edema, and early in-

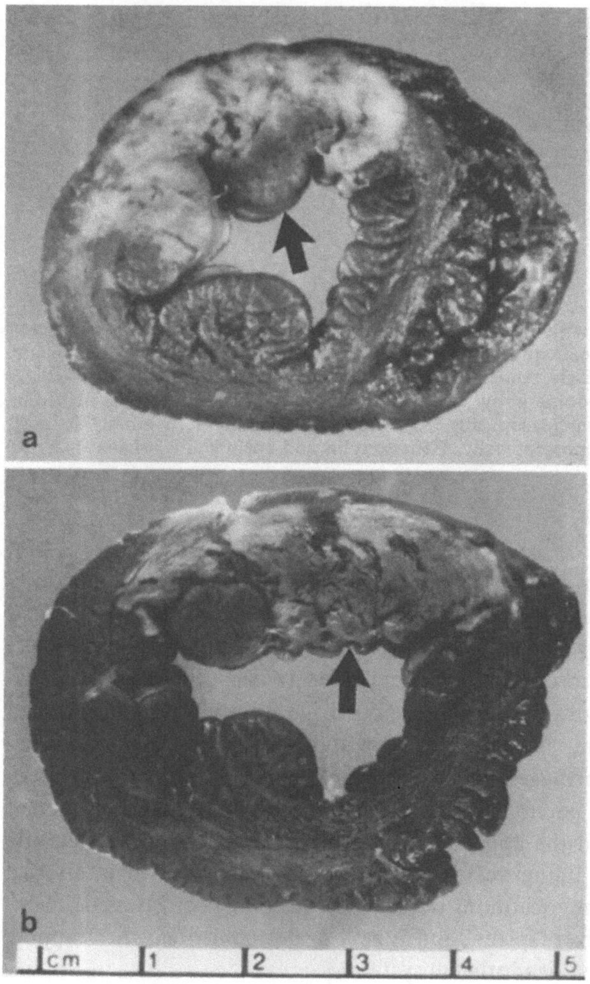

Fig. 2. Transverse slices from two of the hearts studied, stained with TTC. Normal myocardium appears dark, whereas areas of necrosis fail to stain and appear light. The dark areas within the areas of necrosis (*arrows*) represent areas of carbon labeling. Hemorrhages only occurred in these areas. **a** The carbon labeling is predominantly central and subendocardial, with sparing of the lateral and subepicardial portions of the infarcts. **b** The darkened area is also predominantly subendocardial, but there is no sparing of the lateral portions of the infarct

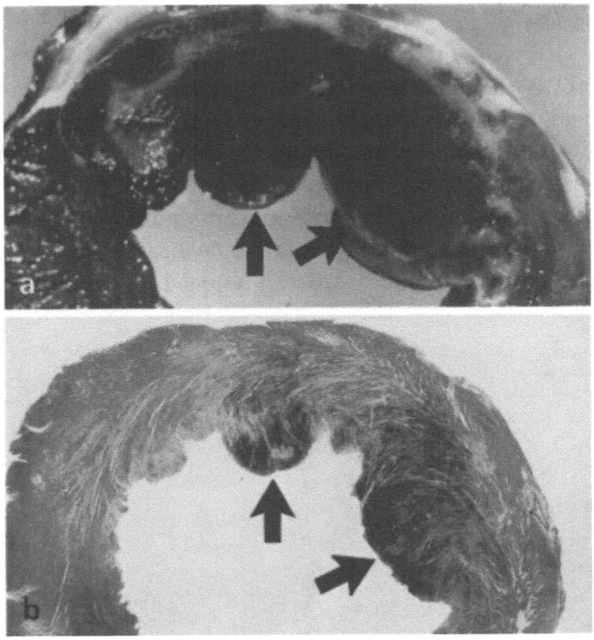

Fig. 3. Slice of heart from the dog with the most extensive carbon labeling and hemorrhage (*arrows*). **a** The areas of blackening almost equals the area of infarction delineated by the TTC technique. **b** A giant whole-mount histologic section of the gross slice shown in **a**. The hemorrhage (*arrows*) that appears darkest is predominantly subendocardial and within the borders of the infarct determined both grossly and microscopically. The area of darkening seen grossly is larger than the area of hemorrhage seen microscopically. Hematoxylin and eosin stain; original magnification × 1

filtration of polymorphonuclear leukocytes at their margins. Areas of hemorrhage were predominantly subendocardial and completely within the areas of necrosis (Fig. 3), as defined both grossly and microscopically. In each slice from each heart, the area of hemorrhage seen microscopically was less extensive than the area of blackening seen grossly (Fig. 3). In addition, areas of hemorrhage were always smaller than the areas of vascular labeling and always occurred within regions containing labeled, injured vessels. Although hemorrhages were severe and confluent in the subendocardium, they were milder and patchy toward the periphery of the zone of vascular injury. Light microscopy showed the appearance of injured vessels within the necrotic areas. Carbon could be found lining vessels, in carbon thrombi, and in interstitial areas. No carbon was found in myocardium outside the areas of necrosis as delineated by TTC. Autopsy study of liver, spleen, and lymph nodes confirmed the trapping of circulating carbon by the reticuloendothelial system.

Planimetry of areas of necrosis and vascular injury in the six dogs showed that the area of necrosis was greater than the area of vascular injury. In all hearts, 52% of the region of necrosis contained labeled, injured, vasculature, but the extent of hemorrhage and vascular injury was less than the extent of necrosis (10.2% ± 4.6% vs 19.8% ± 8.6%, $P < 0.001$). Hemorrhagic areas were more difficult to measure accurately from histologic sections because they were patchy peripherally; they constituted 50%–60% of the regions with injured vessels.

Discussion

Several experimental studies have shown that early reperfusion can salvage jeopardized but viable ischemic myocardium, resulting in infarcts smaller than would be expected with permanent occlusion [5, 7, 10, 13, 19, 28, 29, 30, 32, 34]. If reperfusion is instituted after more than 6 h occlusion, little or no myocardial salvage results in the dog [29, 32].

The present study was specifically designed to determine whether hemorrhage associated with reperfusion causes extension of infarction. Areas of severe vascular injury were labeled with carbon before reflow to determine whether hemorrhage occurred outside as well as inside these areas of vascular injury. The area of ischemic necrosis was identified by use of the TTC technique, a reliable gross indicator of myocardial necrosis [16, 31], with excellent correlation between gross and microscopic measurement of infarct size. In all dogs, hemorrhage occurred only from vessels injured before reperfusion and was confined to the central and subendocardial portions of the infarcts, which are known to be the most severely ischemic and to undergo irreversible damage earliest [27, 30].

Higginson et al. [21], using labeled erythrocytes and microspheres, found that hemorrhages only occurred where myocardial blood flow was less than 21% of control before reperfusion, supporting our data showing that hemorrhages occur only within the infarcts in the most severely ischemic regions. That hemorrhage depends on the severity of preexisting ischemia is also indicated by the fact that the extent of hemorrhage is directly proportional to the duration of the preceding ischemia [8, 12, 14, 17, 18].

Whether reperfusion hemorrhage might interfere with infarct healing and predispose to rupture, aneurysm formation, or infarct expansion [22] must be considered, but cannot be answered by this short-term study. There is, however, some experimental evidence that reperfusion may actually benefit healing by accelerating the proliferation of granulation tissue [1]. Our own ongoing studies, to date, have not shown any detrimental effects of reperfusion on the eventual healing of myocardial infarcts [16a].

The lack of hemorrhage in subepicardial and lateral portions of the infarct observed in this study is of interest. Reimer et al. [30] have shown that there is a wave-front phenomenon of cell death in myocardial infarction with irreversible injury involving the most severely ischemic subendocardium first and then subepicardium. Kloner and associates [25] showed ultrastructurally that within any region of ischemic myocardium, irreversible myocardial cell injury occurs before vascular endothelial injury, and that damaged vessels only occur in regions where there has already been irreversibly ischemic injury to the myocardium. Thus, it is not surprising that toward the subepicardial portion of an infarct, where myocardial cell death evolves later, there is even more delay in the evolution of vascular injury, with less labeling by carbon and less hemorrhage.

In conclusion, in this study hemorrhage with reperfusion occurred only within necrotic tissue where there had been severe vascular injury and irreversible myocardial injury before reperfusion. There is no evidence to suggest that reperfusion per se resulted in an increase in the amount of myocardial necrosis. These findings have an important clinical implication. One potential problem of early reperfusion often discussed is extension of infarction due to reperfusion hemorrhage. The results of this study suggest that hemorrhage after reperfusion is the consequence of preexisting vascular injury, always occurs in already necrotic myocardium, and is not likely to cause infarct extension.

Summary

Early reperfusion may salvage ischemic myocardium; late reperfusion often intensifies morphologic changes of necrosis and causes hemorrhage. To determine whether hemorrhage after reperfusion increases the extent of myocardial infarction, six closed-chest, anesthetized dogs underwent balloon occlusion of the left anterior descending coronary artery for 5½ h, followed by 30 min reflow. Colloidal carbon was injected distal to the balloon before reperfusion to label injured vessels. After death, the area of myocardial necrosis was measured by planimetry of 1-cm thick serial slices of left ventricle stained with TTC. Areas of hemorrhage and vascular injury were also measured. In all hearts, the extent of hemorrhage and vascular injury was less than the extent of necrosis ($10.2\% \pm 4.6\%$ vs $19.8\% \pm 8.6\%$, $P < 0.001$). Further, hemorrhage was always within the area of necrosis, primarily in the subendocardial portion. Hemorrhage after reperfusion occurred only in necrotic tissue where carbon labeling indicated severe vascular injury before reperfusion, suggesting that the hemorrhage was the consequence of preesisting microvascular injury, not its cause.

Acknowledgment. The authors appreciate the expert secretarial assistance of Ms. Patricia King.

References

1. Althaus U, Gurtner HP, Baur H, Hamberger S, Roos B (1977) Consequences of myocardial reperfusion following coronary occlusion in pigs: effects on morphologic, biochemical and hemodynamic findings. Eur J Clin Invest 7:437
2. Boor PJ, Reynolds ES (1977a) A simple planimetric method for determination of left ventricular mass and necrotic myocardial mass in postmortem hearts. Am J Clin Pathol 86:387
3. Boor PH, Reynolds ES (1977b) Myocardial infarct size: clinicopathologic agreement and discordance. Hum Pathol 6:685
4. Bouchardy B, Majno G (1974) Histopathology of early myocardial infarcts. A new approach. Am J Pathol 74:301
5. Bresnahan GF, Roberts R, Shell WE, Ross J Jr, Sobel BE: Deleterious effects due to hemorrhage after myocardial reperfusion. Am J Cardiol 33:82
6. Bulkley BH, Hutchins GM (1977) Myocardial consequences of coronary artery bypass surgery. The paradox of necrosis in areas of revascularization. Circulation 56:906
7. Capone RJ, Most AS (1978) Myocardial hemorrhage after coronary reperfusion in pigs. Am J Cardiol 41:259
8. Cerra FB, Lajos TZ, Montes M, Siegel JH (1975) Hemorrhagic infarction: a reperfusion injury following prolonged myocardial ischemic anoxia. Surgery 78:95
9. Cohn LH (1979) The treatment of acute myocardial ischemia. An integrated medical/surgical approach. Futura, Mt. Kisco

10. Constantini C, Corday E, Lang T et al. (1975) Revascularization after 3 hours of coronary arterial occlusion: effects on regional cardiac metabolic function and infarct size. Am J Cardiol 36:368
11. Cotran RS, Suter ER, Majno G (1967) The use of colloidal carbon as a tracer for vascular injury. A review. Vasc Dis 4:107
12. DeGasperis C, Gonzales-Levin L, Pellegrini A, Ross DN (1971) Ultrastructural aspects of human myocardial capillaries during open heart surgery. Cardiology 56:33
13. Deloche A, Fabiani JN, Camilleri JP et al. (1977) The effect of coronary artery reperfusion on the extent of myocardial infarction. Am Heart J 93:358
14. Engelman RM, Chandra R, Baumann FG, Goldman RA (1976) Myocardial reperfusion, a cause of ischemic injury during cardiopulmonary bypass. Surgery 80:266
15. Fishbein MC, Maclean D, Maroko PR (1978) The histopathologic evolution of myocardial infarction. Chest 73:843
16. Fishbein MC, Meerbaum S, Y-Rit J et al. (to be published) Early phase myocardial infarct size quantification: validation of the triphenyl tetrazolium chloride tissue enzyme staining technique. Am Heart J
16a. Fishbein MC, Geft IL, Hashida J, Ninomya K, Nishizawa S, Venkatesh N, Y-Rit J, Ganz W (1981) Does late reperfusion, after necrosis is complete, have beneficial or detrimental effects on myocardial infarct healing? Circulation 64 (Suppl IV):98
17. Fukuyama T, Roberts R (1979) Detection and quantification of impaired vascular integrity prior to onset of hemorrhage or reduced reflow with ^{125}I-albumin. Circulation 60 [suppl]: II–95
18. Fukuyama T, Sobel BE, Roberts R (1979) Microvascular deterioration: implications for revascularization. (abstr) Circulation 60 [Suppl]: II–240
19. Ginks WR, Sybers HD, Maroko PR, Covell JW, Sobel BE, Ross J Jr: Coronary artery reperfusion. II. Reduction of myocardial infarct size at 1 week after the coronary occlusion. J Clin Invest 51:2717
20. Gruntzig AR, Senning A, Siegenthaler WE (1979) Nonoperative dilatation of coronary stenosis; percutaneous transluminal coronary angioplasty. N Engl J Med 301:61
21. Higginson LAJ, White F, Sanders TM, Bloor CM, Covell JW (1978) Does hemorrhage on reperfusion of the acutely ischemic myocardium cause extension of infarct size? Proc Can Cardiovasc Soc 37:68
22. Hutchins GM, Bulkley BH (1978) Infarct expansion versus extension: two different complications of acute myocardial infarction. Am J Cardiol 41:1127
23. Jennings RB, Ganote CE (1974) Structural changes in myocardium during acute ischemia. Circ Res 35 [Suppl]:III–156
24. Kloner RA, Ganote CE, Whalen DA Jr, Jennings RB (1974) Effect of a transient period of ischemia on myocardial cells. II. Fine structure during the first few minutes of reflow. Am J Pathol 74:399
25. Kloner RA, Rude RE, Carlson N, Maroko PR, DeBoer LWV, Braunwald E (1980) Ultrastructural evidence of microvascular damage and myocardial cell injury after coronary artery occlusion: which comes first? Circulation 62:945
26. Lang T, Corday E, Gold H et al. (1974) Consequences of reperfusion after coronary occlusion. Am J Cardiol 33:69
27. Marcus ML, Kerber RE, Ehrhardt J, Abboud FM (1975) Three dimensional geometry of acutely ischemic myocardium. Circulation 52:254
28. Maroko PR, Libby P, Ginks WR et al. (1972) Coronary artery reperfusion. I. Early effects on local myocardial function and the extent of myocardial necrosis. J Clin Invest 51:2710
29. Mathur VS, Guinn GA, Burris WH (1975) Maximal revascularization (reperfusion) in intact conscious dogs after 2 to 5 hours of coronary occlusion. Am J Cardiol 36:252
30. Reimer KA, Lowe JE, Rasmussen MM, Jennings RB (1977) The wavefront phenomenon of ischemic cell death. I. Myocardial infarct size vs duration of coronary occlusion in dogs. Circulation 56:86
31. Sandritter HW, Jestadt R (1958) Triphenyltetrazoliumchlorid (TTC) als Reduktionsindikator zur makroskopischen Diagnose des frischen Herzinfarktes. Verh Dtsch Ges Pathol 41:165
32. Smith JT, Soeter JR, Haston JJ, McNamera JJ (1974) Coronary reperfusion in primates. Serial electrocardiographic and histologic assessment. J Clin Invest 54:1420
33. Sommers HM, Jennings RB (1964) Experimental acute myocardial infarction. Histologic and histochemical studies of early myocardial infarcts induced by temporary or permanent occlusion of a coronary artery. Lab Invest 13:1496
34. Vatner SF, Baig H, Manders WT, Maroko PR (1978) Effects of coronary artery reperfusion on myocardial infarct size calculated from creatine kinase. J Clin Invest 61.1048

A New Concept in Producing Experimental Myocardial Infarction: Intracoronary Application of Thrombin

M. Hofmann* **, K.R. Karsch***, K.P. Rentrop***, W. Schaper**

* University of Heidelberg, Division of Cardiology, 6900 Heidelberg, FRG
** Max-Planck Institut, Bad Nauheim, FRG
*** Mount Sinai Medical Center, New York, N.Y., USA

Introduction

Recent studies in patients with acute myocardial infarction have shown that occluding coronary artery thrombi can be lysed by local application of streptokinase into the infarct-related coronary artery [9, 17, 22]. Significant improvement of local and global left ventricular function occurred in patients after successful reperfusion in the early stage of myocardial infarction [23]. Experimental studies, however, yielded contradictory results. Some authors found improvement [4, 16, 19], others no change [6, 7, 21] or even deterioration of left ventricular function early after reperfusion [3, 15, 18].

Differences between the results achieved in humans and those from animal experiments could be related predominantly to the mode of reperfusion, which was achieved by sudden and complete release of a mechanical obstruction, resulting in hyperemia [11, 15] in most experimental settings. Therefore a new experimental model for myocardial infarction was developed, based on a thrombotic coronary occlusion at the site of an artificial high-degree stenosis.

Materials and Methods

Twenty-eight mongrel dogs of both sexes and of unknown age, with a mean weight of 31.3 ± 5.6 kg, were studied. After pretreatment with subcutaneous piritramide (5 mg/kg body wt) anesthesia was initiated with i.v. pentobarbital (10 mg/kg body wt) and maintained after intubation with an N_2O/O_2 mixture (3:1) by means of an Engstroem respirator.

Thoracotomy was performed in the fifth intercostal space. After pericardiotomy, the left atrium was ligated and a small 2F catheter inserted. The left anterior descending artery (LAD) and the circumflex artery were prepared and a flow probe was fixed on both proximal arteries. Two ligations 15–20 mm apart were prepared in 20 dogs at the LAD, and in eight dogs at the circumflex artery behind the flow probe (Fig. 1). Directly in front of the distal ligation a stenosis was created by means of a plastic ring with a diameter of 1.4–1.6 mm, which produced a reduction of hyperemia of about 50%. This corresponded to a stenosis of 75%–80% on a length of 5 mm.

Transluminal Coronary Angioplasty and
Intracoronary Thrombolysis. Ed. by Kaltenbach et al.

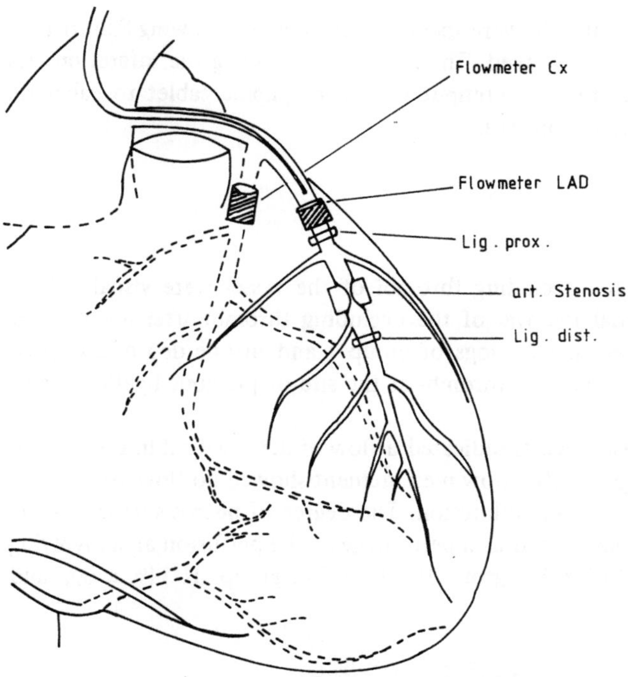

Fig. 1. Illustration of the experimental setting. Two electromagnetic flowmeters and one artificial stenosis either on the LAD or the circumflex artery

Experimental Protocol

Upon completion of the preparation, control measurements were performed.

An 8F Sones catheter was placed selectively in front of the flow probe into either the LAD or the circumflex artery, then the distal ligation was closed. Two IU thrombin in 0.2 ml saline solution was injected directly in front of the proximal ligation. The catheter was withdrawn and the proximal ligation was closed.

In the four 5-dog groups, the occlusion time was 1 h (group I), 2 h (group II), 4 h (group III), and 6 h (group IV). Eight dogs were excluded from the analysis because of prolonged arrhythmias.

At the end of the occlusion time tracer microspheres were injected for the first time. The proximal and the distal ligations were then opened and the occluded vessel was visualized by contrast angiography. Streptokinase (100 000 IU Kabikinase dissolved in 200 ml saline solution) was infused for 1 h into the left main coronary artery. In the dogs with 1 h occlusion time, tracer microspheres were injected a second time at evidence of increased coronary flow, diagnosed by continuous flowmeter recordings. In the other three groups, the second injection of tracer microspheres was performed after removal of both ligations and the third injection at the time of increased flow into the occluded vessel.

At the end of the experiment, the dogs were sacrificed and the coronary arteries were filled with a $BaSO_4$-gelatine mixture under increasing pressure from 70 to 140 mmHg. Six slices of the left ventricle were incubated in p-NBT following Sandritter's method [25], photographed, and X-rayed. The color slide showing the infarction was superimposed on the angiogram on a computer-coupled graphic tablet to calculate infarct size in percentage of perfusion area.

Results

After removal of ligations, the occluding thrombi of the vessel were visualized by angiography in all cases. Initial removal of the occluding thrombi after injection of the contrast medium was seen in two dogs of group I and in one dog of group II. In all other dogs, there were persistent thrombi at the site of previous ligations causing total occlusions.

Electromagnetic flow measurements indicated a flow of 3.8 ± 6.4 ml in the occluded vessel in group I, and in group III a flow measurement showed no flow after occlusion. All dogs had had a myocardial infarction. The degree of necrosis varied in the four groups; infarct size was calculated as a percentage of the perfusion area involving these groups. Group I had 20% ± 4%, group II 50% ± 7%, group III 34% ± 6%, and

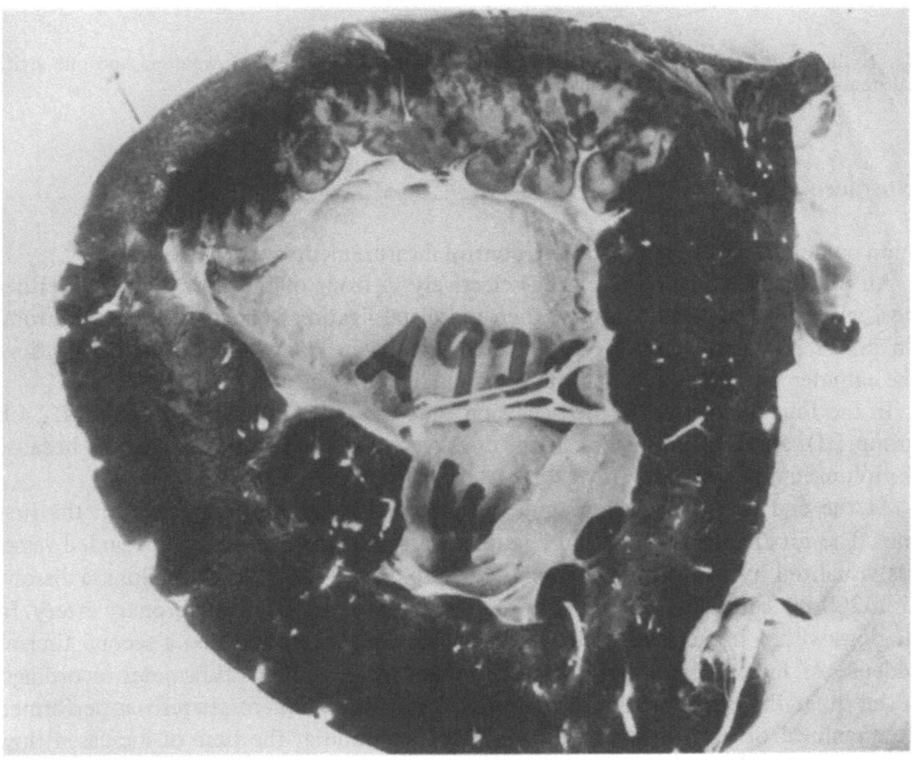

Fig. 2. Slice of the left ventricle of a dog after 1 h occlusion. Incubation with p-NBT. The *pale area* in the subendocardium represents the necrotic tissue of the perfusion are, which is marked by *two needles*

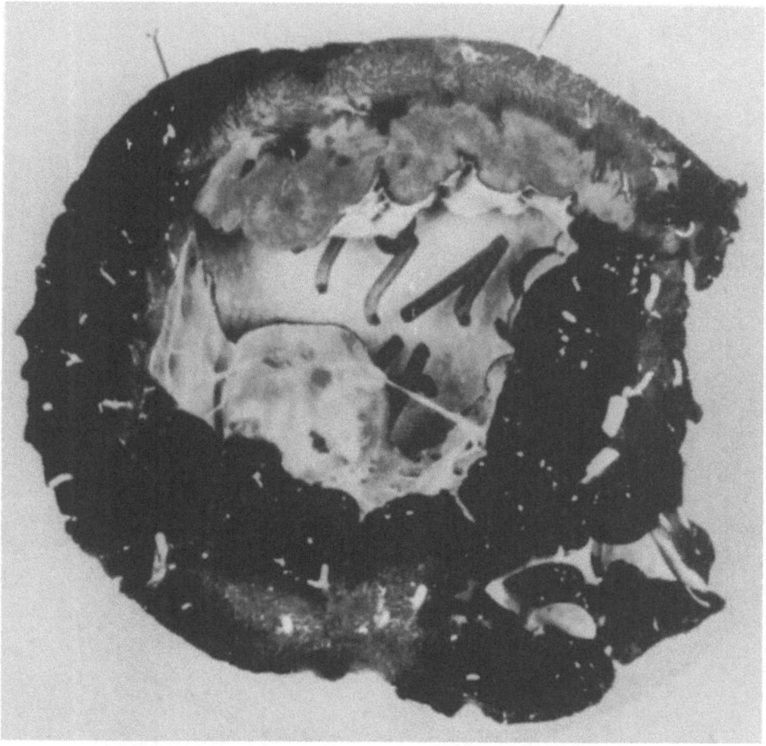

Fig. 3. Slice of the left ventricle of a dog after 2 h occlusion. For details see legend to Fig. 2

group IV 48% ± 7% infarct of the perfusion area of the occluded artery. Macroscopic examination of all the slices of left ventricle, following p-NBT staining, revealed that all animals of group I had had a nonconfluent, patchy infarction, located in the subendocardial myocardium only (Fig. 2). After 2 h occlusion, the infarct area was confluent and involved half of the myocardial tissue in the perfusion area (Fig. 3). In group III the subendocardial layer had a total infarction, but the middle part of the myocardium in the infarct area showed a patchy and nonconfluent necrosis, as demonstrated by Fig. 4. After 6 h occlusion, there was a nearly transmural infarction in some areas, but the necrosis was patchy and nonconfluent in the middle and subepicardial tissue. In all animals of group IV hemorrhage was found, restricted to the center of the necrosis in the subendocardial layer (Fig. 5).

Discussion

Because of the clinical importance of treatment of acute myocardial infarction, much effort has been made to develop a representative animal model. The most common model has been ligation of the LAD, introduced by Harris et al. in 1943 [10]. To avoid thoracotomy, catheter techniques were developed producing obstructions by means of an inflated balloon on the catheter tip [8], or producing a local clot by electrically [24]

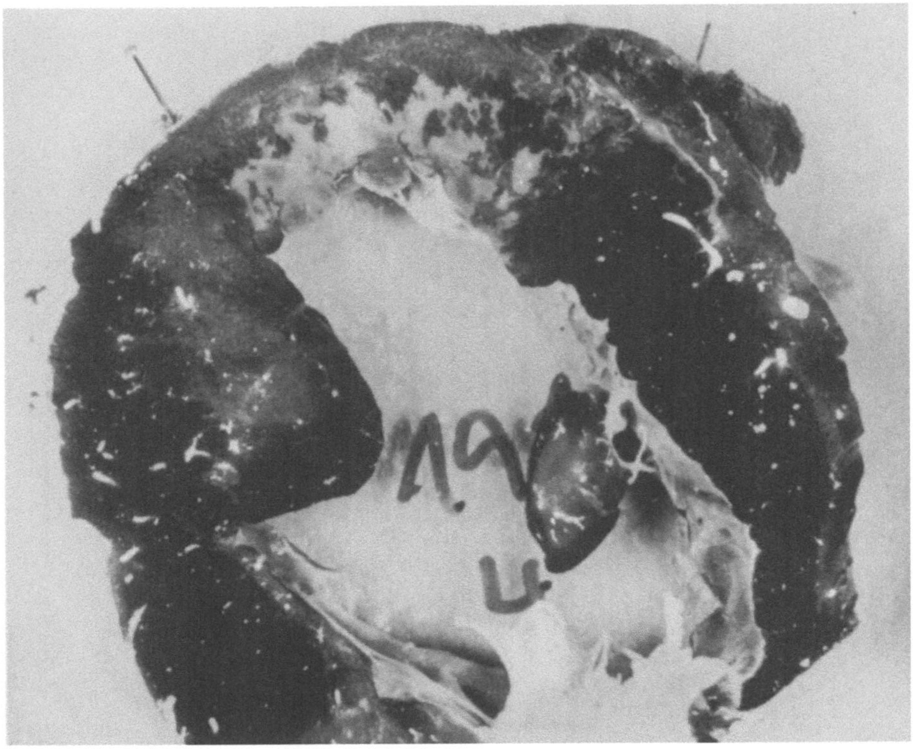

Fig. 4. Slice of the left ventricle of a dog after 4 h occlusion. For details see legend to Fig. 2

or chemically activating coagulation [5]. Using the thrombogenic properties of aluminium-magnesium alloy or copper wires occlusive coronary thrombi can be produced [2, 14]. However, in humans acute coronary artery occlusion is most commonly caused by a thrombosis superimposed upon an atherosclerotic lesion. The fixed atherosclerotic lesion was imitated in our experimental setting by using a constriction corresponding to a lumen reduction of 75%–80%.

Producing thrombi by injection of thrombin was first introduced by Boyles et al. [5]. Histologic studies confirmed the similarity of the experimental thrombus to naturally occurring human arterial thrombus [20].

In all dogs occluding coronary thrombi were found by coronary angiography, which was performed immediately after removal of the ligations. In two dogs of the 1 h occlusion group and one dog of the 2 h group the thrombus was flushed into the peripheral vasculature during the dye injection. This is in accordance with the findings of Mathey and associates, who saw the same effects in patients with short occlusion of the infarct related coronary artery [17]. In patients with a longer interval between onset of symptoms and coronary angiography (longer than 2 h) these effects were not seen. That is in accordance with our experimental results.

Infarct size ranged from 20%–50% in our experiments. Even after 6 h occlusion 52% of the myocardium of the perfusion area was viable. This is in agreement with our results of previously performed experiments in which we found only slightly higher

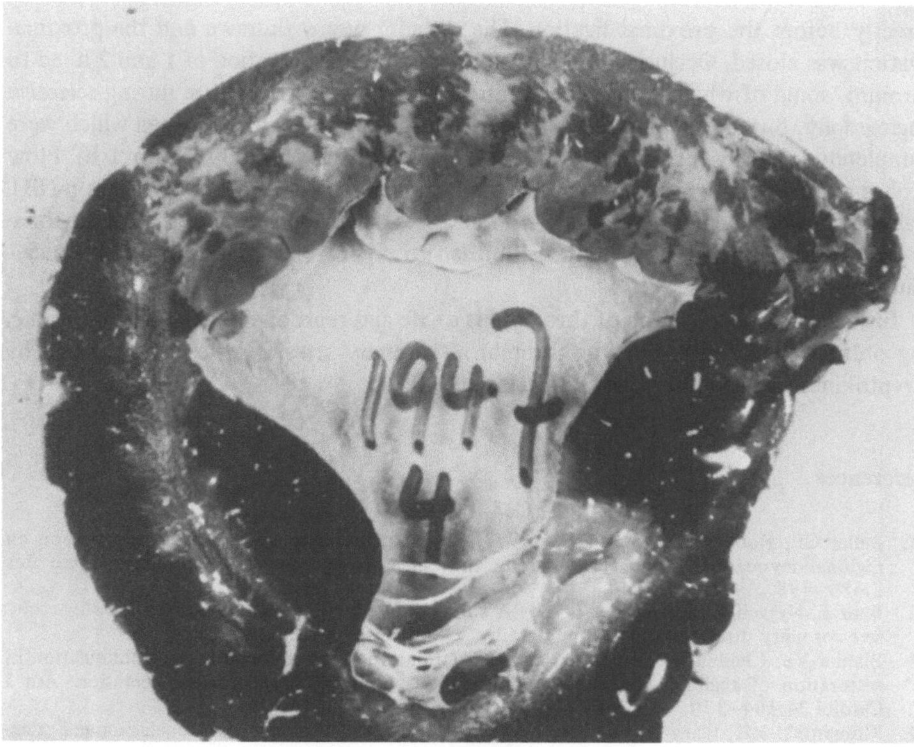

Fig. 5. Slice of the left ventricle of a dog after 6 h occlusion. For details see legend to Fig. 2

infarct sizes with or without reperfusion after 6 h occlusion [12]. Mathur et al. demonstrated a reduction of infarct size when reperfusion was achieved after 2 h occlusion [18]. Especially in this group the incidence of ventricular fibrillation was high (in three of five dogs) and all dogs had to be resuscitated. That might have resulted in a high infarct size in this group.

After 6 h occlusion a considerable amount of myocardium can still be salvaged by reperfusion as indicated by necrosis of only 48% of the perfusion area in our experiments. This is substantiated by our previous results and the experiments of Beller et al., who also found comparable infarct sizes after 6 h occlusion [1, 13].

Summary

Acute myocardial infarction in man is usually due to obturating thrombi in vessels with coronary heart disease. It is therefore desirable to have an experimental model of myocardial ischemia based on a thrombotic coronary occlusion, especially since lysis of thrombi by intracoronary streptokinase application is a new therapeutic approach in man.

In 28 dogs two ligations 15–20 mm apart were prepared at the LAD or at the CX artery. After closure of the distal ligation 2 IU thrombin was injected via a catheter directly before the proximal ligation. The catheter was withdrawn and the proximal ligation was closed. Occlusion time ranged from 1 to 6 h. Ligation of 1 and 2 h led to thrombi, some of which were flushed into the peripheral vasculature during selective angiography, but after 4 and 6 h persistent obturating thrombi were seen which were completely lysed by intracoronary streptokinase infusion (100 000 IU for 1 h). Flow probes and tracer microspheres proved the angiographic findings. Postmortem p-NBT staining showed myocardial infarction in all cases. In five other dogs the intracoronary injection of thrombin without ligation led to myocardial infarction of the epicardium only.

Intracoronary application of thrombin is a safe and reproducible method of producing obturating and disseminating thrombi in coronary arteries which can be lysed by streptokinase infusion into the same vessels.

References

1. Beller GE, Hood WB Jr, Smith TW (1977) Effects of ischemia and coronary reperfusion on regional myocardial blood flow and on the epicardial electrocardiogram. Cardiovasc Res 2:489–498
2. Blair E, Nygren E, Cowley RA (1964) A spiral wire technique for producing gradually occlusive coronary thrombosis. J Thorac Cardiovasc Surg 48:476–485
3. Blanka VS, Chadda KD, Helfant RH (1974) Limitations of myocardial revascularization in restoration of regional contraction abnormalities produced by coronary occlusion. Am J Cardiol 34:164–170
4. Blumenthal MR, Wang H, Liu LMP (1975) Experimental coronary artery occlusion and release. Am J Cardiol 36:225–233
5. Boyles PW, Meyer WH, Graff G, Ashley CC, Ripic RC (1960) Comparative effectiveness of intravenous and intra-arterial Fibrinolyn therapy. Am J Cardiol 6:439–446
6. Capone RJ, Most AS (1978) Myocardial hemorrhage after coronary reperfusion in pigs. Am J Cardiol 41:259–266
7. Constantini C, Corday E, Lang T et al. (1975) Revascularisation after 3 hours of coronary arterial occlusion.: Effects on regional cardial metabolic function and infarct size. Am J Cardiol 36:368–384
8. Corday E, Lang TW, Meerbaum S (1974) Closed chest model intracoronary occlusion for study of regional cardiac function. Am J Cardiol 33:49–59
9. Ganz W, Buchbinder N, Marcus H et al. (1981) Intracoronary thrombolysis in evolving myocardial infarction. Am Heart J 101:4–13
10. Harris AS, Rojas AG (1943) The initiation of ventricular fibrillation due to coronary occlusion. Exp Med Surg 1:105–117
11. Heyndricks GR, Millard RW, McRitchie RH, Maroko PR, Vatner SF (1975) Regional myocardial functional and electrophysiological alterations after brief coronary occlusion in conscious dogs. J Clin Invest 56:978–985
12. Hofmann M, Hofmann M, Genth K, Schaper W (1980) The influence of reperfusion on infarct size after experimental artery occlusion. Basic Res Cardiol 75:572–582
13. Jennings RB, Kaltenbach JP, Sommers HM, Bahr GH, Wartmann WB Studies of the dying myocardial cell. In: James TN, Keyes JW (eds) The etiology of myocardial infarction. Little Brown, Boston, pp 205
14. Kordenat RK, Kezdi P, Stanley EL (1972) A new catheter technique for producing experimental coronary thrombosis and selective visualization. Am Heart J 83:360–364
15. Lang TW, Corday E, Gold H, Meerbaum S (1974) Consequences of reperfusion after coronary occlusion. Effects on hemodynamic and regional myocardial metabolic function. Am J Cardiol 33:69–81
16. Maroko PR, Libby P, Ginks WR et al. (1972) Coronary artery reperfusion. I. Early effects on local myocardial function and the extent of myocardial necrosis. J Clin Invest 51:2710–2716
17. Mathey DG, Kuck KH, Tilsner V, Koebber HJ, Bleifeld W (1981) Nonsurgical coronary artery recanalization in acute transmural myocardial infarction. Circulation 63:489–497

18. Mathur VS, Guinn GA, Buoris WH (1975) Maximal revascularization (reperfusion) in infarct conscious dogs after 2 to 5 hours of coronary occlusion. Am J Cardiol 36:252–261
19. McNamara JJ, Smith GT, Suchiro GT (1974) Myocardial viability after transient ischemia in primates. J Thorac Cardiovasc Surg 68:248–256
20. Oguchi G, Matsuoka M, Ogilkara Y et al. (1956) Experimental studies on thrombosis. Jpn Circ J 23:417–425
21. Puri PS (1975) Contractile and biochemical effects of coronary reperfusion after extended periods of coronary occlusion. Am J Cardiol 36:244–251
22. Rentrop KP, Blanke H, Karsch KR et al. (1979) Acute myocardial infarction: intracoronary application of nitroglycerin and streptokinase in combination with transluminal recanalization. Clin Cardiol 2:354–360
23. Rentrop KP, Blanke H, Karsch KR et al. (1981) Selective intracoronary thrombolysis in acute myocardial infarction and unstable angina pectoris. Circulation 63:307–317
24. Salazar A (1961) Experimental myocardial infarction. Induction of coronary thrombosis in intact closed-chest dog. Circ Res 9:1351–1356
25. Sandritter W, Jestädt R (1958) Triphenyltetrazoliumclorid (TTC) als Reduktionsindikator zur makroskopischen Diagnose des frischen Herzinfarkts. Verh Dtsch Ges Pathol 41:165–172

Thrombolysis in Acute Experimental Myocardial Infarction

K.R. Karsch* **, M. Hofmann***, H. Blanke**, K.P. Rentrop**, W. Schaper***

* Medizinische Klinik, Universität Tübingen, Abt. III, Kardiologie, Otfried-Müller-Str., 7400 Tübingen, FRG
** Mount Sinai Medical Center, New York, N.Y., USA
*** Max Planck Institut, Bad Nauheim, FRG

Introduction

Recent studies in patients with acute myocardial infarction suggested that reduction in infarct size can best be achieved by early recanalization of the infarct-related vessel by means of mechanical or pharmacological intracoronary interventions [12, 23, 31, 32]. Extensive animal experiments were performed to study the effects of early and late coronary artery reperfusion [4, 7, 15, 19, 20, 22, 24, 29]. Jennings and associates [35] had shown that after 20 min occlusion restoration of antegrade flow into the previously occluded artery can prevent myocardial necrosis and the extend of necrosis can vary widely. Nevertheless, less tissue damage was found after transient coronary artery occlusion for a period of up to 3 or 4 h than after permanent coronary artery occlusion [13, 25, 37, 38].

In animal experiments, sudden release of mechanical coronary artery occlusion frequently resulted in dangerous arrhythmias [14]. Additionally, it was speculated that reactive hyperemia after restoration of flow may increase infarct size due to hemorrhage. The objective of the present study was to explore the influence of reperfusion achieved by intracoronary streptokinase on (1) coronary flow, (2) microcirculation, and (3) reperfusion arrhythmias, using a new experimental approach [14].

Materials and Methods

The new experimental approach is described in detail in the preceding article by Hofmann et al. in this volume. After the surgical procedure a 5F Millar catheter-tip manometer was placed in the left ventricle for continuous recording of left ventricular end-diastolic pressure (LVEDP) and systolic pressure. Aortic and right atrial pressure were measured using a Statham pressure transducer. Cardiac index was calculated with a Fischer computer using dye-dilution technique. Left ventricular pressure and LVEDP were used for continuous calculation of myocardial oxygen consumption (MVO_2) according to Bretschneider's equation [6].

In the 5-dog groups, the occlusion time was 1 h (group I), 2 h (group II), 4 h (group III), and 6 h (group IV). At the end of the occlusion time the ligations were opened and streptokinase (100 000 IU Kabikinase dissolved in 200 ml saline solution) was infused for 1 h into the left main coronary artery.

Transluminal Coronary Angioplasty and
Intracoronary Thrombolysis. Ed. by Kaltenbach et al.

Table 1. Hemodynamics ($\overline{X} \pm SD$) before occlusion (time 1), at the end of occlusion (time 2), after withdrawal of ligations (time 3 group II–IV), at reperfusion (time 3 group I, time 4 groups II–IV) after 15 min reperfusion (time 4 group I, time 5 groups II–IV) at the end of streptokinase reperfusion (time 5 group I, time 6 groups II–IV), after 2 hours of reperfusion (time 6 group I, time 7 groups II–IV). LVP, left ventricular pressure; LVEDP, left ventricular end-diastolic pressure; PAO m, mean aortic pressure; CO, cardiac output; HR, heart rate; dp/dt_{max}, maximum rate of LVP rise; dp/dt min, maximum rate of LVP fall; MVO_2, myocardial oxygen consumption

Group	Time	LVP (mmHg)	LVEDP (mmHg)	PAO m (mmHg)	dp/dt max ($mmHg \cdot s^{-1}$)	dp/dt min ($mmHg \cdot s^{-1}$)	CO (liter/min)	HR (beats/ min^{-1})	MVO_2 ($ml\ O_2$/ min • 100 g)
I	1	116 ± 19	18.4 ± 4.4	100 ± 17	1445 ± 348	1741 ± 469	1.4 ± 0.3	75 ± 14	5.3 ± 1.2
	2	109 ± 17	19.1 ± 3.4	96 ± 13	1505 ± 397	1741 ± 464	1.4 ± 0.3	100 ± 40	6.0 ± 2.0
	3	112 ± 16	18.6 ± 1.3	94 ± 9	1478 ± 273	1688 ± 337	1.7 ± 0.5	105 ± 40	6.0 ± 1.8
	4	111 ± 22	18.8 ± 2.5	94 ± 17	1506 ± 508	1596 ± 540	1.4 ± 0.6	105 ± 40	6.0 ± 1.8
	5	101 ± 19	17.8 ± 2.9	84 ± 18	1324 ± 233	1334 ± 378	1.4 ± 0.4	122 ± 31	6.6 ± 0.6
	6	103 ± 17	17.8 ± 3.2	88 ± 15	1393 ± 267	1350 ± 429	1.6 ± 0.6	133 ± 23	7.2 ± 1.1
II	1	100 ± 10	13.9 ± 6.0	79 ± 12	1443 ± 324	1350 ± 120	1.8 ± 0.4	89 ± 28	5.0 ± 0.7
	2	99 ± 14	15.9 ± 4.5	82 ± 17	1463 ± 314	1337 ± 271	1.5 ± 0.6	96 ± 36	5.2 ± 1.3
	3	98 ± 19	15.7 ± 4.3	79 ± 17	1379 ± 272	1239 ± 328	1.5 ± 0.7	101 ± 25	5.5 ± 1.1
	4	101 ± 20	17.5 ± 8.6	78 ± 18	1492 ± 494	1308 ± 435	1.4 ± 0.3	114 ± 35	5.9 ± 1.2
	5	100 ± 18	16.7 ± 7.3	76 ± 20	1512 ± 452	1350 ± 439	1.4 ± 0.3	116 ± 30	6.2 ± 1.6
	6	92 ± 13	17.3 ± 3.7	68 ± 13	1422 ± 243	1098 ± 74	1.4 ± 0.4	99 ± 37	5.2 ± 0.9
	7	90 ± 10	12.6 ± 5.2	64 ± 13	1482 ± 185	1122 ± 249	1.4 ± 0.4	124 ± 22	5.4 ± 1.2
III	1	125 ± 22	16.8 ± 2.8	103 ± 22	1779 ± 532	1847 ± 466	2.3 ± 0.8	92 ± 27	6.6 ± 2.3
	2	113 ± 7	20.5 ± 4.8	92 ± 8	1468 ± 93	1568 ± 286	1.6 ± 0.3	108 ± 42	6.5 ± 1.6
	3	120 ± 22	19.3 ± 4.4	93 ± 25	1739 ± 586	1536 ± 306	1.5 ± 0.4	107 ± 40	6.9 ± 2.5
	4	105 ± 16	19.7 ± 4.1	85 ± 14	1419 ± 366	1326 ± 293	1.6 ± 0.4	122 ± 21	6.8 ± 1.2
	5	105 ± 14	19.8 ± 3.8	78 ± 18	1454 ± 300	1376 ± 260	1.4 ± 0.3	125 ± 20	7.0 ± 1.2
	6	104 ± 14	19.8 ± 3.8	76 ± 16	1446 ± 317	1341 ± 268	1.8 ± 0.8	126 ± 23	6.9 ± 1.2
	7	104 ± 11	19.9 ± 5.8	75 ± 16	1439 ± 361	1275 ± 194	1.7 ± 0.9	134 ± 22	7.1 ± 1.2
IV	1	125 ± 10	15.4 ± 4.1	104 ± 8	1698 ± 659	1757 ± 314	2.7 ± 1.2	106 ± 26	7.2 ± 1.1
	2	125 ± 14	19.5 ± 5.5	100 ± 10	1747 ± 387	1746 ± 387	2.4 ± 0.6	104 ± 27	6.8 ± 1.0
	3	125 ± 19	22.6 ± 5.7	96 ± 18	1680 ± 494	1680 ± 494	2.0 ± 0.7	104 ± 23	6.8 ± 0.9
	4	117 ± 17	20.9 ± 5.1	90 ± 18	1607 ± 463	1607 ± 463	2.2 ± 1.0	130 ± 20	7.6 ± 1.4
	5	114 ± 10	21.0 ± 4.5	85 ± 16	1527 ± 461	1526 ± 461	2.1 ± 1.2	135 ± 22	7.9 ± 1.9
	6	112 ± 24	20.2 ± 4.9	88 ± 23	1458 ± 600	1458 ± 599	1.9 ± 0.6	139 ± 34	8.1 ± 1.2
	7	112 ± 13	19.2 ± 3.6	84 ± 17	1590 ± 345	1590 ± 345	1.7 ± 0.4	136 ± 31	7.4 ± 1.1

Tracer microspheres were injected in all groups at the end of the occlusion time as previously described. The third injection (group I) and the fourth injection (group II–IV) of tracer microspheres were performed 15 min after the increase of flow in the infarct-related vessel.

Tracer microspheres were again injected at the end of streptokinase infusion and after 2 h of the control period in all groups. The catheter was withdrawn and after a control period of 2 h the dogs were sacrificed. The tracer microspheres were 9 μm in diameter and labeled with ^{141}Ce, ^{51}Cr, ^{85}Sc, ^{95}Nb, ^{46}Sc, or ^{113}Sn, 600 000 beads per isotope (3M Company), and injected into the inflow cannula into the left atrium. Two hundred samples per heart were analyzed for radioactivity in a computer-based multichannel gamma spectrometer as described earlier by Schaper et al. [33].

In all four groups, MVO_2 was maintained at a constant level between 5.5 and 8 ml/min/100 g before occlusion and during occlusion, streptokinase infusion, and reperfusion time.

No medication was administered which might have influenced the infarct size, such as nitroglycerin, beta-blockers, or alpha-adrenergic substances.

Results

A total of eight dogs died during the procedure. Five died immediately after closure of the coronary artery, or their resuscitation required more than 5 min. Three died during the reperfusion, two after 1 h and one after 2 h occlusion, due to prolonged episodes of ventricular fibrillation which could not be controlled within 5 min. These dogs were excluded from the following analysis.

Changes of hemodynamic parameters during and after reperfusion are summarized in Table I. Left ventricular end-diastolic pressure decreased slightly from the control measurements to those of reperfusion time in groups I and II with short occlusion time (1 and 2 h respectively). In both groups with longer occlusion times (4 and 6 h occlusion) LVEDP increased significantly ($P < 0.001$) from the time of control measurement to the time of postreperfusion measurement. Contractility showed a marked but not significant decrease in group III only. Cardiac output remained unchanged in both early groups, and decreased significantly in those dogs with prolonged occlusion of the infarct vessel. In all dogs heart rate showed a significant ($P < 0.001$) increase from the preocclusion to the reperfusion period. Myocardial oxygen consumption remained unchanged in groups II, III, and IV and increased significantly in group I only ($P < 0.01$).

Lysis time was defined as the time from the start of streptokinase infusion, and the subsequent increase of flow was measured by electromagnetic flowmeter. Mean lysis time was: group I, 4.6 ± 2.1 min (mean ± SD); group II, 8.4 ± 2.9 min; group III, 15.2 ± 3.9 min; group IV, 30.8 ± 5.5 min ($P < 0.01$).

Electromagnetic flow measurements indicated a flow of 3.8 ± 6.4 ml/min in the occluded vessel in group I, and in group III a flow of 2.4 ± 5.4 ml/min; in groups II and IV the electromagnetic flow measurement showed no flow after occlusion. In all dogs there was an increase of flow directly at the time of partial dissolution of the thrombus: flow increased to 29.6 ± 12.5 ml/min in group I, to 26.2 ± 26.6 ml/min in group II, to 39.4 ± 33.5 ml/min in group III, and to 29.2 ± 19.8 ml/min in group IV. No significant change in coronary flow occurred after reperfusion and during the control period (Table 2).

The changes of microcirculation are depicted in Figs. 1–4. Flow ratio was calculated from microsphere measurements in the ischemic and nonischemic areas from the endo- and epicardial layers. In all groups, a difference between endo- and epicardial flow ratio was found. Both endocardial and epicardial flow increased at the time of reperfusion, and during the period after reperfusion. There was a marked decrease in the endocardial layers during the control period; the epicardial flow appeared nearly unchanged.

After closure of the LAD/Cx in the 20 dogs remaining in the study, three dogs had immediate ventricular fibrillation at the time of occlusion. Defibrillation was successful in all animals at once. Six dogs developed transient multifocal ventricular

Table 2. Mean value and standard deviation of coronary electromagnetic flow measurement (C flow) and microcirculation determined by tracer microspheres at the different time intervals (see Table 1)

Group	Time	C flow		Microspheres	
		Infarct vessel (ml/min)	Control (ml/min)	Endocardial p/n ratio	Epicardial p/n ratio
I	1	25 ± 5	28 ± 3	–	–
	2	3 ± 3	37 ± 11	0.2	0.37
	3	25 ± 8	35 ± 11	0.87	1.2
	4	30 ± 6	42 ± 15	0.95	1.03
	5	29 ± 4	33 ± 8	0.72	0.96
	6	30 ± 7	30 ± 5	0.68	1.01
II	1	78 ± 3	28 ± 3	–	–
	2	0	39 ± 9	0.26	0.32
	3	1 ± 1	44 ± 8	0.31	0.47
	4	26 ± 11	49 ± 18	0.54	0.97
	5	40 ± 9	42 ± 13	0.72	0.85
	6	22 ± 3	46 ± 11	0.62	0.79
	7	20 ± 5	38 ± 10	0.44	0.96
III	1	37 ± 7	45 ± 15	–	–
	2	2 ± 2	36 ± 7	0.11	0.31
	3	5 ± 3	35 ± 8	0.14	0.37
	4	39 ± 15	63 ± 18	0.42	0.71
	5	40 ± 8	49 ± 12	0.72	0.97
	6	40 ± 8	46 ± 10	0.6	0.83
	7	35 ± 8	58 ± 15	0.61	0.77
IV	1	27 ± 5	58 ± 18	–	–
	2	0	38 ± 7	0.16	0.28
	3	3 ± 2	43 ± 8	0.17	0.41
	4	29 ± 9	49 ± 13	0.90	0.96
	5	32 ± 10	45 ± 9	0.71	1.03
	6	38 ± 10	58 ± 14	0.47	0.95
	7	33 ± 15	56 ± 18	0.37	1.08

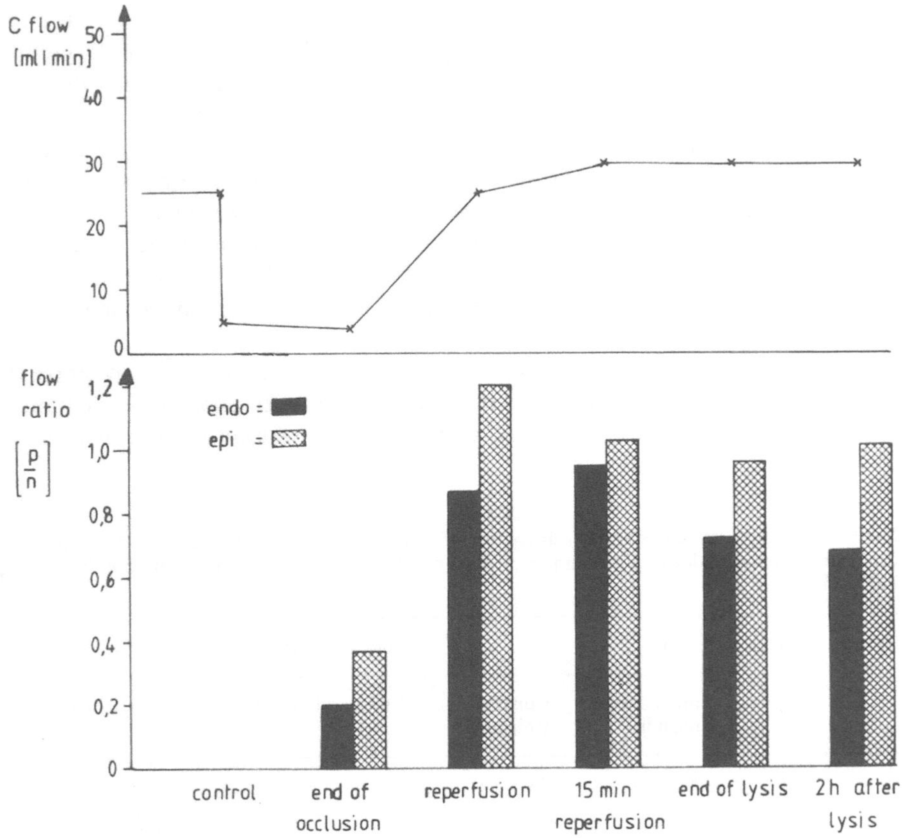

Fig. 1. Comparison of electromagnetic flow (*upper panel*) and tracer microsphere flow (*lower panel*) in group I

premature beats. In one dog, ventricular tachycardia occurred for 5 min. Ventricular fibrillation, which could easily be managed after one countershock with 50 Ws occurred at the time of increased flow in the previously occluded artery in two dogs in group I, three dogs in group II, and one dog in group III. Three dogs in group developed multifocal persistent premature ventricular beats after reperfusion; one dog developed a new left bundle branch block 5 min after reperfusion, and one an AV block I. In group II, three dogs showed persistent multifocal ventricular beat; one dog developed a bigeminus for 40 min. In group III, all dogs had transient premature ventricular beats after reperfusion; in one dog a bigeminus occurred. In group IV, no ventricular fibrillation occurred; one dog developed a left bundle branch block, and three dogs had transient premature ventricular beats.

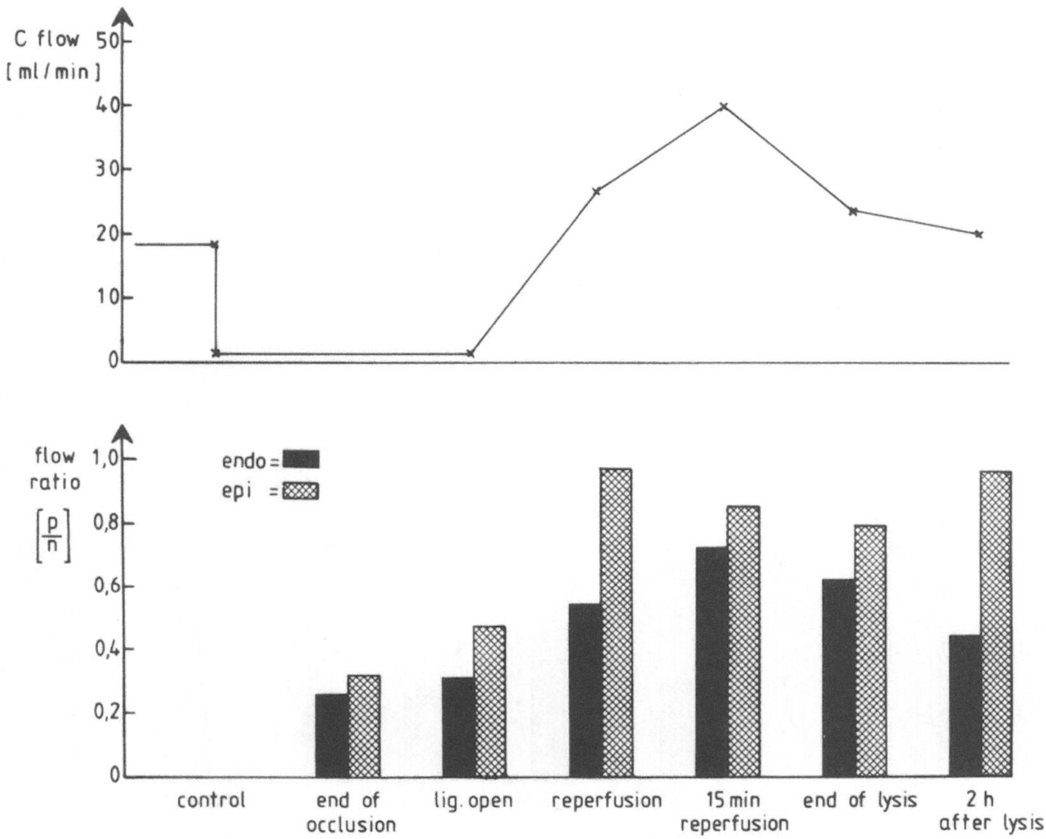

Fig. 2. Electromagnetic coronary flow (*upper panel*) and tracer microsphere flow (*lower panel*) in group II

Discussion

Restoration of blood flow to the ischemic myocardium was achieved by selective infusion of streptokinase directly into the occluded coronary artery. The effectiveness of lysis of intracoronary thrombi by fibronolytic substances was first demonstrated by Boyles et al. in 1960: however, the drug was administered semiselectively into the root of the aorta [5].

In all dogs, rapid lysis was achieved even after 6 h occlusion. Our findings suggest that lysis time is dependent upon the previous occlusion time. These findings are in concordance with the results of Kordenat et al., who found a linear relationship between the age of the thrombus and the time required to attain complete lysis [18].

Fischbein et al. have demonstrated that hemorrhage is caused by disruption of endothelium of large intramyocardial arteries [11]. Kloner et al. demonstrated that endothelial injury occurs 4–6 h after occlusion [17]. As indicated by our results, the minimal occlusion time required for occurrence of hemorrhage is not altered if reperfusion is achieved by local application of streptokinase.

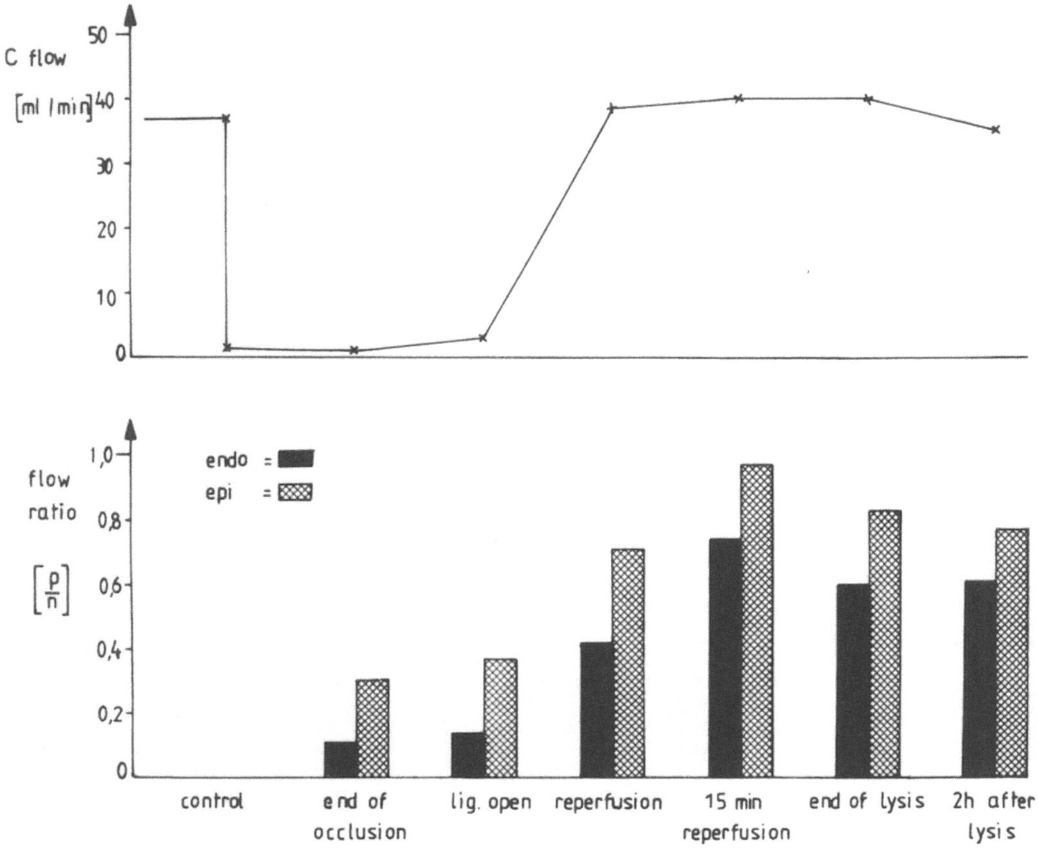

Fig. 3. Electromagnetic coronary flow (*upper panel*) and tracer microsphere flow (*lower panel*) in group III

The effects on coronary flow and microcirculation during and after intracoronary lysis of thrombi by streptokinase are unknown. The efficacy of total occlusion by a clot was demonstrated by microspheres which showed minimal flow in the perfusion area of the occluded artery in all dogs and was not different to the flow after withdrawal of the ligations.

At the time of reperfusion, myocardial blood flow in the epicardial layer showed an immediate significant increase to normal levels in all groups, whereas endocardial flow normalized only in group IV at once. The slow increase of endocardial flow after reperfusion was possibly due to further lysis of thrombotic material at the site of the stenosis or in the periphery of the occluded artery in groups I–III, or to slow flow phenomena resulting from ischemic changes in the coronary vascular beds. However, this seems to be unlikely since Bloor et al. found significant changes only after more than 6 h occlusion [3].

The immediate normalization of myocardial blood flow in the endocardial layer at the time of reperfusion, which occurred only in group IV after 6 h occlusion, coincides with the macroscopic findings of central hemorrhage in this group. Thus, the

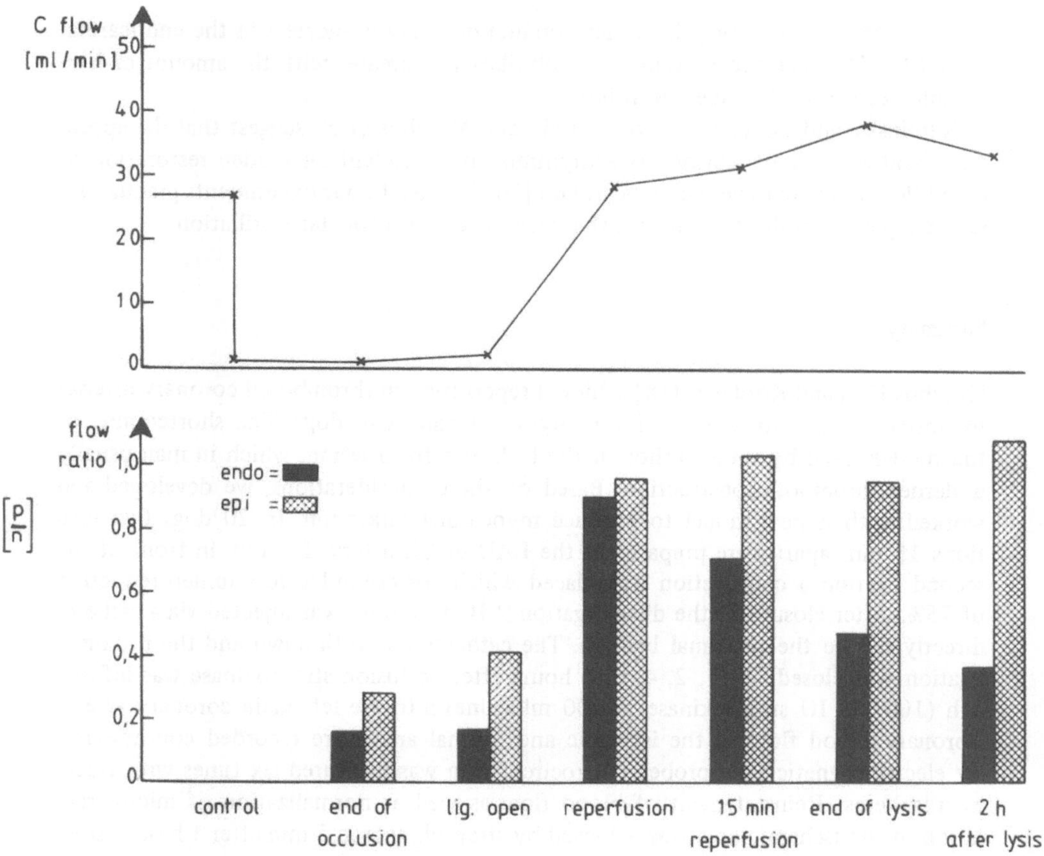

Fig. 4. Electromagnetic coronary flow (*upper panel*) and tracer microsphere flow (*lower panel*) in group IV

myocardial blood flow increase after 6 h occlusion is more likely due to hemorrhage into the myocardium resulting from endothelial injury of the peripheral vasculature.

Malignant ventricular arrhythmias after occlusion and during reperfusion are reported to be the other major hazard in early recanalization of the infarct vessel in animal experiments [1, 2, 8, 27, 30, 36, 39]. In 1960 Stephenson reported ventricular fibrillation after occlusion of the left anterior descending artery in 91 of 330 dogs [36]. After 30 min occlusion, reperfusion was performed and ventricular fibrillation occurred after sudden relief of the ligation in 169 of 239 dogs. The proportion of ventricular fibrillations after occlusion found in our dogs (13/28) is similar to the results of Stephenson. Ventricular fibrillation occurred after reperfusion in ten of eighteen dogs with occlusion of 1 or 2 h. Only one dog in the two groups with longer occlusion times developed ventricular fibrillation after reperfusion. Therefore, occurrence of reperfusion arrhythmias seems to be dependent on the duration of previous occlusion. Since reperfusion promptly restores electrical activity in fibers rendered unresponsive by ischemia, as demonstrated by Downar et al. [10], it is likely that reperfusion may also transiently reestablish the conductions necessary for reentry, resulting in the reemergence of ectopic activity [28]. Since conduction delay is shortest in the endocardial layer [9, 34], incidence of ventricular fibrillation decreases with the amount of irreversible necrosis in the subendocardium.

Kaplinsky and associates, Levites et al., and Moschos et al. suggest that the appearance and severity of ventricular arrhythmias is dependent on sudden restoration of blood flow to acute ischemic myocardium [16, 21, 26]. In our experiments gradual onset of reperfusion did not prevent the occurence of ventricular fibrillation.

Summary

Moschos [26] and Kordenat [18] achieved reperfusion in thrombosed coronary arteries by intracoronary infusion of thrombolytic substances in dogs. The shortcoming of the models used by these authors is the lack of a fixed lesion, which in man usually underlies thrombotic obstruction. Based on these considerations, we developed and worked with a new model to produce myocardial infarction. In 20 dogs two ligations 15 mm apart were prepared at the LAD or CX artery. Directly in front of the second ligation a constriction was placed which corresponded to a lumen reduction of 75%. After closure of the distal ligation 2 IU thrombin was injected via a catheter directly before the proximal ligation. The catheter was withdrawn and the proximal ligation was closed. At 1, 2, 4, or 6 hours after occlusion streptokinase was infused 1 h (100 000 IU streptokinase in 200 ml saline) into the left main coronary artery. Coronary blood flow to the ischemic and normal area were recorded continuously by electromagnetic flow probes. Microcirculation was measured six times with tracer microspheres. Reinstatement of blood flow as well as normalization of microcirculation in the ischemic area was achieved by streptokinase in 5 min after 1 h occlusion, 8 min after 2 h, 15 min after 4 h, and 31 min after 6 h.

At the time of reopening of the coronary artery, flow increased slowly; no hyperemic response was noted by the flow probe measurements. Microsphere measurements showed an initial normalization of flow directly after reperfusion in all myocardial layers and a slow decrease of flow in the endocardial layers during the control period. Hemorrhage occurred only after 6 h occlusion and was limited to the central area of necrosis.

In the presence of a high-degree fixed stenosis and thrombotic occlusion, local infusion of streptokinase resulted in a slow restoration of antegrade flow without hyperemia. Furthermore, recanalization by thrombolytic substances does not increase the extent of reperfusion hemorrhage. Serious reperfusion arrhythmias occurred only after 1 and 2 h occlusion and seemed to be independent of the mode of reperfusion.

References

1. Axelrod PJ, Verrier RL, Lown B (1975) Vulnerability to ventricular fibrillation during acute coronary occlusion and release. Am J Cardiol 36:776–782
2. Battle WE, Naimi S, Avitall B et al. (1974) Distinctive time cause of ventricular vulnerability to fibrillation during and after release of coronary ligation. Am J Cardiol 34:42–47
3. Bloor CM, White FC (1975) Coronary artery reperfusion. Effects of occlusion duration on reactive hyperemia responses. Basic Res Cardiol 70:148–158
4. Bolooki H, Golkar RR, Morales A, Kaiser GA (1973) Effects of direct myocardial revascularization on infarct size: a clinical and experimental correlation. Surg Forum 24:137–139
5. Boyles PW, Meyer WH, Graff J, Ashley CC, Ripic RG (1960) Comparative effectiveness of intravenous and intraarterial fibrinolysin therapy. Am J Cardiol 6:439–455
6. Bretschneider HJ (1971) Determinanten des myokardialen Sauerstoffverbrauchs. In: Dengler HJ (ed) Die therapeutische Anwendung betasympathicolytischer Stoffe. Stuttgart New York
7. Constantini C, Corday E, Lang TW et al. (1975) Revascularization after 3 hours of coronary arterial occlusion: Effects on regional cardiac metabolic function and infarct size. Am J Cardiol 36:368–384
8. Corbalan R, Verrier RL, Lown B (1976) Differing mechanisms for ventricular vulnerability during coronary artery occlusion and release. Am Heart J 92:223–230
9. Cox JL, Daniel TM, Boineau JP (1973) The electrophysiologic time course of acute myocardial ischemia and the effects of early coronary artery reperfusion. Circulation 48:971–979
10. Doronar E, Janse MK, Durreo D (1977) The effect of acute coronary artery occlusion on subepicardial transmembrane potentials in the intact porcine heart. Circulation 56:217–224
11. Fishbein MC, Y-Rit J, Lando U, Kanamatsuse K, Mercier JC, Ganz W (1980) The relationship of vascular injury and myocardial hemorrhage to necrosis after reperfusion. Circulation 62:1274–1279
12. Ganz W, Buchbinder N, Marcus H et al. (1981) Intracoronary thrombolysis in evolving myocardial infarction. Am Heart J 101:4–13
13. Ginks WR, Sybers HD, Maroko PR, Corvell JW, Sober BE, Ross J (1972) Coronary artery reperfusion. J Clin Invest 51:2717–2723
14. Hofmann M, Hofmann M, Genth K, Schaper W (to be published) The influence of reperfusion on infarct size after experimental artery occlusion. Basic Res Cardiol
15. Jarmakani JM, Limbird L, Graham TC, Marks RA (1976) Effects of reperfusion on myocardial infarct, and the accuracy of estimating infarct size from serum creatine phosphokinase in the dog. Cardiovasc Res 10:245–253
16. Kaplinski E, Ogawa S, Michelson EL, Dreifus LS (1981) Instantaneous and delayed ventricular arrhythmias after reperfusion of acutely ischemic myocardium: evidence for multiple mechanisms. Circulation 63:333–340
17. Kloner RA, Rude RE, Carlson N et al. (1980) Ultrastructural evidence of microvascular damage and myocardial cell injury after coronary artery occlusion: which comes first. Circulation 6:945–952
18. Kordenat RK, Kezdi P, Stanley EL (1972) A new catheter technique for producing experimental coronary thrombosis and selective visualization. Am Heart J 83:360–364
19. Krug A (1970) The extent of ischemic damage in the myocardium of the cat after permanent and temporary coronary occlusion. J Thorac Cardiovasc Surg 60:242–247
20. Lang TW, Corday E, Gold H et al. (1974) Consequences of reperfusion after coronary occlusion. Am J Cardiol 33:69–81
21. Levites R, Banka VS, Helfant RH (1975) Electrophysiologic effects of coronary occlusion and reperfusion. Circulation 52:760–765
22. Maroko PR, Libby P, Ginks WR et al. (1972) Coronary artery reperfusion. I. Early effects on local myocardial function and the extent of myocardial necrosis. J Clin Invest 51:2710–2716
23. Mathey DG, Kuck KH, Tilsner V, Koebbler HJ, Bleifeld W (1981) Nonsurgical coronary artery recanalization in acute transmural myocardial infarction. Circulation 63:489–497
24. Mathur VS, Guinn GA, Burris WH (1975) Maximal revascularization (reperfusion) in intact conscious dogs after 2 to 5 hours of coronary occlusion. Am J Cardiol 36:252–261
25. McNamara JJ, Smith GT, Suehiro GT (1974) Myocardial viability after transient ischemia in primates. J Thorac Cardiovasc Surg 68:248–256
26. Moschos CB, Burke WM, Lenau PH, Oldewurtel HA, Regan TJ (1970) Thrombolytic agents and lysis of coronary artery thrombosis. Cardiovasc Res 4:228–234

27. Murdock DK, Loeb JM, Euler DE, Randall WC (1979) Electrophysiology of coronary reperfusion. Circulation 61:175–182
28. Naimi S, Avital B, Levine HJ (1974) Abrupt shortening of effective refraction period (ERP) following coronary ligation: possible mechanism of reperfusion arrhythmias. Circulation 50 [Suppl]:III–385
29. O'Brien C, Caroll M, O'Rouke PT et al. (1972) The reversibility of acute ischemic injury to the myocardium by restoration of coronary flow. J Thorac Cardiovasc Surg 64:840–846
30. Penskoe PA, Sobel BE, Corr PB (1978) Disparate electrophysiological alterations accompanying dysrhythmia due to coronary occlusion and reperfusion in the cat. Circulation 58:1023–1035
31. Rentrop KP, Blanke H, Karsch KR et al. (1979) Acute myocardial infarction: intracoronary application of nitroglycerin and streptokinase in combination with transluminal recanalization. Clin Cardiol 2:354–360
32. Rentrop KP, Blanke H, Karsch KR et al. (1981) Selective intracoronary thrombolysis in acute myocardial infarction and unstable angina pectoris. Circulation 63:307–317
33. Schaper W (1971) The collateral circulation of the heart. Elsevier, Amsterdam London New York
34. Scheelag BJ, El-Sherif N, Hope RR, Lazzara R (1974) Characterisation and localisation of ventricular arrhythmias resulting from myocardial ischemia and infarction. Circ Res 35:372–380
35. Sommers HM, Kennings RB (1964) Experimental acute myocardial infarction. Histological and histochemical studies of early myocardial infarcts induced by temporary or permanent occlusion of a coronary artery. Lab Invest 13:1491–1503
36. Stephenson SE, Cole PK, Parrish FF (1960) Ventricular fibrillation during and after coronary artery occlusion. Incidence and protection afforded by various drugs. Am J Cardiol 5:77–84
37. Theroux P, Franklin D, Ross J, Kemper W Jr (1974) Regional myocardial function during acute coronary artery occlusion and its modification by pharmacologic agents in the dog. Circ Res 35:896–908
38. Theroux P, Ross J, Franklin D, Kemper WS, Sasayama S (1976) Coronary arterial reperfusion. III. Early and late effects on regional myocardial function and dimensions in conscious dogs. Am J Cardiol 38:599–606
39. Waldo AL, Kaiser GA (1973) A study of ventricular arrhythmias associated with acute myocardial infarction in the canine heart. Circulation 47:1222–1228

Serum Creatine Kinase Values in the Course of Acute Myocardial Infarction Following Local Fibrinolytic Therapy

A. Ryzlewicz, F. Martens, Th. Schirop, K. Ibe

Resuscitation Center of the Medical Clinic and Outpatient Department of the Free University of Berlin at the Charlottenburg Clinic

Local application of streptokinase into the stenosed coronary artery was introduced in our department of cardiology at the beginning of 1980. The criteria which must be fulfilled before the procedure may be performed are:

1. Time since onset of chest pain 3 hours or less
2. Typical myocardial infarction findings on ECG
3. No absolute contraindication to streptokinase or anticoagulant therapy.

After ventriculography and coronarography in which the stenosed coronary artery was located, streptokinase was administered to a mean total dose of 300 000 units. After transfer to the intensive care unit serial measurements of creatine kinase (CK) concentration were made every 4 h for about 3 days in order to estimate the extent of myocardial infarction.

Figure 1 shows the composition of the two groups. Fifty-five patients were treated conservatively as a control group. Twenty-eight patients underwent local fibrinolytic therapy with positive results in 21 cases.

Figure 2 shows the serum CK levels of these groups averaged at corresponding times. There is a difference in maximum CK levels. A maximum was found at 16 h after

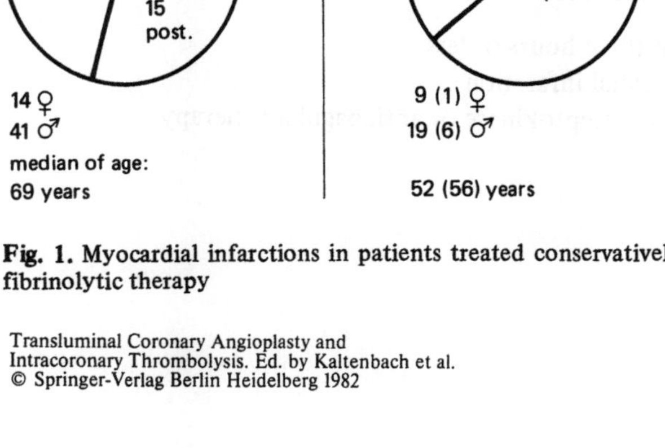

Fig. 1. Myocardial infarctions in patients treated conservatively and in patients treated with local fibrinolytic therapy

Transluminal Coronary Angioplasty and
Intracoronary Thrombolysis. Ed. by Kaltenbach et al.

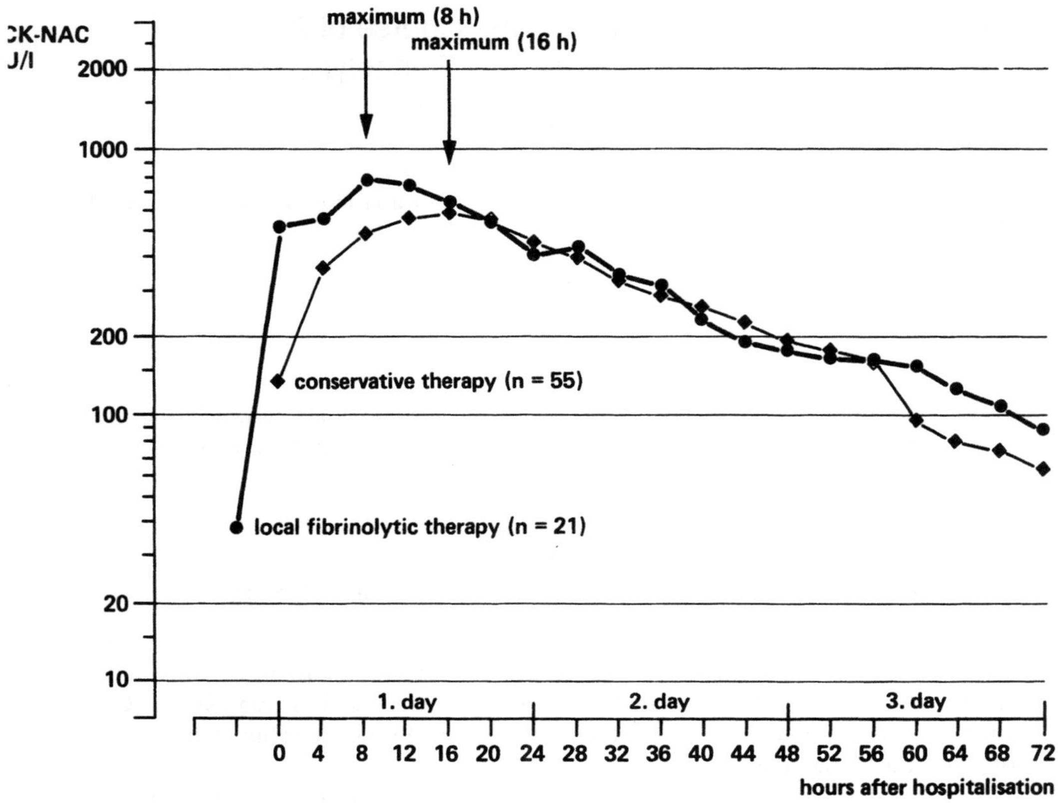

Fig. 2. Average serum CK levels in the two groups. (*NAC* = N-acetyl cysteine activated test)

admission in the conservatively treated patients; the maximum in the streptokinase group occurred at 8 h after terminating local therapy.

If equal total amounts of CK are measured in the course of myocardial infarction then the higher maximum must occur earlier. If an earlier maximum is found in a lower curve, one may deduce that this represents a smaller infarction. Comparing the average CK levels we could not find this constellation and suspect that local fibrinolytic therapy – in our cases and from the evidence of CK measurements – could not reduce the size of myocardial infarction.

Criteria for coronary recanalisation with streptokinase are:

1. Time since onset of chest pain three hours or less
2. ECG findings typical of myocardial infarction
3. No absolute contraindication to streptokinase or anticoagulant therapy.

Literature from the authors

Effects of Coronary Artery Reperfusion on Myocardial Infarct Size in Conscious Dogs

G.R. Heyndrickx, P.R. Maroko, K. Baughman, S.F. Vatner

Department of Cardiology, Akademisch Ziekenhuis, University of Gent, Belgium, and the Department of Medicine, Harvard Medical School, Peter Bent Brigham Hospital, Boston, USA

Introduction

Since Kjekshus and Sobel [8] and Shell et al. [12] observed a quantitative relationship between the size of experimental myocardial infarction and the depletion of creatine kinase (CK) in the myocardium and demonstrated a linear relationship between the size of experimental myocardial infarction – determined by myocardial CK depletion – and the amount of CK appearing in the blood, the determination of the extent of necrosis during the acute phase of myocardial infarction has become an important point in the clinical evaluation and management of patients with acute infarction.

Coronary artery reperfusion during the acute phase of infarction using intracoronary streptokinase infusion is now currently performed in several centers, infarct size usually being calculated from the amount of CK appearing in the blood over a 24-h period.

Since prior studies examining the effects of reperfusion on the calculation of infarct size from the appearance of CK in blood have been conflicting [3, 6] the goals of this study were to evaluate (a) the relationship between CK appearance in blood and myocardial infarct size as determined by myocardial CK depletion after a 24-h coronary occlusion; (b) this relationship in a separate series of dogs, in which reperfusion intervened; and (c) the relationship between myocardial infarct size determined by gross (pathology (and confirmed by histology) and by myocardial CK depletion. Experiments were conducted in conscious dogs to avoid the effects of anesthesia on enzyme kinetics [12] and also because these animals remain hemodynamically stable after coronary occlusion [5].

Methods

Thirty-six mongrel dogs (19–35 kg) were anesthetized with 30 mg/kg sodium pentobarbital for implantation of a Doppler ultrasonic flow transducer and a hydraulic occluding cuff on either the left anterior descending or circumflex coronary artery and heparin-filled Tygon catheters (Norton Co., Tallmadge, Ohio) in the left atrium and aorta [5].

Experiments were conducted 3–6 weeks after recovery from operation. The occluding cuff was inflated for 24 h in 19 dogs. Reperfusion was carried out 1 h after occlu-

Transluminal Coronary Angioplasty and
Intracoronary Thrombolysis. Ed. by Kaltenbach et al.

sion in nine dogs and 3 h after occlusion in eight dogs. Serial samples of blood were withdrawn from each dog over a 24-h period. After 24 h all dogs were anesthetized with sodium pentobarbital and killed. The heart was excised and prepared for myocardial CK determination and pathology.

In all dogs infarct size (IS) was determined by gross pathological inspection (IS_p) and compared with calculated infarct size from CK appearance in the blood samples (IS_s). Infarct size was also determined by myocardial CK depletion (IS_m) in 11 dogs with 24-h occlusion and 14 dogs with reperfusion. CK was assayed using CK n-1 reagent while protein contents of homogenates and of tissue fraction were determined by the biuret procedure [4]. Creatine kinase in plasma and tissue fractions was assayed spectrophotometrically as described by Rosalki [11]. Results were expressed as international units per milliliter, international units per milligram protein, or international units per milliliter per gram myocardium. The techniques and formulas described by Shell et al. [12] were used to calculated IS_m and IS_s.

Linear regression analysis was used to examine relationship among infarct size measurements. The slopes were compared by calculating residual variances and using the t distribution to test for significant differences [1].

Results

Effects of Reperfusion on Gross Appearance of Infarct

The infarct size determined by gross pathology was similar in the 24-h occlusion group (23.2 ± 4.6 g) (mean ± SEM) and the 1- and 3-h occlusion groups (24.1 ± 5.2 g). However, all groups showed marked variability in infarct size, e.g., left circumflex occlusion produced infarct ranging from 0–51.5 g. Hemorrhagic infarcts were present in 23% of dogs with 24-h occlusion compared with 83% of the reperfused dogs.

Effects of Reperfusion on Serial Blood CK Curve

Reperfusion both at 1 h and 3 h resulted in a significant alteration of the configuration of the blood CK curves from those obtained from dogs with 24-h occlusions (Fig. 1). After 1-h, 3-h, and 24-h occlusion CK reached a peak respectively at 4.2 ± 0.4 h, 6.8 ± 0.5 h, and 11.4 ± 0.5 h.

Relationship Between IS_s and IS_m

Twenty-four Hour Occlusion. A linear relationship was observed ($IS_s = 14.26 \pm 1.18 \times IS_m$, $r = 0.92$) (Fig. 2).

Reperfusion. While the relationship remained linear, it was altered ($IS_s = 15.33 + 2.07 \times IS_m$, $r = 0.89$). The slope was significantly greater ($P < 0.05$) than observed for dogs

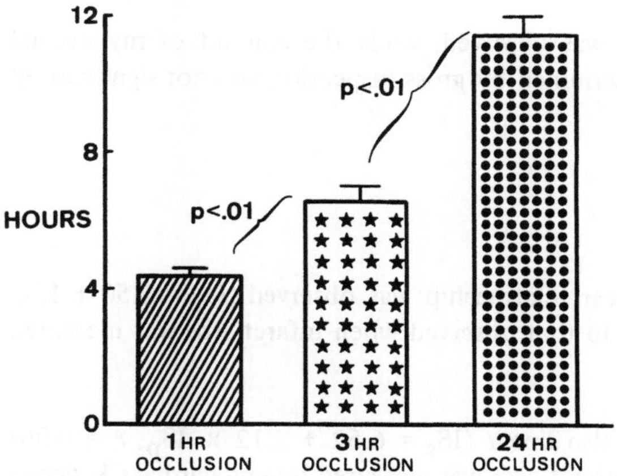

Fig. 1. The average time to peak blood CK activity is compared for dogs perfused at either 1 or 3 h and dogs with permanent occlusion. The time to peak blood CK activity was significantly different in the three groups ($P < 0.01$)

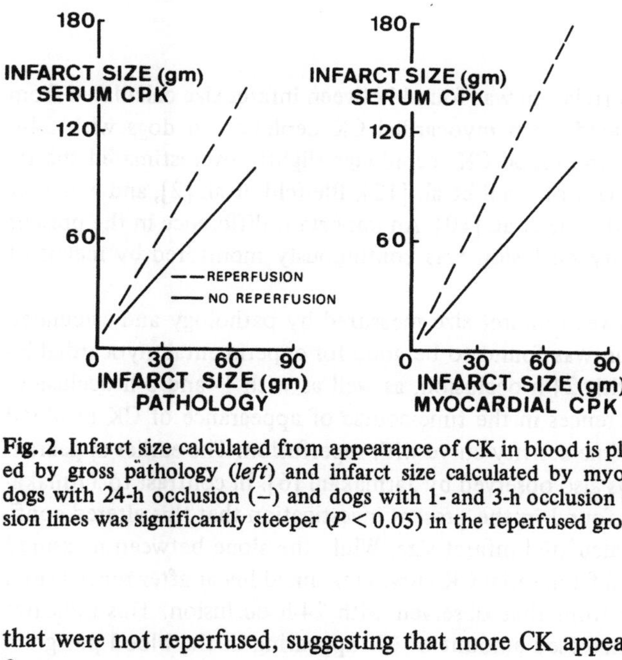

Fig. 2. Infarct size calculated from appearance of CK in blood is plotted against infarct size measured by gross pathology (*left*) and infarct size calculated by myocardial CK depletion (*right*) for dogs with 24-h occlusion (–) and dogs with 1- and 3-h occlusion (– – –). The slope of both regression lines was significantly steeper ($P < 0.05$) in the reperfused group

that were not reperfused, suggesting that more CK appeared in blood per gram of infarct.

Relationship Between IS_p and IS_m

Twenty-four Hour Occlusion. A linear relationship was observed ($IS_p = 12.64 + 0.69 \times IS_m$, $r = 0.87$). The amount of myocardial CK depleted per gram of infarct determined by gross inspection was 26.8 ± 2.61 IU/mg protein/g infarct.

Reperfusion. A similar relationship was observed, while the amount of myocardial CK depleted per gram of infarct determined by gross inspection was not significantly different.

Relationship Between IS_S and IS_P

Twenty-four Hour Occlusion. A linear relationship was observed ($IS_S = 2.50 + 1.38 \times IS_P$, $r = 0.94$) which was similar to that observed when infarct size was measured by myocardial CK depletion.

Reperfusion. This relationship was also linear ($IS_S = 6.52 + 2.12 \times IS_P$, $r = 0.90$) and similar to that observed when infarct size was measured by myocardial CK depletion, but significantly different from that observed in dogs with 24-h occlusion ($P < 0.02$) (Fig. 2).

Discussion

In the present study a good correlation was found between infarct size calculated from blood CK curves and calculated from myocardial CK depletion in dogs with 24-h coronary occlusion, although the blood CK techniques slightly overestimated the infarct size. This confirms the data of Shell et al. [12], Bleifeld et al. [2], and Norris et al. [9], but is inconsistent with Roe et al. [10]. An important difference in the present investigation was that coronary occlusion was continuously monitored by means of the implanted flow probe.

The linear relationship between infarct size measured by pathology and calculated from myocardial CK depletion was found to be good for experimental myocardial infarction in conscious dogs with 24-h occlusion, as well as with 1- and 3-h occlusion. We observed significant differences in the time-course of appearance of CK in blood and configuration of the CK-time activity curve with reperfusion. The earlier appearance of CK after reperfusion was also observed by Jarmakani [6]. In contrast to Jarmakani [6] and Bresnahan [3] we found in the present investigation that this altered configuration did influence the calculated infarct size. While the slope between measured infarct size and that calculated from serial CK curves remained linear after reperfusion, it was significantly different from that observed with 24-h occlusion. This indicates that reperfusion led to an increased amount of CK appearing in the blood per gram of infarct or per unit of CK depleted from myocardium. This could be explained by a decreased local degradation of CK in the myocardium due to a washout phenomenon of CK into the systemic circulation after release of the occlusion.

Another important finding is the variability in infarct size observed in conscious dogs in either the presence or absence of reperfusion, which is in contrast with a recent study by Jennings and Wartman in anesthetized dogs [7].

The finding that reperfusion alters the relationship between calculated and measured infarct size is an important consideration when using the blood CK method to calculate infarct size both in experimental animals and in patients.

Since in animals partial release of occlusion can always happen, flow monitoring during such experiment seems mandatory.

Patients with evolving myocardial infarction may present (a) subtotal coronary occlusion, (b) temporary coronary spasm on a fixed lesion, or (c) a dynamic process with clot formation and lysis. Reperfusion occurs under all these conditions which would result in an altered relationship between calculated and measured infarct size.

More importantly, however, in patients with acute myocardial infarction in whom reperfusion is achieved either by intracoronary thrombolysis with streptokinase or by emergency aortocoronary bypass surgery, the application of the formula as used in nontreated patients may also result in overestimation of infarct size and thus erroneously suggest that the intervention extended the infarction. Finally it is conceivable that any intervention that increases perfusion of the ischemic myocardium may increase washout of CK into the blood.

Summary

The major findings of the present investigation are:

1. Reperfusion alters the configuration of the serial blood CK curve and results in a different linear relationship between calculated and measured infarct size, resulting in greater recovery of CK in blood per unit of infarcted myocardium.
2. Infarct size measured by gross pathology correlates well with infarct size calculated with the technique of Kjekshus and Sobel [8].
3. Left circumflex occlusion in the conscious dogs results in a wide range of infarct sizes.

References

1. Armitage P (1973) Statistical methods in medical research. Blackwell, Oxford
2. Bleifeld W, Mathey D, Hanrath P, Buss H, Effert S (1977) Infarct size estimated from serial creatine phosphokinase in relation to left ventricular hemodynamics. Circulation 55:303–311
3. Bresnahan GF, Roberts R, Shell WE, Ross J, Sobel BE (1974) Deleterious effects due to hemorrhage after myocardial reperfusion. Am J Cardiol 33:82–86
4. Gornall AG, Bardawill CJ, David MM (1949) Determination of serum protein by means of the biuret reaction. J Biol Chem 177:751–766
5. Heyndrickx GR, Millard RW, McRitchie RJ, Maroko PR, Vatner SF (1975) Regional myocardial functional and electrophysiological alterations following brief coronary artery occlusion in conscious dogs. J Clin Invest 56:978–985
6. Jarmakani JM, Limbird L, Graham RC, Marks RA (1976) Effect of reperfusion on myocardial infarct, and the accuracy of estimating infarct size from serum creatine phosphokinase in the dog. Cardiovasc Res 10:245–253
7. Jennings RB, Wartman WB (1957) Production of an area of homogeneous myocardial infarction in the dog. Arch Pathol 63:580–585
8. Kjekshus JK, Sobel BE (1970) Depressed myocardial creatine phosphokinase activity following experimental myocardial infarction in rabbit. Circ Res 27:403–414
9. Norris RM, Whitlock RML, Barratt-Boyes C, Small CW (1975) Clinical measurement of myocardial infarct size. Modification of a method for the estimation of total creatine phosphokinase release after myocardial infarction. Circulation 51:614–620

10. Roe CR, Cobb FR, Starmer CF (1977) The relationship between enzymatic and histologic estimates of the extent of myocardial infarction in conscious dogs with permanent coronary occlusion. Circulation 55 (3):438–448
11. Rosalki SB (1967) An improved procedure for serum creatine phosphokinase determination. J Lab Clin Med 69:696–705
12. Shell WE, Kjekshus JK, Sobel BE (1971) Quantitative assessment of the extent of myocardial infarction in the conscious dog by means of analysis of serial changes in serum creatine phosphokinase activity. J Clin Invest 50:2614–2625

Coronary Artery Recanalization and Subsequent Aortocoronary Bypass Surgery in Acute Myocardial Infarction

D.G. Mathey*, G. Rodewald, P. Rentrop, K. Leitz, W. Merx, B.J. Messmer, W. Rutsch, E.S. Bücherl

Departments of Cardiology and Cardiac Surgery of the University Hospitals Hamburg, Göttingen, Aachen, FRG, and Berlin

A significant arteriosclerotic stenosis remains after successful coronary artery recanalization, implying the risk of reinfarction [2]. Aortocoronary bypass surgery (ACBS) following recanalization is meant to prevent reinfarction and to provide adequate myocardial perfusion. To evaluate the feasibility of such an approach and to determine its efficacy in terms of mortality, morbidity, and ventricular function, we have reviewed our experience with early and elective bypass surgery following successful recanalization.

Methods

Forty-eight of 188 successfully recanalized patients were included in this study. In 34 patients, ACBS was performed acutely within 10 days of the onset of infarct; in 14 patients, ACBS was performed later on an elective basis. Three of the four University Centers involved in this cooperative study favoured early bypass surgery, one elective surgery.

In the 34 patients with early bypass surgery, the indications for surgery were: recurrent angina pectoris in seven patients, the severity of the remaining stenosis in 12 patients, the remaining stenosis and stenoses in other coronary arteries in 13 patients, and recurrent coronary artery spasm in addition a significant stenosis in two patients.

The 14 patients who had elective ACBS had surgery because of angina pectoris in six cases the remaining stenosis in seven cases, and the remaining stenosis plus stenoses in other coronary arteries in one case.

Global and regional ejection fraction were determined from the RAO left ventricular angiogram (Fig. 1). In order to correlate the different regions of the left ventricle with blood supply, segments 2 and 3 were defined to receive their blood from the LAD and segments 4 and 5 from the right or circumflex coronary artery.

* Department of Cardiology, University Hospital Eppendorf, Martinistr. 52, 2000 Hamburg 20, FRG

Transluminal Coronary Angioplasty and
Intracoronary Thrombolysis. Ed. by Kaltenbach et al.

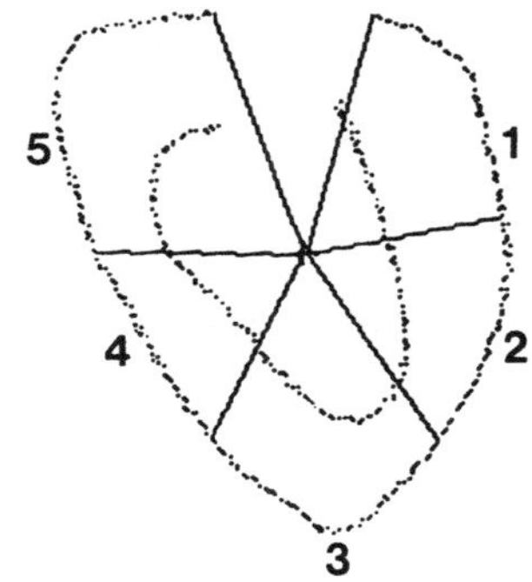

Segment #	Reg. Change of Area (normal values*) %	± 2 S.D. %
1	68	18
2	61	28
3	59	22
4	72	22
5	48	20

*obtained from 40 normal subjects

Fig. 1. Analysis of regional left ventricular wall motion from the monoplane RAO angiogram

Results

Coronary angiography revealed a total occlusion of a major artery in 42 patients and a subtotal occlusion in six patients. The average occlusion time from the onset of symptoms to reperfusion was 2.6 h in the acute group and 4.4 h in the elective group. In 8 patients of the acute group, ACBS was performed on the day of recanalization, on the average 3.4 days later. The patients of the elective group were operated on after an average interval of 61 days. At the time of surgery, subepicardial hemorrhage was observed in five of the 34 patients operated on acutely. The average number of grafts per patient was 2.1 in the acute group and 1.6 in the elective group.

In 29 of the 34 acute patients, graft patency was examined postoperatively. The graft to the infarct vessel was patent in 24 of the 29 patients, yielding a patency rate of 83%. Twenty of 23 bypass grafts to other coronary arteries were patent, corresponding to a patency rate of 87%. In the elective group, the bypass graft to the infarct vessel was patent in all 13 patients. Only one of the other grafts was found to be occluded.

Left ventricular segments supplied by the infarct vessel were called ischemic segments, those supplied by other coronary arteries non-ischemic. Figure 2 summarizes the changes in regional wall motion following recanalization and acute bypass surgery from the acute state immediately after recanalization to the postoperative state. There was marked improvement in regional wall motion from an average values of 14% to 40% ($P < 0.001$). The improvement was not dependent on whether the graft to the infarct vessel was patent or not. In contrast to the ischemic segments, mechanical function of non-ischemic segments did not change significantly.

Global lèft ventricular ejection fraction as the net result of regional wall motion of the ischemic and nonischemic segments also improved significantly by an average of 26%, but remained just below the normal range (Fig. 2). Again, there was no difference between patients with a patent or closed graft to the infarct vessel.

Figure 3 illustrates the improvement in regional anterior wall motion following recanalization of the LAD and acute ACBS in a 32-year-old patient with acute anterior myocardial infarction. In contrast, the 28-year-old patient whose LV angiograms are shown in Fig. 4 experienced reinfarction 3 months after recanalization and ACBS

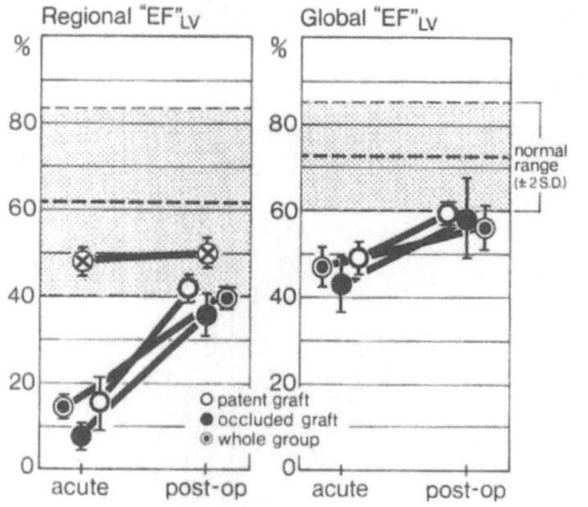

Fig. 2. Mean changes in regional (*left*) and global (*right*) ejection fraction (EF) following reanalization and early ACBS from the acute to the postoperative stage. Significant improvement ($P < 0.001$) in regional EF was observed in ischemic left ventricular segments (○, ○, ●), whereas in nonischemic segments (●) no difference was noted. Global EF also improved significantly ($P < 0.001$)

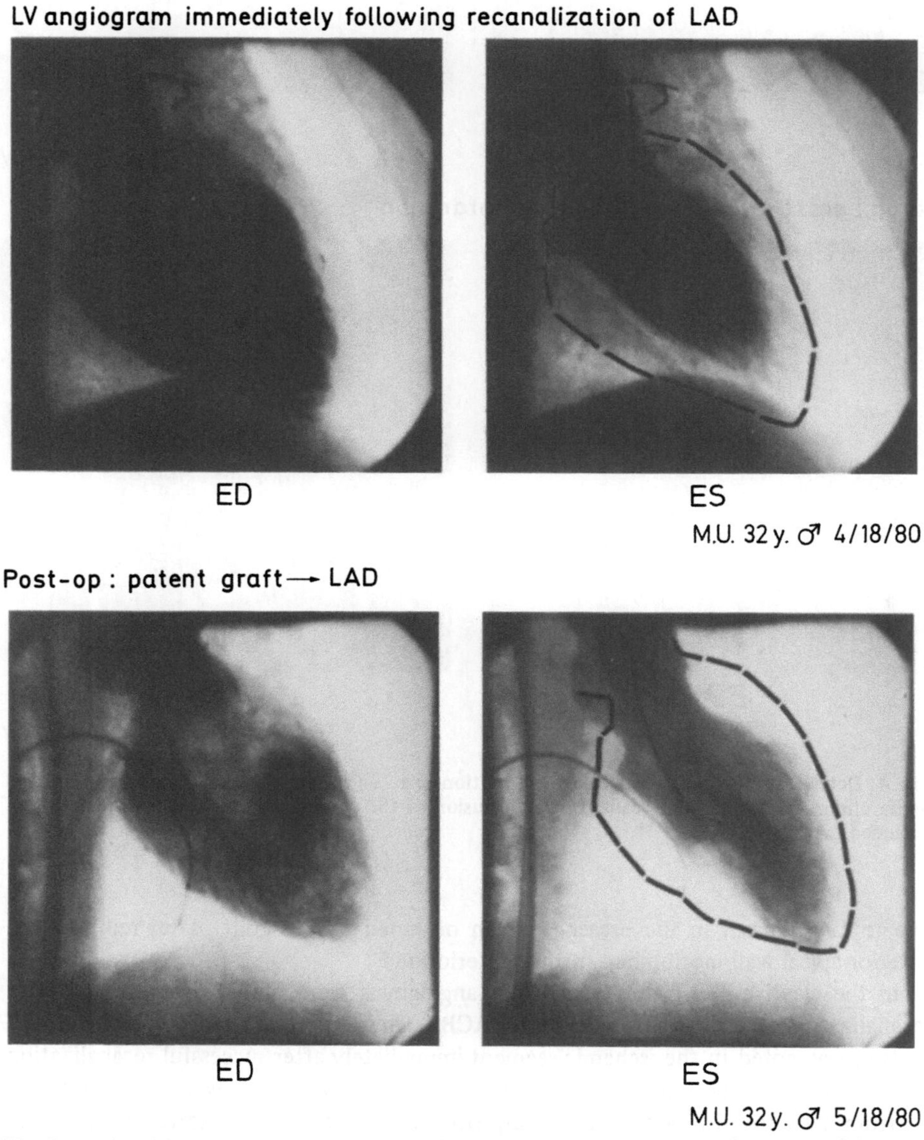

Fig. 3. Marked improvement in anterior-apical wall motion postoperatively after successful recanalization and ACBS in a 32-year-old male patient with a patent graft to the infarct vessel

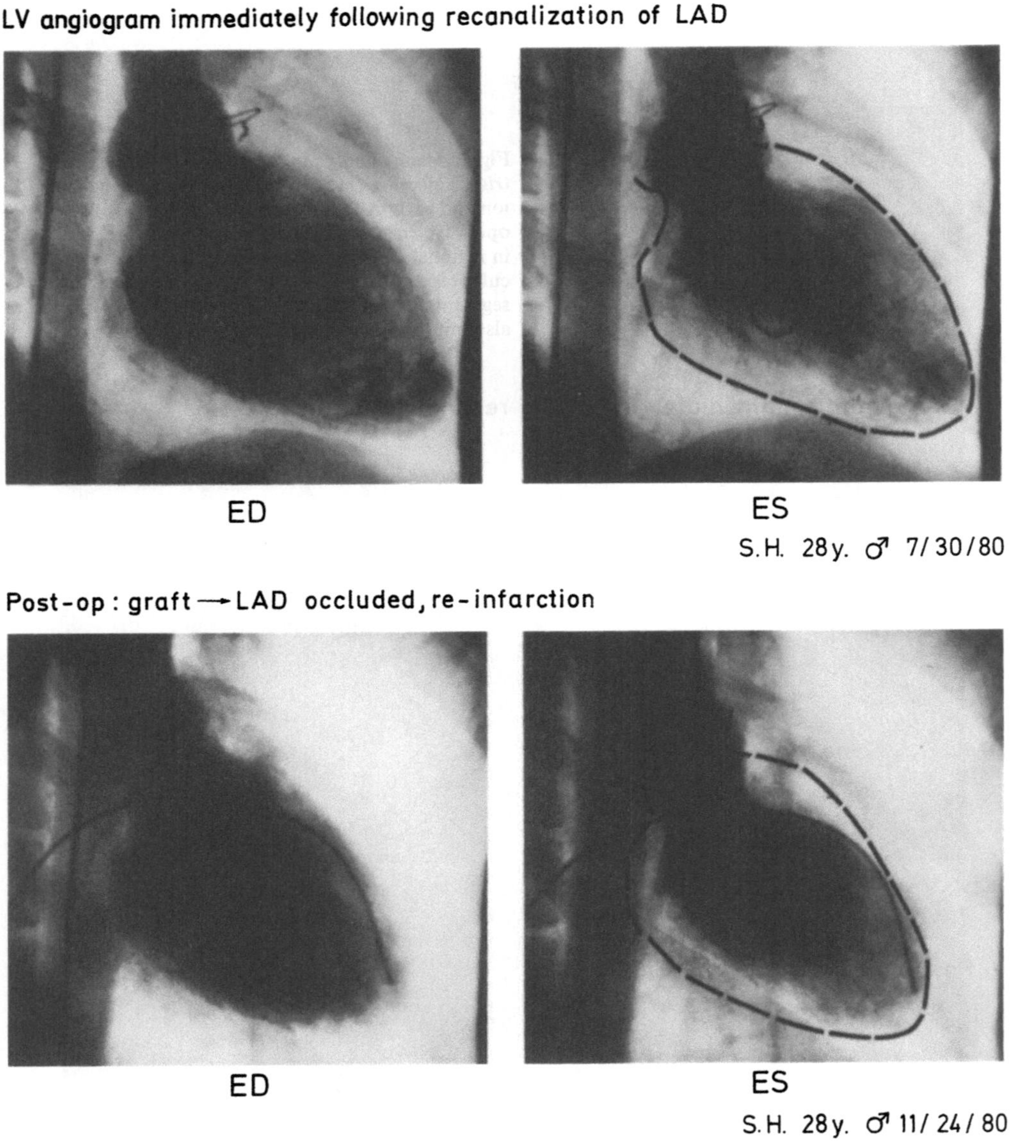

Fig. 4. Deterioration in left ventricular wall motion in a 28-year-old patient with graft closure and reinfarction. Reinfarction was caused by reocclusion of the recanalized LAD in the presence of an occluded LAD graft

due to LAD spasm in the presence of an occluded bypass graft. After reinfarction, anterior-apical wall motion had further deteriorated.

In the elective group, left ventricular angiograms were obtained before and after recanalization as well as before and after ACBS. On average, no change in regional wall motion was noted in the ischemic segment immediately after successful recanalization (Fig. 5). Wall motion remained depressed. Chronically, however, wall motion improved from 19% to 34%, with further improvement to 48% postoperatively. Again, no significant change in wall motion was noted in nonischemic segments.

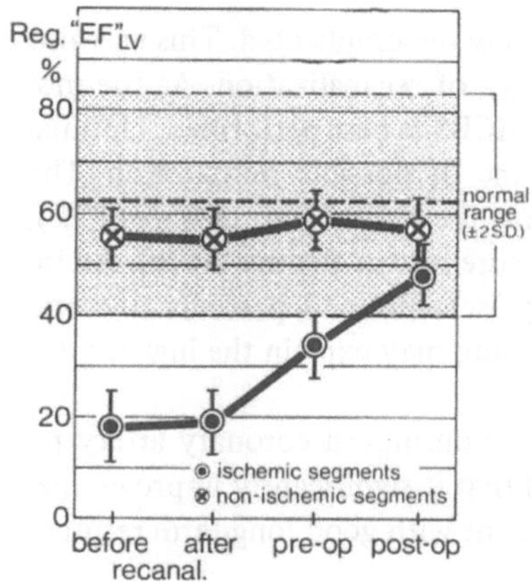

Fig. 5. Improvement in regional wall motion of the ischemic left ventricular segment following recanalization with a tendency towards further improvement postoperatively. Immediately after recanalization, no change in wall motion was noted

So far we have been able to follow the 48 patients for 3–12 months. In the acute group of 34 patients, there was one late death. This patient, a 52-year-old man in whom both bypass grafts were occluded, died suddenly 4 months after ACBS. Another patient had a nonfatal reinfarction. One patient had occasional mild angina pectoris. Thirty-one patients were completely asymptomatic. In the elective group, one patient died suddenly, one suffered reinfarction, one had angina pectoris, and one remained in mild heart failure.

Discussion

Following coronary artery recanalization and ACBS, we found substantial, consistent improvement in regional wall motion in the area supplied by the recanalized and revascularized infarct vessel. This strongly suggests that early reperfusion converted ischemic, nonfunctioning myocardium into nonischemic and functioning myocardium. The improvement in ventricular function was not dependent on whether the graft to the infarct vessel was patent, indicating that reperfusion achieved by recanalization alone was mainly sufficient to restore myocardial function at rest. Regional wall motion did not become normal, however, suggesting that myocardial infarction was not completely prevented.

The ACBS following successful recanalization was meant to reduce the risk of reinfarction and to further improve myocardial blood flow, particularly during exercise, since a significant arteriosclerotic stenosis usually remains after recanalization. As reported by Merx et al. elsewhere in this book, reinfarction occurred after recanalization in 20% of the patients, whereas in our series reinfarction was observed in only two of 48 patients (4%). The frequency of angina pectoris following acute myocardial infarction has been well documented, being 61% for subendocardial and 35% for transmural myocardial infarction [1]. Following recanalization, angina pectoris was the indication for acute ACBS in seven of 34 patients and the indication for elective ACBS in six of 14 patients. Following recanalization and ACBS, only two of the 48 patients had mild angina pectoris.

Acute ACBS following recanalization was completely uncomplicated. This was also true for those cases undergoing operation on the day of recanalization. At the moment, it is not clear at what time after recanalization ACBS is best performed. Optimal timing will largely depend on the frequency and time of possible reinfarction. The risk of reinfarction, however, has to be weighed against the risk of graft closure (17%), which appears to be higher than the regular graft closure rate in elective ACBS. An increased resistance to bypass blood flow in acutely ischemic and partially necrotic tissue secondary to capillary damage and/or cell swelling may explain the higher graft closure rate.

We conclude that the complementary approach of nonsurgical coronary artery recanalization and ACBS can be performed safely and that it significantly improves mechanical function of the ischemic left ventricular segment with good long-term results.

References

1. Levy WK, Cannon DS, Cohen LS (1975) Prognosis of subendocardial myocardial infarction. Circulation 52 [Suppl]:II–107
2. Mathey DG, Kuck KH, Tilsner V, Krebber HJ, Bleifeld W (1981) Non-surgical coronary artery recanalization in acute transmural myocardial infarction. Circulation 63:489

Combined Intracoronary Fibrinolysis And Early Aortocoronary Bypass Graft

B.J. Messmer, W. Merx, P. Bardos, S. Effert

Department of Thoracic and Cardiovascular Surgery and the Department of Internal Medicine I, Klinikum of the RWTH, Aachen, FRG

Selective intracoronary thrombolysis has proved to be an effective therapeutic procedure during the early phase of acute myocardial infarct [1, 2]. The ischemic damage may be reduced or even reversed depending upon the time elapsed between the onset of ischemia and the restitution of blood flow.

Clinical Material and Method

Between March 1980 and March 1981 a total of 63 patients (51 men and 12 women) with an average age of 60 years underwent selective intracoronary thrombolysis for acute myocardial infarct at the University Hospital in Aachen. Coronary angiography demonstrated complete occlusion of the coronary artery corresponding to the infarct area in 45 patients and severe but incomplete obstruction in the remaining 18 patients. Since the latter group of patients are rather inhomogeneous with regard to the exact cause and the degree of stenosis they will not be included into the present study.

The artery responsible for the acute infarct in 45 patients (36 men and 9 women) with complete occlusion was the left anterior descending branch in 19, the right coronary artery in 15, and the circumflex artery in 11 patients.

Intracoronary application of an infusion of 500 ml Rheomacrodex containing 200 000 units streptokinase and 1 mg nitroglycerin was started as soon as the infarct vessel had been identified, with an infusion rate of 5–8 ml/min which corresponds to 2000–3200 units streptokinase/min. Prior to intracoronary application of streptokinase each patient received 10 000 units heparin and 1 g acetylsalicylic acid intravenously as well as an infusion with nitroglycerin at a dosage of 1–5 mg/h. If necessary ß-blocking agents, Xylocaine or calcium antagonists were added to the acute treatment.

The infusion time for streptokinase ranged between 40 and 1000 min. After recanalization the infusion was continued for at least another 20 min.

Results

Intracoronary thrombolysis was successful in 37 of 45 patients, which amounts to a success rate of 82%. Infusion time for streptokinase until recanalization was 29.4 ± 20.3 min (mean ± SD) and the time between onset of acute symptoms and recanali-

Transluminal Coronary Angioplasty and
Intracoronary Thrombolysis. Ed. by Kaltenbach et al.

zation of the artery averaged 4.1 ± 1.7 h. In eight patients (18%) intracoronary application of streptokinase was not successful and two of these patients died in persistent cardiogenic shock.

Of 37 patients with successful lysis 14 (12 males and two females) underwent aortocoronary bypass surgery at an average age of 56 years, while for various reasons 23 patients were found not be candidates for surgery. In this medically treated group three patients died within 1 month of successful lysis, and even though it has not been proved but in one patient death was most likely due to reocclusion of the primarily affected artery. Another five early reocclusions with definite but nonfatal myocardial infarct occurred in the medically treated group of patients.

Of the 14 surgically treated patients, 11 had early bypass operation at an average of 3 days (range 6 h–11 days) after successful thrombolysis. An average of 2.6 vein grafts were inserted in these patients. In three patients surgery was performed after an interval of 3–5 months. In this subgroup an average of 1.6 grafts were necessary.

None of the surgically treated patients died. Three major but nonfatal complications were encountered after early operations. In one case reintervention was necessary for late tamponade 2 weeks after the operation, one patient was in need of circulatory support with the intra-aortic balloon pump for 2 days, and in one case a transient hemiparesis occured 5 days after the operation.

Follow-up was achieved in 13 of the 14 patients who underwent the combined medicosurgical procedure. The average postoperative follow-up time was 6 months and ranged between 1 and 13 months. According to the New York Heart Association classification 11 patients are functional class I, and there is one patient each in functional classes II and III. Six patients had control angiocardiography during the follow-up period. All vein grafts were open and the ejection fraction averaged 62.2% ± 10.4% compared to 52% ± 3.2% at the time of hospital admission.

Discussion

Selective intracoronary thrombolysis by direct infusion of streptokinase represents a promising alternative in treatment of acute myocardial infarct during its early phase. Necessary, however, are a catheterization laboratory working around the clock on an emergency basis and an experienced cardiology staff.

Based on the present experience 30% of the patients selected for intracoronary fibrinolysis become candidates for subsequent aortocoronary bypass surgery. Early in our series intervention was postponed for 3–5 months after the acute phase, allowing the heart to recover from the ischemic episode. The high reocclusion rate among the medically treated patients, however, made us change our policy from late to early surgical revascularization, which nowadays takes place within 72 h of successful intracoronary fibrinolysis in patients suitable for surgery.

Heparinization and administration of streptokinase do not represent a contraindication for early bypass surgery even if performed only a few hours after successful medical revascularization. The dosage of streptokinase is low and increased bleeding due to coagulation problems has never been observed. The postoperative complications seen in three patients are not unusual after major cardiac procedures and they are hardly related to the early timing of the operation. The only bleeding complication occured several days after surgery when the patient was already on Coumadin, a prophylactic medication which at our institution is given as a routine for 6 months in all patients with aortocoronary bypass grafts.

Considered that each patient entered the hospital with severe transmural myocardial ischemia the late results after the combined treatment are excellent. The majority of patients are absolutely free of symptoms and without any medical therapy. One patient, however, developed a large anterolateral aneurysm in spite of successful medical revascularization within 4 1/2 h of onset of symptoms and bypass surgery within the following 24 h. Late control shows a patent and well-functioning vein graft. This case illustrates once more the unsolved basic problem of the heart's unpredictable tolerance for acute ischemia.

In order to reduce the high early reocclusion rate in patients not amenable to secondary surgical revascularization, percutaneous transluminal balloon dilatation has been done simultaneously in a recent series of patients. This procedure may also be helpful in patients with single-vessel occlusion where intracoronary fibrinolysis and transluminal balloon dilatation may even prevent subsequent surgery.

Conclusions

1. Selective intracoronary fibrinolysis represents an effective therapeutic procedure during the early phase of acute myocardial infarct.
2. The risk of reocclusion after successful thrombolysis seems to be high.
3. Early bypass surgery after successful thrombolysis is therefore mandatory in order to assure a good long-term result.
4. Patients not suitable for coronary bypass surgery and patients with single-vessel disease may profit from simultaneous transluminal balloon dilatation.

References

1. Rentrop P, Blanke H, Köstering K, Karsch KR (1979) Acute myocardial infarction: intracoronary application of nitroglycerin and streptokinase in combination with transluminal recanalization. Clin Cardiol 5:354
2. Rentrop P, Blanke H, Karsch KR, Kaiser H, Köstering H, Leitz K (1981) Selective intracoronary thrombolysis in acute myocardial infarction and unstable angina pectoris. Circulation 63:307

Surgical Revascularization after Intracoronary Lysis

K.H. Leitz*, P. Rentrop, H. Oster, H. Blanke, K. Karsch

Department of Thoracic and Cardiovascular Surgery,
Department of Cardiology, University of Göttingen, FRG

The main principle of medical therapy of acute myocardial infarction consists in lowering the oxygen demand of the jeopardized myocardium [3]. Saving myocardium by reperfusion, as done in the experimental animal, has not yet been tried in the clinical state, disregarding the few mostly unsuccessful surgical attempts [7]. By injection of streptokinase into the occluded coronary artery right after the diagnostic catheterization Rentrop succeeded first in nonsurgical coronary artery recanalization and reperfusion of myocardium in an early state of infarction [8]. Meanwhile other groups confirmed his results [5, 6].

In the following we review our results with this new therapeutic concept. We would like to limit this communication to those patients in whom lytic therapy and myocardial revascularization were applied.

Method

The study group consisted of 26 patients who were admitted to hospital because of chest pain. All patients underwent cardiological evaluation including angiography, ventriculography, and standard hemodynamic measurements. After angiographic determination of the ischemia-related coronary artery an opening of the totally or subtotally occluded vessels was attempted with catheters or guide wires. Thereafter streptokinase was injected into the coronary artery. The exact method as well as the clinical course of these patients is the subject of separate papers [9]. According to the success of the lytic therapy the 26 patients were divided into 2 groups:

Group 1. Nineteen patients with acute myocardial infarction and successful lysis
Group 2. Seven patients with acute myocardial infarction and unsuccessful lysis.

All 26 patients were regarded as surgical candidates. The standard technique of cardiopulmonary bypass included mild body hypothermia, left ventricular venting, and the application of the cardioplegic solution of Bretschneider et al. [1]. All coronary arterial anastomoses were performed during a single aortic cross-clamping.

Supported by the Deutsche Forschungsgemeinschaft SFB 89 – Cardiology Göttingen

* Zentrum Chirurgie II, Abteilung für Koronarchirurgie, Medizinische Einrichtungen der Universität Göttingen, Robert-Koch-Str. 40, 3400 Göttingen, FRG

Transluminal Coronary Angioplasty and
Intracoronary Thrombolysis. Ed. by Kaltenbach et al.

Twenty patients had postoperative recatheter studies 14 days–3 months after the operation. Special emphasis was put on the akinetic zone which was measured according to Feild et al. [4].

Results

The 19 patients in group 1, 16 male and three female, with a mean age (± SD) of 59.2 ± 7.8 years, had successful reopening of their ischemia-related coronary arteries after a mean duration of symptoms of 5.8 ± 5.7 h. The infarct vessel was in 13 cases the left anterior descending, in five cases the right coronary artery and once the circumflex branch. Sixteen patients had total occlusion of the infarct vessel, three subtotal. Seven patients had single-vessel disease, six double- and six triple-vessel disease.

Six patients were operated on urgently (1–8 days after successful reperfusion). The operation was indicated because of new chest pain in combination with ECG changes as well as because of rhythmic instability (one patient). Thirteen patients had surgery on a scheduled basis with a mean interval of 60 days after reopening. The indication for operation in these patients was continous angina in spite of intensive medical therapy. In 18 cases the ischemia-related coronary artery could be revascularized. In one instance the right coronary artery was too calcified and small, and therefore an anastomosis was not attempted. Five patients had single-vessel revascularization, the average number of grafts per patient was 2.2, and the surgical degree of revascularization 100%.

Intraoperatively there have been no problems. The intra-aortic balloon pump was not necessary in any patient. No hemorrhage could be found after opening of the pericardium as well as after the surgical revascularization. In seven patients biopsies were taken from the myocardium corresponding to the occluded vessels. In patients operated on acutely these biopsies revealed no abnormalities. Biopsies of patients operated on after an interval demonstrated subendocardial fibrotic zones of 300–1300 μm. One patient died 8 days after operation (group 1 mortality rate: 5.3%). He was found dead in his bed. At autopsy one of his four constructed bypasses was occluded. Eighteen patients with 39 grafts had reangiography (patency rate 97%). Comparing the pre- and postoperative hemodynamic states, a significant improvement of the ejection fraction as well as a significant decrease of the akinetic segment was demonstrated (Fig. 1).

A typical example of our therapeutic protocol is a 42-year-old lady who was sent to our hospital with signs of inferior infarction. The angiographic picture demonstrated an occluded right coronary artery (Fig. 2a). After 14 min intracoronary infusion of streptokinase the distal part of the vessel was visible, but the critical stenosis causing the acute occlusion persisted (Fig. 2b). Because of persistent chest pain not responding to intensive medical therapy the lady was operated on 14 days after the successful reperfusion. She received four bypasses, and on control angiography the vein bypass to the infarct vessel was open (Fig. 2c). She had an uneventful recovery.

All seven patients (mean age 59.0 ± 3 years) in whom the reopening failed had surgical therapy within 24 h of angiography and came to surgery because of persisting signs of myocardial ischemia. The ischemia-related coronary artery in these group 2 patients was in six cases the left anterior descending and once the main stem of the

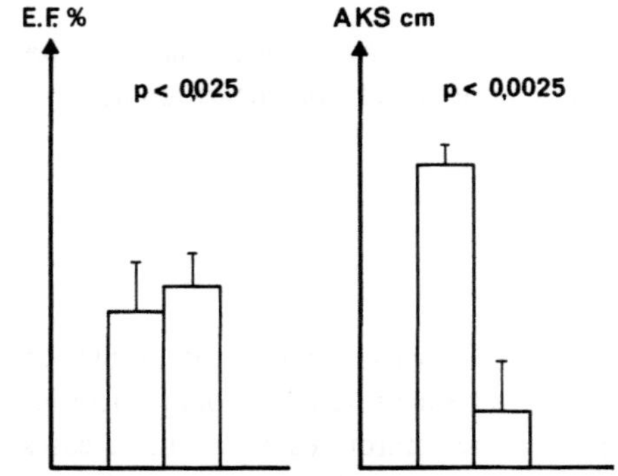

Fig. 1. Comparison of pre- and postoperative ejection fraction (*left*) and length of the akinetic segment (*right*)

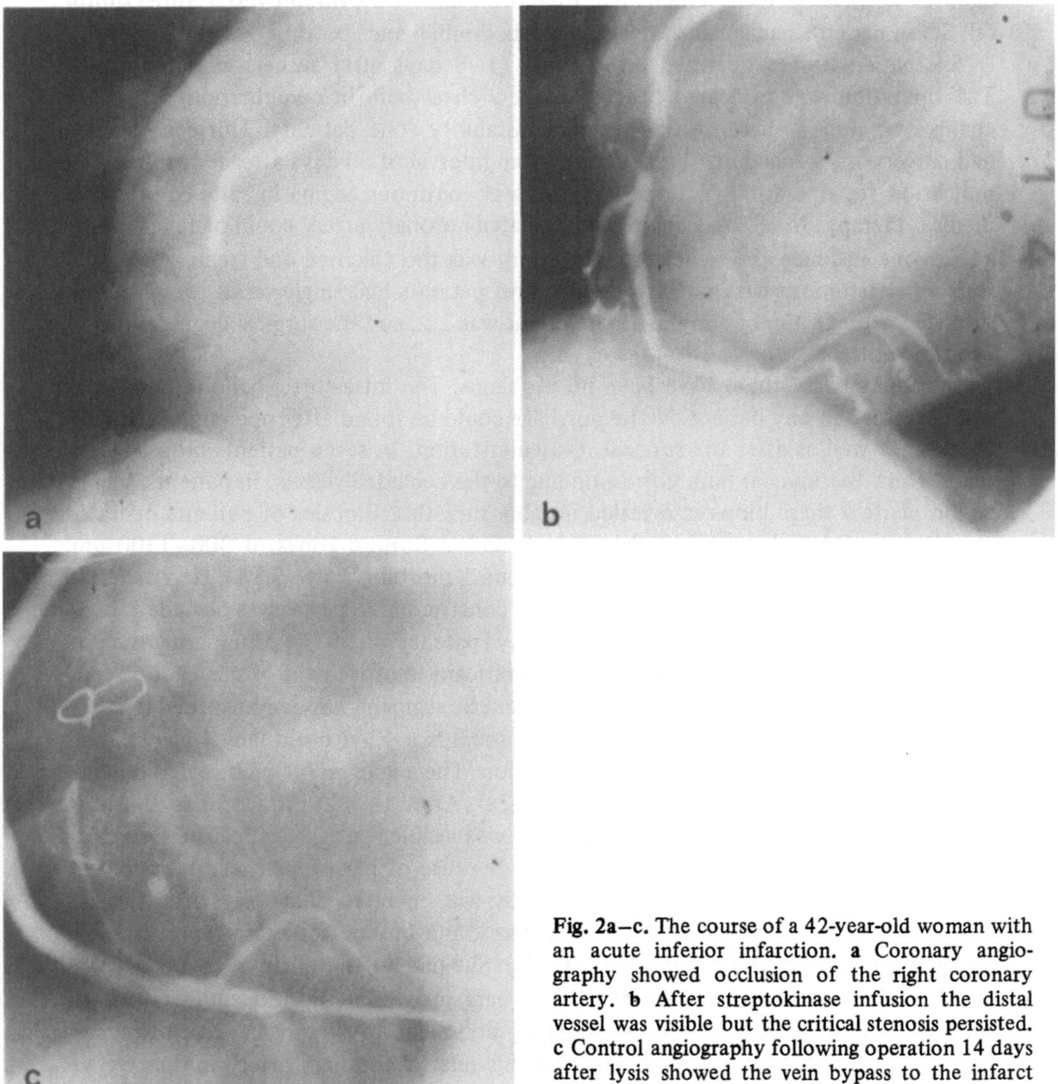

Fig. 2a–c. The course of a 42-year-old woman with an acute inferior infarction. **a** Coronary angiography showed occlusion of the right coronary artery. **b** After streptokinase infusion the distal vessel was visible but the critical stenosis persisted. **c** Control angiography following operation 14 days after lysis showed the vein bypass to the infarct vessel to be open

left coronary artery. Three patients had single-vessel disease, one patient double-vessel disease, and three patients triple-vessel disease. The mean ejection fraction was 48.2% ± 13.3%. One patient died of ventricular fibrillation on the way to surgery despite attempts of resuscitation. Of the six patients operated on one died 3 days after operation due to consumption coagulopathy. At autopsy all three constructed vein grafts were open (group 2 mortality rate: 17%). Only in two patients has control angiography performed. All three vein grafts were open.

Discussion

The concept of vascular occlusion resulting from fresh thrombus formation in coronary arteries with critical or subcritical stenosis is well documented [2]. Since fresh thrombotic material is lysable by streptokinase, this drug was used to induce nonsurgical reperfusion [8]. However, the underlying critical or subcritical coronary narrowing causing the thrombosis is expected to persist. Surgical revascularization in these patients therefore appears to be the logical step after selective intracoronary thrombolysis. From a surgical standpoint three question remain unsolved:

a) Should every patient with successful reopening be operated on?
b) At what time should the operation be performed?
c) What should be done with the patients in whom the lytic therapy failed to induce reperfusion?

After reopening of occluded coronary arteries every patient should be put on anticoagulation therapy. Under this therapeutic regime reocclusion of newly opened coronary vessels in our hands was low. Therefore the indication for operation is only given in those patients who continue to have anginal pain. That means the indication for operation is the same as for patients with stable angina pectoris, since these patients have been converted from an unstable state to a stable one by the nonsurgical reperfusion. An asymptomatic patient is only a surgical candidate if he has triple-vessel disease or a left main stem lesion. Since reinfarction and reocclusion of reopened coronary vessels in our hands was low, the large part of our patient underwent operation on a semiurgent base. Only if anginal pain or rhythmic instability continue right after recanalisation would we operate on a emergency base. If reperfusion was successful, we are not afraid of reperfusion damage, even if the preoperative creatine phosphokinase levels are high. If reperfusion is unsuccessful the prognosis for the patient is poorer. So we had to operate on all seven patients with unsuccessful lysis because of failure of medical therapy as well as worsening of the hemodynamic state. The operative mortality in these patients was high, as had been expected from the study of the literature [7], but we lost none of these patients due to reperfusion damage.

We conclude that the complementary approach of nonsurgical reperfusion and surgical revascularization can be performed safely and that it significantly improves left ventricular function. Further controlled studies are needed to determine optimal timing for surgery.

References

1. Bretschneider HJ, Huber G, Knoll D, Lohr B, Nordbeck H, Spieckermann PG (1975) Myocardial resistance and tolerance to ischemia. Physiology and biochemical basis. J Cardiovasc Surg 16:241
2. Chandler AB, Chapmann J. Erhardt LR et al. (1974) Coronary thrombosis in myocardial infarction. Am J Cardiol 34:823
3. Cyran J (1980) Die Therapie des akuten Myocardinfarktes. Internist (Berlin) 21:675
4. Feild BJ, Russel O, Dowling JT, Rackley CE (1972) Regional left ventricular performance in the year following myocardial infarction. Circulation 46:679
5. Huhmann W, Nieth H, Duangphung K (1980) Ursachen des Herzinfarktes. Koronarangiographische Beobachtungen bei Patienten mit frischem Herzinfarkt. Conference of the German Assoc of Heart and Circ Res, Muenster.
6. Mathey DG, Rodewald G, Rentrop P et al. (to be published) Non-surgical coronary artery recanalisation and bypass grafting of the remaining stenosis – a complementary approach to reduce infarct size and prevent re-infarction. Am Heart J
7. Mundth ED, Buckley MJ, Leinbach RC, Gold HK, Dagett WM, Austen WG (1973) Surgical intervention for the complications of acute myocardial ischemia. Ann Surg 178:379
8. Rentrop P, Blanke H, Karsch KR et al. (1979) Wiedereröffnung des Infarktgefäßes durch transluminale Rekanalisation und intrakoronare Streptokinaseapplikation. Dtsch Med Wochenschr 104:1438
9. Rentrop P, Blanke H, Karsch KR, Kaiser H, Köstering H, Leitz KH (1981) Selective intrakoronary thrombolysis in acute myocardial infarction and unstable angina pectoris. Circulation 63: 307

Systemic Short-Time Thrombolysis in Acute Myocardial Infarction

R. Schröder*, G. Biamino, E.-R. von Leitner

Kardio-Pulmonologische Abteilung der Medizinischen Klinik und Poliklinik im Klinikum Steglitz der Freien Universität Berlin

Introduction

In a recent study, Rentrop et al. [3] demonstrated that intracoronary application of streptokinase in patients with acute myocardial infarction led to reopening of a thrombotic occluded coronary artery in the majority of cases. These results were confirmed by Ganz et al. [1], Mathey et al. [2], and Rutsch et al. [4]. Early restoration of blood flow could be the most effective way of limiting myocardial necrosis. However, the necessary prerequisite, acute coronary angiography, limits this mode of therapy to a small proportion of the total number of patients with acute myocardial infarction. Furthermore, the possible beneficial effects of a reopening of an occluded coronary artery will very much depend on the time for which the vessel was actually occluded. Applying an intracoronary thrombolysis must inevitably lead to a considerable delay between onset of symptoms and beginning of therapy.

The advantage of intracoronary streptokinase infusion was seen in the established reopening of the infarcted vessel within 1–2 h. However, it has not been proven that systemic intravenous fibrinolytic therapy in patients with acute myocardial infarction does not also lead to a recanalization of the thrombotic occluded vessel in a comparably short time. The aim of our study was to test this, using a short-time infusion of 500 000 units streptokinase or 1 000 000 units urokinase. The proposition and the nature of the procedure were explained to the patient and his relatives and informed consent was obtained. The Ethical Committee of the Berlin Steglitz Free University Hospital had previously approved the study.

Procedure

Within 8 h of the onset of chest pain patients under the age of 71 years with symptoms and an ECG typical of evolving myocardial infarction were selected for acute angiography. Nitroglycerin infusion was started in patients with signs of lung congestion. Diazepam and if necessary pethidine were injected intravenously. In the catheter lab, a Judkins catheter was inserted by means of a 7F catheter sheath introducer system

* Medizinische Klinik und Poliklinik im Klinikum Steglitz der Freien Universität, Hindenburgdamm 30, 1000 Berlin 45

Transluminal Coronary Angioplasty and
Intracoronary Thrombolysis. Ed. by Kaltenbach et al.

via the femoral artery. After injection of 5000 units heparin, the coronary artery corresponding to the ECG location of the myocardial injury was visualized before and after the intracoronary injection of 0.3 mg nitroglycerin. Thereafter, 0.5 g acetylsalicylic acid and 0.25 g methylprednisolone were injected intravenously, and 500 000 units streptokinase, dissolved in 36 ml levulose, were infused intravenously within 30 minutes. At commencement of the intravenous streptokinase infusion, a Ducor pigtail catheter was placed into the left ventricle and ventriculography was performed in RAO position. Thereafter, selective coronary angiography of the noninfarcted coronary artery was performed and a Swan-Ganz catheter inserted into the pulmonary artery.

If 60 min after beginning the intravenous streptokinase infusion an occluded artery was not reopened, recanalization with a soft guide wire was attempted, and then an intracoronary infusion of 2000–4000 units/min streptokinase over 1 h performed.

After this procedure, the patient was transferred to the coronary care unit with the Swan-Ganz catheter placed in the pulmonary artery and a Ducor pigtail catheter in the abdominal aorta. For the following 72 h heparin was infused intravenously according to thrombin time, and a phenprocoumon treatment was initiated and continued for the next 3 weeks. Left ventricular and coronary angiography were repeated after 24 h, the catheters inserted through the introducer still placed in the femoral artery. The arterial catheters then were removed. After 3–4 weeks another angiographic control was performed.

In patients older than 70 years, no angiography before thrombolysis was performed. In order to keep the bleeding risk low, 500 000 units urokinase were infused within 10–20 min and a second infusion of 500 000 units urokinase was given 1 h thereafter. Acetylsalicylic acid, heparin infusion, and phenprocoumon were administered as in the younger age-group. If clinically warranted and if informed consent from the patient was obtained, coronary angiography was performed during the 4th week after the beginning of the acute event.

For serial creatine phosphokinase (CK) and MB-CK determinations, in all patients blood samples were taken hourly for at least 24 h and at 2 h intervals thereafter.

Results and Discussion

In 31 patients, coronary angiography was performed before and up to 3 h after the beginning of a short-time intravenous infusion of 500 000 units streptokinase over 30 min (Fig. 1). In six patients only subtotal occlusion of the coronaty artery, corresponding to the ECG location of the myocardial injury, was seen on first angiography. A thrombus demonstrated in four cases could be lysed. A better flow was achieved during the acute phase and there was no evidence of a thrombus after 24 h or 3–4 weeks respectively. In one patient without a thrombus, a 90% stenosis of the circumflex artery remained unaffected. On angiography 25 days later, this vessel was occluded but showed good peripheral filling through collaterals. Clinically, there was no corresponding event during recovery.

In 25 patients, on first angiography complete occlusion of the infarcted artery was found. In one patient with dissection of the vessel wall and a false aneurysm no streptokinase infusion was performed. Two patients had an intracoronary infusion of 2000

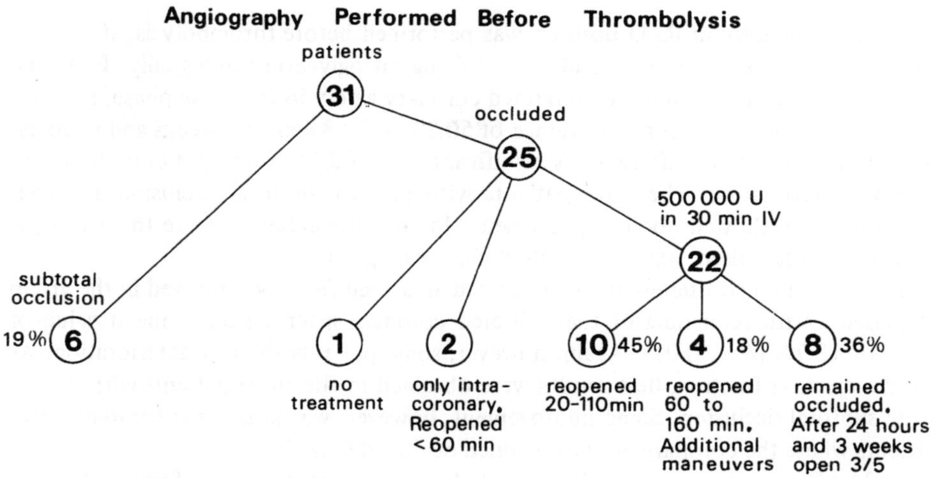

Fig. 1. Findings at first angiography and results of thrombolytic treatment in 31 patients with evolving myocardial infarction

units streptokinase per minute only. In both cases the coronary artery was recanalized within 60 min.

In 22 patients, first a 30 min systemic streptokinase infusion was performed. In ten of these patients patency was achieved within 60 min. Complete and fast flow to the periphery occurred between 20 and 110 min after the beginning of the streptokinase infusion.

In the other 12 patients, no patency was achieved 60 min after commencement of the 30 min intravenous streptokinase infusion. Recanalization and immediate fast flow to the periphery was achieved by the guide wire procedure in one patient. In three further patients, patency occurred during intracoronary streptokinase infusion. Complete and fast flow to the periphery was observed in one patient 1 h after commencement of the intracoronary streptokinase infusion. In the other two patients, slow flow to the periphery remained up to 1 h and 1 h 35 min respectively after the beginning of the intracoronary streptokinase infusion. On angiography 24 h later, there was fast and complete opacification of the infarcted coronary artery in all three patients.

In eight of the 22 patients (36%), neither with intravenous nor with subsequent intracoronary streptokinase infusion patency of the infarcted coronary artery could be achieved in the acute phase. In two of these patients no angiographic follow-up investigations were done. A third patient died from ventricular rupture 3 h after the intracoronary streptokinase infusion was finished. In three of the five patients with angiographic follow-up, the infarcted artery was found recanalized after 24 h and after 3–4 weeks.

In 18 patients with total and four with subtotal occlusion of the infarcted coronary artery, angiographic control was performed after 24 h. Patency of the infarcted coronary artery could be demonstrated in 20 cases (91%). The corresponding figures after 3–4 weeks are 18 of 22 (82%) angiographically controlled patients (one reocclusion only).

Ventriculography in RAO position was performed before thrombolysis, after 24 h, and after 3–4 weeks without and after 1.6 mg nitroglycerin sublingually. In 14 patients with recanalization of the infarcted coronary artery in the acute phase, the ejection fraction increased from an average of 50.2% to 59.8% after 3 weeks and nitroglycerin treatment. This difference is significant ($P < 0.05$). Some patients, however, showed deterioration. The three patients with primary subtotal occlusion and lysis of a thrombus showed good improvement. In the five patients where the artery remained occluded, there was no consistent change (Fig. 2).

The segmental shortening of the infarcted areas significantly improved in the group of patients with reopening of the infarcted coronary artery, from a mean value of 9.4% to 18.7% ($P < 0.01$). Again, however, some patients showed deterioration. As for the ejection fraction, best results were obtained in the three patients with thrombotic subtotal occlusion. Some improvement, however, was also demonstrated in five patients where the coronary artery remained occluded (Fig. 3).

In 34 of our patients, no angiography before thrombolysis was performed. Most of them were over 70 years old and in order to keep the bleeding risk low, urokinase was infused (Fig. 4). We grouped these patients into those with an early MB-CK enzyme peak (less than 15 h after beginning of the acute event), those with a peak after 22–24 h as expected, where the coronary artery remained occluded, and an intermediate group with a MB-CK peak between 16 and 19 h after the onset of symptoms.

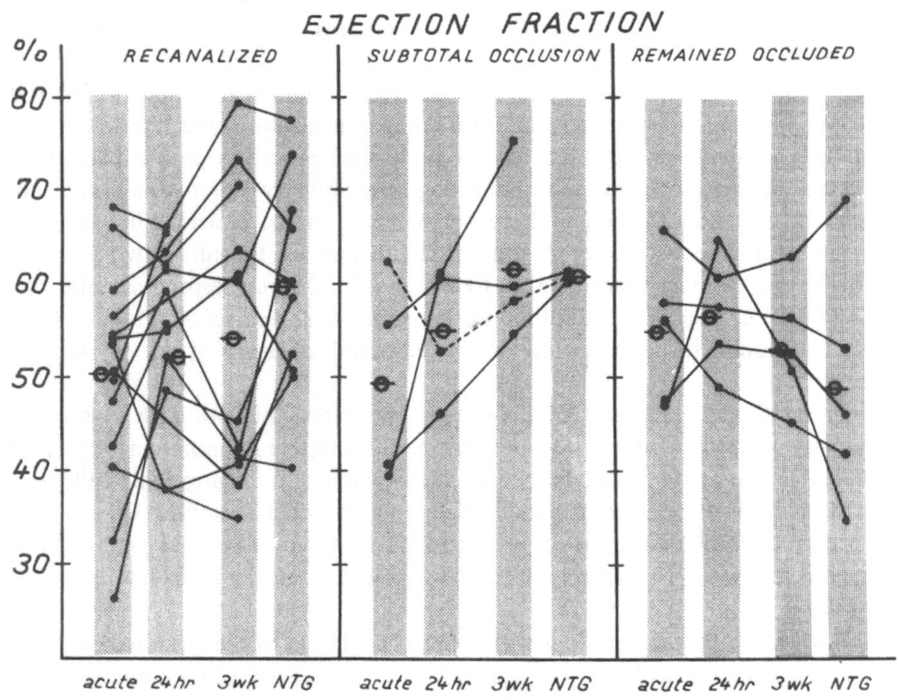

Fig. 2. Individual data and mean values of the ejection fraction in 23 patients before thrombolysis (*acute*), after 24 h, and after 3–4 weeks without and after 1.6 mg nitroglycerin (NTG) sublingually

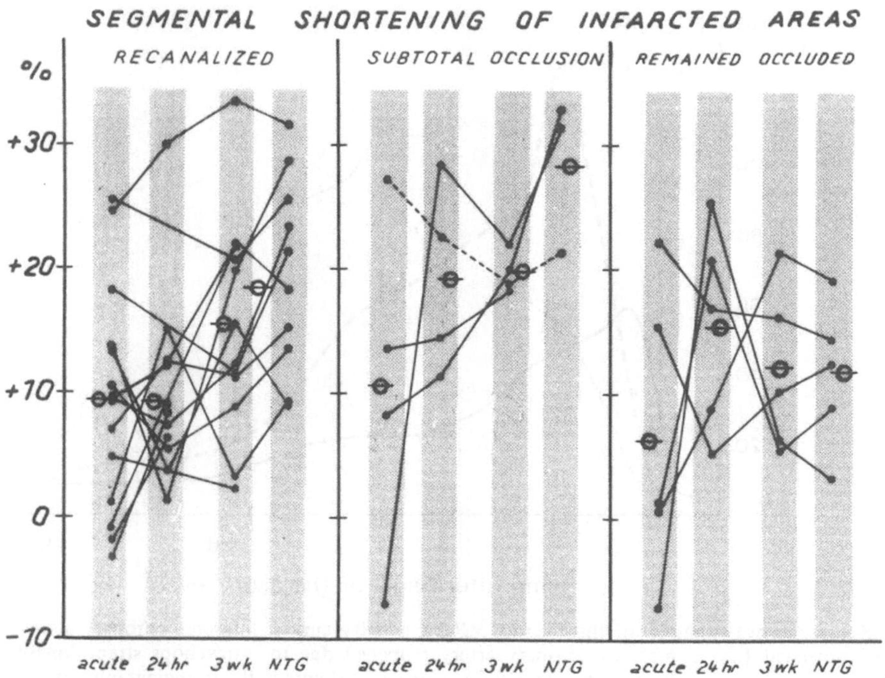

Fig. 3. Individual data and mean values of segmental shortening of the infarcted areas in 23 patients before thrombolysis (*acute*), after 24 h, and after 3–4 weeks without and after 1.6 mg nitroglycerin (NTG) sublingually

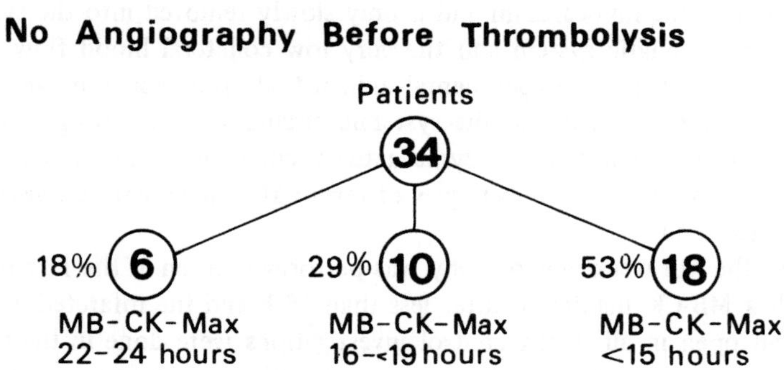

Angiography 3-4 weeks			
Infarct-artery occluded	3	1*	0
Infarct-artery open	1	7	10
Angiography not performed	2	2	8

*Reinfarction 5th day

Fig. 4. Thirty-four patients without angiography in the acute phase, grouped according to the time the peak in the serial serum MB-CK activity curve is reached after onset of symptoms, and results of angiography at the 4th week

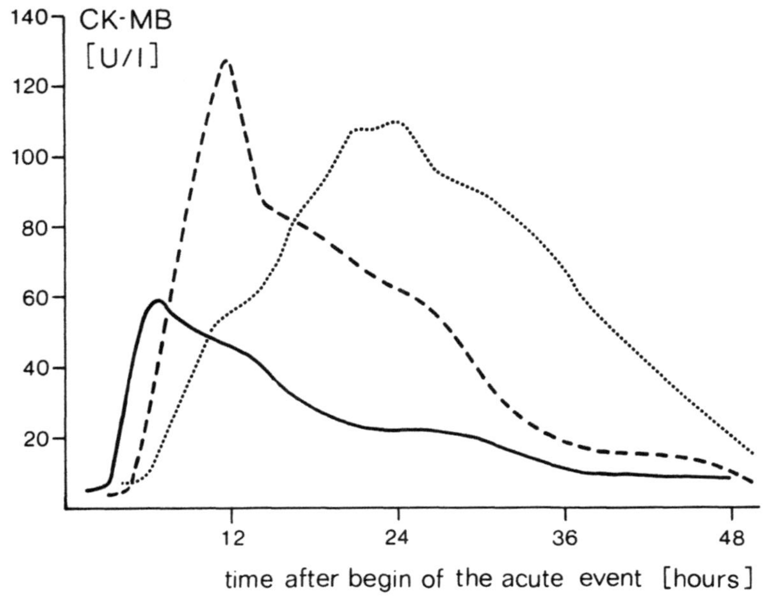

Fig. 5. Representative examples of three serum MB-CK activity curves: infarcted coronary artery remained occluded (......), infarcted coronary artery reopened due to intravenous streptokinase infusion (– – – – –), and early peak in the MB-CK curve in patients without angiography in the acute phase (———). See Fig 3 and Table 2

Creatine phosphokinase is released from irreversibly damaged myocardial cells but remains in the myocardium and is only slowly removed into the systemic circulation by the lymphatic system and the very low collateral blood flow. Vatner et al. [6] demonstrated in the experimental animal that after reopening an occluded coronary artery CK rose sharply in the systemic circulation, exhibiting a significantly earlier peak in the serial serum enzyme activity curve suggesting a washout phenomenon. In Fig. 5, representative examples of serum MB-CK activity curves of our patients are demonstrated.

In the 4th week, angiography was performed in ten of the 18 patients of the group with a MB-CK maximum after less than 15 h and the infarcted coronary artery was found open in all. Eight control investigations were done in the ten patients of the intermediate group. Only in one patient with a reinfarction – probably reocclusion – the circumflex artery was occluded. Even in the group with a late MB-CK maximum, in one of four angiographically controlled patients the coronary artery was not occluded. In summary, in 18 of 22 patients (82%) a nonoccluded infarcted coronary artery could be demonstrated in the 4th week after myocardial infarction.

In Table 1, time after onset and height of the maximum of the MB-CK serum curves as well as time between onset of symptoms and beginning of thrombolysis are listed for the patients with angiography before thrombolysis. In three patients, the vessel remained occluded in the acute phase and after 24 h and 3 weeks. The maximum in the serial serum enzyme curve was reached after 23 h with a peak value of 87 units (curve 1 in Fig. 5). In those patients with reopening of an occluded coron-

Table 1. Time after onset of symptoms and height of the maximum of the MB-CK serum curves, and time between onset of symptoms and beginning of thrombolysis in 24 patients with angiography before thrombolysis (mean SD)

	Number of patients	Peak MB-CK level after onset of symptoms (h)	Peak MB-CK level (units/liter)	Time between onset of symptoms and beginning of thrombolysis (h)
Subtotal occlusion	5	12.9 ± 3.3	45.7 ± 16	3.5 ± 1.2
Reopened with intracoronary infusion	2	12.5 ± 0.7	113.2 ± 59	4.3 ± 2.7
Reopened with intravenous infusion	14	14.4 ± 2.8	115.0 ± 57	4.0 ± 1.4
Artery remained occluded	3	23.2 ± 1.8	86.6 ± 35	5.7 ± 1.8

ary artery the peak was reached about 10 h earlier. The maximum value was considerably higher, as expected, due to washout of MB-CK (curve 2 in Fig. 5). The three patients where the infarcted coronary artery remained occluded in the acute phase but was found reopened after 24 h and 3 weeks are not included in this table. They had peak MB-CK levels 15, 15.5, and 25.5 h respectively after onset and maximum values of 100, 237, and 72 units respectively. The time between onset of symptoms and beginning of thrombolysis was 6.5, 2.25, and 6.25 h respectively.

Table 2 shows the corresponding figures for the 34 patients without angiography before thrombolysis. Of special interest are the results in the group with a maximum in the serial serum enzyme curve less than 15 h after the onset of symptoms. These patients not only showed a very early maximum with an average of 11.5 h, they also had the lowest maximum (curve 3 in Fig. 5). Thus, the total amount of MB-CK released in the serum is lower than in all the other groups although due to reperfusion more

Table 2. Time after onset of symptoms and height of the maximum of the MB-CK serum curves, and time between onset of symptoms and beginning of thrombolysis in 34 patients without angiography in the acute phase

Peak MB-CK	Number of patients	Peak MB-CK level after onset of symptoms (h)	Peak MB-CK level (units/liter)	Time between onset of symptoms and beginning of thrombolysis (h)
Peak MB-CK < 15 h	18	11.5 ± 2.3	46.5 ± 20	3.0 ± 1.3
Peak MB-CK 16–19 h	10	17.0 ± 1.0	85.2 ± 56	4.2 ± 1.3
Peak MB-CK 22–24 h	6	23.0 ± 1.1	64.6 ± 21	5.0 ± 2.1

MB-CK per g necrotic myocardium should be expected than without reperfusion [6]. This gives support to the assumption that a considerable amount of myocardium was salvaged in these cases. It cannot be ruled out, however, that the majority of these patients primarily had smaller infarcts.

What differentiates these patients from the others? The time between onset of symptoms and beginning of thrombolysis is the lowest – 3.1 h mean. In the group of patients with angiography in the acute phase it was more than 4 h (Tables 1 and 2). This difference is mostly explained by the delay due to angiography.

Second and probably more important, these older patients more often had two- and three-vessel disease and more collaterals. It could be that these patients will benefit most from a thrombolytic therapy whereas in younger patients with sudden occlusion of one major artery in most cases the time until the vessel is reopened is too long.

Complications and Clinical Course

In the 31 patients with angiography before thrombolysis, there were no deaths during the acute intervention. One patient had a blood pressure drop following the first intracoronary visualizing of the noninfarcted coronary with subsequent ventricular fibrillation. He could be defibrillated promptly and had an uneventful recovery. There was only one hospital death in this group, due to ventricular rupture in a patient where the infarcted coronary artery remained occluded. One patient developed a somewhat larger hematoma from bleeding at the femoral artery puncture site.

In the older age-group of 34 patients without angiography in the acute phase, four patients died during hospital follow-up due to: one ventricular wall rupture, one reinfarction not corresponding to the primarily affected vessel, one left heart failure, and one sudden death on the 18th day, following preceding resuscitation from ventricular fibrillation on the 14th day. On autopsy, the coronary artery corresponding to the primary myocardial injury was found not occluded in the patient with ventricular rupture or the one with sudden death. No autopsy was performed on the other two patients.

Two patients developed serious hemorrhage during heparin infusion on the 3rd day. In both cases, puncture of the subclavian vein was done or had been tried in an external hospital.

In summary, five of the 65 patients (7.7%) died and serious hemorrhage was seen in three patients (4.6%).

Conclusions

The aim of our study was to prove whether, how often, and in what time an occluded coronary artery could be reopened by an intravenous short-time streptokinase or urokinase infusion. A direct comparison between the efficacy of intracoronary and intravenous thrombolysis is not possible. We could, however, demonstrate that intracoronary thrombi can be lysed safely and relatively quickly in a significant amount of cases.

If and under which clinical conditions patients with evolving myocardial infarction will benefit from an early intravenous short-time fibrinolytic therapy remains to be proven by a controlled prospective randomized trial.

References

1. Ganz W, Buchbinder N, Marcus H et al. (1981) Intracoronary thrombolysis in evolving myocardial infarction. Am Heart J 101:4–13
2. Mathey D, Kuck KH, Rose HJ, Tilsner V, Bleifeld W (1980) Lyse der akuten Koronararterien-Thrombose durch intrakoronare Streptokinase. Z Kardiol 69:229
3. Rentrop P, Blanke H, Kostering H, Karsch KR (1980) Intrakoronare Streptokinase-Applikation bei akutem Infarkt und instabiler Angina pectoris. Dtsch Med Wochenschr 105:221
4. Rutsch W, Weber H, Paeprer H, Schmutzler H (1980) Maßnahmen zur Myokardreperfusion beim akuten Myokardinfarkt: Transluminale, mechanische Rekanalisation und koronarselektive Thrombolyse mit Streptokinase. Z Kardiol 69:230
5. Schröder R, Biamino G, Von Leitner E-R, Linderer T (1981) Intravenöse Streptokinase-Infusion bei akutem Myokardinfarkt. Dtsch Med Wochenschr 106:294
6. Vatner S, Baig H, Manders WT, Maroko P (1978) Effects of coronary artery reperfusion on myocardial infarct size calculated from creatine kinase. J Clin Invest 61:1048–1056

The Use of Plasminogen in Intracoronary Lysis

V. Tilsner, K.H. Kuck, D. Mathey

Department of Blood Coagulation Disorders and Medical Clinic Department of Cardiology, University Hospital, 2000 Hamburg-Eppendorf, FRG

The duration of intracoronary lysis is of importance for the success as well as for the side effects of the treatment. The shorter the duration of lysis needed the quicker reperfusion occurs, thereby increasing the survival changes of the myocardium and minimizing the effect on the blood coagulation due to the accompanying systemic lysis, i.e., the risk of bleeding is reduced. We found the mean duration of lysis to be 29 ± 15 min (mean ± SD).

Three criteria are important for the success of intracoronary lysis:

1. The thrombus must consist of lysable material.
2. The lytic drug must reach the thrombus in sufficient concentration. The distance from the catheter tip to the thrombus is decisive.
3. The thrombus must contain sufficient plasminogen, in order to be quickly lyseable. As plasminogen has a high affinity to thrombi, we give an intracoronary injection of 5000 CTA units plasminogen before starting lysis, in order to achieve a local enrichment of plasminogen. The plasminogen flowing off into the circulation is so small with this dosage that the systemic lysis is not measurably potentiated.

Table 1 shows the dependence of the fibrinogen decrease on the duration of lysis. The lysis acceleration by plasminogen is evident in Fig. 1. In the beginning the three patients were not given an initial plasminogen dose, but this was carried out subsequently.

Table 1. The influence of intra-coronary lysis with 2000 units streptokinase/min on fibrinogen

	Before lysis	After lysis
n	69	69
x	307,16	181,65
s	124,91	141,95

Thereof dependent upon the duration of lysis

	Upto 30′	Upto 45′	Upto 60′	Upto 90′
n	43	16	7	3
x	280,42	220,64	150,56	90,23
s	114,35	108,41	65,21	54,17

Transluminal Coronary Angioplasty and Intracoronary Thrombolysis. Ed. by Kaltenbach et al.

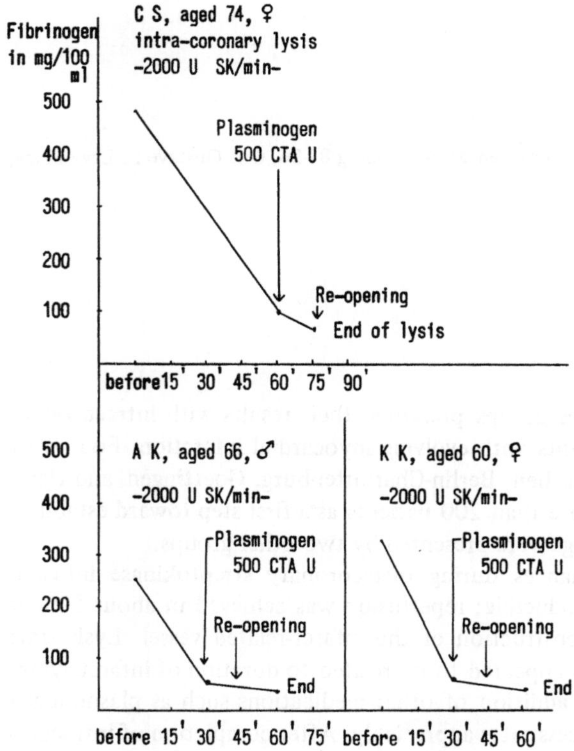

Fig. 1. The reaction of fibrinogen to application of plasminogen in intracoronary lysis with streptokinase (SK)

We did not undertake a comparison with the series of patients who were lysed without plasminogen, due to the small number of cases and the improved techniques now available.

Fibrinogen can also be reduced by shock complications independently of fibrinolysis. This effect can best be recognised by the thrombocytopenia either existing before the start of lysis or occurring during lysis. The fibrin degradation products are usually more or less raised before lysis as a result of shock with a mean titer or 2^3 in the staphylococcus clumping test. They increase systemically during lysis and in the coronary sinus reach values around 2^9 and 40 μg/ml in the latex test.

Overview

Peter Rentrop

Division of Cardiology, Mount Sinai Medical Center, Annenberg 8–26, One Gustave L. Levy Place, New York, N.Y. 10029, USA

Eight European and United States groups presented their results with intracoronary infusion of streptokinase in patients with evolving myocardial infarction. Four West German groups (Universities of Aachen, Berlin-Charlottenburg, Goettingen, and Hamburg) have pooled the data of more than 200 patients as a first step toward establishing a registry. Experimental findings were presented by two other groups.

The coronary-angiographic changes during intracoronary streptokinase infusion have been found to be quite reproducible: reperfusion was achieved in about 80% of patients with initially complete obstruction of the infarct-related vessel. Lysis time required to achieve recanalization appeared to be related to duration of infarct symptoms. Modification of dosage or addition of other medications such as plasminogen or nitroglycerin did not alter success rates appreciably. After completion of intracoronary lysis, significant lesions of more than 50% persisted in 94% of the registry patients.

These findings are well explained by pathoanatomic studies which were presented by Fulton. Severe atherosclerotic disease was found at the site of coronary thrombosis in the majority of cases. Of the occluding thrombi, 90% were less than 1 cm in length. In 75% of the cases Fulton found tears in the intimal lining at the site of thrombotic obstruction.

Significant improvement of left ventricular function was found in the chronic stage in patients treated successfully within 4 h after onset of pain. In addition, presence of collaterals prior to reperfusion correlated positively with functional improvement. In some patients reperfused after more than 4 h of chest pain, ejection fraction was worse at the time of chronic angiography.

In experimental studies myocardial hemorrhage was seen after reperfusion. Since hemorrhage appears to be confined to necrotic myocardium, it is unlikely to cause infarct extension. Other potentially negative effects of reperfusion, such as compromised collateral supply due to cell swelling, remain to be examined.

In no patient was there acute deterioration of left ventricular function after reperfusion. Reperfusion was associated with premature ventricular contractions in about 30% of the registry patients. Ventricular tachycardia or ventricular fibrillation were rare and responded to standard therapy. Reperfusion arrhythmias were much more benign in the clinical setting than in many previously reported animal experiments. Experimental data reported at this meeting suggest that the incidence of dangerous reperfusion arrhythmias may be reduced by gradual restoration of flow.

Transluminal Coronary Angioplasty and
Intracoronary Thrombolysis. Ed. by Kaltenbach et al.

Serious hemorrhage requiring transfusion occurred in 7.4% of the registry patients. In the majority of cases it was associated with use of the transfemoral technique and a drop of fibrinogen concentration below 100 mg%.

Death was not attributed to the acute intervention by any of the groups. Hospital mortality was 10.3% (21/204) in the registry patients; reinfarction occurred in 13.7% (32/204). In the absence of well-matched or randomized control groups it is impossible to assess the impact of the intervention upon hospital mortality or reinfarction rate.

In recanalized patients reinfarction usually occurred at the site of the initial infarction. Since repeat angiography revealed a complete or subtotal reocclusion in almost all of the patients, some groups advocated early bypass surgery. Other groups, however, reported very low reinfarction rates, which they attributed to an aggressive effort to lyse all thrombotic material in the acute stage and to meticulous anticoagulation in the follow-up period.

The techniques of lysing coronary artery thrombi appear to be in evolution. On the one hand, efforts are being made to evaluate modified conventional intravenous streptokinase infusion by angiography; recanalization was reported to occur within 22–110 min after rapid systemic application of 500.000 units of streptokinase or urokinase in 45% of the patients. On the other hand, superselective techniques are being developed in several centers which report reperfusion rates of about 90%.

Borderline Indications for TCA

Preliminary Experience with Percutaneous Transluminal Coronary Angioplasty in Patients with Coronary Spasm

L.G. Bentivoglio, N.W. Wolf, S.G. Meister, L.R. Leo

Medical College of Pennsylvania, Philadelphia, PA 19129, USA

The existence of coronary spasm and spasm-induced angina pectoris are well established facts. Coronary spasm may occur at a coronary site with no detectable fixed stenosis or contribute a time-varying component to an organic obstruction.

In the context of percutaneous transluminal coronary angioplasty (PTCA), coronary spasm occupies a position of particular interest for three main reasons: (1) by location, focal character, symmetry and usual absence of wall calcification it mimics the very type of organic coronary stenosis considered ideal for PTCA; (2) being unpredictable, it may occur during PTCA and possibly affect the immediate results; (3) being recurrent, it can be expected to outlast the PTCA relief of the organic component of a mixed stenosis, reproducing blockage and symptoms at a later time. The practical importance of these issues would be marginal if coronary spasm were rare in candidates for PTCA, and the National Institutes of Health registry is in fact consistent with a very minor role for spasm: less than 1% in over 1300 cases. However, our experience of nine cases of coronary spasm in 44 potential candidates for PTCA (a 20% prevalence) suggests that spasm is frequently either not reported or not looked for.

If the prevalence of coronary spasm in candidates for PTCA and its effects on risks and immediate and long-term results are to be established, efforts must be made to detect its chance occurrence during diagnostic coronary angiography. Three rules should be followed to unmask coronary spasm in potential candidates for PTCA:

1. Whenever possible, coronary vasodilators of any type should be withheld for a long enough period to assure their absence from body tissues during diagnostic angiography.
2. When a critical, seemingly organic stenosis is discovered, coronary angiography should be repeated after the administration of coronary vasodilators. Sublingual nitroglycerin (NTG) is usually effective, but in one of our nine patients intracoronary (IC) NTG reduced an 80% stenosis to a subcritical 45% stenosis where sublingual NTG had failed (Fig. 1).
3. We therefore suggest that NTG, and Ca^{++} blocking agents when available, be employed by the IC route before concluding that a critical stenosis is purely organic. It should be recognized that by this method coronary spasm can be detected only in those patients in whom it happens to be present during coronary angiography; its observed prevalence, therefore, is likely to be lower than its true prevalence.

Table 1 shows some of the clinical features in the nine patients of our series, with coronary spasm. Patient 1, mentioned above, and patient 2 were not subjected to

Transluminal Coronary Angioplasty and Intracoronary Thrombolysis. Ed. by Kaltenbach et al.

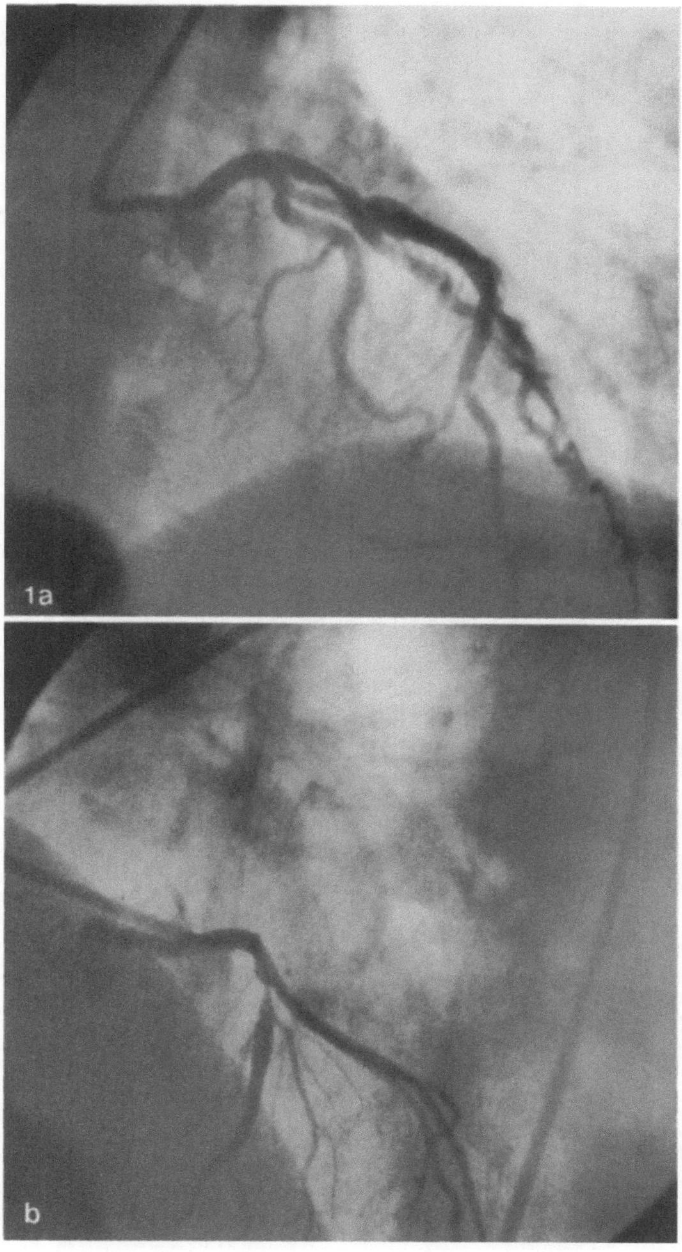
1a
b

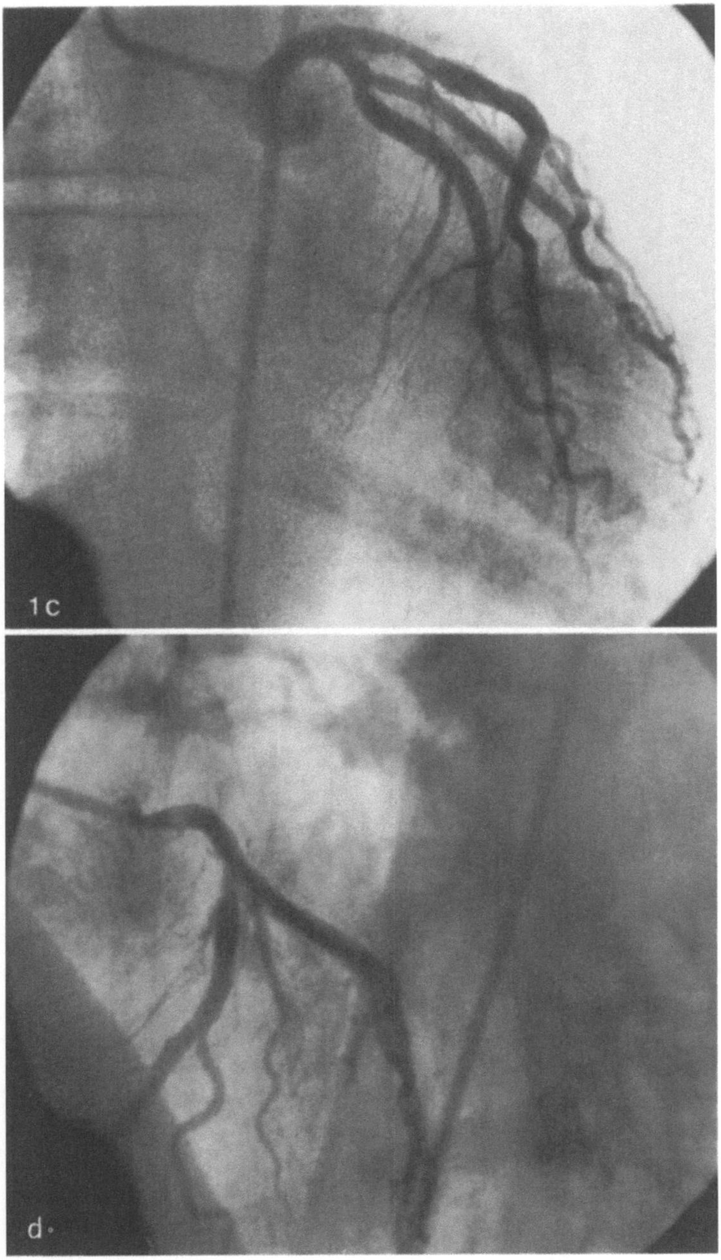

Fig. 1a–d. Left coronary artery (LCA). **a** 30° RAO projection after the sublingual administration of 0.8 mg NTG. **b** 45° LAO projection with additional 30° craniocaudal (CC) rotation after 0.8 mg NTG sublingually. An 80% proximal stenosis of the anterior descending artery (ADA) is noted. **c** and **d** LCA in the same projection as in *a* and *b* after 100 μg IC NTG. The fixed component of the mixed stenosis is seen to represent only 45% of the lumen diameter

Table 1. Some clinical features of nine patients with coronary spasm

Patient	Age	Sex	Chest pain		Coronary stenosis (%)				Medication after angiography (mg/day)		Follow-up
			Pattern	Duration	Before PTCA			After PTCA			
					Coronary artery	Control	After IC NTG				
1	52	F	Exercise, rest → threatened MI → hospitalization	5 months	ADA	80	45	–	Nifedipine	40	No chest pain.
2	48	M	Unheralded, treatened MI → hospitalization	1 week	ADA	80	24	–	Nifedipine Isosorbide dinitrate	40 120	Recurrent attacks of pain during rest and exercise, 8–10/month. Inferior MI 7 months later. On repeat angio, ADA 60%, RCA 100%. Elective CABG surgery to ADA & RCA.
3	45	F	Exercise → rest → sleep; lately up to 20 attacks/day	14 months	ADA	90	66	40	Isosorbide dinitrate	40	Mild, rare attacks after nifedipine 40 mg/day was started 2 months following PTCA.
4	34	M	Unheralded MI → hospitalization	2 months	ADA	70	70	30	Nitroglycerin		Attacks of pain during rest and exercise resumed 2 months after PTCA. On repeat angio, spasm (70%) relieved by IC NTG (40%). Mild, rare attacks after nifedipine was started.
5	31	M	Rest & Exercise → hospitalization	3 weeks	ADA	90	70	70 (failure)	Isosorbide dinitrate	80	Unable to dilate because of abnormal catheter path. Coronary spasm during catheter advancement relieved by IC NTG. Elective CABG surgery to ADA.

6	54	M	Rest & exercise severe → threatened MI → hospitalization	1 week	RCA	100	90 streptokinase ↓ 60	95 (complicated failure)	Isosorbide dinitrate	80	Emergency CABG surgery to RCA. Inferior MI. Well after discharge.
7	64	F	Unheralded developing MI → hospitalization; recurrent ST ↑ Q wave in lead III, AVF	1 hour	RCA	80	80	35	None		No chest pain after PTCA.
8	60	M	Sleep & rest	10 days	ADA	68 78	26 78	– 17	None		Development of exertional chest pain 1 month after first catheterization. On repeat study, ADA 78%, fixed. Successful PTCA. No chest pain since.
9	43	F	Rest & exercise; lately, many episodes/day	34 months	ADA	90	80	20	Nifedipine Isosorbide dinitrate	40 40	Minimal chest pain

PTCA because of subcritical fixed stenoses. Both were put on nifedipine, with good results in one and unfavorable results in the other.

In patients 3–6 the fixed stenoses were moderately severe, ranging from 60% to 70% of the lumen diameter. In patients 3 and 4, both with ADA obstructions, PTCA was successful, with reduction of the organic component to 40% and 30% respectively. However, in both patients chest pain at rest and with exercise recurred after discharge. In both it responded favorably to nifedipine but some chest pain persisted. Patient 5, with ADA stenosis, developed chest pain and ST segment changes during unsuccessful PTCA due to inability to reach the lesion. The pain responded quickly to IC NTG with no detectable damage to the vessel. He underwent successful elective CABG surgery a few days later. In patient 6 the RCA was found to be occluded on diagnostic angiography but flow resumed after IC NTG, revealing a 90% obstruction. The stenosis further reduced to 60% after 300 000 units IC streptokinase. One week later, PTCA was complicated by coronary dissection and the patient underwent emergency CABG surgery with a residual inferior MI.

Finally, in patients 7–9 with the most severe fixed stenotic components (80%, 78%, and 80% of the lumen diameter respectively), the stenoses were reduced to 35%, 17%, and 20% respectively by PTCA. Two patients are asymptomatic over a year after PTCA on no coronary medication; the third has minimal symptoms 1 month after PTCA on nifedipine and nitrates.

Patients 2 and 8 are of particular interest because of the rapid progression of an initially subcritical fixed component of the mixed stenosis in both. During their first study, IC NTG reduced the stenoses from 70% to 23% in patient 2 (Fig. 2a–d) and from 68% to 26% in patient 8 (Fig. 3a–d). Despite nifedipine and nitrates, patient 2 continued to experience attacks of chest pain at rest and exercise at the rate of 8–10 per month and suffered an inferior MI 6 months after the first cardiac catheterization. A repeat study a month later showed the fixed stenosis of the ADA to have progressed from 23% to 60% of the lumen diameter (Fig. 2e, f). The RCA, formerly showing only small and focal aneurysmal dilatations in its proximal half, was now occluded near its origin (Fig. 2g, h). This marked progression of the disease took place in a period of only 6 months. The patient underwent uneventful elective CABG surgery of the ADA and RCA and is presently asymptomatic on Persantine 150 mg/day.

Following discharge on nifedipine and nitrates, patient 8 also experienced the recurrence of moderately severe episodes of chest pain 3 months later, and coronary angiography had to be repeated. The new study revealed the stenosis to be severe and fixed, having increased from 26% to 78% of the lumen diameter in just 4 months (Fig. 3e, f). In this patient, PTCA was very successful and he has remained asymptomatic on a medical program which initially included nifedipine 40 mg/day. Presently he is on no medication. The course of events in these two patients suggests a cause-and-effect relationship between coronary spasm superimposed on a subcritical organic stenosis and its subsequent rapid progression. In the limit, pure coronary spasm in patients prone to it might be the precursor of an obstructing atheroma at its site of occurrence.

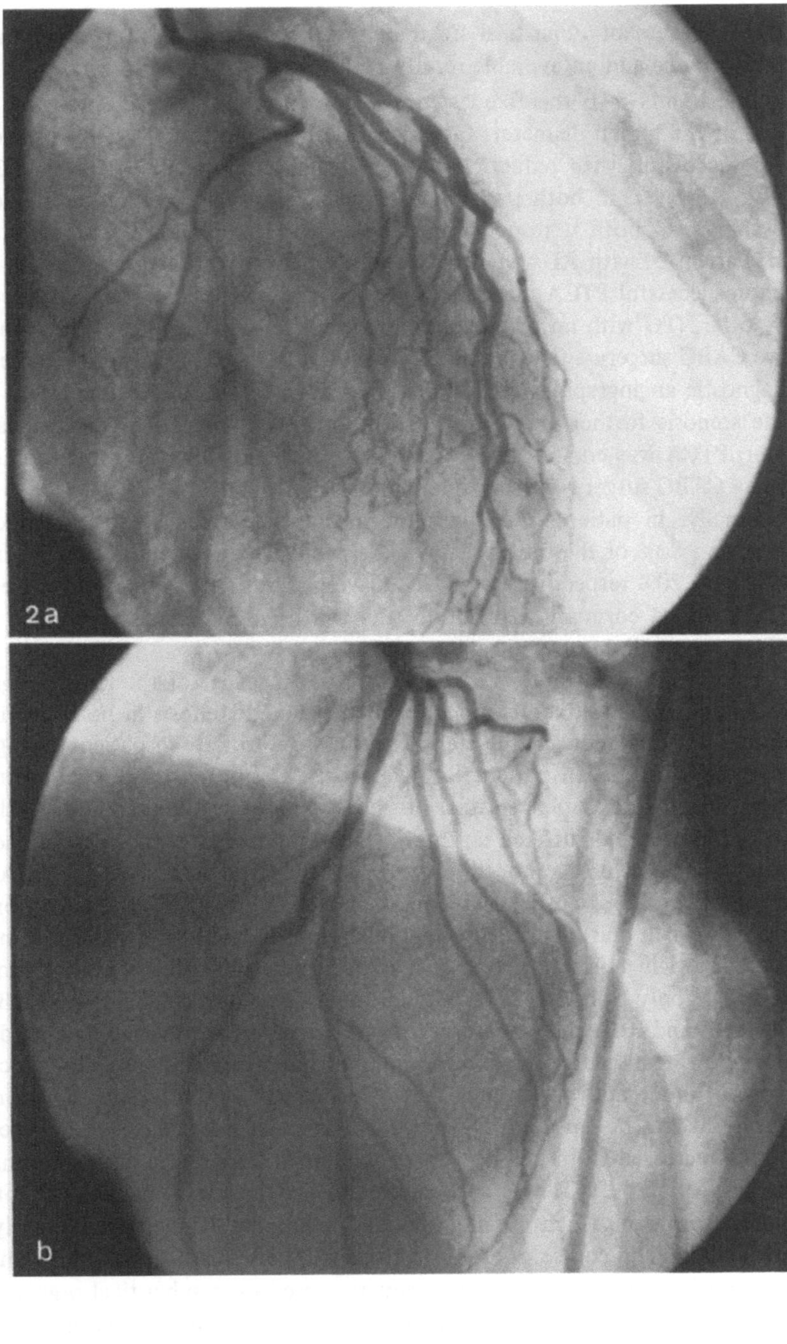
2a
b

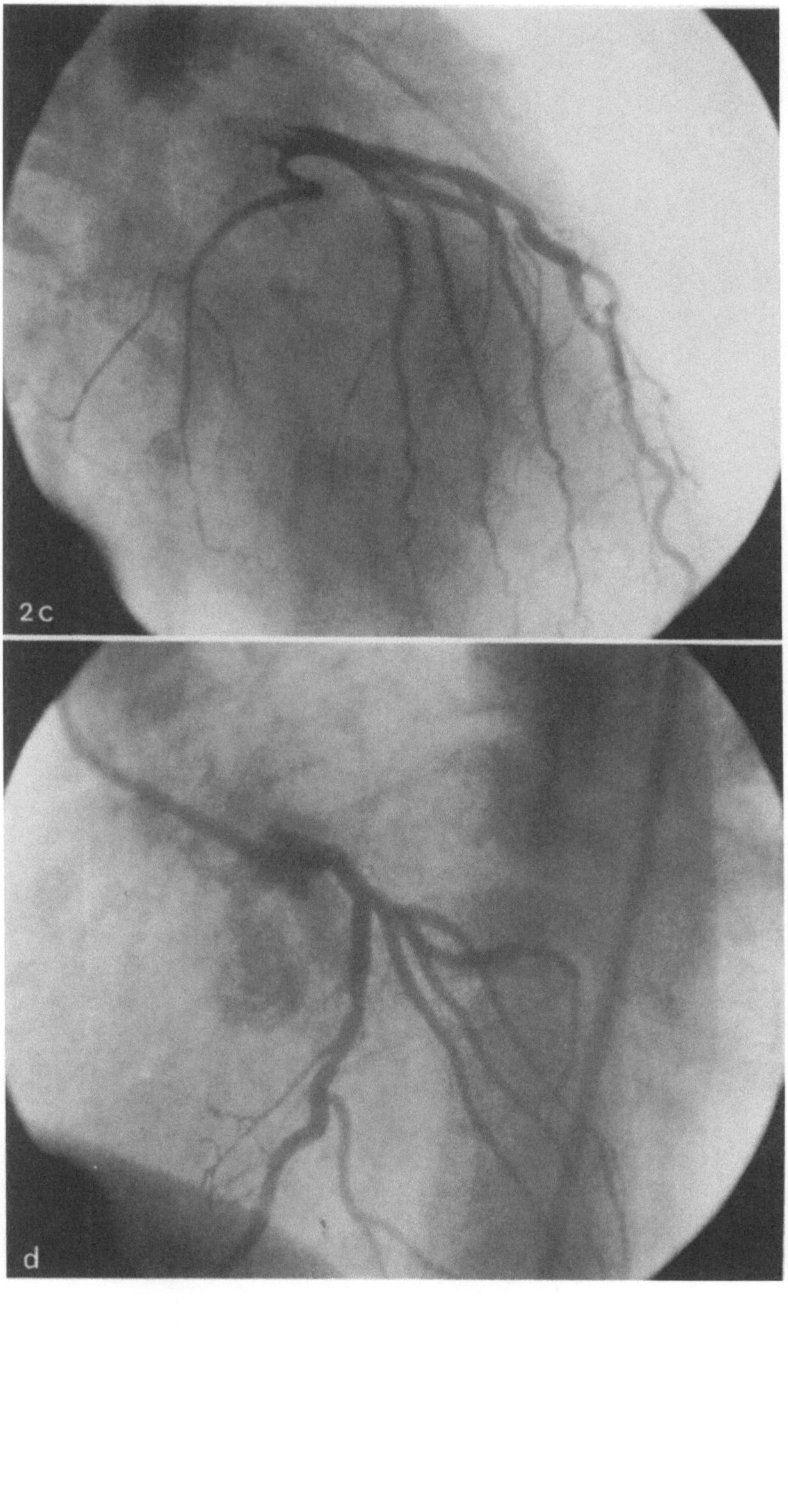
2c
d

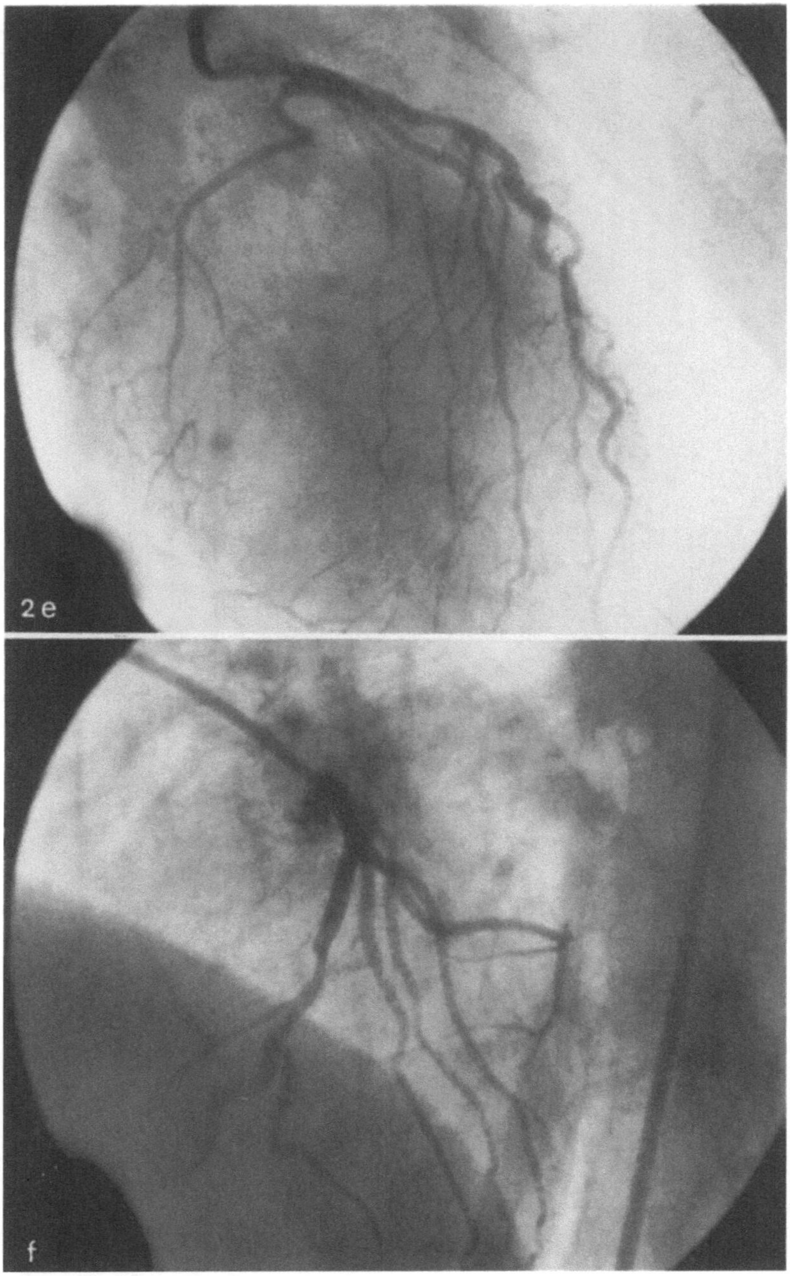
2e
f

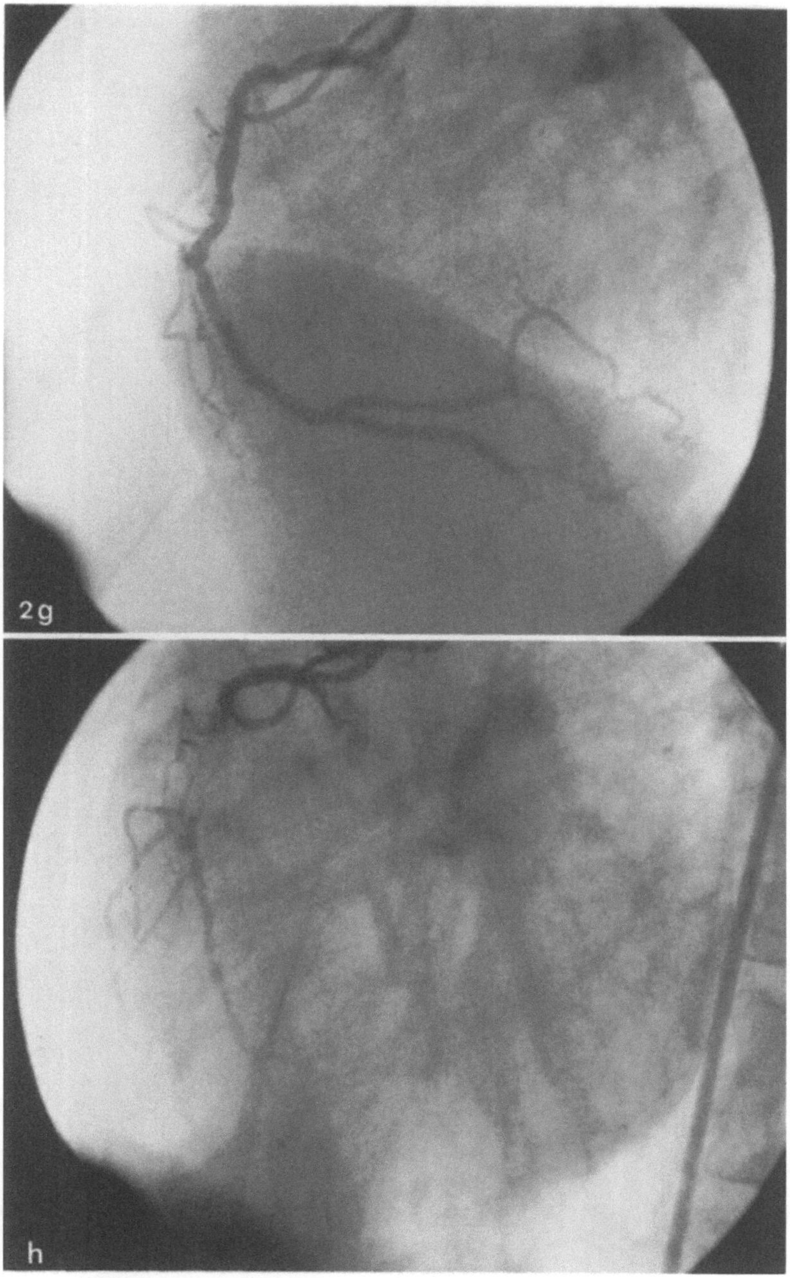

Fig. 2. a Control LCA angiogram in the 30° RAO projection. **b** Control LCA angiogram in the 45° LAO projection with additional 30° CC rotation. A 70% proximal stenosis of the ADA is present. **c** and **d** LCA in the same projection as in **a** and **b** after 100 μg IC NTG. The stenosis has decreased to 23% of the lumen diameter. **e** and **f** LCA 7 months later in the same projections after 100 μg IC NTG. The fixed component of the mixed stenosis has increased to 60%. **g** RCA in the 35° LAO projection; control. No stenosis is present but small focal aneurysmal dilatations are noted in the proximal and middle thirds. **h** Seven months later the RCA is occluded

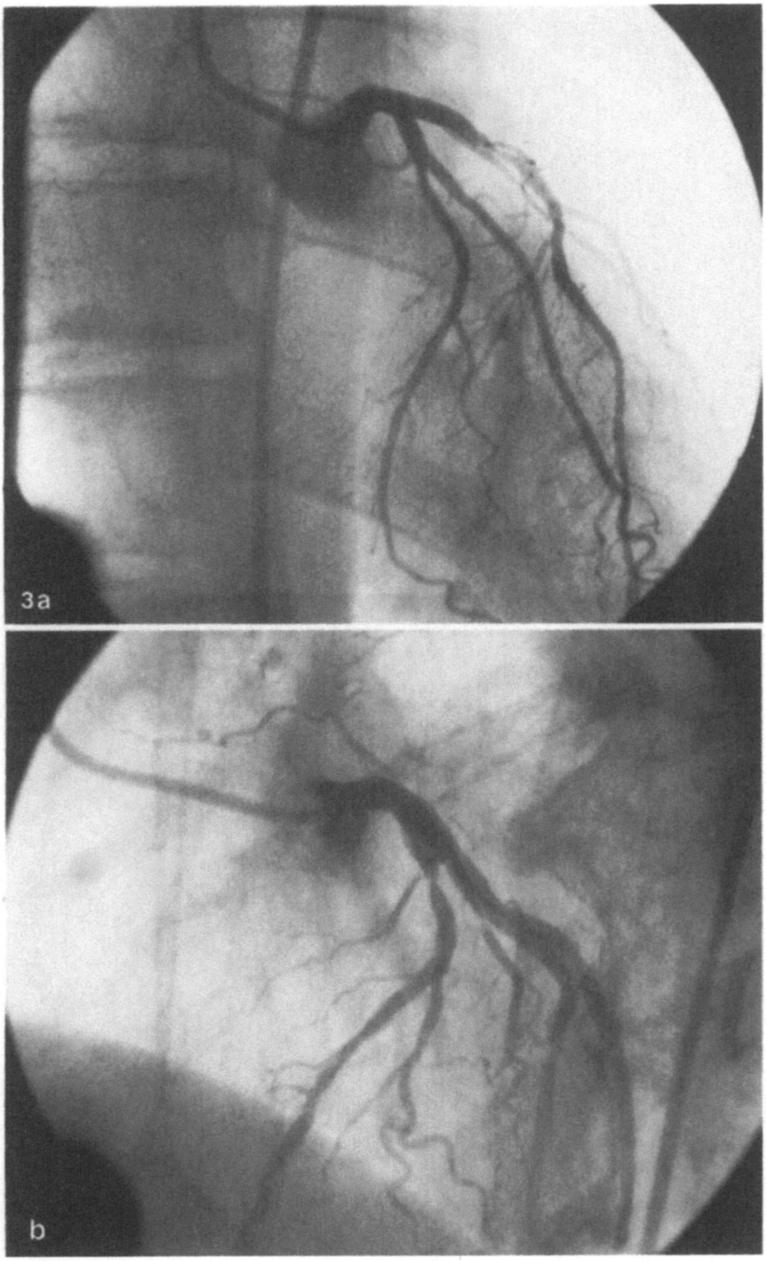
3a
b

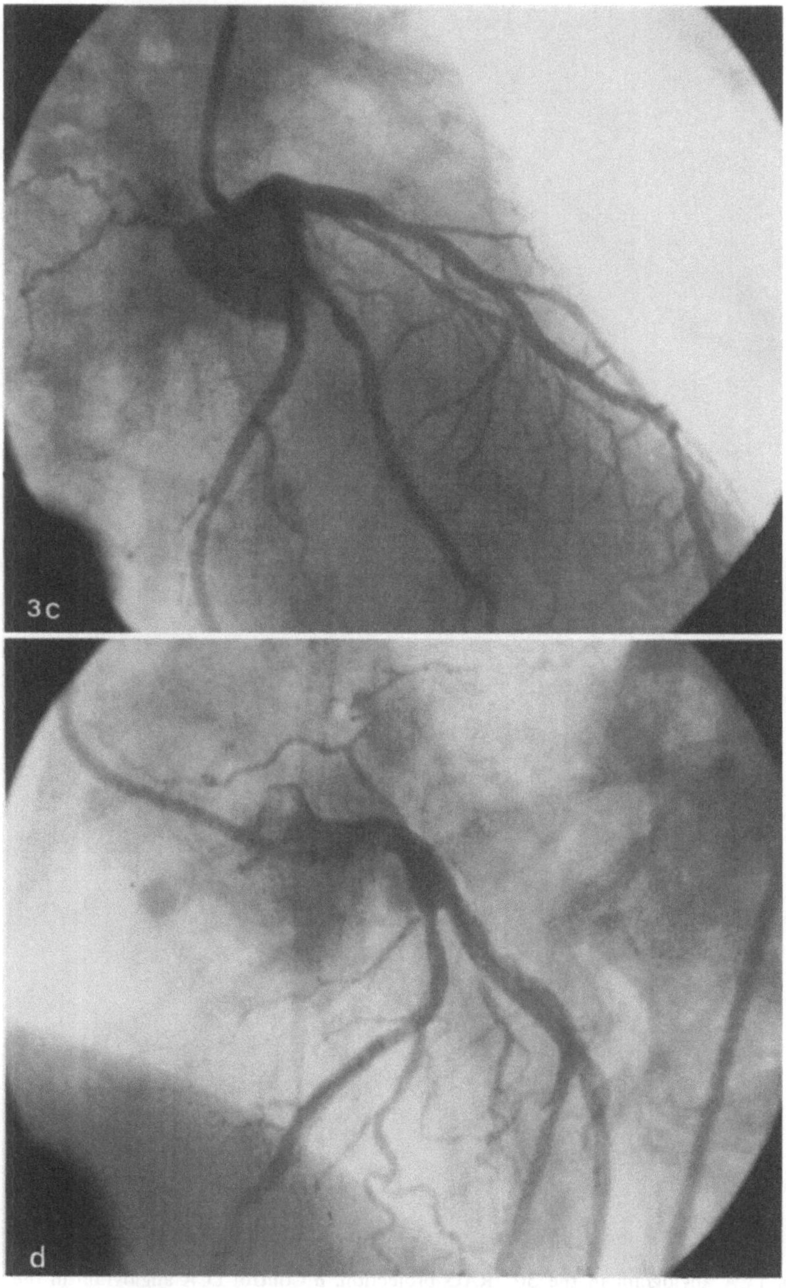
3c
d

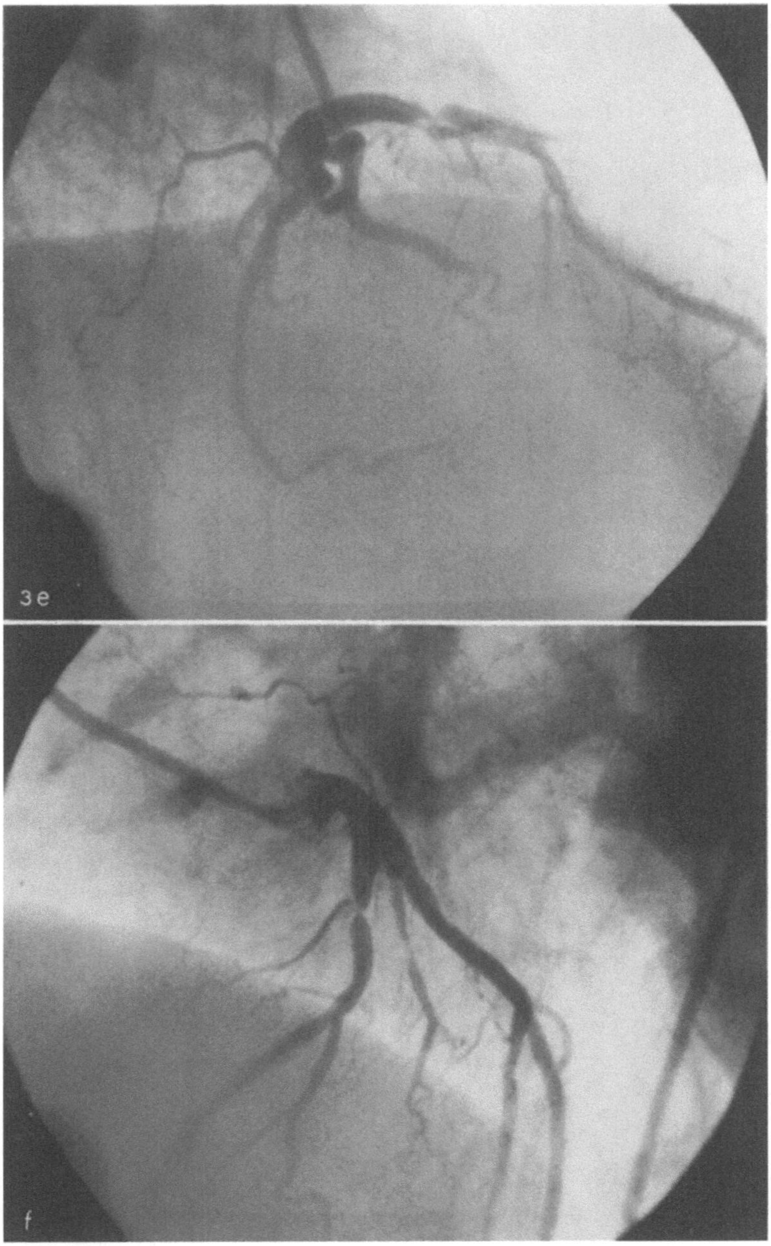

Fig. 3. **a** Control LCA angiogram in the 30° RAO projection. **b** Control LCA angiogram in the 45° LAO projection with additional 30° CC rotation. A 68% proximal stenoses of the ADA is noted. **c** and **d** LCA in the same projections after 100 μg IC NTG. The fixed component of the mixed stenosis amounts to only 26% of the lumen diameter. **e** and **f** LCA in the same projections after 100 μg of IC NTG 3 months later. The fixed component of the stenosis has grown to 78% of the lumen diameter

On the basis of our limited experience we would like to draw the following tentative conclusions:

1. Vasospastic angina is common in potential candidates for PTCA.
2. To unmask spasm, angiograms schould be taken before and after coronary vasodilators whenever possible.
3. Intracoronary NTG sometimes relieves spasm resistant to sublingual NTG.
4. The results of PTCA appear to be better when the fixed component of a mixed stenosis is very severe.
5. Mixed coronary lesions can progress rapidly to severe, fixed stenoses.

This presentation is aimed primarily at calling attention to and stimulating interest in the occurrence of coronary spasm in potential candidates for PTCA, and in its influence on immediate and late results and on complications. Our conclusions, based as they are on a small series, are tentative and may prove incorrect.

Transluminal Coronary Angioplasty and Coronary Spasm

Remark to the paper of Dr. Bentivoglio by M. Kaltenbach

Department of Cardiology, Centre of Internal Medicine, J.W. Goethe University, Theodor-Stern-Kai 7, 6000 Frankfurt a.M., FRG

The observations of Dr. Bentivoglio have important clinical implications, among them:

1. The coexistence of organic atherosclerosis and coronary spasm may influence the indication for transluminal coronary angioplasty (TCA).
2. The presence of coronary spasm in the same patient may be a changing pattern which can appear and disappear in the course of the disease.

In regard to the combination of atherosclerosis with spasm we made an interesting observation in a patient in whom TCA was performed as early as 1977. This young man presented with angina predominantly occurring during exercise and showed angiographically a 70% left main stenosis. The result of TCA was an almost completely opened vessel; the patient experienced prompt relief of symptoms. Several weeks later, however, angina reoccurred and this time was much more pronounced during rest. By administration of ergonovine angina could be provoked. Several weeks after TCA the patient suffered an anterior myocardial infarction and 2 weeks later he died of cerebral damage caused by ventricular fibrillation. Postmortem examination revealed a smooth, nonstenosing atheroma in the left main coronary artery. Thus, coronary spasm was apparently superimposed on atherosclerosis and deteriorated after TCA despite successful dilatation of the atheroma.

On the other hand, we have seen several patients with coronary spasm which later, in the course of the disease, disappeared. Apparently the coronary spasm occurred during a period of rapid progression of coronary atherosclerosis. The timing of transluminal angioplasty in these patients has to be adjusted to the stage of the disease. Two female patients presented with unstable angina and a 60% LAD stenosis. In both TCA was performed with good primary results. Several weeks later symptoms reoccurred; one patient had repeated TCA with good long-term results, the other patient experienced an uncomplicated anterior myocardial infarction. Two other patients with similar conditions were not exposed to TCA but carefully observed. They both showed rapid progression within a few months; angiographically the stenoses progressed from 60% to 80% and 90% respectively. During the same period the symptoms changed from unstable angina to severe stable angina pectoris. In this stage of the disease TCA was thought to be indicated, and was performed with good results.

Thus, the combination of organic and functional coronary arterial narrowing can provide problems in regard to angioplasty. With predominant spasm and only mild or no organic disease TCA is clearly not indicated. If spasm is superimposed on a

Transluminal Coronary Angioplasty and
Intracoronary Thrombolysis. Ed. by Kaltenbach et al.

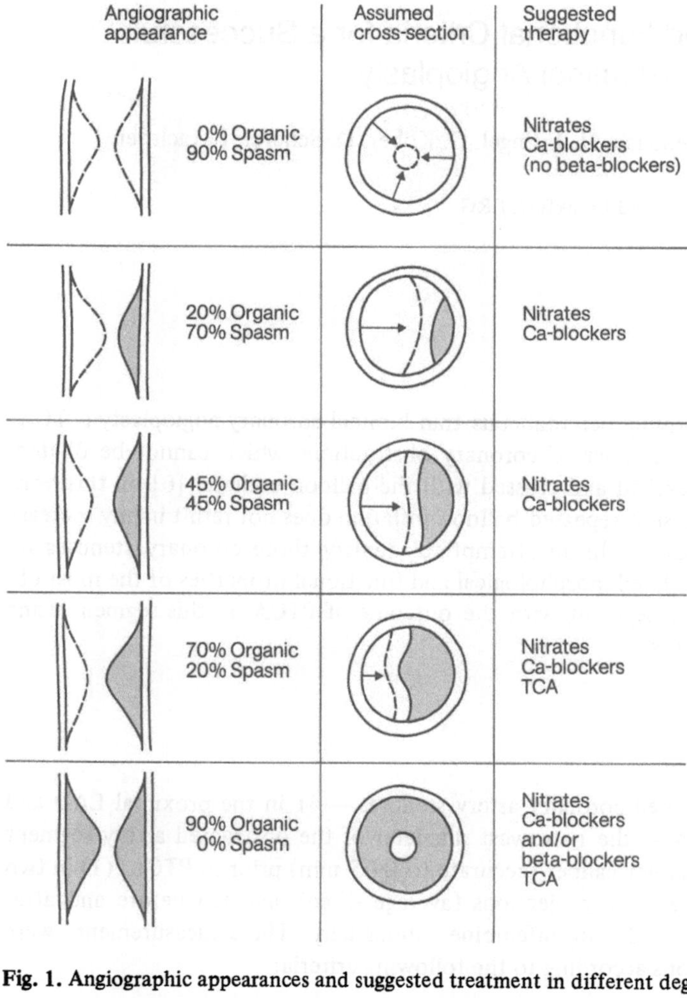

Fig. 1. Angiographic appearances and suggested treatment in different degrees of stenosis

50%–60% organic stenosis we assume that TCA can be postponed, but the patient has to be carefully followed up. Good results can in general be achieved if the organic part of the stenosis is 70% or more. In Fig. 1 the different findings and therapeutic considerations are summarized.

Morphological and Functional Criteria for a Successful Percutaneous Transluminal Angioplasty

W. Rafflenbeul, M. Kaltenbach, H.-J. Engel, G. Kober, D. Scherer, P. Lichtlen

University Hospitals Hannover and Frankfurt, FRG

Most laboratories performing percutaneous transluminal coronary angioplasty (PTCA) encounter a reasonable number of coronary obstructions which cannot be dilated, although they can be reached and crossed with the balloon catheter [6]. In this resistant type of coronary lesion repeated balloon inflation does not result in any increase of the residual vessel lumen. In an attempt to identify those coronary stenoses resistant to PTCA we correlated morphological and functional properties of the most obstructed coronary artery segment with the outcome of PTCA on this segment using quantitative measurements.

Methods

In 50 isolated, well-defined coronary artery stenoses – 41 in the proximal LAD and 9 in the proximal RCA – the narrowest diameter of the obstructed artery segment was measured with a vernier caliper (accurate to 0.05 mm) prior to PTCA: (1) in two to five different angiographic projections (average three), and (2) before and after 0.8 mg nitroglycerin plus 20 mg nifedipine sublingually. These measurements were used to classify the lesions according to the following criteria:

1. Morphological configuration: if the narrowest diameter of the stenosis differed by more than 25% in various projections the lesion was defined as an eccentric lesion, if by less than 25% as a concentric lesion.
2. Functional changes (vasomobility): an increase of the smallest diameter of greater than 15% in at least one projection after nitroglycerin and nifedipine was considered as pharmacologically induced vasodilation.
3. The subsequent PTCA was regarded successful with a diameter increase of the most obstructed vessel segment of more than 25% in at least one projection after the dilatation procedure.

To assess intraobserver variability a pilot study was conducted. Repeated measurements of the same coronary artery diameters – ranging from 0.65 mm to 4.07 mm – revealed an average difference between the measurements of 7.9% ± 2.5%. All measurements were performed by the same observer and the results are expressed as arithmetic mean ± standard deviation. The significance of differences was assessed by the t test, and P values < 0.05 were considered significant.

Transluminal Coronary Angioplasty and
Intracoronary Thrombolysis. Ed. by Kaltenbach et al.

Results

According to these criteria 18 of 50 coronary obstructions (36%) were considered concentric and 32 (64%) eccentric lesions. The severity of the obstructions was similar in both groups with a mean degree of area stenosis of 82% ± 9% and 80% ± 12% respectively.

Of 18 concentric lesions, 16 showed no change of the narrowest diameter after administration of the vasodilatory drugs (Fig. 1): the average stenotic diameter was 1.27 ± 0.20 mm before and 1.32 ± 0.21 mm after nitroglycerin and nifedipine ($P > 0.10$). All 16 of these lesions and one of the two concentric lesions responsive to vasodilators were successfully dilated with PTCA, increasing the average diameter from 1.27 ± 0.20 mm to 2.04 ± 0.18 mm (Fig. 2).

In contrast, 29 of 32 eccentric lesions demonstrated a significant increase of the smallest diameter after nitroglycerin and nifedipine from an average diameter of 1.29 ± 0.22 mm to 1.92 ± 0.21 mm (Fig. 1). However, the response of eccentric lesions to PTCA was less uniform (Fig. 2): whereas 22 stenoses showed a significant increase of the mean narrowest diameter from 1.29 ± 0.22 mm to 1.75 ± 0.20 mm, in ten of 32 stenoses (31%) PTCA left the smallest diameter nearly unchanged (1.43 ± 0.23 mm and 1.51 ± 0.21 mm respectively; not significant).

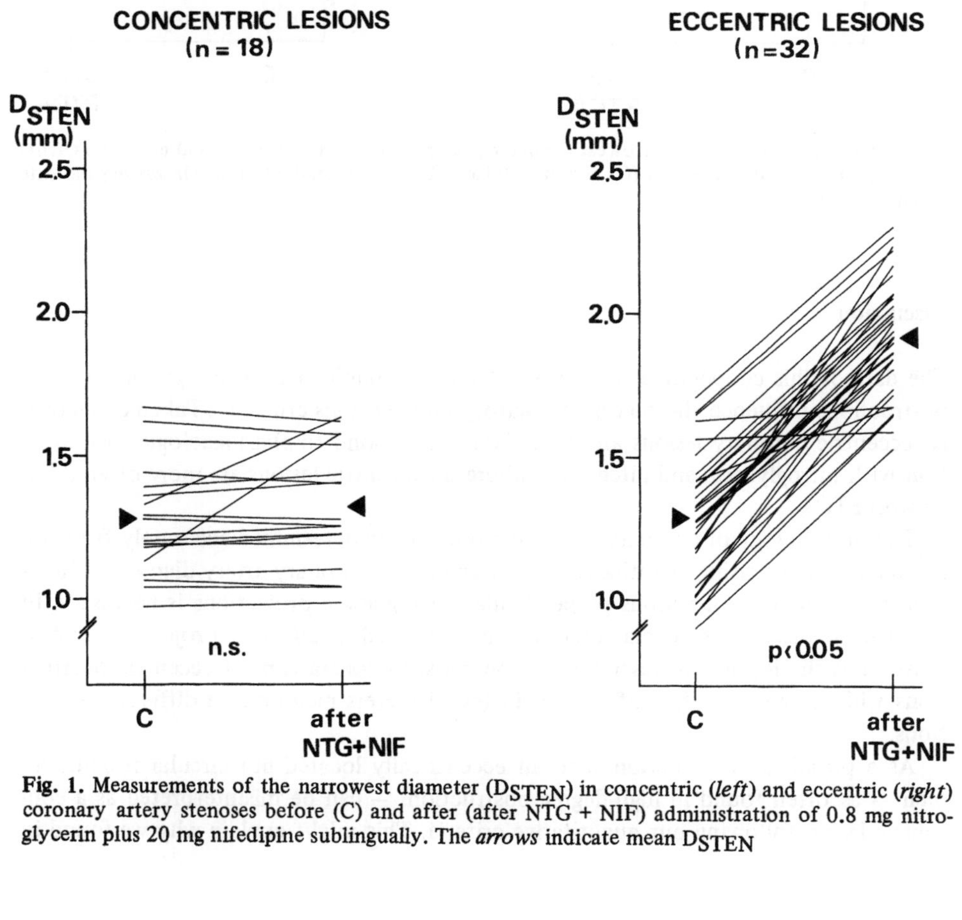

Fig. 1. Measurements of the narrowest diameter (D_{STEN}) in concentric (*left*) and eccentric (*right*) coronary artery stenoses before (C) and after (after NTG + NIF) administration of 0.8 mg nitroglycerin plus 20 mg nifedipine sublingually. The *arrows* indicate mean D_{STEN}

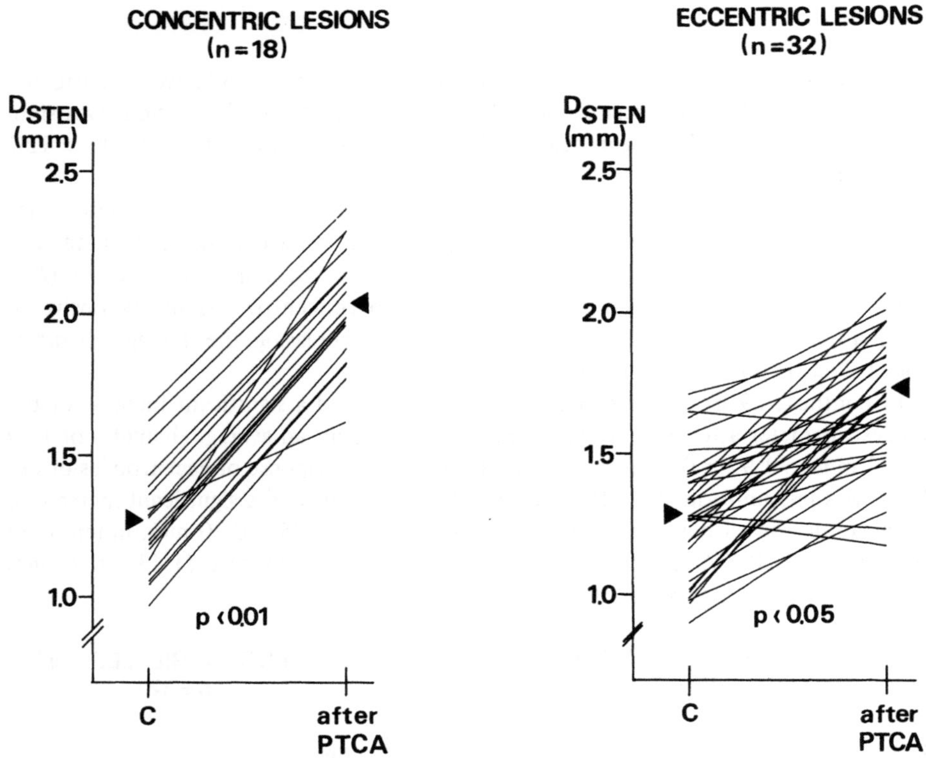

Fig. 2. Measurements of the narrowest diameter (D_{STEN}) in concentric (*left*) and eccentric (*right*) coronary artery stenoses before (C) and after (after PTCA) balloon dilatation. The *arrows* indicate mean D_{STEN}

Discussion

The data of this cooperative study suggest that morphological properties of coronary obstructions influence the success of dilatory interventions crucially. Taken collectively, eccentric coronary lesions are more likely to respond to pharmacological vasodilation with nitroglycerin and nifedipine, whereas concentric lesions are more often dilated with PTCA.

The morphology of coronary artery stenoses can be determined accurately from angiographic frames using quantitative measurements of coronary artery diameters. However, the evaluation of various perpendicular angiographic projections is necessary. In a concentric lesion similar diameters will be measured in different projections and in most cases the lesion will resemble an hourglass. In contrast, most eccentric obstructions will show substantial differences in the diameters measured in different projections.

As a pitfall, an obstruction with an eccentrically located but circular residual lumen – as often found in high-degree obstructions – can be misinterpreted as a concentric lesion following our quantitative criteria. This might explain why we found in our study a higher number of concentric lesions than previously reported in postmortem [2]. Furthermore, the range of deviation in measured diameters allocating obstructions to either concentric or eccentric morphology was arbitrarily selected in our study.

Dilatation of extramural coronary arteries with nitroglycerin and – more recently – with Ca^{++} – antagonists has been demonstrated in several studies [1, 3, 4]. Both drugs cause relaxation of vascular smooth muscle by different mechanisms. In most eccentric lesions the normal vessel wall is left intact segmentally [5] with smooth muscle cells still capable of relaxation. This might explain why we found a measurable increase in the residual luminal diameter in most eccentric lesions after nitroglycerin and nifedipine. On the other hand, the "soft" relaxed vessel wall might give to the pressure of the inflating balloon and by this mechanism prevent an effective PTCA in some patients.

In concentric lesions *circumferential* degeneration of the vessel wall along with fibrosis and/or calcification creates "tight" lesions and might prevent a pharmacologically induced vasodilation. This intramural circular rigidity, however, should represent an ideal opposing force for the distending balloon, accounting for the successful pressure impact on atherosclerotic material in many coronary obstructions. In addition, our results indicate that stenosis morphology traced from angiographic frames is not the sole characteristic determining the efficacy of PTCA once the stenosis is crossed with the balloon catheter. Other factors like the vintage of the lesion concomitant with degenerative changes in the plaque as well as the elasticity of the residual normal wall segment may influence the acute success of PTCA.

References

1. Gensini GG, Kelly AE, DaCosta BCB, Huntington PP (1971) Quantitative angiography: the measurement of coronary vasomobility in the intact animal and man. Chest 60:522
2. Hort W, Moosdorf R, Kalbfleisch H, Köhler F, Milzner-Schwarz U, Frenzel H (1977) Postmortale Untersuchungen über Lokalisation und Form der stärksten Stenosen in den Koronararterien und ihre Beziehung zu den Risikofaktoren. Z Kardiol 66:333
3. Leutenegger F, Rafflenbeul W, Gahl K, Walpurger G, Engel H-J, Lichtlen P (1980) Quantitative Koronarangiographie: Dilatation von Koronarstenosen nach Nifedipin. Schweiz Med Wochenschr 110:1703
4. Rafflenbeul W, Urthaler F, Russell RO, Lichtlen P, James TN (1980) Dilatation of coronary artery stenoses after isosorbide dinitrate in man. Br Heart J 43:546
5. Ross R, Glomset JA (1976) The pathogenesis of atherosclerosis. N Engl J Med 295:369
6. Williams DO, Riley RS, Singh AK, Most AS (1982) Unsuccessful percutaneous transluminal coronary angioplasty: identification of remedial causes. In this volume, pp 91–94

Transluminal Angioplasty in Patients with Unstable Angina Pectoris

J. Meyer*, H. Schmitz, R. Erbel, B. Böcker-Josephs, H. Grenner, W. Krebs, W. Merx, P. Bardos, C. Minale, B.J. Messmer, S. Effert

Dept. Internal Medicine I and Dept. Cardiovascular Surgery Klinikum RWTH Aachen, FRG

Percutaneous transluminal coronary angioplasty (PTCA) has been performed in 101 patients in our department since October 1978 (Table 1). Initially we selected only patients iwith stable angina pectoris. These patients were transferred to the Department of Internal Medicine or to the Department of Surgery for considerations of bypass surgery because of their severe, medically not sufficiently treatable angina pectoris. Their clinical symptoms were stable over a period of more than 3 months. All had proximal, isolated coronary stenoses. This group represents the normal population for PTCA according to the indication initially set by Grüntzig.

Since our hospital is the referral centre for a larger area and cooperates closely with several other hospitals and rehabilitation centres, patients with unstable angina pectoris, with preinfarction syndrome, and with signs of a nontransmural myocardial infarction are admitted rather often. In some of them coronary angiography has already been performed in the referring hospital. The history of 47 such patients (Table 1) was significantly shorter (3.1 ± 2.3 months) than that of the 47 patients with chronic stable angina (22.7 ± 28.6 months). The normal waiting time for bypass surgery at the moment is up to 4 months. However, as these patients had clear symptoms of an unstable angina or an impending infarction with transient ST-T changes and/or slight MB-CK changes but no Q waves we performed PTCA in the 47 patients with proximal isolated coronary stenoses within 36 h of admission.

The premedication consisted of 3 × 10 mg nifedipine and 3 × 500 mg acetylsalicylic acid on the preceding day and 20 mg nifedipine and 500 mg acetylsalicylic acid at the beginning of the procedure in both groups. In addition 100 ml/h dextran was infused intravenously. To rule out coronary spasms 0.1–0.2 mg nitroclycerin was addi-

Table 1. Data of 101 patients treated with PTCA

	Stable angina	Unstable angina	After lysis
No. of patients	47	47	7
Age (years)	47.7 ± 7.8	50 ± 7.7	59.7 ± 11.7
Duration of symptoms (months)	22.7 ± 28.6	3.1 ± 2.3	18.8 ± 27.9
Success rate (%)	68	72	71 (5/7)

* Dept. Internal Medicine I, Klinikum RWTH, Goethestr. 27, 5100 Aachen, FRG

Transluminal Coronary Angioplasty and Intracoronary Thrombolysis. Ed. by Kaltenbach et al.

tionally injected into the diseased coronary vessel before the introduction of the balloon catheter.

A third group of seven patients (Table 1) had been admitted to our hospital with acute transmural myocardial infarction. Selective intracoronary streptolysis with streptokinase was able to reopen the occluded vessel within 8 h of the acute event. Control coronary angiogram in these patients revealed a severe isolated stenosis at the site of the previous thrombotic occlusion. These seven patients are part of a total of 70 patients with an acute infarction treated with selective thrombolysis. From our experience with these patients we knew that a reocclusion at the same coronary site quite often occurs within the next 72 h. We therefore decided to dilate the underlying stenosis if it was isolated and proximal. In five patients PTCA was performed in the same session as intracoronary streptolysis after the vessel was patent again. We used the same introducing sheath in the groin. The patients had received 150 000–300 000 units streptokinase, 10 000 units heparin, 1 g acetylsalicylic acid, 1–5 mg/h nitroglycerin, and 250 mg prednisone during the 60–90 min of streptolysis. In one patient PTCA was performed 30 h later and in one patient 4 weeks later.

The distribution of the localization of stenoses in patients with chronic stable and unstable angina and in those after lysis was quite similar (Table 2). Both main stem stenoses were unsuccessfully treated. Stenoses in the left anterior descending artery (LAD) occurred more frequently than in the right coronary artery (RCA). Both in stable and in unstable angina the success rate in LAD (74% and 77%) exceeded that in RCA stenoses (58% and 67%). The overall success rate in patients with unstable angina (72%) was slightly but not significantly higher than in patients with the chronic stable form (68%). In the group of seven patients with infarction the procedure was successful in dilating the underlying, severe organic stenosis in five cases immediately after successful reopening of the totally occluded vessel by streptolysis.

Table 2. Localization of stenoses and success rate of treatment by PTCA in stable and in unstable angina as well as after successful intracoronary streptolysis of an acute myocardial infarction

Stable Angina pectoris		
Localization	No. of patients	Success rate
Main stem	1	–
LAD	34	25 (74%)
RCA	12	7 (58%)
Total	47	32 (68%)
Unstable angina		
Main stem	1	–
LAD	31	24 (77%)
RCA	15	10 (67%)
Total	47	34 (72%)
After lysis		
LAD	5	4
RCA	2	1
Total	7	5

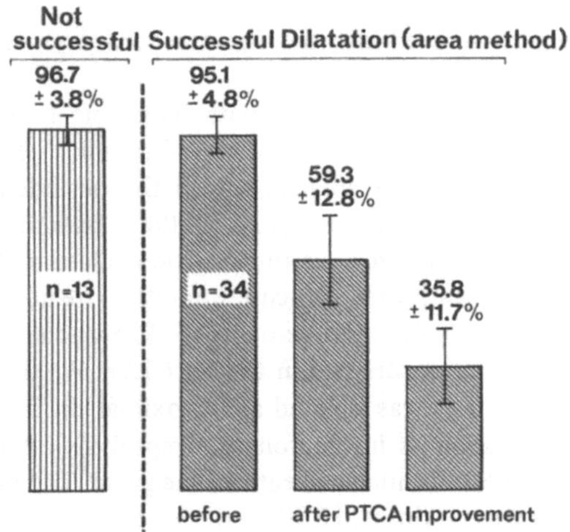

Fig. 1. Degree of stenosis (area method) before and after PTCA and amount of improvement in 47 patients with chronic stable angina pectoris. Comparison of the degree of stenosis in successfully and unsuccessfully treated patients

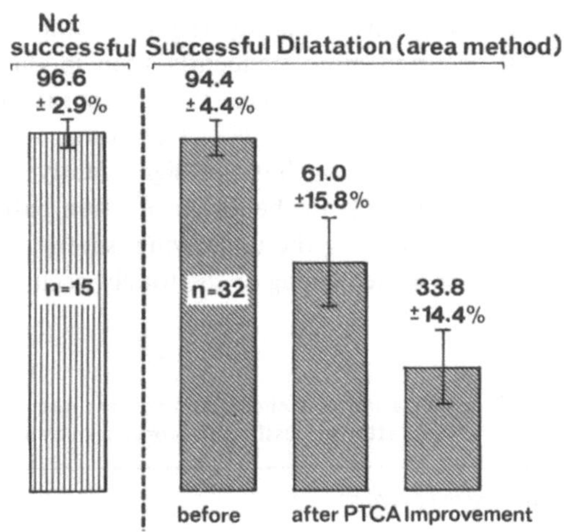

Fig. 2. Degree of stenosis (area method) before and after PTCA and amount of improvement in 47 patients with unstable angina pectoris. Comparison of the degree of stenosis in successfully and unsuccessfully treated patients

The degree of the stenoses (area method) measured in two to five different projections, including the craniocaudal in the main stem and the LAD stenoses, was similar in patients with stable angina (Fig. 1) and in those with unstable angina (Fig. 2). In both groups the degree of stenosis in those patients who were not successfully treated was slightly, but not significantly higher than in those who were successfully treated. In the stable group (Fig. 1) the degree of stenosis was diminished from 94.4% ± 4.4% to 61.0% ± 15.8%, the improvement being 33.8% ± 14.4%. In the group with unstable angina the initial degree of 95.1% ± 4.8% was diminished to 59.3% ± 12.8%.

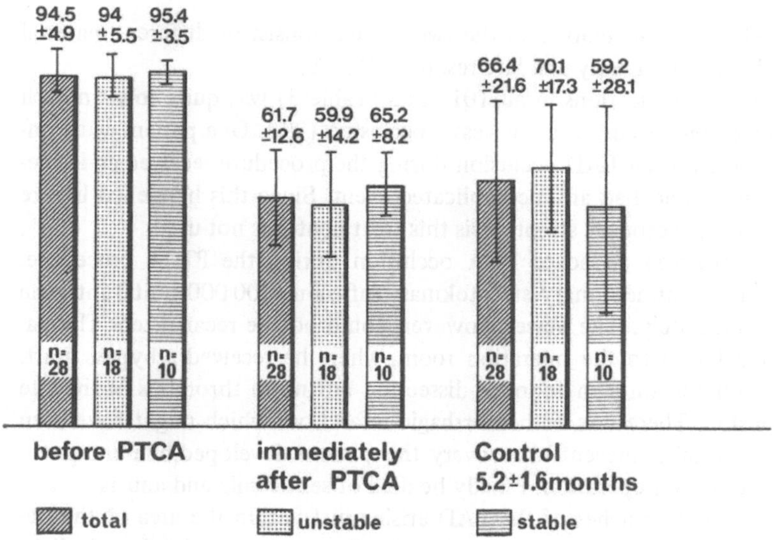

Fig. 3. Comparison of the degree of stenosis (area method) before and immediately after PTCA as well as at the control study 5.2 ± 1.6 months later in 28 successfully treated patients

Thus the improvement in the unstable group was slightly, but not significantly better (35.8% ± 11.7%) than in the stable group (33.8% ± 14.4%).

In 28 of the 101 patients (18 patients with previously unstable and ten with stable angina) a control study was performed 5.2 ± 1.6 months after PTCA. The overall degree of stenosis (Fig. 3) had risen slightly to 66.4% ± 21.6%. While the primary success in the group of 18 patients with unstable angina immediately after PTCA (59.9% ± 14.2%) was slightly better than in the group of ten patients with stable angina (65.2% ± 8.2%), the results in the control study showed the reverse situation. In the unstable group the mean resting degree of stenoses (70.1% ± 17.3%) was higher than in the stable group (59.2% ± 28.1%). Because of the wide variety in the individual cases and the considerable overlap the differences in this limited group were not significant. The tendency, however, should be followed and be controlled in the future. It may

Table 3. Complications during and immediately after PTCA in 101 patients

Disease	Complications
Unstable angina	One LAD occlusion – immediate bypass surgery Two LAD septal branch occlusions – conservative treatment, CPK +, ECG ϕ
Stable angina	One RCA occlusion – unsuccessful intracoronary streptolysis, bypass surgery, pneumonia, sepsis, anuria, death One ventricular fibrillation at control angiography – defibrillation

come out eventually that the stenoses in the two groups consist of different material and may show quite different early and late results in PTCA.

The rate of major complications in all 101 cases (Table 3) was quite low. In each group one patient experienced an acute vessel occlusion (2%). One patient with unstable angina who had a total LAD occlusion during the procedure received an immediate bypass operation and had an uncomplicated event. Since this happened before our experience with intracoronary streptolysis this treatment was not used.

One patient experienced an acute RCA occlusion during the PTCA procedure. We installed a selective intracoronary streptokinase infusion (300 000 units) into the occluded vessel immediately. The vessel, however, could not be recanalized. The patient was then transferred to the operation room, where he received a bypass graft. During the operation the surgeon found a dissection but not a thrombus at the site of the vessel occlusion. There was no hemorrhagic infarction, which might have been expected. After an initially uneventful recovery this patient developed bilateral pneumonia in the 3rd week after operation. Finally he died of septicemia and anuria.

In two patients septal branches of the LAD arising just within the area of the stenosis were occluded by the compressed material. These patients developed slight MB-CK changes but no Q waves. No bypass operation was necessary or even possible in these small intraseptal vessels. Another patient went into ventricular fibrillation during the control coronary angiography at the end of a successful dilatation. He was immediately defibrillated. In the group of patients treated after intracoronary streptolysis there was no complication attributable to PTCA. No reocclusion and no sign of a hemorrhagic infarction occurred.

Conclusion

In summary we can say that PTCA can be performed in patients with stable as well as unstable angina with similar good early results. The complication rate in the two groups is similar. It will have to be analyzed quite carefully in the future whether the early and late results differ in patients with stable and unstable angina. In this limited series there is at least a tendency to better results in the stable group. Because of the sometimes very urgent situation we try to perform PTCA in patients with unstable angina in the same session as the initial coronary angiography if these patients are primarily admitted to our hospital. The angiographic procedure in those patients is always scheduled when one operating room is available for an emergency operation.

Our experience with intracoronary streptolysis in acute transmural infarction has shown that a reocclusion of the vessel at the site of the previous thrombosis occurs quite often within the next days. We therefore strive for an early revascularization whenever possible. In patients with multivessel diseases we prefer early bypass operation. In some patients with an isolated stenosis, however, PTCA can be performed successfully with good results and a low complication rate the same session as streptolysis. In two of our seven patients a cardiogenic shock, which developed despite reopening of the vessel by streptokinase, could be reversed by the successful dilatation of the high-grade proximal coronary stenosis.

Adrenergic Coronary Vasoconstriction with Coronary Stenosis

E.O. Feigl, C.W. Buffington

University of Washington, Seattle, WA 98195, USA

Clinical studies suggest that alpha-receptor-mediated (alpha-mediated) coronary vasoconstriction may play a role in the genesis of myocardial ischemia in patients with coronary artery stenoses. Mudge et al. [11, 12] have demonstrated an inappropriate increase in coronary vascular resistance in response to the cold pressor test in patients with coronary artery disease. Since previous studies in dogs have shown that alpha-mediated coronary vasoconstriction competes with local metabolic vasodilation during sympathetic activation [9], the idea that a similar competition exists in the presence of coronary stenosis was tested [3].

Methods

Thirteen dogs were anesthetized with morphine sulfate and chloralose. Ventilation was controlled and arterial oxygen tension kept between 125 and 150 mmHg. Arterial and pulmonary wedge pressures were measured. A cannula-tip flow transducer was inserted into the ascending aorta via the right carotid artery. A balloon at the tip was inflated and the cannula wedged into the left coronary artery. Coronary flow (ultrasonic Doppler shift method) and pressure distal to an adjustable stenosis were measured. The stenosis produced a 70% area reduction of the cannula and sharply limited reactive hyperemia (Fig. 1).

Coronary sinus and arterial blood were sampled for oxygen content, oxygen tension, and plasma lactate determinations. Myocardial oxygen consumption, oxygen extraction, and lactate extraction were calculated.

The experiment involved intracoronary infusion of norepinephrine in graded doses (1–3 μg/min) before and after intracoronary phenoxybenzamine (0.25 mg/kg) administration. The experiment was terminated at the onset of left ventricular failure, as manifested by a fall in arterial pressure or rise in pulmonary artery wedge pressure.

Coronary resistance was calculated as the quotient of mean coronary pressure distal to the stenosis and coronary flow. Coronary resistance, myocardial oxygen extraction, and myocardial lactate extraction were plotted against myocardial oxygen consumption. Data from each dog were fit with an appropriate equation by means of the least squares method and interpolated values of the dependent variables at uniform values of oxygen consumption were compared using a paired t test.

Transluminal Coronary Angioplasty and
Intracoronary Thrombolysis. Ed. by Kaltenbach et al.

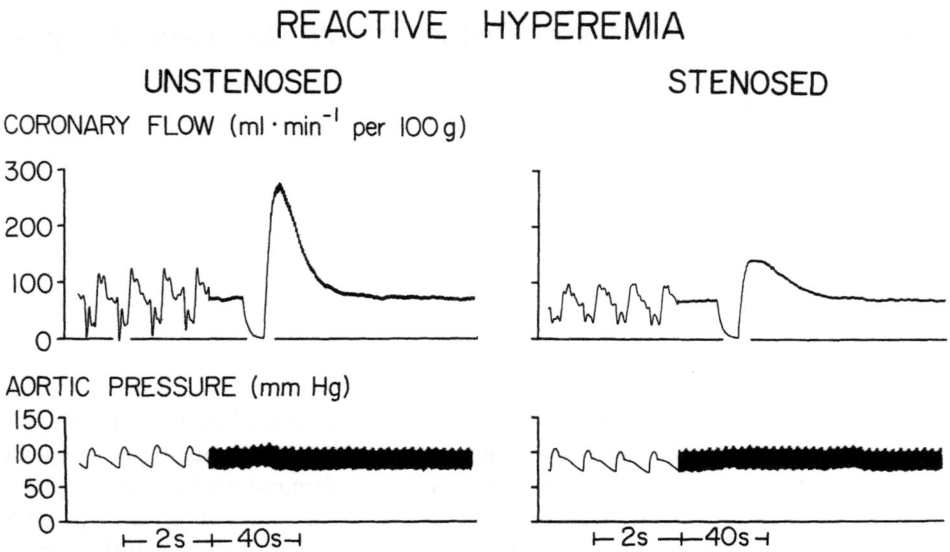

Fig. 1. Reactive hyperemia following complete occlusion for 10 s is blunted by the 70% area reduction stenosis used in these experiments [3]

Results

This experiment was designed to assess the contribution of alpha-mediated coronary vasoconstriction to the relationship between myocardial oxygen delivery and consumption in the presence of an inflow restriction. Coronary resistance was lower at equivalent levels of oxygen consumption following elimination of adrenergic vasoconstriction with phenoxybenzamine (Fig. 2). Measurements of myocardial oxygen extraction indicate that alpha-receptor blockade increased oxygen delivery at any given level of myocardial metabolism (Fig. 3).

It is possible that alpha-mediated vasoconstriction in the presence of a coronary stenosis could impair oxygen delivery sufficiently to cause anaerobic metabolism. However, the data do not support this hypothesis, since myocardial lactate extraction was unchanged by phenoxybenzamine at all levels of sympathetic stimulation studied (Fig. 4).

Discussion

These results indicate that alpha-mediated coronary vasoconstriction exists in the presence of a moderate coronary artery stenosis. The imposition of a stenosis elicits a compensatory vasodilation of the distal coronary bed [6]. A superimposed sympathetic stimulus which activates myocardial beta-receptors results in a further decrease in coronary resistance by a local metabolic mechanism. It is noteworthy that alpha-mediated vasoconstriction can effectively compete with local metabolic vasodilation up to the point of cardiac failure.

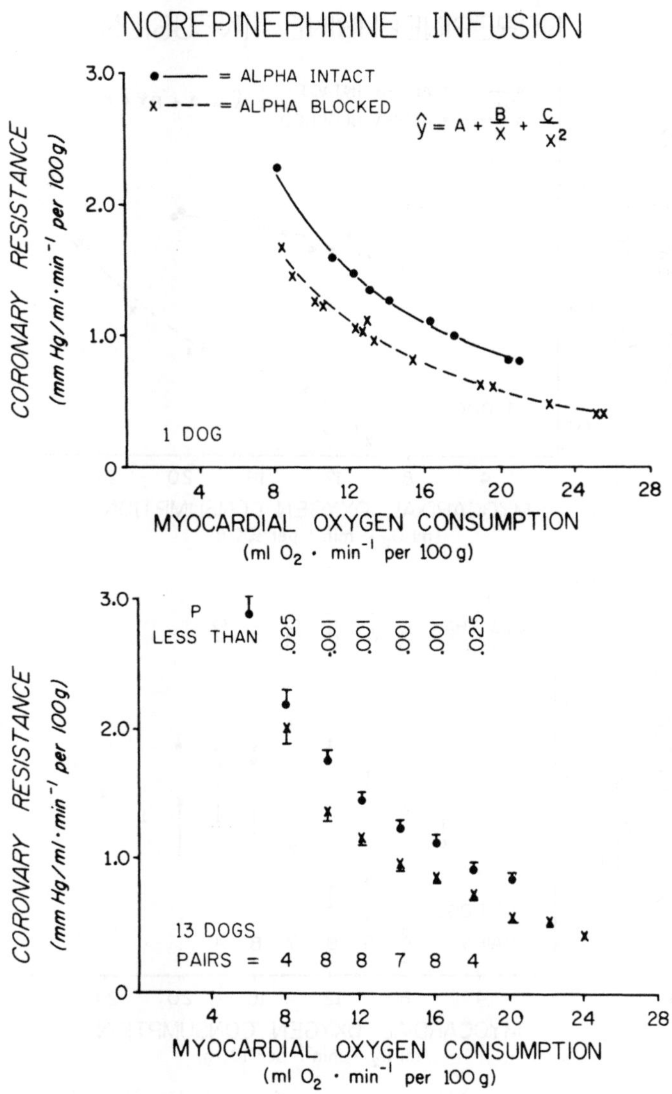

Fig. 2. During norepinephrine infusion, coronary resistance is higher at equivalent levels of myocardial oxygen consumption with vascular alpha-receptors intact than following phenoxybenzamine, indicating sympathetic vasoconstriction. The data from one animal are given in the *upper* panel, and the average data from 13 animals are given in the *lower* panel. The number of paired t comparisons and probability values are given. The *bars* indicate 1 SEM [3]

Given this competition in the presence of a stenosis, it is logical to suppose that a small reduction in oxygen delivery might have dire consequences. This possibility was assessed by measurement of myocardial lactate extraction, a commonly used indicator of anaerobic myocardial metabolism [2]. Although lactate extraction decreased at high levels of sympathetic stimulation, no differences were demonstrated following blockade of alpha-mediated vasoconstriction.

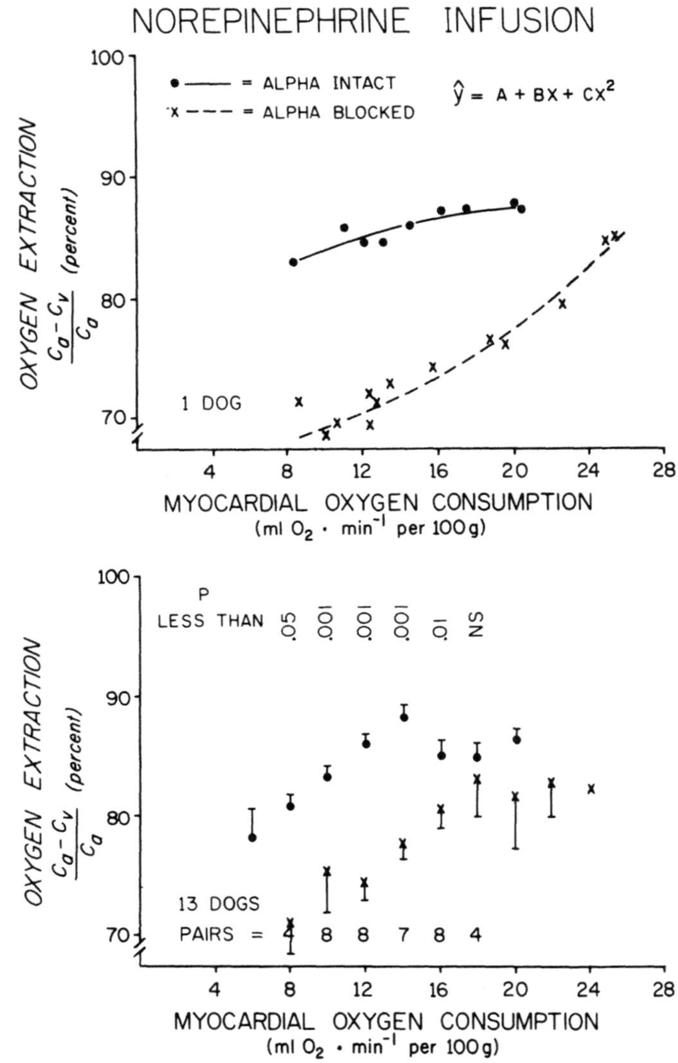

Fig. 3. During norepinephrine infusion, myocardial oxygen extraction is higher at equivalent levels of myocardial oxygen consumption with vascular alpha-receptors intact than following phenoxybenzamine. This indicates a competition between alpha-receptor coronary vasoconstriction and local metabolic vasodilation in the presence of a 70% coronary stenosis. The data from one animal are given in the *upper* panel and the average data from 13 animals are given in the *lower* panel. The number of paired t comparisons and probability values are given. The *bars* indicate 1 SEM [3]

This study does not address the role of alpha-mediated vasoconstriction during frank myocardial ischemia, since the experiments were terminated at the onset of left ventricular failure. The impairment of contractile function and cardiac failure that accompanies severe ischemia [5, 8] precluded steady-state measurements. Use of a regional rather than a global model of myocardial ischemia may have avoided this

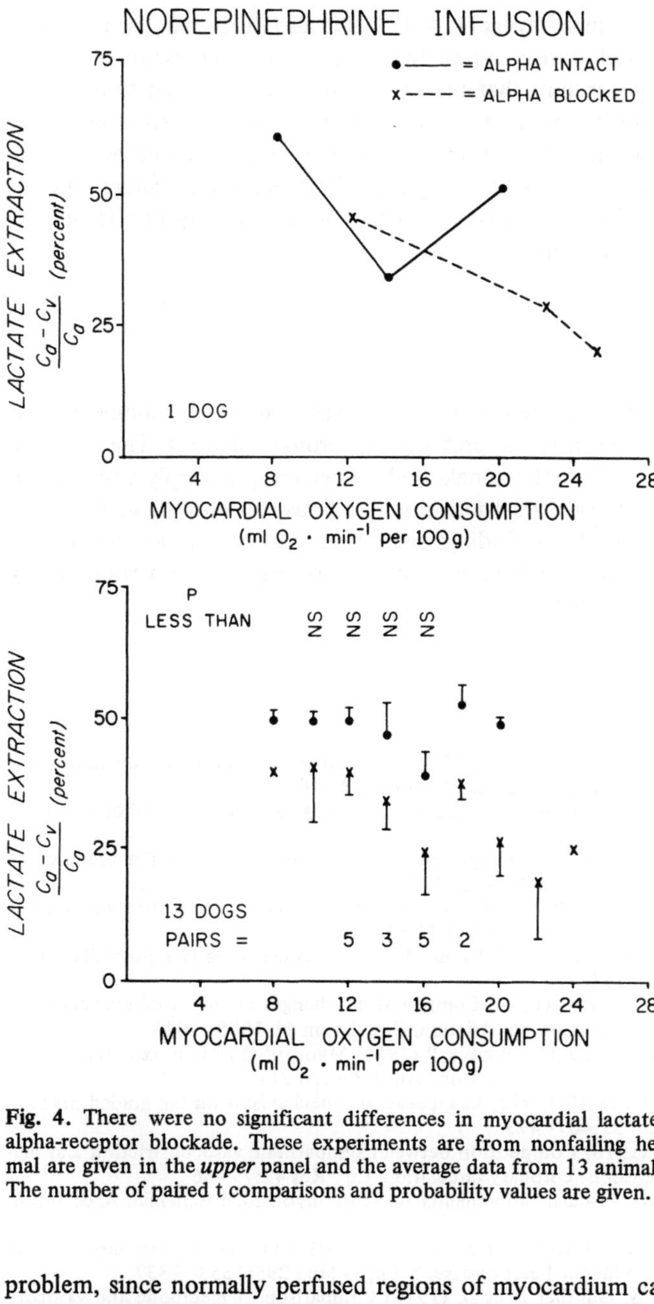

Fig. 4. There were no significant differences in myocardial lactate extraction before and after alpha-receptor blockade. These experiments are from nonfailing hearts. The data from one animal are given in the *upper* panel and the average data from 13 animals are given in the *lower* panel. The number of paired t comparisons and probability values are given. The *bars* indicate 1 SEM [3]

problem, since normally perfused regions of myocardium can compensate for the loss of contractile function in an ischemic region [10]. A regional model, however, would result in inhomogeneous coronary sinus blood oxygen and lactate concentrations and invalidate myocardial oxygen consumption and lactate extraction measurements.

It is possible that most of the vasodilation observed following alpha-receptor blockade occurred in the subepicardial layers of the ventricular wall. This would be particularly likely at higher levels of sympathetic stimulation, since coronary vascular reserve is exhausted first in the inner layers [1, 4, 13]. It is also likely that the reduction in lactate extraction observed during sympathetic stimulation represents a balance between regions of the myocardium that receive adequate oxygen and those where anaerobic metabolism occurred because metabolism exceeded oxygen availability. Griggs et al. [7] have shown that lactate uptake may persist despite net lactate production when coronary flow is lowered to the point of left ventricular failure, indicating that aerobic and anaerobic metabolism can occur simultaneously in different regions of the contracting myocardium.

Summary and Conclusions

This study demonstrates that alpha-mediated coronary vasoconstriction competes with local metabolic vasodilation even in the presence of coronary stenosis. The competition persists up to the point where the imbalance between oxygen supply and demand produces cardiac failure. This vasoconstriction is not powerful enough to cause net myocardial lactate production. These findings support clinical observations in humans with coronary artery disease that an "inappropriate" adrenergic vasoconstriction may play a role in the production of angina.

References

1. Bache RJ, McHale PA, Greenfield JC Jr (1977) Transmural myocardial perfusion during restricted coronary inflow in the awake dog. Am J Physiol 232:H645–H651
2. Brachfeld N (1976) Characterization of the ischemic process by regional metabolism. Am J Cardiol 37:467–473
3. Buffington CW, Feigl EO (1981) Adrenergic coronary vasoconstriction in the presence of coronary stenosis in the dog. Circ Res 48:416–423
4. Buss D, Wüsten B, Schaper W (1978) Effects of coronary stenoses and ventricular loading conditions on coronary flow. Basic Res Cardiol 73:571–583
5. Case RB, Nasser MG, Crampton RS (1969) Biochemical aspects of early myocardial ischemia. Am J Cardiol 24:766–775
6. Gould KL, Lipscomb K, Calvert C (1975) Compensatory changes of the distal coronary vascular bed during progressive coronary constriction. Circulation 51:1085–1094
7. Griggs DM Jr, Nagano S, Lipana JG, Novack P (1966) Myocardial lactate oxidation in situ and the effect thereon of reduced coronary flow. Am J Physiol 211:335–340
8. Lekven J, Miøs OD, Kjekshus JK (1973) Compensatory mechanisms during graded myocardial ischemia. Am J Cardiol 31:467–473
9. Mohrman DE, Feigl EO (1978) Competition between sympathetic vasoconstriction and metabolic vasodilation in the canine coronary circulation. Circ Res 42:79–86
10. Moir TW (1972) Coronary vascular adjustments to acute myocardial ischemia. Arch Intern Med 129:799–807
11. Mudge GH Jr, Grossman W, Mills RM Jr et al. (1976) Reflex increase in coronary vascular resistance in patients with ischemic heart disease. N Engl J Med 295:1333–1337
12. Mudge GH Jr, Goldberg S, Gunther S et al. (1979) Comparison of metabolic and vasoconstrictor stimuli on coronary vascular resistance in man. Circulation 59:544–550
13. Wirth RH, Brückner UB, Keller K et al. (1979) Effects of moderate coronary stenosis on myocardial flow reserve in man and in the dog. Basic Res Cardiol 74:351–360

Variant Angina: The Role of Thromboxane A_2 with Observations on the Importance of Study Design

G.C. Friesinger, R.M.S. Robertson, D. Robertson, G. Fitzgerald, J. Roberts, R. Moss, J. Oates

Divisions of Cardiology and Clinical Pharmacology, Vanderbilt Medical School, Nashville, Tennessee, USA

The principal focus of this symposium is on the relief of acute coronary artery obstruction, but it seems appropriate to be concerned with the mechanisms by which an acute occlusion may occur. Data are extremely fragmentary and incomplete concerning events immediately preceding and responsible for acute myocardial infarction, although the evidence that they result in acute obstruction in a large portion of patients now seems convincing.

The clinical course of many patients with unstable angina and/or variant angina (which we choose to call vasotonic angina) indicate that coronary spasm can result in myocardial infarction [19, 20, 21, 26, 31]. Actual demonstration of such is rare, although it has been unequivocally shown in a few patients. It is conceivable that occlusion is the consequence of intense, prolonged spasm. Hence, the study of coronary artery spasm may be a particularly fruitful area for investigation of the events immediately preceding coronary occlusion and myocardial infarction.

The mechanism(s) underlying coronary spasm is unknown [6, 7, 27, 30, 32, 42] but the suggestion that thromboxane A_2 (Tx A_2) may provoke coronary artery spasm in humans has attracted great interest. Elevated levels of its inactive hydration product thromboxane B_2 (Tx B_2) have been found in the peripheral blood [16] and coronary sinus blood [14] of patients with vasotonic angina. Some patients with vasotonic angina have appeared to benefit from antiplatelet therapy [17]. In addition, circulating platelet aggregates are increased in the peripheral blood of patients with unstable angina and myocardial infarction [36] and in the coronary sinus blood of patients with vasotonic angina during attacks but not between attacks [33].

To test the hypothesis that Tx A_2 is the cause of coronary spasm, we measured arterial and coronary sinus Tx B_2 levels in seven patients during spontaneous episodes of spasm. We then selected a group of patients chronically affected with coronary vasospasm and conducted double-blind cross-over trials of indomethacin and aspirin in this group.

During the course of these and other studied we have performed on vasotonic angina, it has become apparent that the variability and unpredictability of the phenomenon make it particularly complicated to design, carry out, and interpret trials to eva-

* Much of data included in this manuscript was published in the *New England Journal of Medicine*, Vol. 304:17; 998, April 23, 1981

Transluminal Coronary Angioplasty and
Intracoronary Thrombolysis. Ed. by Kaltenbach et al.

luate therapy. This matter is of such importance that a brief resume of our experience in 17 patients in whom we have attempted to evaluate the variability of the course of the syndrome is also included.

Methods and Study Design

Evaluation of the Course of Vasotonic Angina

Patient Selection. To evaluate the variability in the course of vasotonic angina, 17 consecutive patients seen at the Vanderbilt Hospital with the diagnosis of variant angina were studied. Twelve were male and five female; ages ranged from 32 to 82 years (mean 55 years). Diagnostic criteria included angina at rest associated with more than 1 mm of transient ST segment elevation. Fifteen had evidence of recurrent spontaneous or ergonovine-provoked transient coronary occlusion at catheterization and no rise in intra-arterial pressure or heart rate preceding ST segment elevation during hemodynamic monitoring. The other two patients, who did not undergo hemodynamic monitoring, had angiographically normal coronary arteries with the typical clinical and electrocardiographic abnormalities of the rest of the group. Angiographic findings were highly variable but most patients had mild to moderate arteriographically apparent atherosclerosis. Only a single patient with the most severe narrowing (90% in one vessel) had exertional angina as well as the rest angina syndrome.

Study Design. All patients entered into a series of double-blind, random-order, crossover protocols to test the efficacy of a number of therapeutic agents. These began with a 2–4 day placebo run-in period after all drugs had been stopped, and then drug periods of 3–5 days were alternated with further placebo periods. All periods were determined by one of us not involved with the direct care of the patient and were of sufficient length to allow a full 2–4 day placebo period more than five half-lives removed from the active drug. For drugs with a long physiologic effect, such as aspirin, the placebo period lies beyond the known duration of effect. Sublingual nitroglycerin was constantly available for use with chest pain, but no nitrates were taken prophylactically.

Throughout these trials continuous electrocardiographic recording was performed, using an ICR 2-channel recorder with leads chosen to best demonstrate the episodes of ST elevation. All recordings were calibrated, and multiple patient positions were recorded to ensure that ST changes seen could not be accounted for by changes in position. In addition, patients kept daily diaries noting all episodes of chest pain, their length and severity as well as the number of nitroglycerin required for relief. We tabulated the frequency of all episodes of ST elevation which lasted 1 min or more and were 1 mm or more over baseline. We then analyzed the number of ischemia episodes for each 24-h period. For the initial placebo run-in period, we examined the number of episodes daily; to compare the initial period with later placebo periods, we used the average number of episodes daily for each period.

Patients were allowed to be ambulatory in the Clinical Research Center or the Coronary Care Stepdown Unit if their ischemic episodes were not associated with significant alterations in hemodynamics due either to arrhythmias or to the mass of muscle ischemia. Patients were telemetered for greater safety. Patients with serious hemodynamic consequences of their ischemia were studied in the Coronary Care Unit.

Evaluation of the Role of Thromboxane A_2 and Antiplatelet Agents

Patient Selection. Some of the patients in the above study were also included in these additional studies. Seven patients (four men and three women) with spontaneous episodes of angina at rest were chosen because their ischemic episodes were sufficiently frequent to allow study of spontaneous ischemia rather than provoked ischemia. These patients will be designated group 1. Three patients were subsequently restudied when the disease had become inactive. In five of the seven patients, only mild lesions (less than 30% diameter narrowing) were present on arteriography. None of the patients had exertional angina. One patient progressed to infarction within 1 day of hospitalization.

Nine patients (four men and five women) experienced episodes of vasotonic angina pectoris over long periods of time, at least 2 months of disease activity, and constituted a group in whom antiplatelet agents could be tried during control and constituted a group in whom antiplatelet agents could be tried during control and treatment periods. All patients had multiple daily episodes of angina at rest accompanied by ST segment elevation. These patients will be designated group 2.

Eleven healthy volunteers (eight men and three women) who had abstained from all medications, including aspirin, for 7 days before evaluation served to provide control data for the thromboxane assays.

Study Design. We collected urine from the 11 normal control patients for estimation of 2,3-dinor Tx B_2, the principal urinary metabolite of Tx A_2 in human beings [29]. A 15-ml sample of peripheral venous blood was also drawn from these subjects for measurement of Tx B_2.

For direçt measurement of thromboxane metabolites in vasotonic angina, five patients in group 1 had a 7F Wilton-Webster catheter placed in the coronary sinus under fluoroscopic visualization after coronary arteriography. The position of the catheter's sampling orifice was determined by gentle hand injection of contrast material and by measurements of oxygen saturation. A 20 gauge Teflon needle was placed in the radial artery, and the coronary sinus and arterial lines were both flushed with a Sorensen continuous-flush device with 2500 units heparin in 500 ml 5% dextrose in water at a rate of 3 ml/h, with additional brief hand flushes every 15 min. The patient who had a myocardial infarction on the day following hospitalization did not undergo these procedures.

We observed the electrocardiogram at the bedside and withdrew blood samples at a baseline (ischemic time), which was always at least 20 min from the most recent ischemic episode. We then resampled during ST segment elevation, usually within the first 30 s of an ischemic episode. During prolonged episodes several samples could be drawn. Additional samples were collected after the ST segment elevation had resolved and at various intervals thereafter. Samples were drawn during a total of eight ischemic episodes in five patients. More than one sample was drawn during six of these episodes. One sample was drawn during the minute before ST segment elevation when a sample planned for a baseline determination was rapidly followed by an ischemic episode.

One patient had taken aspirin 5 days before the sampling. This patient had a 24-h urine sample collected and analyzed for 2,3-dinor Tx B_2 2 days after sampling, with no interim change in his condition. The patient who had a myocardial infarction had no plasma samples drawn but did have a 24-h urine specimen collected and analyzed in the same manner during the day on which she had vasotonic angina and infarction.

We also evaluated the effect of antiplatelet agents in group 2 who had relatively stable chronic complaints.

All trials were performed in a random-order, double-blind, placebo-controlled fashion. Patients were allowed to remain ambulatory if their episodes of pain were not frequent, severe, or associated with serious ventricular arrhythmias. All patients had free access to sublingual nitroglycerin (0.4 mg) for anginal episodes but did not take it prophylactically. Patients with very painful episodes or arrhythmias associated with ischemia received intermittent intravenous nitroglycerin in bolus doses of 0.4 mg for these episodes. Intermittent doses of sublingual or intravenous nitroglycerin were also given for any episode of ischemia noted by nursing personnel, whether it was painful or not (three patients sensed only 10%–20% of their ischemic episodes).

Electrocardiographic monitoring was performed as described in the study of the patients who were evaluated for the natural course of vasotonic angina. There was wide variability between patients in the frequency of ischemic episodes during the trials, from 1 to 42 episodes/day (mean 18 episodes/day).

Indomethacin was given in oral doses of 50 mg every 8 h for 3–4 days. Platelet aggregation was studied on the 1st day of placebo therapy and on the 1st day of indomethacin therapy to ensure inhibition of prostaglandin synthetase. For these studies, 18 ml blood was drawn without a tourniquet through a 23 gauge siliconized needle into a plastic syringe containing 2 ml 3.2% aqueous sodium citrate. Platelet-rich plasma was prepared by centrifugation at 140 *g* for 15 min at room temperature. The platelet count determined by phase microscopy was 250 000–320 000/ml and was standardized to 300 000/ml. Platelet aggregation studies were performed in a Payton dual-channel aggregation module (Payton Associates, Buffalo, N.Y.) with 250 μl platelet-rich plasma as previously described [25]. The effects of two to four concentrations each of adenosine diphosphate, epinephrine, and sodium arachidonate were tested, always in the same sequence. Inhibition of the second wave of platelet aggregation was evident in all three patients while they were taking indomethacin but in none during placebo administration.

Aspirin was given in doses of 150 mg on day 1 and 300 mg on days 2 and 3. Twenty-four hour collections of urine for measurements of 2,3 dinor Tx B_2 were analyzed in three patients during this trial and in one patient 5 days after a single dose of 150 mg of aspirin as well.

Biochemical Analyses. The assay of urinary 2,3-dinor Tx B_2 was accomplished with stable-isotope dilution and combined gas chromatography-mass spectrometry with a chemically synthesized internal standard carrying three deuterium atoms on the ω-carbon [39]. We added 345 ng tri-deutero internal standard (tritium-labeled at 220 000 disintegrations/min) to 10% aliquots of 24-h urine samples and refrigerated them: the samples were desalted on Amberlite XAD-2 [12], extracted with ethyl acetate, chromatographed on an open silicic acid column in ethyl acetate, filtered, and subjected to further purification by both reverse and straight-phase high-pressure liquid chromatography with solvent systems previously described [41]. After derivatization as the methyl ester, *tert*-butyldimethylsilylether, with excess ethereal diazomethane and *tert*-butyldimethyl-chlorsilane imidazole, the samples were applied to silica gel thin-layer, chromatographic plates (4 by 15 cm) and developed in heptane, combined with ethyl acetate (9:1, vol/vol; rate of flow, 0.4), eluted, and concentrated. The gas chromatographic-mass spectrometric analysis was performed on a standard 3% OV-1 column isothermally at 270 °C with monitoring of the (M-57) positive ions at m/c 641 (nondeuterated) and 644 (deuterated) by a Hewlett-Packard 5980A mass spectrometer. Urinary levels were determined by reference to a standard curve and normalized to creatinine levels [37]. The accuracy and precision of the assay are of the order of ± 15%. Normal levels range from 143 to 295 pg/mg creatinine (mean ± SD 206 ± 58). Plasma samples were analyzed for Tx B_2 in a similar fashion with a tri-deutero Tx B_2 standard with selected ion monitoring at m/c 669 (nondeuterated) and 673 (deuterated).

In determining Tx B_2 in plasma, we first addressed the problem of the appropriate anticoagulant. In the normal controls, venous plasma samples were divided among three tubes. Tube contained an anticoagulant mixture (sodium citrate $2H_2O$, 43 mg; soybean trypsin inhibitor, 0.5 mg; ϵ-aminocaproic acid, 131.2 μg; heparin, 500 units; and indomethacin, 1 mg/ml). Tube B contained the same anticoagulant mixture without heparin, and tube C contained EDTA alone. On four further occasions, samples were divided only between tubes B and C.

Samples drawn into EDTA tubes had consistently higher levels than the same samples drawn into tubes A or B; there was no significant difference between samples in anticoagulants A and B. No peripheral venous sample from a normal subject in these anticoagulants had a level above 399 pg/ml, and 89% of the levels were below 200 pg/ml. Samples from patients in group 1 were all drawn into the original anticoagulant mixture containing heparin.

All plasma samples were immediately placed on ice and then centrifuged at 0 °C and 1000 *g* for 10 min, and the supernatant was analyzed for Tx B_2. Levels of Tx B_2 were determined by radioimmunoassay except in the coronary sinus and arterial samples designated in Table 1, which were analyzed by stable-isotope dilution assay. Radioimmunoassays of Tx B_2 were performed with a highly specific anti-Tx B_2 antibody obtained from Dr. F. Fitzpatrick of the Upjohn Company [8] and a procedure previously described by Boeynaems et al. [3]. The coefficient of variation of this assay is less than 6%.

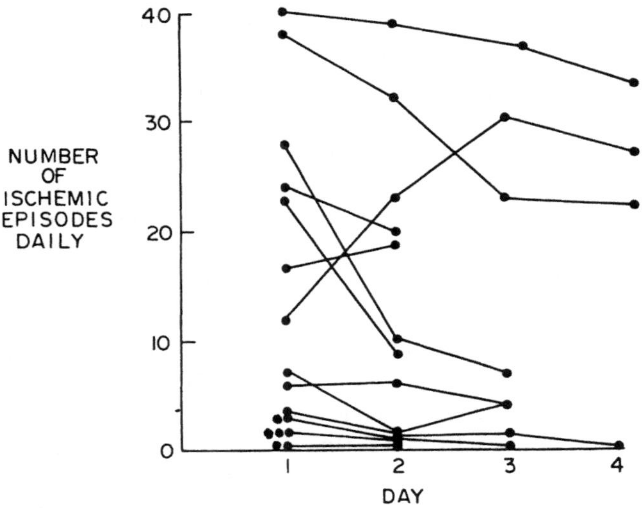

Fig. 1. The number of ischemic episodes during the first placebo period

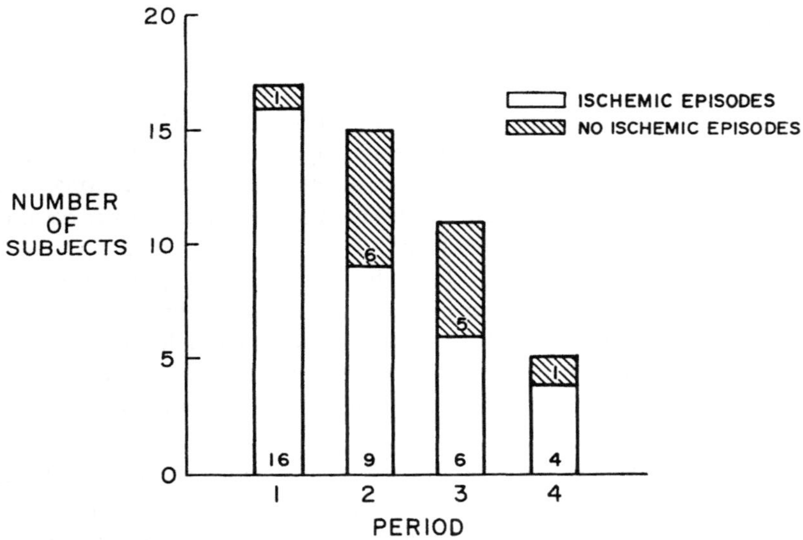

Fig. 2. Ischemic episodes in the four placebo periods

Results

Studies on the Course of Vasotonic Angina

Figure 1 illustrates the number of ischemic episodes during the first placebo period. Over the 4-day period, only two patients showed an increase in episodes. Two patients had no episodes on the 1st day. For the 15 patients with episodes on the 1st day, nine had a decrease to less than 40% of the frequency of episodes by the 2nd day.

Figure 2 compares the four placebo periods, which were obtained over about a 30-day span, the placebo periods being interspersed with drug trial periods. The steady diminution in patients remaining in each placebo period represents the removal of patients from further study when the patient experienced totally asymptomatic placebo period. By the fourth placebo period, only four of the original 17 patients had continuing ischemic episodes.

Direct Measurements of Thromboxane Metabolites

Peripheral venous samples drawn during a quiescent phase of the disease in three patients in group 1 all had metabolite levels below 200 pg/ml. Although two of these patients had elevated levels of 2,3 dinor Tx B_2 in 24-h urine collections (547 and 460 pg/mg creatinine) during the active phase of the diasease, the patients who had taken aspirin 7 days before had a normal 24-h urinary level of 2,3-dinor Tx B_2 (198 pg/mg creatinine) despite frequent and severe vasotonic angina. Elevated urinary levels of 2,3-dinor Tx B_2 (647 pg/mg creatinine) were also found in the patient with myocardial infarction during the 24 h of collection.

Coronary sinus and arterial levels of Tx B_2 drawn in group 1 patients are presented in Table 1. Patients 1–4 had mild atherosclerosis only; the involved artery was the right artery in patient 1, the anterior descending artery in patients 2 and 3, and the circumflex marginal artery in patient 4. Patient 5 had a severe fixed narrowing in the anterior descending artery. In patients 1–4, all but one baseline value in coronary sinus blood and all arterial baseline levels were within the range of the peripheral venous levels obtained in group 1. Arterial concentration were generally unaltered by ischemia, although one of the four patients had a delayed rise in plasma Tx B_2. Coronary sinus values increased with ischemia, but early samples did not show a change from the baseline in the patients with mild disease. In fact, the level in the sample fortuitously drawn within the minute before an ischemic episode in patient 3 was also within the normal range. Samples drawn later in the course of an episode often rose tenfold, but the highest levels were observed in the first several minutes after the onset of ischemia.

Patient 5, with severe atherosclerosis localized in the left anterior descending artery, had continuously elevated Tx B_2 levels in both coronary sinus and arterial blood. She had no consistent rise in arterial levels, but her coronary sinus levels rose with ischemia. Unlike those of the other patients, however, samples taken before ischemia already had elevated levels of Tx B_2. Coronary sinus levels measured in patient 4, with the lesion in the circumflex marginal artery, were normal throughout the sampling period.

Inhibitor Trials of Antiplatelet Drugs

These trials were done in the patients who constituted group 2. Three patients received indomethacin. Despite inhibition of platelet aggregation in vitro, there was no change in the frequency of chest pain or in its severity in these three patients. Nitroclycerin consumption did not differ from that in the placebo period. In addition, review of the

Table 1. Coronary sinus and arterial levels of thromboxane B_2 in vasotonic angina

Thromboxane B_2 levels (pg/ml)								
Patient	Baseline	Before ischemia	During ST segment elevation			After ischemia		
			First 30 s	1–2 min	3–4 min	1 min	2 min	8 min
Coronary sinus								
1[a]	< 50	–	–	< 50				
	< 50	–	–	66	160	–	–	
2	65	–	52	720	–	–	–	
	328			850				
3	<200	<200	200	500	1500, 2000	1500	2500	600
4	<200	–	–	260	200	200	–	
5	400	-	780		520	620	–	
	600		1380	740		1500		
Arterial								
1	<200	–	<200	<200	<200	–	–	
2	< 50	–	54	< 50	698	–	–	
				< 50				
3	–	–	–	–		–	–	
4	<200	–	–	<200	<200	<200	–	
5	820	–	580	–	740	900	–	
			940			2080		

A dash indicates that no sample was drawn during this time period in this patient. Coronary sinus samples for patients 1 and 2, and arterial samples from patient 2 were analyzed by GC-MS stable-isotope dilution assay; all other samples were analyzed by radioimmunoassay. When there is more than one line for a patient, each line represents a separate episode. The corresponding lines for each patient under the coronary sinus and arterial headings represent samples drawn from the same episodes.

[a] Patient 1 had taken aspirin 5 days prior to sampling.

continuously recorded electrocardiogram showed no change in the magnitude of ST segment elevation, the duration of the elvation, or the incidence of associated arrhythmias. The frequency of episodes was also unaltered (Table 2).

Six patients received aspirin. Urinary 2,3-dinor Tx B_2 levels were reduced by more than 75% after 150 mg aspirin and then to normal (less than 295 pg/mg creatinine) after 300 mg aspirin in the three patients in whom they were measured. In two patients, repeat 24-h urine samples 5 and 7 days after cessation of aspirin continued to show suppression of thromboxane production (Table 3).

Despite this effect, there was no decrease in the frequency of severity of chest pain with aspirin was compared with placebo, and the use of nitroglycerin was not changed. As in the patients given indomethacin, there was no decrease in episodes of ischemia (as documented by electrocardiogram) in terms of frequency, duration, or magnitude (Table 4). Placebo periods after aspirin therapy were also analyzed, but there was no significant decrease in the number of ischemic episodes during these periods.

Table 2. Total episodes of ischemia during the indomethacin trial

Patient	Episodes of ischemia									
	Placebo					Indomethacin				
	Day				Total	Day				Total
	1	2	3	4		1	2	3	4	
1[a]	42	40	32	–	114	30	12	26	–	68
2	12	2	2	15	31	11	12	13	8	44
3	13	9	16	6	44	7	7	11	16	41

Numbers represent episodes of ST elevation more than 1 mm over baseline.
[a] Patient 1 had 3-day trials rather than 4-day trials.

Table 3. Twenty-four hour urinary 2,3-dinor thromboxane B_2 production during aspirin trial

Patient	Thromboxane B_2 production (pg/mg creatinine)		
	Placebo	Aspirin	After aspirin
1	547	68	
2	460	69	66 (5 days after)
3	930	140	188 (7 days after)

Table 4. Total episodes of ischemia during the aspirin trial

Patient	Placebo Day		Aspirin		
	1	2	150 mg	300 mg	300 mg
1	5	8	8	6	5
2	13	9	24	15	16
3	24	21	20	16	14
4	5	5	5	5	6
5	4	3	0	2	–
6	0	0	0	1	0

Numbers represent episodes of ST elevation more than 1 mm over baseline. Patient 5 did not receive a second 300 mg dose. One-way analysis of variance shows that the frequency of episodes is not significantly different during aspirin therapy than during placebo ($F_{4,24} = 0.059; P > 0.25$).

Discussion

Evidence that the platelet may have a role in ischemic syndromes comes from a number of sources. In a canine model with an externally applied coronary constrictor to produce severe narrowing, spontaneous cyclic decreases in coronary flow have been observed [10, 40]. These alterations in flow are prevented by aspirin [10] or by prostacyclin [1], a potent vasodilator and antiaggregatory agent; platelet aggregates can be recovered from the area of constriction at the time of flow reduction [9]. These aggregates may either physically obstruct flow or release enough Tx A_2 to cause occlusion by vasospasm.

In human beings, an atherosclerotic coronary circulation could provide a favorable site for platelet aggregation. The production of prostacyclin by the vessel wall may well be attenuated by the presence of lipid peroxides in the atherosclerotic plaque, leaving the effect of Tx A_2 relatively unopposed [38]. Mehta and Metha [23] have found that generation of malondialdehyde, an indirect index of platelet prostaglandin production, is elevated in patients with classical exertional angina. In other studies, they demonstrated a decrease in platelet aggregation and platelet counts across the coronary bed in patients with atherosclerosis [24] and postulated that platelets are "activated" and perhaps deposited as they pass through atherosclerotic vessels. Several of our patients also had elevated circulating platelet aggregates in the coronary sinus during ischemic episodes [33], although sequential samples throughout the course of ischemic episodes were not drawn for those determinations.

Although local thromboxane release in the coronary artery itself is widely held to be the cause of coronary spasm, our data do not show a rise in Tx B_2 coincident with the onset of ischemia. Since the half-life of Tx A_2 in serum is approximately 30 s [13], measurements of Tx B_2 in the coronary sinus – only a few seconds downstream in circulation time – should provide a sensitive index of levels in the coronary artery in the absence of alterations in metabolism. Of course, if coronary occlusion is rapid and complete it could prevent any thromboxane released from reaching the coronary sinus. The sample drawn fortuitously in the minute before ST elevation is of particular importance in this regard. At this time, just before coronary occlusion, the Tx B_2 level was not elevated. In addition, levels of Tx B_2 often remain elevated (in the range of 500–1000 pg/ml) for 6–10 min after ST elevation resolves before returning to baseline values. If an elevation in Tx A_2 alone were sufficient to cause coronary spasm, spasm should persist at this time.

The marked elevation in Tx B_2 levels occurring later in ischemia could be secondary to the ischemia itself or to turbulent flow in a transiently occluded artery. Although in our sampling system there is no way to prevent some Tx A_2 from being generated by aggregating platelets during passage through the sampling catheters, this generation should be constant, since Tx B_2 levels return to the baseline between ischemic episodes. Several groups [14, 18] have found that coronary sinus Tx B_2 levels increase with pacing-induced ischemia in patients with classical angina but not vasotonic angina. This finding suggests that ischemia itself may produce an invironment in which Tx A_2 is released, and supports the hypothesis that this release may be a secondary phenomenon. Once Tx A_2 is released, of course, its effects of the coronary vasculature may lead to further vasoconstriction.

Only one other group has measured coronary sinus levels of Tx B_2 with spontaneous episodes of vasotonic angina [14], and their results differed from ours. In samples drawn within the first 30 s after ST segment elevation, these authors found that Tx B_2 levels were already elevated. However, simultaneously measured coronary sinus flow was also elevated at that time – a finding that is difficult to explain. A reduction in flow, as demonstrated by Chierchia et al. [4], would be expected in most patients, although the region of coronary sinus flow measured could be important. We did not perform simultaneous coronary sinus flow measurements in our patients. It is also possible that Tx A_2 levels were in fact elevated at a time when levels of its hydration product, Tx B_2, did not reflect that elevation. Because of these discrepancies, the precise role of Tx A_2 in vasotonic angina may be further clarified through therapeutic trials of thromboxane synthesis inhibitors. Specific inhibitors are not available for clinical use, although a newly synthesized thromboxane analogue, pinane Tx A_2, is under investigation in animal models of ischemia [35].

Cyclic illnesses present special problems in study design. Our experience [31] and that of others [19] suggests that cycles of disease activity are the rule in vasotonic angina. Data collected with placebo before and after the trials of active drugs helped to confirm that any observed changes in disease activity were related to drugs rather than to the cycle. For example, the data on indomethacin in patient 1 (Table 2) appear to suggest a partial benefit from the active drug. However, in this case randomization had led to initial administration of placebo; continued Holter monitoring in the period after the indomethacin trial showed a continuing decrease in disease activity. Within 2 weeks of the indomethacin trial in patient 1, subjective and electrocardiographic evidence of ischemia ceased for several months. The data from our group of 17 patients make it obvious that drug studies are particularly difficult to design and interpret in the syndrome of vasospastic angina.

In this study, indomethacin did not benefit a group of patients with well-characterized vasotonic angina. Similar negative results were seen with aspirin at a dose that reduced urinary 2,3-dinor Tx B_2 excretion by at least 85%. We interpret this result to mean that platelet Tx A_2 alone provides an insufficient explanation for coronary artery spasm in these patients. Recent data from Chierchia et al. [5] support this hypothesis. These researchers gave patients with coronary artery spasm enough aspirin to prevent the generation of Tx B_2 in whole blood in vitro. Despite this inhibition of production of Tx B_2 (and by inference Tx A_2) the episodes of spasm were not prevented. Since the inhibition of prostacyclin should reverse before that of thromboxane [22, 28], our observation that there is no benefit in the period after aspirin therapy is also important. Although nitroglycerin may also affect prostaglandin metabolism by inhibiting arachidonic acid oxygenation in platelets [34] and enhancing prostacyclin production by the vascular endothelium [15], its use did not vary from the placebo period to the drug period and could not account for the lack of therapeutic effect.

Cautious interpretation of these results is necessary. Since vasotonic angina represents an extreme end of the spectrum of coronary artery spasm, these data cannot be extrapolated to unstable angina or myocardial infarction. In addition, our results do not prove that aspirin and indomethacin are without effect on the ultimate prognosis, even in vasotonic angina. Because our studies were conducted over a short term, potential benefit in preventing myocardial infarction or arrhythmias could not be assessed. Finally, the recent demonstrations that Tx A_2 can be found in vessel walls [2] and can be generated be leukocytes [11] as well as by platelets raise the possibility that vascular or leukocytic Tx A_2, though limited in quantity, may nevertheless be functionally important. Despite the marked reduction in total production of Tx B_2 achieved in the aspirin and indomethacin trials described it is possible, though unlikely, that a critical quantity of intracoronary Tx A_2, escaped inhibition.

Although these data do not eliminate Tx A_2 as a causative factor in vasotonic angina, they strongly suggest that the key to the enigma of coronary vasospasm may lie elsewhere.

References

1. Aiken JW, Gorman RR, Shebuski RJ (1979) Prevention of blockage of partially obstructed coronary arteries with prostacyclin correlated with inhibition of platelet aggregation. Prostaglandins 17:483–494
2. Ally AI, Horrobin DF (1980) Thromboxane A_2 in blood vessel walls and its physiological significance: relevance to thrombosis and hypertension. Prostaglandins Med 4:431–438
3. Boeynaems JM, Waelbroeck M, Dumont JE (1979) Cholinergic and β-adrenergic stimulation of prostaglandin release by dog thyroid *in vitro*. Endocrinology 105:988–995
4. Chierchia S, Brunnelli C, Simonetti I, Lazzari M, Maseri A (1980a) Sequence of events in angina at rest: primary reduction in coronary flow. Circulation 61:759–768
5. Chierchia S, Decaterina R, Brunelli S, Crea F, Patrono C, Maseri A (1980b) Lose-dose aspirin prevents thromboxane A_2 synthesis by platelets but not attacks of Prinzmetal angina. Circulation 62 [Suppl]:III–215
6. Dagenais G, Gundel W, Conti C (1979) Peripheral venospasm associated with signs of transient myocardial ischemia. Am Heart J 80:544–546
7. Endo M, Hirosawa K, Kameko N, Hase K, Inoue Y, Konna S (1976) Prinzmetal's variant angina: coronary arteriogram and left ventriculogram during angina induced by methacholine. N Engl J Med 294:252–255
8. Fitzpatrick F, Gorman R, McGuire J, Kelly R, Wynalda M, Sun F (1977) Radioimmunoassay for thromboxane B_2. Anal Biochem 82:1–7
9. Folts JD, Rowe GC (1980) Cyclical blood flow reductions in stenosed arteries: vasospasm or platelet aggregates? Clin Res 28:170A
10. Folts JD, Crowell EB, Rowe GG (1976) Platelet aggregation in partially obstructed vessels and its elimination with aspirin. Circulation 54:365–370
11. Goldstein IM, Malmsten CL, Kindahl H et al. (1978) Thromboxane generation by human peripheral blood polymorphonuclear leukocytes. J Exp Med 148:787–792
12. Hamberg M, Samuelsson B (1971) On the metabolism of prostaglandins E_1 and E_2 in man. J Biol Chem 246:6713–6721
13. Hamberg M, Svensson J, Samuelsson B (1975) Thromboxanes: A new group of biologically active compounds derived from prostaglandin endoperoxides. Proc Natl Acad Sci USA 72: 2994–2998
14. Kuzuya T, Tada M, Inoue M et al. (1980) Increased levels of thromboxane A_2 in peripheral and coronary circulation in patients with angina pectoris. Am J Cardiol 45:454
15. Levin RI, Weksler BB, Jaffe EA (1980) Nitroglycerin induces production of prostacyclin by human endothelial cells. Clin Res 28:471A
16. Lewy RI, Wiener L, Smith JB, Walinsky P, Silver MJ, Saia J (1979a) Comparison of plasma concentrations of thromboxane B_2 in Prinzmetal's variant angina and classical angina pectoris. Clin Cardiol 2:404–406
17. Lewy RI, Smith JB, Silver MJ, Saia J, Walinsky P, Wiener L (1979b) Detection of thromboxane B_2 (TB_2) in peripheral blood of patients with Prinzmetal's angina. Clin Res 27:462A
18. Lewi RI, Wiener L, Walinsky P, Lefer AM, Silver MJ, Smith JB (1980) Thromboxane release during pacing-induced angina pectoris: Possible vasoconstrictor influence on the coronary vasculature. Circulation 61:1165–1171
19. MacAlpin RN, Kattus AA, Alvaro AB (1973) Angina pectoris at rest with preservation of exercise capacity: Prinzmetal's variant angina. Circulation 47:946–958

20. Maseri A, Severi S, DeNes M et al. (1978a) 'Variant' angina: one aspect of a continuous spectrum of vasospastic myocardial ischemia. Am J Cardiol 42:1019–1035
21. Maseri A, L'Abbate A, Baroldi G et al. (1978b) Coronary vasospasm as a possible cause of myocardial infarction: a conclusion derived from the study of 'preinfarction' angina. N Engl J Med 299:1271–1277
22. Masotti G, Poggesi L, Galanti G, Abbate R, Neri S, Severi GG (1979) Differential inhibition of prostacyclin production and platelet aggregation by aspirin. Lancet 2:1213–1216
23. Mehta J, Mehta P (1980) Increased platelet prostaglandin generation and abnormal platelet sensitivity to prostacyclin and thromboxane A_2 in angina pectoris. Am J Cardiol 45:454
24. Nehta J, Mehta P, Pepine C, Conti CR (1980) Platelet function studies in coronary artery disease. VII, Effect of aspirin and tachycardia stress on aortic and coronary venous blood. Am J Cardiol 45:945–951
25. Oelz O, Seyberth HW, Knapp HR, Sweetman BJ, Oates JA (1976) Effects of feeding ethyl-dihomogramma-lenolenate on prostaglandin biosynthesis and platelet aggregation in the rabbit. Biochem Biophys Acta 431:268–277
26. Oliva PV, Potts DE, Pluss RG (1973) Coronary arterial spasm in Prinzmetal angina; documentation by coronary arteriography. N Engl J Med 288:745–751
27. Osler W (1893) The principles and practice of medicine, 1st edn Appleton, New York
28. Preston F, Whipps S, Jackson CK, French AJ, Wyld PJ, Stoddard J (1981) Inhibition of prostacyclin and platelet thromboxane after low-dose aspirin. N Engl J Med 304:76–79
29. Roberts LJ II, Sweetman BJ, Payne NA, Oates JA (1977) Metabolism of thromboxane B_2 in man. J Biol Chem 252:7414–7417
30. Robertson D, Oates JA (1978) Variant angina and Raynaud's phenomenon. Lancet 1:452
31. Robertson RM, Breinig JB, Robertson D (1979a) Chronic recurrent variant angina. Southern Med 72:1297–1303
32. Robertson D, Robertson RM, Nies AS, Oates JA, Friesinger GC (1979b) Variant angina pectoris: investigation of indexes of sympathetic nervous system function. Am J Cardiol 43: 1080–1085
33. Robertson RM, Robertson D, Friesinger GC, Timmons S, Hawiger J (1980) Platelet aggregates in peripheral and coronary sinus blood in patients with spontaneous coronary astery spasm. Lancet 2:829–831
34. Schafer AI, Alexander RW, Handin RI (1980) Inhibition of platelet function by organic nitrate vasodilators. Blood 55:649–654
35. Schror K, Smith EF, Bickerton M et al. (1980) Preservation of ischemic myocardium by pinane thromboxane A_2. Am J Physiol 238:H87–92
36. Schwartz MB, Hawiger J, Timmons S, Friesinger GC (1980) Platelet aggregation in ischemic heart disease. Thromb Haemost 43:185–188
37. Seyberth MW, Sweetman BJ, Frolich JC, Oates JA (1976) Quantification of the major urinary metabolite of the E prostaglandins by mass-spectrometry. Evaluation of the methods application to clinical studies. Prostaglandins 11:381–397
38. Sinzinger H, Feigl W, Silberbauer K (1979) Prostacyclin generation in atherosclerotic arteries. Lancet 2:469
39. Taber DF, Lee CH (1978) The preparation of Dimethyl (7–$^2H_3$ 2-oxoheptyl) phosphonate. J Labelled Comp & Radiopharm 14:599–602
40. Uchida Y, Yoshimoto N, Murao S (1978) Effects of anti-anginal agents on cyclical reductions of coronary blood flow. Jpn Heart J 19:904–912
41. Whorton AR, Carr K, Smigel M, Walter L, Ellis K, Oates JA (1979) Reversed phase high performance liquid chromatography of prostaglandins – biological applications. J Chromatogr 163:64–71
42. Yasue H, Touyama M, Kato H, Tanaka S, Akiyama F (1976) Prinzmetal's variant form of angina as a manifestation of alpha-adrenergic receptor-mediated coronary artery spasm: documentation by coronary arteriography. Am Heart J 90:148–155

Prostaglandin Derivatives and Platelet-specific Proteins During Transluminal Coronary Angioplasty

K. Silberbauer, H. Sinzinger, G. Kober

2nd Dept. of Internal Medicine, University of Vienna, Austria
and Dept. of Cardiology, University of Frankfurt a.M., FRG

Introduction

There is much speculation about the role of prostaglandins and thromboxanes in ischemic heart disease. These endogenous compounds are potent modulators of vascular smooth muscle tone and platelet aggregability. During platelet activation platelets generate a potent vasoconstrictor, thromboxane A_2 (TXA_2), whereas prostaglandin I_2 (PGI_2), produced by the vessel wall, is a potent vasodilator and inhibits platelet aggregation [5]. Both PGI_2 and TXA_2 are unstable and spontaneously convert to the inactive metabolites 6-Oxo-prostaglandin F_1 α (6-Oxo-PGF_1 α) and thromboxane B_2 (TXB_2), respectively [2, 7]. In addition, the measurement of plasma concentrations of β-thromboglobulin (βTG), a specific protein, which is extruded from well-defined platelet granules into the surrounding medium, might reflect in vivo platelet activation [4].

Therefore, we assessed whether transluminal coronary angioplasty (TCA) might influence platelet count (PL) and plasma concentrations of TXB_2, 6-Oxo-PGF_1 α, and βTG in coronary sinus blood.

Patients and Methods

In five patients (two females, three males, age 39–60 years) with severe LAD stenosis ($>$ 75% narrowing) blood was drawn simultaneously from the coronary sinus and from the aorta immediately before and 5 min after TCA. Coronary sinus blood was also sampled 15 s after intracoronary balloon deflation. Before the insertion of the catheter (Sones technique), the patients received 10000 IU heparin (Heparin Novo) in the brachial artery. Blood was sampled about 40 min after heparin application. Platelet count was performed by phase contrast microscopy. The blood samples for prostaglandin analysis were drawn into plastic syringes and transferred quickly into iced 10-ml tubes containing EDTA (2%) and aspirin (0.5 mg/ml). They were immediately centrifuged at 2000 *g* for 30 min at 4 °C. The supernatants were separated and stored at −20 °C for subsequent analysis. We measured 6-Oxo-PGF_1 α and TXB_2 by radioimmunoassay in unextracted plasma [3]. The antibodies for the radioimmunoassay were produced in our laboratory in rabbits.

Transluminal Coronary Angioplasty and
Intracoronary Thrombolysis. Ed. by Kaltenbach et al.

The levels of sensitivity of the assays are less than 70 pg for 6-Oxo-PGF$_1$ α and TXB_2. The levels of βTG were determined with a commercially available radioimmunoassay (Radiochemical Center Amersham). All values are expressed as mean ± SEM. The statistical analysis was performed by the two-tailed Student's t test of paired data.

Results

No influence of TCA on PL was found. However, TXB_2 and βTG increased significantly in coronary sinus blood after deflation of the obstructing balloon; 5 min after TCA, TXB_2 reached baseline values, whereas βTG remained high (Fig. 1). We could not detect measurable levels of 6-Oxo-PGF$_1$ α before or after TCA.

Ratios of PL, TXB_2 and βTG in the coronary sinus and in the ascending aorta (CS/AO) before TCA and 5 min thereafter are shown in Fig. 2. The CS/AO ratio of PL and TXB_2 was about 1 and did not change 5 min after TCA, whereas the CS/AO ratio of βTG increased significantly after TCA.

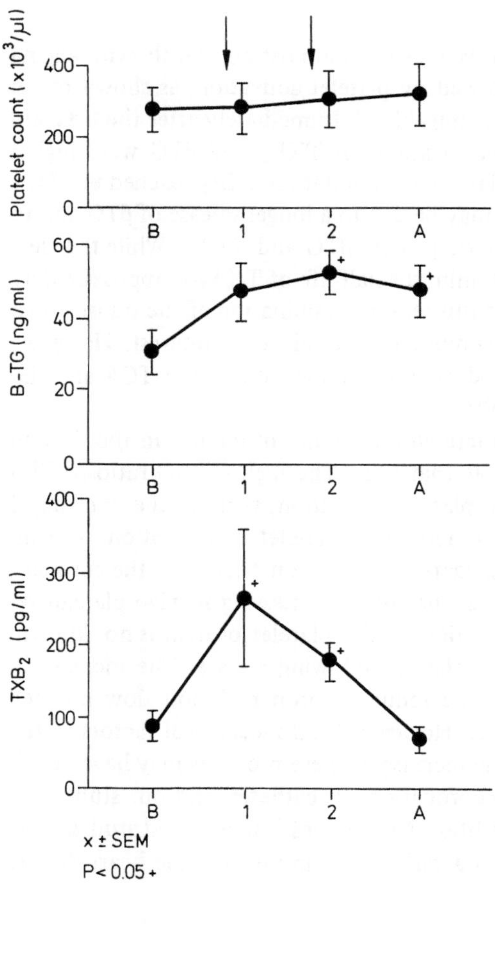

Fig. 1. Platelet count, βTG and TXB_2 in coronary sinus before TCA (B), 15 s after the first (*1*) and second (*2*) balloon deflation, and 5 min thereafter (*A*)

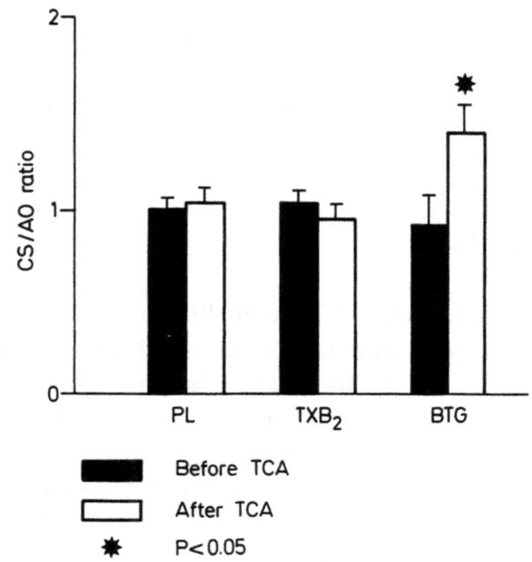

Fig. 2. Ratios of PL (TXB_2), and βTG in coronary sinus and in ascending aorta before and 5 min after TCA

Discussion

Transluminal coronary angioplasty, which is associated almost constantly with angina pectoris and/or ECG alterations, was followed by platelet activation, as shown by an increase of TXB_2 and βTG in the coronary sinus blood. Immediately after the first and the second balloon deflation plasma concentrations of TXB_2 and βTG were higher than before TCA. Five minutes after the last balloon deflation TXB_2 reached pre-TCA values, whereas βTG remained high. This may be due to a longer release of βTG and to the different half-lives of the platelet-specific protein βTG and TXA_2. While the clearance of βTG had a half-life of about 100 min, the half-life of TXA_2 is approximately 30 s, being converted to TXB_2 [1, 5]. For this reason, examination of the transcardiac changes in the concentrations of these compounds would be of interest. However, the catheter technique did not allow blood sampling immediately after TCA and the aorta and the coronary sinus simultaneously.

Therefore, we do not know whether there would be any difference in the PL and TXB_2 across the myocardial circulation at that time. The high CS/AO ratio of βTG 5 min after TCA indicates intracoronary platelet activation, whereas the unchanged CS/AO ratio of PL excludes a severe intracoronary platelet consumption. The increase in TXA_2 might induce platelet aggregates and vasoconstriction in the coronary circulation. While plasma levels of βTG can be used in assessing in vivo platelet release, it must be remembered that the function of this platelet protein is not known, either in the platelet granules or in the plasma following release. The increase in platelet products could be secondary to the reduced coronary blood flow induced by the obstructing balloon and to hypoxia. However, local mechanical factors in the vessel wall may be of significance too. The increase of these products may have occurred in the coronary circulation or in the coronary sinus catheter, and our study cannot distinguish between these two possibilities. Nevertheless, since recent studies have shown intracoronary platelet aggregates in a variety of clinical ischemic heart disease syndromes, it seems possible that sensitized platelets release TXA_2 into the coronary circulation with a resultant intracoronary aggregation. We could not detect measurable concentrations of 6-Oxo-PGF_1 α, the stable metabolite of PGI_2, which, synthesized in coronary vascular tissue, may serve as a physiological TXA_2 antagonist [5]. Although an endogenous balance between TXA_2 and PGI_2 has been postulated there has been no previous systematic investigation dealing with this possibility in patients with cardiac disease.

On the other hand, metabolic products of PGI_2 other than 6-Oxo-$PGF_1\alpha$ have been described [6], and under certain conditions 6-Oxo-$PGF_1\alpha$ may not reflect the total changes in PGI_2. Furthermore, localized alterations in PGI_2 may exert important effects without altering the PGI_2 concentrations in coronary sinus blood, at least as measured with current techniques.

Therefore, low local concentrations of PGI_2 could prevent or disturb platelet aggregation under certain circumstances such as TCA. Thus selective inhibition of thromboxane synthetase could be of clinical significance for TCA.

Summary

In five patients with severe LAD-stenosis TCA was followed by a significant increase of TXB_2 and βTG in the coronary sinus blood, indicating transient platelet activation. The platelet count remained unchanged and excluded intracoronary platelet consumption. These data show that TCA is associated with thromboxane and βTG release into the coronary circulation.

References

1. Dawes J, Smith RC, Pepper DS (1978) The release, distribution and clearance of human β-thromboglobulin and platelet factor. 4. Thromb Res 12:851–859
2. Hamberg M, Svensson J, Samuelsson B (1975) Thromboxanes: a new of biologically active compounds derived from prostaglandin endoperoxides. Proc Natl Acad Sci USA 72:2994–2998
3. Leithner C, Sinzinger H, Stummvoll HK, Klein K, Silberbauer K, Peskar BA (1980) Enhanced 6-oxo-$PGF_1\alpha$ levels in plasma during hemodialysis. Prostaglandins Med 5:425–427
4. Ludlam CA, Bolton AE, Moore S, Cash JD (1975) New rapid method for diagnosis of deep vein thrombosis. Lancet II:259–260
5. Moncada S, Vane JR (1979) Pharmacology and endogenous roles of prostaglandin endoperoxides, thromboxane A_2, and prostacyclin. Pharmacol Rev 30:293–331
6. Oates JA, Roberts LJ, Sweetnam BJ, Maas RL, Gerkens JF, Taber DF (1980) Metabolism of the prostaglandins and thromboxanes. In: Samuelson B, Ramwell PW, Paoletti R (eds) Advances in prostaglandin and thromboxane research. Raven Press, New York pp 35–41
7. Wong PV-K, Sun FF, McGiff JC (1978) Metabolism of prostacyclin in blood vessels. J Biol Chem 253:5555–5557

Persistent Angina After Transmural Infarction due to High-grade Single-vessel Stenosis

W.-D. Bussmann, D. Scherer, H. Klepzig jn., G. Kober, F.D. Maul, W. Schneider, M. Kaltenbach

Center of Internal Medicine, Department of Cardiology, Clinic of University Frankfurt, Theodor-Stern-Kai 7, 6000 Frankfurt am Main, FRG

In patients with large akinetic segments due to transmural myocardial infarction, revascularization procedures are not indicated. In a recent study, however, we observed improvement of formerly akinetic segments following bypass surgery in seven of 21 patients [2]. Function normalized or improved to at least a hypokinetic pattern [1].

With these results in mind, balloon dilatation was performed in nine patients who had transmural myocardial infarction and akinesis related to a stenosis in the supplying vessel. These cases constitute 6% of the 150 patients who have undergone TCA in Frankfurt.

Angina pectoris was present in eight of nine patients and ST segment depression in five of them. Exercise tolerance was 3.7 min at 110 watts. Following successful dilatation in nearly all patients the degree of stenosis diminished (from 87% to 40%). Angina pectoris, ST segment depression, and exercise tolerance improved remarkably (Table 1).

Two examples are shown in Fig. 1. The first patient with ventriculographic evidence of extensive anterior myocardial infarction and aneurysm had dyspnea and angina pectoris during exertion. Evidence of myocardial ischemia was difficult to confirm, at least by exercise ECG. Following successful dilatation of a 90% stenosis in the LAD, the patient became asymptomatic. Exercise tolerance increased from 50 to 170 watts. The ventriculographic pattern did not change markedly. Thallium scan and nuclear ejection fraction during exercise, however, showed improvement. The second patient had evidence of posterior wall infarction with corresponding akinetic segments which were completely reversible following dilation.

Table 1. Transmural myocardial infarction in nine patients

Criterion	Before TCA	After TCA
Degree of stenosis (%)	87	40
Angina pectoris (*n*)	8	2
ST segment depression (*n*)	5	1
Exercise tolerance (min)	3.7	5.7
Exercise work load (watts)	110	130

Transluminal Coronary Angioplasty and Intracoronary Thrombolysis. Ed. by Kaltenbach et al.

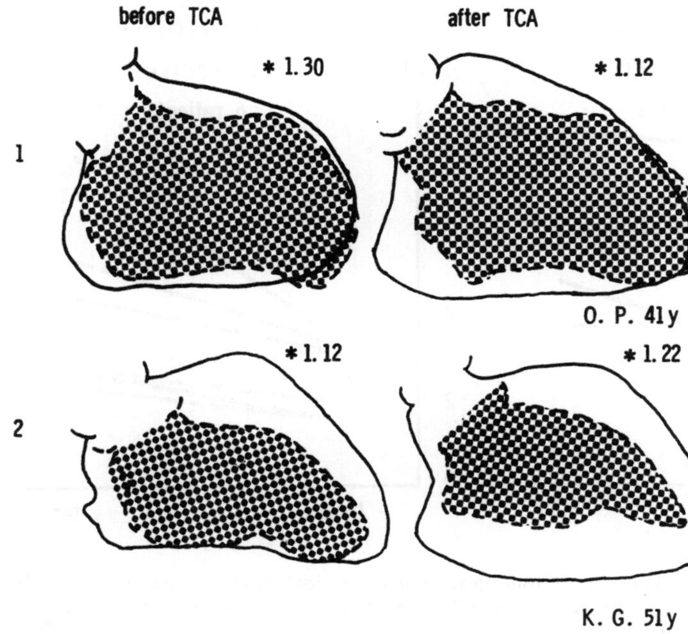

Fig. 1. Ventriculographic patterns before and after TCA in two representative cases. In case 1 ventricular function following TCA did not improve very much, but ejection fraction during exercise increased and angina during exertion disappeared. In case 2 akinetic inferior wall segments improved markedly following reopening of the right coronary artery during the TCA procedure. (* magnification factor)

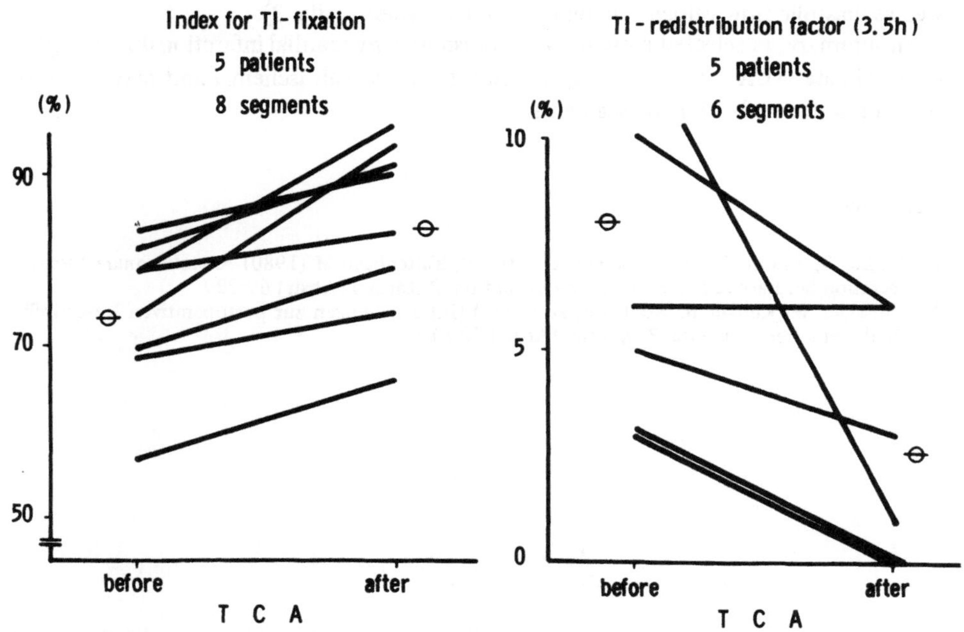

Fig. 2. Thallium fixation indices and redistribution factors during exercise increased following TCA in the area and distribution of the involved vessel. All patients had transmural myocardial infarction in the same region

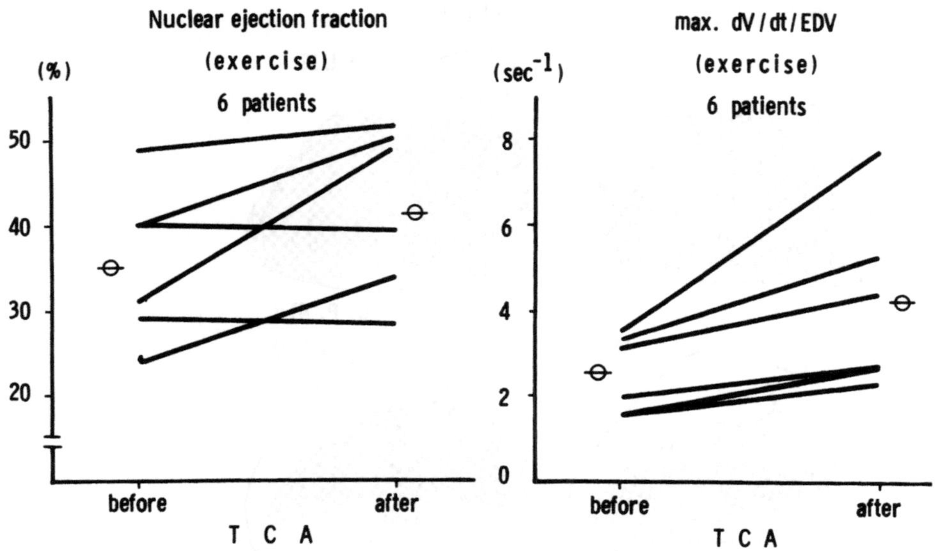

Fig. 3. Nuclear ejection fraction and diastolic flow velocity (dV/dt/EDV) increased in nearly all patients with transmural myocardial infarction following TCA in the supplying vessel. Function in the infarcted area is improved

Scintigraphic studies in these patients revealed improvement of myocardial ischemia. Thallium fixation increased and redistribution regressed (Fig. 2). Ejection fraction as well as diastolic flow velocity increased in most patients (Fig. 3).

In summary, in selected patients with transmural myocardial infarction due to single-vessel disease, TCA can relieve angina, reduce myocardial, ischemia and may improve function in formerly akinetic segments.

References

1. Kunkel B, Krause E, Schöneberger A, Satter P, Kaltenbach M (1980) Aortokoronare Bypass-operation bei stark reduzierter Ventrikelfunktion. Z Kardiol [Abstr] 69:229
2. Schneider W, Kunkel B, Kohl S et al. (1981) Untersuchungen zur postoperativen Reversibilität akinetischer Segmente. Z. Kardiol [Abstr] 70:617

Prognosis of Nontransmural Myocardial Infarction

K. Schnellbacher, Th. Cerchez, P. Stürzenhofecker, H. Roskamm

Rehabilitationszentrum für Herz- und Kreislaufkranke Bad Krozingen, FRG

Many patients with nontransmural myocardial infarction suffer from angina pectoris after the infarction [4]. Thus the long-term prognosis remains controversial [1, 2, 3, 5].

From 1973 to 1977, 332 patients were admitted to our clinic with the diagnosis of nontransmural myocardial infarction. Coronary angiography was performed 2–3 months following the clinical event. The average follow-up period was 4.08 years.

From these patients, 122 had zero-vessel disease and are characterized by a high exercise tolerance (110 watts), a high percentage without angina pectoris (79.8%), and a good prognosis (cardiac mortality was 0.2% per year). Most of these patients probably had not had a myocardial infarction.

The remaining 210 patients had positive coronary angiograms with stenoses exceeding 50%. Most of the montransmural myocardial infarctions were in the anterior wall with a stenosis in the LAD in 78.3% of the patients. With greater vessel involvement prognosis deteriorates (Table 1).

Of the reinfarctions, 79% were transmural and 63% occurred in the area of the previous nontransmural infarction. Of the patients with one-vessel disease, 85 had lesions in the LAD (79% a severe stenosis, 21% an occlusion). The patients with one-vessel disease had postinfarction angina pectoris in 46.2%, a maximum exercise tolerance of 88.3 watts (range 12.5–150 watts), a maximum ST segment depression of 0.09 mV (range 0–0.5 mV) and a maximum increase of pulmonary capillary wedge pressure of 22.5 mmHg (range 7–44 mmHg).

Table 1. Mortality and reinfarction in 210 patients after nontransmural myocardial infarction

	No. of vessels diseased		
	One	Two	Three
No. of patients	112	55	43
Total mortality/year (%)	2.2	1.3	4.6
Cardiac mortality/year (%)	1.1	1.3	4.1
Reinfarctions/year (%)	2.8	5.8	5.1
Cardiac death and reinfarction in 4.08 years follow-up (%)	16.0	30.0	37.2

Transluminal Coronary Angioplasty and
Intracoronary Thrombolysis. Ed. by Kaltenbach et al.

Due to severe angina pectoris and considerable functional impairment, 17 patients received bypass surgery. None of these patients died or suffered a reinfarction. Retrospectively 71% of these patients would have benefitted from angioplasty.

In spite of this, there is a rather poor prognosis for the remaining 95 patients with one-vessel disease. The total mortality rate is, at 2.6% per year, five times higher than the mortality rate in the age-matched normal population in West Germany. The cardiac mortality rate was 1.3% per year, the reinfarction rate 3.4% per year. Cardiac death or reinfarction occurred in 18.9% during the follow-up period of 4.08 years.

Of the 18 patients with one-vessel disease who died or had a reinfarction, 89% had lesions in the LAD. In the exercise test 61% had no angina pectoris at the maximal exercise level, 56% had no ST segment depression, and 50% no pathologic increase of pulmonary capillary wedge pressure.

Summary

Nontransmural myocardial infarction is in most cases characterized by:

1. Anterior wall location with severe stenosis of the proximal LAD
2. Pre- and especially postinfarction angina pectoris
3. A relatively high rate of mortality and later transmural myocardial infarction in the area of the nontransmural infarction.

For these reasons it can be said that many of these patients are good candidates for angioplasty.

References.

1. Bemiller CR, Pepine CJ, Rogers A (1973) Long-term observations in patients with angina and normal coronary angiograms. Circulation 47:36
2. Cannon DS, Levy W, Cohen LS (1976) The short- and long-term prognosis of patients with transmural and non transmural myocardial infarction. Am J Med 61:452
3. Madias JE, Chahine RA, Gorlin R, Blacklow DJ (1974) A comparison of transmural and nontransmural acute myocardial infarction. Circulation 49:488
4. Roskamm H, Samek L, Cerchez T et al. (1978) Der nicht transmurale Herzinfarkt – ein diagnostisches Problem. Dtsch Med Wochenschr 12:497
5. Strauss H, Sobel BE, Roberts R (1978) Acute and long-term prognosis in patients with transmural versus subendocardial infarction. Circulation 59[Suppl]:II–193

Overview

W.-D. Bussmann

Center of Internal Medicine, Department of Cardiology and Nephrology, University Clinic of Frankfurt a.M, Theodor-Stern-Kai 7, 6000 Frankfurt a.M. 70, FRG

Percutaneous transluminal coronary angioplasty (PTCA) of coronary artery stenosis is primarily indicated in patients with angina pectoris on exertion and fixed coronary artery lesions. However, the use of the method can now be discussed in patients with suspicion of coronary spasm and in those experiencing transmural or nontransmural myocardial infarction with persisting angina pectoris in the follow-up period.

Bentivoglio and co-workers demonstrate on a limited number of patients that PTCA can successfully be performed when coronary spasm is superimposed on fixed stenoses of a moderate degree. Intracoronary nitroglycerin or calcium antagonists should be given to unmask true coronary spasm without an organic stenosis. Most variable stenoses with superimposed coronary spasm tend to progress later on to fixed stenosis. Angioplasty in this situation can be successful in many patients.

As suggested by Rafflenbeul and co-workers, eccentric stenoses react less favourably to angioplasty than concentric stenoses. This might be due to the fact that the pressure of the inflation balloon dilates the "soft" normal vessel proportion, with the result that less pressure is imposed on the area of plaque within the stenosis. On the other hand, there is from the clinical point of view no major difference in the success of PTCA in patients with stable or unstable angina pectoris (Meyer and co-workers).

In general, the pathophysiologic mechanism of coronary spasm is unresolved, as shown by Feigl and co-workers and Friesinger and Silberbauer. Alpha-adrenergic vasoconstriction is seen as the neurogenic component, and the role of thromboxane A_2, mediated by platelets or the vessel wall itself, seems to be the biochemical component of the mechanism.

In a subgroup of patients after transmural myocardial infarction, typical angina pectoris persists even in single-vessel disease. Viable myocardium is present in the perfusion area. The vessel might have been primarily closed but partially reopened, as in cases after fibrinolysis, or there was only a primary high-grade stenosis, leading to a small infarction. PTCA in this situation can be effective in abolition of angina pectoris and improvement of myocardial function during exercise (Bussmann et al.).

Patients with nontransmural anterior myocardial infarction often show severe stenosis in the proximal left anterior descending coronary artery. Cardiac mortality during a 4-year follow-up period ranges between 16% and 37%. Therefore, these patients with nontransmural anterior myocardial infarction may form another group of candidates for PTCA (Schnellbacher et al.).

Transluminal Coronary Angioplasty and
Intracoronary Thrombolysis. Ed. by Kaltenbach et al.

Angioplasty in Peripheral and Renal Arteries

Percutaneous Transluminal Recanalization (Angioplasty) in Leg Arteries

W. Seyferth, E. Zeitler

Radiological Center, Klinikum Nürnberg, Flurstr. 17, 8500 Nürnberg, FRG

Percutaneous transluminal recanalization/angioplasty (PTA) in lower extremities can be performed in the vascular section between pelvic bifurcation and tibiofibular trunk.

Technique

The site of the arterial puncture is determined by the vascular section to be treated. The mode of advancing the catheter from the contralateral vascular section in the pelvic region that Roth and Bachmann [1, 3] have introduced is also used more and more for dilatation of femoral artery stenoses. Proximal compression of the treated vascular section following the examination is thereby avoided.

Today, only three catheter types are used for PTA in our Department:

1. The sidewinder catheter which is necessary for safe positioning of the guide wire when proceeding from the contralateral side.
2. The teflon step catheter after Zeitler [5, 6], which is a modified van Andel catheter [4] with side holes arranged 10 cm proximal to the catheter tip. The advantage of this catheter is that contrast material can be applied in each phase of the dilation procedure.
3. The dilatation balloon catheters after Grüntzig [2] in different lengths and different balloon diameters for adaptation to the lumen diameter.

The pathologic vascular section must be passed with the Zeitler catheter and simultaneously be treated with a bougie. Subsequently, a balloon catheter can be advanced. Sometimes, in case of distant stenoses, one can advance again a Zeitler or van Andel catheter with a larger diameter for smoothing the vascular wall.

Results

Since July 1976 we have performed 719 treatments in 569 patients. The mean age was 65 years (28–87 years); 71% were male and 29% female. Of the treatments, 59% were carried out in stage II after Fontaine (Table 1), and 41% in stage III and IV (Table 2) of the arterial vascular disease. In 3.3% (24 cases) the treatment was given up because the puncture failed or because of a false indication.

Transluminal Coronary Angioplasty and
Intracoronary Thrombolysis. Ed. by Kaltenbach et al.

Table 1. Leg artery PTA in patients with intermittent claudication (stage II)

Stenoses/occlusions	Successful	Doubtful	Unsuccess-ful	Total	Successes as proportion of total (%)
Aortic stenosis	5	–	–	5	
Iliac artery stenoses	122	4	6	132	3
Iliac artery occlusions	1	–	1	2	
Femoropopliteal artery stenosis	127	9	4	140	91
Deep femoral artery stenoses	5	1	–	6	
Femoropopliteal artery occlusions < 10 cm	94	3	7	104	90
> 10 cm	20	6	8	34	59
Total	374	23	26	423	

Eight patients (1.9%) showed recidivation at 2 weeks. Seven patients (1.7%) underwent operation for complications. In addition, there were eleven successful PTAs of concomitant lower leg obliterations.

Table 2. Leg artery PTA in patients with rest pain (stage III) and gangrene (stage IV)

Stenoses/occlusions	Successful	Doubtful	Unsuccess-ful	Total	Successes as proportion of total (%)
Iliac artery stenoses	33	2	5	40	82.5
Femoral comm. deep femoral artery stenoses	9	–	3	12	
Femoropopliteal artery stenosis	62	5	6	73	85.0
Femoropopliteal artery occlusions < 10 cm	64	10	14	88	73
> 10 cm	30	5	25	60	50
Lower leg obliterations (isolated)	11	1	10	22	50
Total	209	23	63	295	71

18 patients (6.1%) showed recidivation at 2 weeks. 2 (3.04%) underwent operation or repeat PTA.
[a] Also 3 successful PTAs in 4 attempts at concomitant lower leg obliterations

Based on the angiographic assessment of the primary results, the success rates in stage II were nearly equally good in iliac artery stenoses, femoropopliteal stenoses, and femoropopliteal occlusions not longer than 10 cm. The pressure gradient, however, measured with the ultrasound Doppler technique (Fig. 1), indicates that a significant difference exists between the treatment of a near occlusion and that of a stenosis in the femoropopliteal region. We attribute this to the fact that the near stage II occlusion is commonly a singular wall lesion, whereas stenoses are often multilocular so that subintimal dissections, being the cause of a dilatation over a long distance, occur

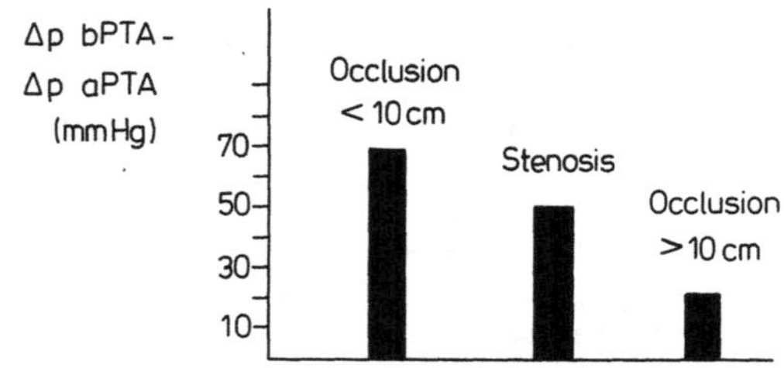

Fig. 1. Results of ultrasound Doppler measurements in stage II patients, showing change in arterial pressure after PTA

more often. Decrease of the pressure gradient was much more evident after PTA of occlusions than after PTA of stenoses.

On the whole, the results in stage III and IV – with the exception of femoropopliteal stenoses (85%) – are less favorable, the reason being the more severe atherosclerosis. Complications, surgical intervention in stage II and stages III/IV are nearly equal, whereas the early recidivation rate is significantly higher in stage III/IV (6.1%) than in stage II (1.9%). The reasons are both the worse pathologic situation in the vascular section to be treated and the more severe obliterations in the run-off.

Discussion

The introduction of the Grüntzig dilatation catheter [2] brought about improvement in the results obtained in the iliac artery. Additionally, the kissing balloon technique made possible treatment of stenoses above the bifurcation, which we have successfully carried out in five cases. The experience of the team and the course of the treatment play a much more important role in the result of PTA in femoropopliteal stenoses (Fig. 2a, b) than does the choice of a special balloon-catheter type.

In spite of a refinement of routine techniques in recent years, the present method of treatment in the tibiofibular trunk (Fig. 3a, b) could not essentially be extended to peripheral vessels.

It is remarkable that the number of stage II patients admitted to our hospital has increased in recent months. We ascribe this phenomenon to the fact that the indications for PTA are increasingly accepted among surgeons, and that the treatment procedure is becoming more widely known among those doctors who refer the patients directly to us.

Summary

We have performed 719 treatment procedures in leg arteries so far, with a success rate of 87% in iliac arteries and 85% in the femoropopliteal region. Consequently, PTA can be considered as the method of choice for stenoses and occlusions shorter than 10 cm.

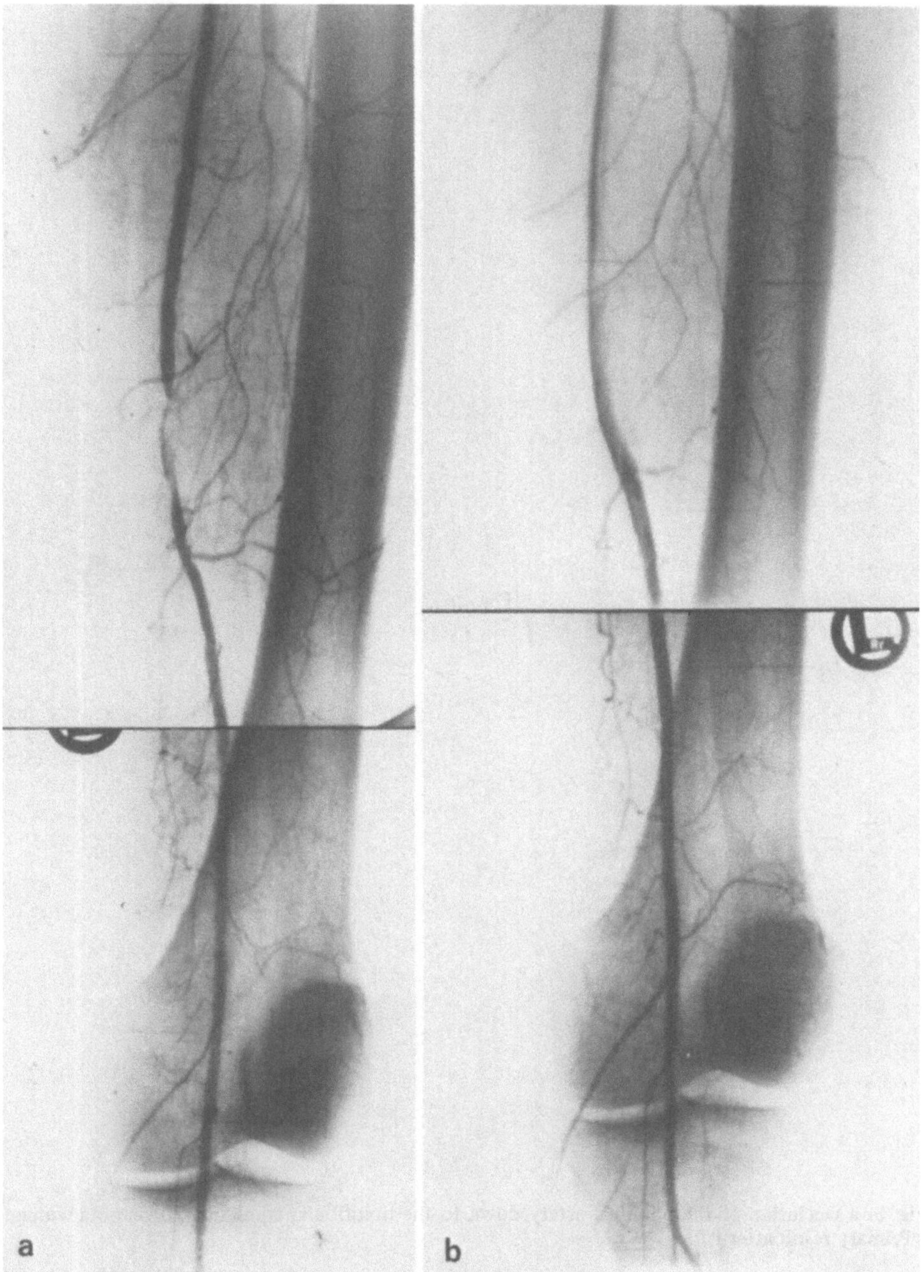

Fig. 2. a Short occlusion of the left femoral artery in a 62-year-old woman. **b** Primary result after PTA

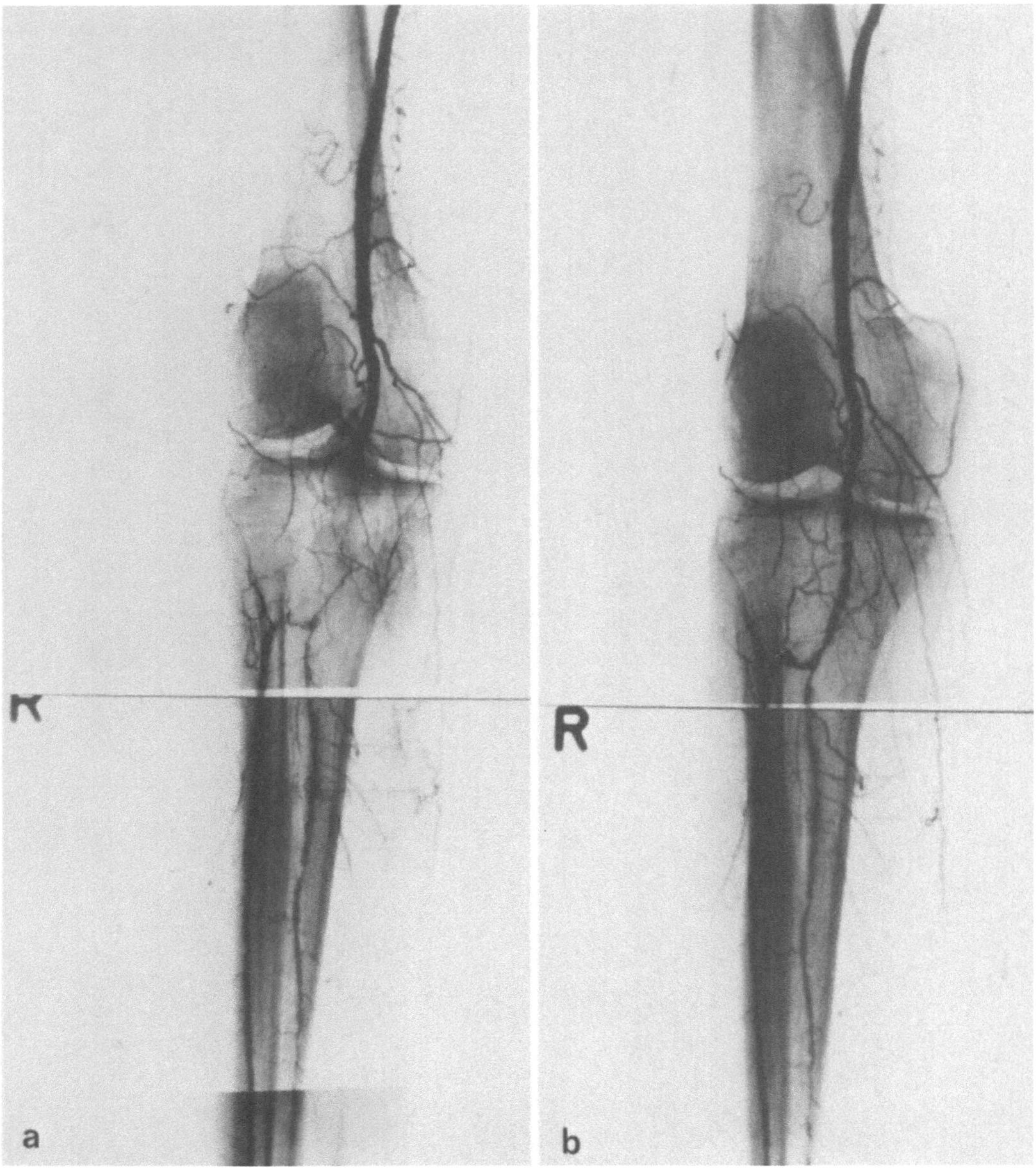

Fig. 3. a Occlusion of the popliteal artery down to the tibiofibular trunk in a 70-year-old woman. **b** Primary result after PTA

Stenoses stage IIa–IV in iliac arteries, in the superficial and deep femoral artery, in the popliteal artery, and the rare cases in the lower leg should be submitted primarily to PTA. Occlusions in the superficial femoral artery shorter than 10 cm, in the popliteal artery, and in the tibiofibular trunk are an indication for PTA in all stages of the arterial vascular disease.

The Fate of "No Angioplasty" in Peripheral Vascular Disease

R. Sörensen, A. Grassot, H.V. Zühlke

Abteilung für Röntgendiagnostik und Chirurgische Klinik der Freien Universität Berlin im Klinikum Steglitz, Berlin

Percutaneous transluminal angioplasty (PTA) and recanalization (PTR) are well-documented procedures, successfully used now for nearly 20 years, but still there are many places where this technique is not performed to the extent which seems to be necessary.

During a period of 2 years (1978–1980) 40 of our patients were thought to have an indication for PTA or PTR judged by arteriographic findings. These patients did not undergo PTA for various reasons and the fate of their disease was investigated in retrospect. Clinically 20 patients had stage II, seven stage III, and eight stage IV disease. No clinical data were available on five patients.

The angiographic findings were stated for each leg separately (Table 1). Patients with a lesion treatable by surgery on one leg were suggested for PTA of the other side if stenoses or occlusions up to 10 cm in length were demonstrated angiographically. In 40 patients 51 treatable lesions of iliac, superficial femoral, and popliteal arteries, and arteries distal to the trifurcation were found. Included are two patients with stenoses at the anastomoses of a femoropopliteal bypass and four who were thought to be candidates for a trial of angioplasty prior to amputation.

Of 40 lesions in the femoropopliteal region 25 were treated conservatively or had no treatment in spite of the fact that occlusions were less than 10 cm in length. Ten of these patients had surgical repair of an artery on the opposite side. Eight lesions were treated by revascularization surgery and on seven lesions no further information was available. The eight stenoses of the iliac arteries had surgery. Of the three patients with disease below the trifurcation two had amputation following the diagnosis and one refused surgery and was treated conservatively (Table 2).

Table 1. Angiographic findings in 51 lesions treatable by angioplasty

Lesion and site	No. of lesions
Stenoses of the femoropopliteal arteries	23
Occlusions of the femoropopliteal arteries	15
Stenoses of bypass anastomoses	2
Stenoses of the iliac arteries	8
Arteries below the trifurcation	3

Transluminal Coronary Angioplasty and
Intracoronary Thrombolysis. Ed. by Kaltenbach et al.

Table 2. Follow-up of 51 lesions considered for angioplasty

Site of lesions	No. of occurences
Lesions of the femoropopliteal arteries	40
Conservative treatment or no treatment	25
Surgical treatment	8
No information	7
Lesions of the iliac arteries	8
Surgical treatment	8
Lesions distal to the trifurcation	3
Conservative treatment	1
Surgical treatment (amputation)	2

The surgical therapy included aortobifemoral bypasses, femoropopliteal bypasses, patch plastics, sympathectomies, thrombendarterectomies, and combinations of these operations. Of 16 revascularization procedures three patients had to have amputations during the time of observation and four had postsurgical complications (infection, pneumonia, or occluded bypass graft) which were not fatal.

Six patients had a second arteriogram during the 2 years of this retrospective study. One was found to have an occluded femoropopliteal bypass graft. Four stenoses had become occlusions, two of them longer than 12 cm. Two patients had an amputation following the second angiogram and one had an amputation without reangiography. Twenty patients were left without treatment or with conservative treatment at the end of this study.

The idea of following up the outcome and the complications in patients who did not undergo an invasive procedure was originated by Baum [2] in 1964. He evaluated incidents due to the disease of patients awaiting an angiographic examination. He compared those incidents to the complications of the procedures itself. The results were almost identical. Although PTA and PTR were successfully performed following the first description by Dotter and Judkins [4] in 1964, surgeons are still reluctant to use them. There is no doubt that patients with intermittent claudication of stage II and occlusions less than 10 cm in length should have PTR – conservative management is not enough. Severe occlusive disease on one side often masks symptoms of a treatable lesion on the opposite side neglected by patient and doctor. There is discussion whether lesions without symptoms should be treated or not: however, the progression of the disease is known and short stenoses may change rapidly into long occlusions [5, 7].

The treatment for inoperable patients with stage III or IV disease should not only be sympathectomy. Extremities can be saved in a high percentage of cases by a trial of PTA before an amputation [3, 5, 6, 7]. Dilatations of stenoses occuring in grafts of femoropopliteal or femorotibial bypasses can also be successfully treated according to the literature [1].

In our opinion amenable lesions should be treated as soon as possible even if the patient had no symptoms at the time of angiography.

References

1. Alpert JR, Ring EJ, Berkowitz HD et al. (1979) Treatment of vein graft stenosis by balloon chatheter dilatation. JAMA 242:2769–2771
2. Baum S, Stein GN, Kuroda KK (1965) Complications of "no arteriography." Radiology 85: 835–838
3. Colapinto RF, Harries-Jones EP, Johnston KW (1980) Percutaneous transluminal dilatation and recanalisation in the treatment of peripheral vascular disease. Radiology 135:583–587
4. Dotter CT, Judkins MP (1964) Transluminal treatment of arteriosclerotic obstruction. Circulation 30:654–670
5. Mortajeme A, Keifer JW, Zuska AJ (1980) Percutaneous transluminal angioplasty and case selection. Radiology 135:573–581
6. Zarins CK, Lu C, McDonnell AE, Whitehouse WM (1980) Limb salvage by percutaneous transluminal recanalisation of the occluded superficial femoral artery. Surgery : 701–708
7. Zeitler E, Schoop W, Zahnow W (1971) The treatment of occlusive arterial disease by transluminal catheter angioplasty. Radiology 99:19–26

Percutaneous Transluminal Renal Angioplasty: Experience in Over 100 Arteries

T.A. Sos*, K.W. Sniderman*, T. Pickering**, E.D. Vaughan, Jr.***, D. Case **, J.H. Laragh**

* Department of Radiology, New York Hospital – Cornell Medical Center, 525 E. 68th St., New York, NY 10021, USA
** Department of Medicine, Division of Cardiovascular Medicine, New York Hospital – Cornell Medical Center
*** Department of Surgery, Division of Urology, New York Hospital – Cornell Medical Center

Percutaneous Transluminal Angioplasty

In a visionary paper in 1964 Dotter and Judkins [1] first described percutaneous transluminal angioplasty, and predicted that the technique would be applicable to proximal segments of the renal and coronary arteries. History proved them correct. The development of the double-lumen balloon dilating catheter by Grüntzig and Hopff [3] in 1974 has made renal and coronary artery dilatation not only possible but an accomplished fact; since the late 1970s many centers all over the world have performed at least a thousand and possibly several thousand such procedures [4, 6, 7, 9, 10, 11, 12, 14].

We wish to describe our experience in percutaneous transluminal renal angioplasty (PTRA) of over 100 arteries in 87 patients.

Materials and Methods

Patient Selection

Since 1978 at the New York Hospital we have performed PTRA on 94 native renal arteries in 78 patients (Table 1) aged 50 ± 15 years (mean ± SD). There were 37 males and 41 females; of the females 18 had fibromuscular dysplasia (FMD). Forty-seven patients (mean age 58 ± 9 years) with 60 arteries had atherosclerotic disease and 24 patients (mean age 38 ± 17 years) had FMD. Nine patients had stenosis at or near the

Table 1. Patient population for renal angioplasty

Etiology	No. of arteries	No. of patients	Age (years)
Atherosclerosis	60	47	58 ± 9
Fibromuscular dysplasia	26	24	38 ± 17
Arteritis	6	5	21 ± 7
Post-transplantation	9	9	–
Postsurgical stenosis	2	2	–
Total	103	87	50 ± 15

Transluminal Coronary Angioplasty and
Intracoronary Thrombolysis. Ed. by Kaltenbach et al.

anastomotic site following renal transplantation. Five young patients with six arteries had probable though not histologically proven arteridites. Two patients had post-surgical stenoses, one in a renal artery venous bypass graft, and one following inadvertent ligation of the main renal artery. Two atherosclerotic hypertensive patients had severe coexistent renal failure prior to PTRA with BUN of 80 mg/dl and 69 mg/dl, and creatinine of 4.4 mg/dl and 4.5 mg/dl respectively. Nine patients underwent PTRA of multiple arteries, either simultaneously or at a subsequent catheterization. Successful repeat PTRA of three arteries was performed in one atherosclerotic patients, and a transplant renal artery restenosis was also redilated.

Patients with native renal artery disease were selected for PTRA if they fulfilled the criteria for curability of renovascular hypertension which have been reported in detail elsewhere [15]. These investigations, including selective renal vein renin sampling, were performed on an outpatient basis. Briefly, the criteria were:

1. High level of peripheral plasma renin activity indexed against 24 h urinary sodium levels.
2. Hypersecretion of renin from the ipsilateral kidney (stenotic side) reflecting decreased renal blood flow and ischemia.
3. Suppression of renin secretion from the contralateral (uninvolved) side.
4. Angiotensin dependence of the hypertension documented by blockage of the conversion of angiotensin I to angiotensin II by a converting enzyme inhibitor (Captopril).

In addition a few patients with angiographically documented severe renal artery stenosis (greater than 70% diameter stenosis), who had either renal failure or bilateral renal artery stenosis but did not meet the above criteria, underwent PTRA if otherwise they would have been considered candidates for renal artery surgery. Hospitalization and arteriography were usually carried out only after the above tests were performed on an outpatient basis. Informed consent for PTRA was obtained prior to arteriography, and PTRA was frequently performed immediately following the diagnostic arteriogram if a severe stenosis was found. No patient who fulfilled the above criteria and had an angiographically documented severe renal artery stenosis was turned down for PTRA because of coexistent medical problems.

Renal transplant patients were considered candidates for PTRA if their blood pressure was greater than 160/95 mmHg and difficult to control and if a greater than 70% diameter luminal stenosis was angiographically documented. We did not find plasma renin activity and radionuclide studies to be consistently helpful in patients who had undergone renal transplants.

Methods

Catheterization

Catheters for PTRA were generally introduced from the femoral arteries though in a few instances, especially with caudally oriented renal arteries in younger patients, the axillary route was preferred.

In all but two instances (with vessels less than 2 mm in diameter) double-lumen balloon catheters were used. In the other two cases a 6.5F or 7F catheter was introduced into the artery a la Dotter.

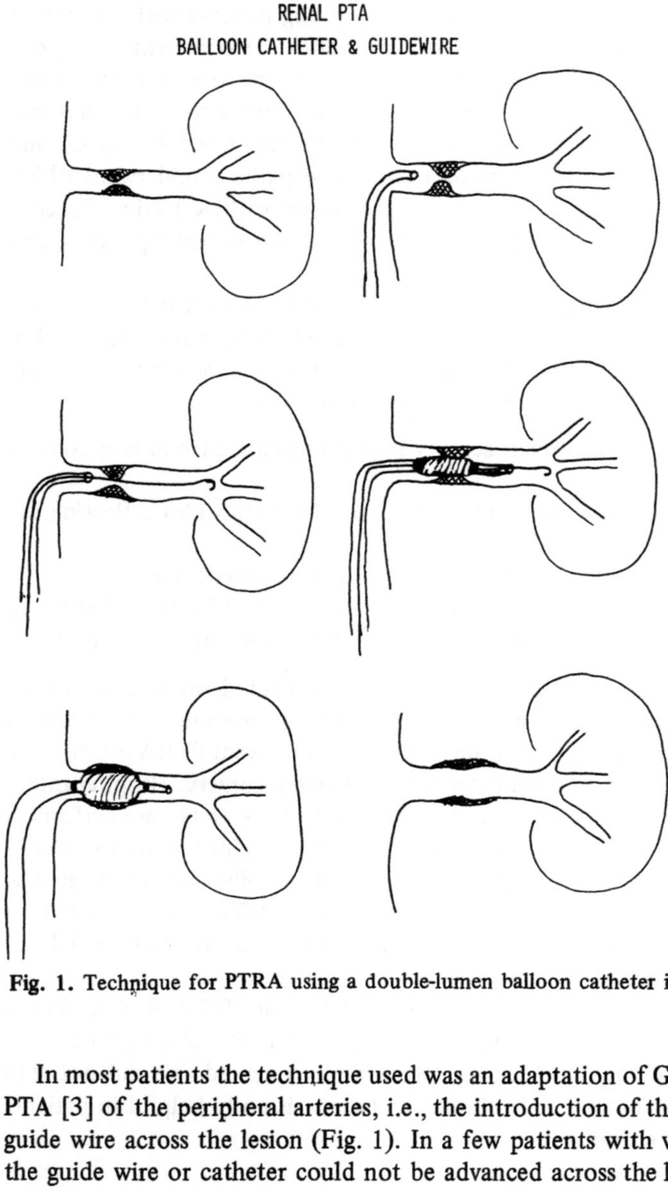

Fig. 1. Technique for PTRA using a double-lumen balloon catheter introduced over a guide wire

In most patients the technique used was an adaptation of Grüntzig's original one for PTA [3] of the peripheral arteries, i.e., the introduction of the dilating catheter over a guide wire across the lesion (Fig. 1). In a few patients with very tight stenoses where the guide wire or catheter could not be advanced across the lesion, we used our adaptation of Grüntzig's coaxial technique using an 8F teflon outer guiding catheter to engage the ostium of the artery and to advance a 4.5F double-lumen catheter across the lesion without a wire guide [13] (Fig. 2). In most of the patients with FMD, neither of these techniques was successful in crossing long segments of stenoses, and in these patients as well as in a few atherosclerotic ones, the lesions were crossed by carefully advancing a Simmons (shepherd's crook-shaped) catheter [13] across the lesion without a guide wire while constantly injecting a dilute contrast-saline solution to monitor the course of the catheter and perhaps to push the arterial wall away from the catheter tip (Fig. 3).

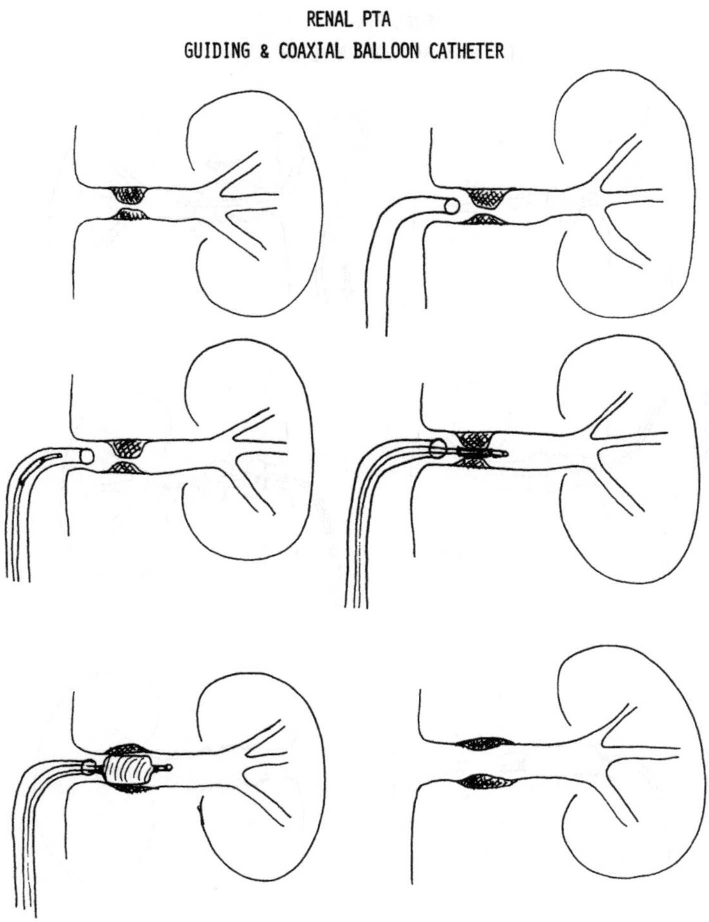

Fig. 2. Technique for PTRA using a guiding catheter to introduce a miniature double-lumen balloon catheter without a guide wire

Pressure Measurements

Proximal renal artery or aortic pressure was always obtained just before advancing the catheter across the lesion. Renal artery pressure distal to the stenosis was recorded in every patient, and a simultaneous systemic pressure was obtained by a peripheral arterial catheter, the sidearm of an introducing arterial sheath, or cuff pressure. In every instance following PTRA a pullback pressure across the dilated area was obtained, and in no case was this performed with a catheter smaller in diameter than the one used to measure the initial pressure distal to the lesion. Pressures were recorded on calibrated paper on an Electronics for Medicine monitor.

Severity of Stenosis

The severity of each lesion was graded on all pre- and post-PTRA angiograms by estimating visually the percentage of luminal diameter stenosis, since evaluation of the cross-sectional area is unreliable from a single-plane angiogram.

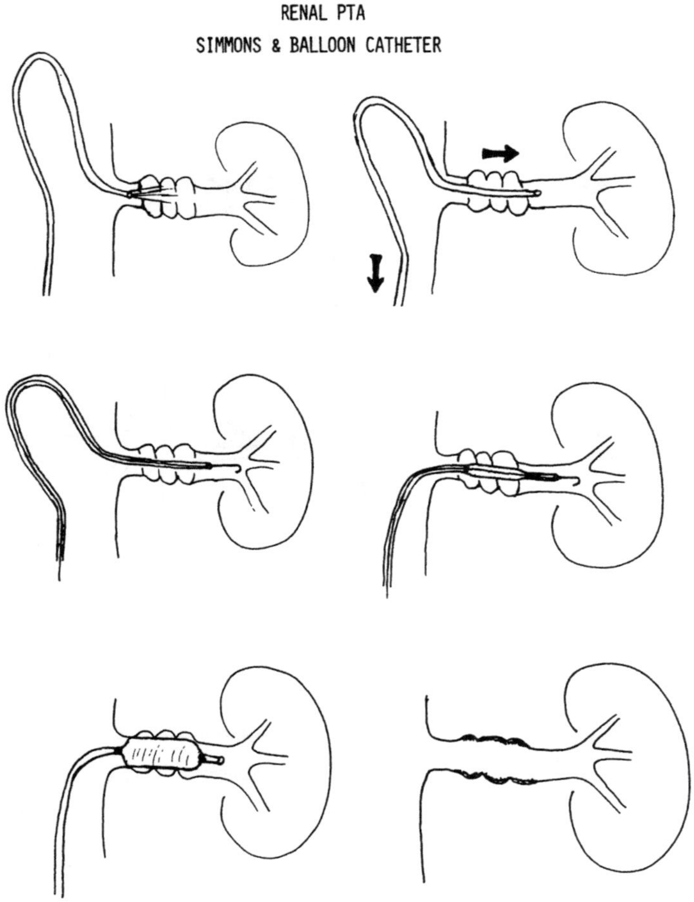

Fig. 3. Technique for PTRA using a Simmons catheter for initially crossing the stenosis

Laboratory Tests

Renin

In each patient selective renal vein and IVC renin samples were obtained immediately before and 15–30 min following PTRA. Patients who had technically successful PTRAs were scheduled for repeat renal vein renin measurements at 6-month intervals, though the patients often did not return.

Radionuclide Flow Studies

Some but not all patients underwent pre- and post-PTRA radionuclide studies.

Renal Function

All patients had pre- and post-PTRA measurements of BUN and creatinine levels.

Adjunctive Medications

Anticoagulants

Pre-PTRA. Most though not all patients take aspirin 300 mg/day orally for 2–3 days prior to PTRA.

During PTRA. Heparinization is carried out with approximately 5000 units heparin intravenously from the start of the procedure. An additional 2000 units heparin is often injected into the proximal renal artery just before crossing the stenosis.

Post-PTRA. Heparin is not reversed by protamine at the end of PTRA, but additional heparin is not given. No systematic attempt was made to keep patients on coumarin following PTRA, though in patients who have had a difficult PTRA of an atherosclerotic lesion, we give coumarin to achieve anticoagulant levels of approximately two times normal for approximately 3–6 months. In most patients aspirin 300 mg/day is continued for the rest of the patient's life, unless contraindicated.

Antispasmodics

Immediately prior to crossing a renal artery stenosis we inject a "cocktail" of tolazoline hydrochloride (Priscoline) 25 mg and lidocaine 40 mg, one ingredient at a time, to prevent renal artery spasm (which we have frequently documented angiographically during PTRA), in addition to the 2000 units heparin previously described. Intraarterial, sublingual, or paste applications of nitroglycerin may also be useful, and we have used it occasionally.

Results

Initial technical success (greater than 25% increase in luminal diameter and greater than 20% reduction of the aortorenal pressure gradient) was obtained in 82% of all arteries (Table 2). In atherosclerosis we were successful in 45/60 (75%) arteries (Figs. 4 and 5) including 4/8 with complete occlusion; in 23/26 (89%) arteries with FMD (Fig. 6); in 6/6 arteries in patients with arteridites; in 2/2 postsurgical stenoses; and in 8/9 (90%) stenoses following renal transplantation (Fig. 7).

Table 2. Technical success in PTRA

Etiology	No. of arteries	No. of technical successes
Atherosclerosis	60	45 (75%)
Fibromuscular dysplasia	26	23 (89%)
Arteritis	6	6 (100%)
Post-transplantation	9	8 (90%)
Postsurgical stenosis	2	2 (100%)
Total	103	84 (82%)

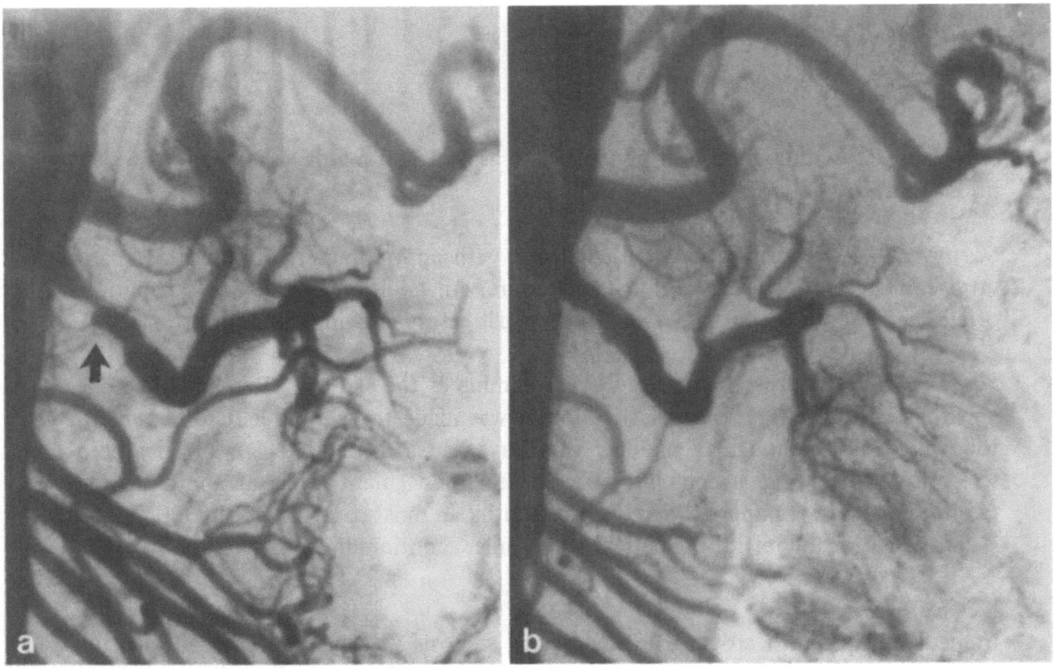

Fig. 4 a, b. Aortograms in atherosclerotic renal artery stenosis. a prior to PTRA (*arrow* shows stenosis); b following PTRA

Following technically successful PTRA of native renal arteries the aortorenal pressure gradient dropped from 118 ± 42 mmHg to 13 ± 18 mmHg ($P < 0.001$) and the mean diameter of the stenoses decreased from 91% ± 9% to 27% ± 24% ($P < 0.001$).

In the two patients with renal failure, following successful PTRA BUN fell from 80 mg/dl and 69 mg/dl to 30 mg/dl and 34 mg/dl, and creatinine fell from 4.4 mg/dl and 4.5 mg/dl to 1.7 mg/dl and 2.6 mg/dl within a week and stayed at these levels for 1½ and 2 years respectively.

In the initial 45 patients, following technically successful PTRA blood pressure fell from 192 ± 3 / 113 ± 13 mmHg to 141 ± 16 / 84 ± 7 mmHg ($P < 0.001$) on no or decreased medication at a follow-up of up to 24 months, average 10 months (Fig. 8). Ninety percent of the patients with FMD required no medication, whereas approximately 50% of those with atherosclerosis were on some antihypertensive medication. Following technically successful post-transplant PTRA in eight patients blood pressure fell from 195 ± 5 / 121 ± 6 mmHg to 132 ± 15 / 85 ± 7 mmHg on no or reduced medication.

Complications

There were no deaths or kidneys lost directly related to PTRA (within 1 month). Emergency surgery was not necessary in any patient. Nonocclusive dissection of a main or branch renal artery occurred three times. In two instances a successful bypass

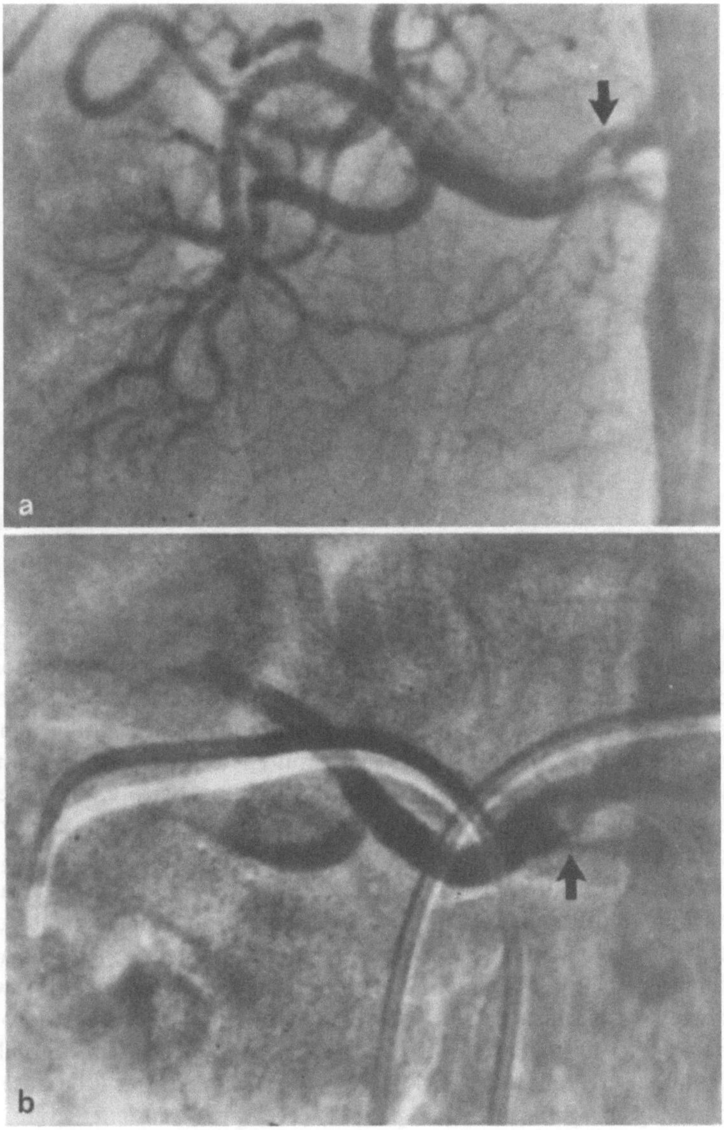

Fig. 5a–c. Renal arteriograms in a 65-year-old man with atherosclerotic renal artery stenosis (*black arrows*). **a** prior to PTRA; **b** immediately after PTRA; **c** 30 months after PTRA

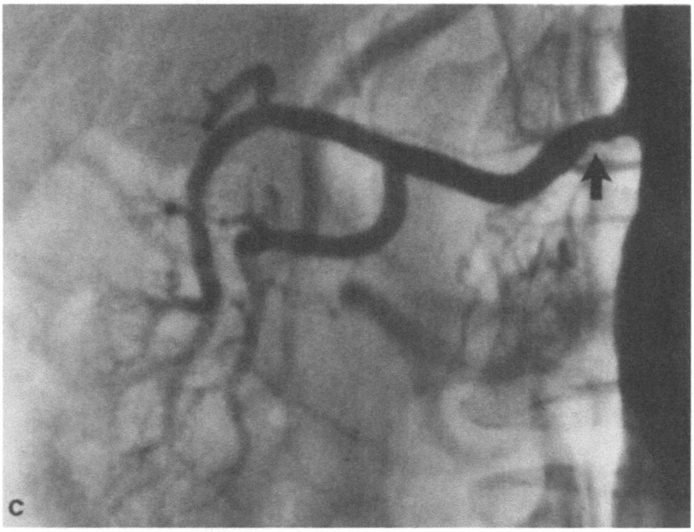

Fig. 5c

was performed within the next few days; one patient with severe diffuse atherosclerosis was judged too ill to undergo surgery (neither his blood pressure nor his renal function changed immediately or at the 2-year follow-up). Occlusive dissection of a lower pole renal artery occurred in one patient; this too was successfully bypassed. The balloon ruptured in one patient during successful PTRA of a very resistant main renal artery lesion of the intimal form of FMD; the main renal artery was successfully dilated, but a small lower pole branch supplying less than 20% of the kidney was dissected and occluded by the jet from the ruptured balloon. Several months later, this patient underwent an attempted resection of the lower pole at another hospital where they encountered "technical problems" during surgery and a nephrectomy became necessary. Two patients developed large puncture site hematomata which required surgical repair. Two patients developed transient renal failure. Two small peripheral branches (one in a patient with complete renal artery occlusion) were occluded on post-PTRA angiograms. Whether these were due to spasm, thrombosis, or dissection is not clear: follow-up angiography was not performed because they were judged clinically insignificant. One patient developed transient severe thrombocytopenia and hemolytic anemia following successful recanalization of a completely occluded artery. In this patient a hypersensitivity reaction to cholesterol microembolization is postulated.

Discussion

Eighty-two percent of native and transplant renal artery stenoses were successfully dilated with no mortality and little morbidity. The greater success with FMD is due to the lesser extent of coexistent vascular disease (aortic aneurysm, iliac stenosis, etc.), and also to two special subsets of patients in the atherosclerotic group. Eight

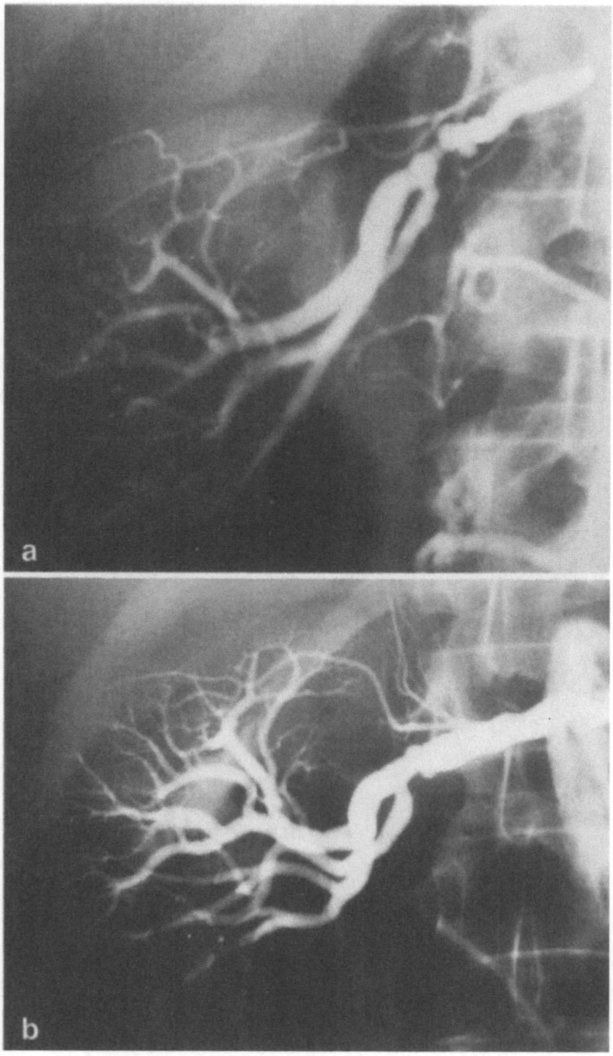

Fig. 6a, b. Angiograms in a 30-year-old hypertensive woman with fibromuscular dysplasia. **a** pre-PTRA; **b** post-PTRA

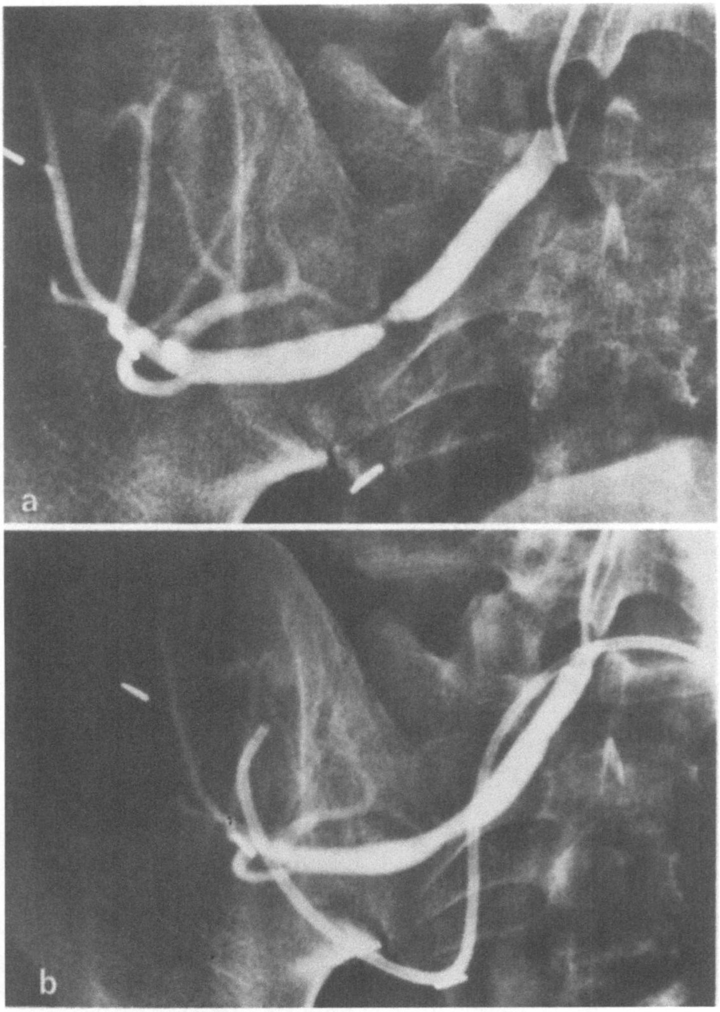

Fig. 7. a A hypertensive young man with renal transplant arterial stenosis. **b** successful PTRA. Patient is normotensive two years after PTRA

patients with atherosclerosis had complete renal artery occlusion and we were successful in dilating four (50%). A second intriguing subset of atherosclerotics were patients with "ostial" renal artery stenosis. Of 17 such lesions PTRA was judged excellent in only two (greater than 50% increase in luminal diameter), 14 were improved (20%–50% increase in diameter), and in one we failed. Ostial lesions were either extremely resistant to inflation of the balloon or were elastic and returned to the same or slightly greater diameter as they were prior to PTRA. These stenoses are in fact probably lesions of the thickened atherosclerotic aortic wall through which the "ostial" portion of these renal arteries courses (Fig. 9). The relative rigidity and the different vector of the force of the compressing balloon in this area may explain our relatively poor results at this site.

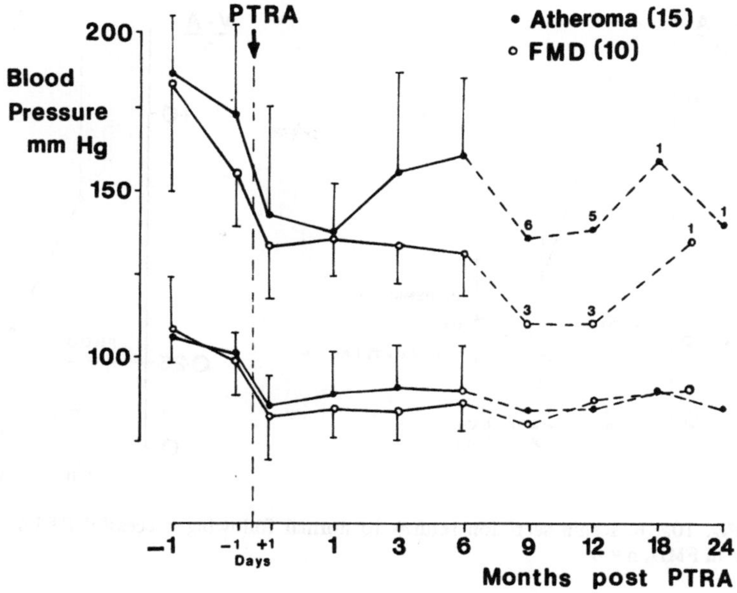

Fig. 8. Blood pressure response following PTRA

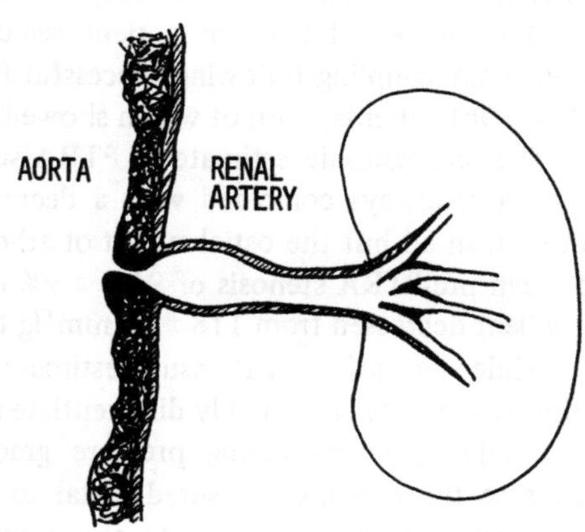

Fig. 9. Ostial renal artery stenosis is really a lesion of the thickened atherosclerotic aortic wall

We have adhered to relatively rigid criteria for patient selection for PTRA because angiographic [2] and pathologic [5] data indicate that patients with severe renal artery stenosis can be normotensive. Since the long-term results of PTRA are not yet available, this caution seems prudent.

Reports of successful blood pressure control in patients who do not have lateralizing renins prior to successful PTRA vary [8]. In a recent report 15 of 22 patients without renin-dependent hypertension reported as "clinical successes" were followed for only 48 h after PTRA, whereas a second group of 36 renin-dependent patients in the same study were followed for up to 1 year [10].

In our experience, changes in blood pressure in the initial 1–7 days after PTRA were not reliable indicators of long-term sustained relief of hypertension. Many pa-

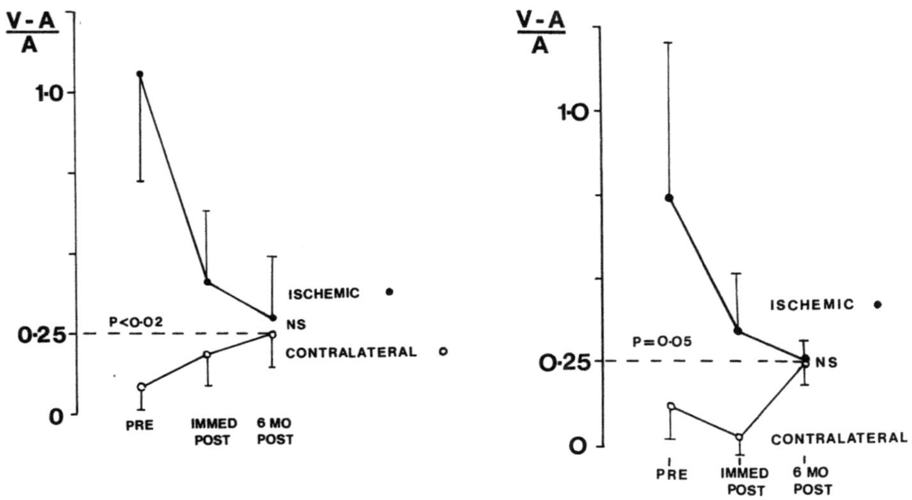

Fig. 10a, b. Renin secretion returns to normal following successful PTRA. **a** in atherosclerosis; **b** in FMD; n = 6

tients including those with technically unsuccessful PTRA experienced transient lowering of blood pressure probably due to bed rest.

Our theoretical basis of patient selection is supported by repeat selective renal vein renin sampling following successful PTRA in atherosclerotic (Fig. 10a) and FMD (Fig. 10b) patients, both of which showed normalization of renin secretion.

The angiographic estimate of PTRA success (greater than 25% increase in luminal diameter) always coincided with a decrease of at least 20% in the pressure gradient. In fact, in all but the ostial subset of atherosclerostics luminal diameter changed from a mean pre-PTRA stenosis of 91% ± 9% to 27% ± 24% ($P < 0.001$) and the pressure gradient decreased from 118 ± 42 mmHg to 13 ± 18 mmHg ($P < 0.001$).

While we realize that visual estimates may be somewhat inaccurate, few would dispute that one can reliably differentiate a 90% stenosis from a 25% stenosis.

Similarly, in measuring pressure gradients we realize that collateral flow may increase the pressure measured distal to a severe stenosis, though the catheter itself may significantly contribute to the occlusion. It is also true, however, that the pullback pressure was never obtained following PTRA with a catheter smaller in diameter than the one used to measure the initial gradient. Thus, while the pre-PTRA pressure may be inaccurate, if on pullback little or no gradient is found PTRA can be considered successful.

In many patients, especially in young women, spasm of the renal artery was seen during and after PTRA; in these cases, intra-arterial injections of 30–40 mg lidocaine relieved the spasm and made it possible to continue the procedure. We now routinely use an intrarenal artery injection of lidocaine prior to crossing the lesion.

Although only long-term results can and will determine the future role of PTRA, we are encouraged on the basis of our 2½-year experience. We have attempted PTRA on over 100 arteries with a high rate of technical success with no mortality, no loss of kidneys, and little morbidity. The early results show successful relief of hypertension in patients following successful PTRA. Patients can be out of bed the same day or the day after PTRA, and are discharged in a few days. If restenosis develops it can be successfully redilated, and the few complications did not preclude subsequent successful surgery.

In our institution currently all patients with documented renovascular hypertension undergo PTRA. Surgery is reserved for the few in whom PTRA has failed or resulted in a surgically correctable complication.

References

1. Dotter CT, Judkins MP (1964) Transluminal treatment of arteriosclerotic obstruction. Description of a new technic and a preliminary report of its application. Circulation 30:654–670
2. Eyler WR, Clark MD, Garmann JE et al. (1962) Angiography of the renal areas including a comparative study of renal arterial stenosis in patients with and without hypertension. Radiology 78:879–891
3. Grüntzig A, Hopff H (1974) Perkutane rekanalisation chronischer arterieller Verschlüsse mit einem neuen Dilatationskatheter. Modifikation der Dotter-Technik. Dtsch Med Wochenschr 99:2502–2511
4. Grüntzig A, Kuhlmann U, Vetter W et al. (1978) Treatment of renovascular hypertension with percutaneous transluminal dilatation of renal-artery stenosis. Lancet 1:801–802
5. Holley KE, Hunt JC, Brown AL et al. (1964) Renal artery stenosis: a clinical-pathologic study in normotensive and hypertensive patients. Am J Med 37:14–22
6. Katzen BT, Chang J, Lukowsky GH et al. (1979) Percutaneous transluminal angioplasty for treatment of renovascular hypertension. Radiology 131:53–58
7. Millan VG, Mast WE, Madias NE (1979) Nonsurgical treatment of severe hypertension due to renal-artery intimal fibroplasia by percutaneous transluminal angioplasty. N Engl J Med 300:1371–1373
8. Russell RP Renal hypertension. Surg Clin North Am 54:349–361
9. Saddekni S, Sniderman KW, Hilton S et al. (1980) Percutaneous transluminal angioplasty of non-atherosclerotic lesions. Am J Roentgenol 135:975–982
10. Schwarten DE (1980) Transluminal angioplasty of renal artery stenosis: 70 experiences. Am J Roentgenol 135:969–974
11. Sniderman KW, Sprayregen S, Sos TA et al. (1980) Percutaneous transluminal dilation in renal transplant arterial stenosis. Transplantation 30:440–444
12. Sos TA (1980) Angioplasty in renal artery stenosis. In: Symposium on interventional angiography. Am Heart Assoc 53rd Annu Sci Sess Nov. 17, 1980
13. Sos TA, Sniderman KW (1981) Percutaneous transluminal angioplasty. Semin Roentgenol 16:26–41
14. Tegtmeyer CJ, Dyer R, Teates CD, et al. (1980) Percutaneous transluminal dilatation of the renal arteries. Techniques and results. Radiology 135:589–599
15. Vaughan ED, Bühler FR, Laragh JH et al. (1973) Renovascular hypertension: renin measurements to indicate hypersecretion and contralateral suppression, estimate renal plasma flow and score for surgical curability. Am J Med 55:402

Percutaneous Transluminal Dilatation (Angioplasty) in Renal Arteries

E. Zeitler*, R. Grosse-Vorholt*, U. Gessler**, E. Krönert*, E. Lux**

Radiological Center* and the 4th Medical Clinic**, Flurstr. 17, 8500 Nürnberg, FRG

Percutaneous transluminal renal dilatation (PTRD) as a useful clinical method could be more strongly advocated after development of the coaxial double-lumen balloon catheters by Grüntzig for iliac and coronary artery dilatation [2, 3, 4, 5, 6, 7, 8, 9, 10, 11]. Only a safe technique of passing the stenosis and dilatation with balloon could be an alternative to vascular surgery.

From January 1978 to April 1981, we examined in Nürnberg 38 patients (24 male, 13 female) with suspected renovascular hypertension, with the aim of submitting them to PTRD [6, 9].

Seven patients of the original 38 did not eventually undergo PTRD. In two cases (both male) angiography revealed a renal artery occlusion which had developed from a renal artery stenosis in the interval between previous and new angiography. Three patients (two male, one female) had no pressure gradient between aorta and peripheral renal artery. In a 21-year-old male patient with fibromuscular renal artery stenosis after right nephrectomy, an angiography demonstrated a high-grade left renal artery stenosis which was impossible to pass, and he also had a stenosis in the superior mesenteric artery. This patient underwent vascular surgery. Catheter passage also failed in one female patient with high-grade renal artery stenosis. This patient had an atrophic kidney.

Of the 31 patients who did undergo PTRD, 19 were male (mean age 49 years, range 17–60 years) and 12 were female (mean age 44 years, range 28–70 years). There were 40 renal artery stenoses; these could be passed with a catheter, and balloon dilatation was possible. Results show that in 95% of the cases, dilatation of the angiographically proven and hemodynamically effective stenoses was possible.

Eight patients (five women, three men) on whom we performed PTRD had fibromuscular stenosis (five right, one left, and two bilateral). One patient developed an acute thrombosis which was successfully treated by vascular surgery, and one 70-year-old woman had an atrophic left kidney. Six of the eight had naturally normal blood pressure and in the other two normal pressure was achieved with medication.The mean age was 38 years (range 28–50 years). Two patients subsequently underwent a second PTRD.

The example in Fig. 1 shows that high-grade stenoses can also be submitted to PTRD. A 38-year-old man had a high-grade right renal artery stenosis. The renin quotient had increased to 4.5. Blood pressure was about 190/120 mmHg under antihypertensive medication. The stenosis could be passed with the sidewinder catheter II.

Transluminal Coronary Angioplasty and
Intracoronary Thrombolysis. Ed. by Kaltenbach et al.

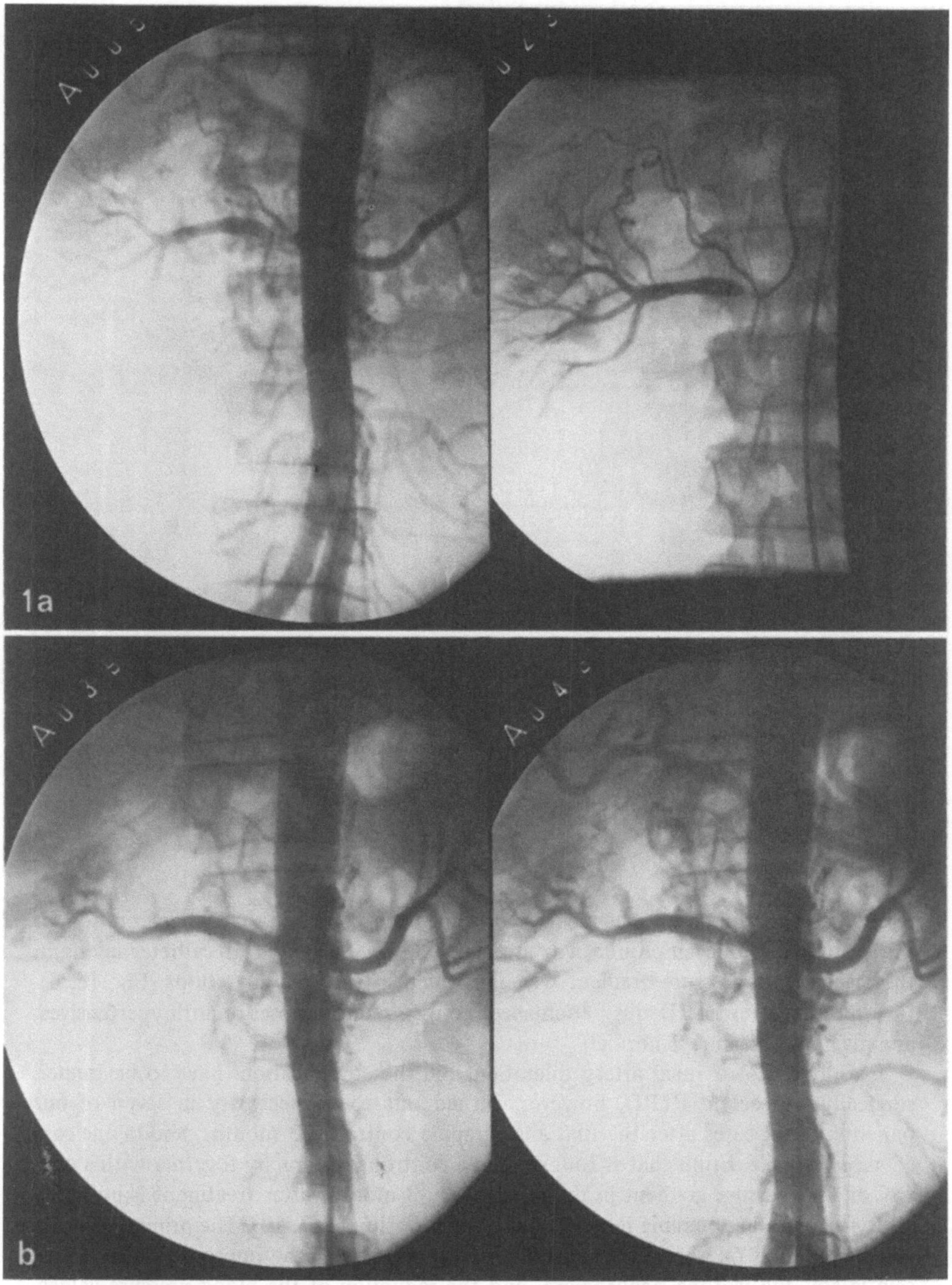

Fig. 1. Patient with renovascular hypertension. **a** renal artery stenoses right before PTRD; **b** control angiography after PTRD; **c** blood pressure before PTRD; **d** blood pressure after PTRD

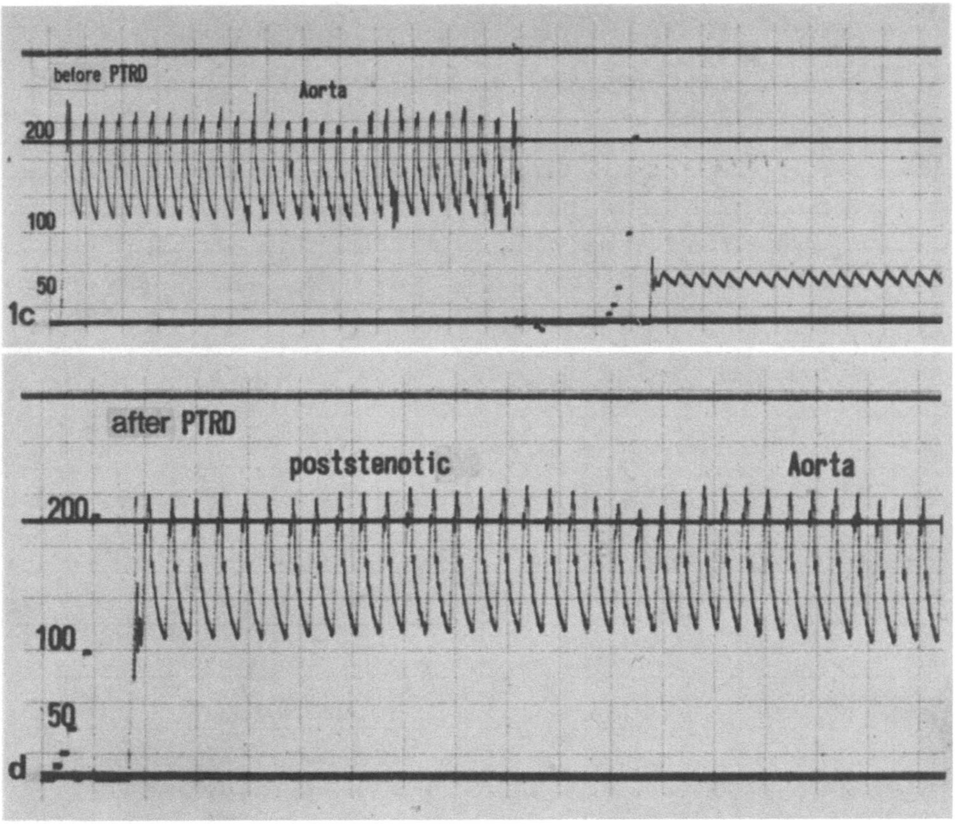

After the first dilatation, the poststenotic pressure increased, and augmentation of the systolic-diastolic amplitude was ascertainable on the graph at catheter laying in the artery. The pressure gradient was eliminated after three dilatations (Fig. 1c, d). Five months after PTRD this patient needs only a reduced doses of antihypertensives, and his blood pressure is normal.

In only 2.5% of renal artery dilatations did the complications have to be treated surgically. A second PTRD, however, turned out to be necessary in seven of our patients; in six cases after the first angiographic control at 3 months, and in one case 19 months later. From that it follows that a control angiography together with a control of the pressure gradient in the renal artery 3 months after treatment is indispensable for revealing possible rest stenoses or recidivation [5, 7, 10]. The primary success can be assessed on the decrease of the pressure gradient, the improved radionuclide scintigram, the isotope nephrogram, and the reduction of the blood pressure values. On an average the systolic pressure gradient could be reduced by PTRD from 125 mmHg to 28 mmHg (Fig. 2).

In 25 patients, the renal function had been controlled before PTRD and repeatedly afterwards with radionuclides. In 11 cases regression of the initial improvement was

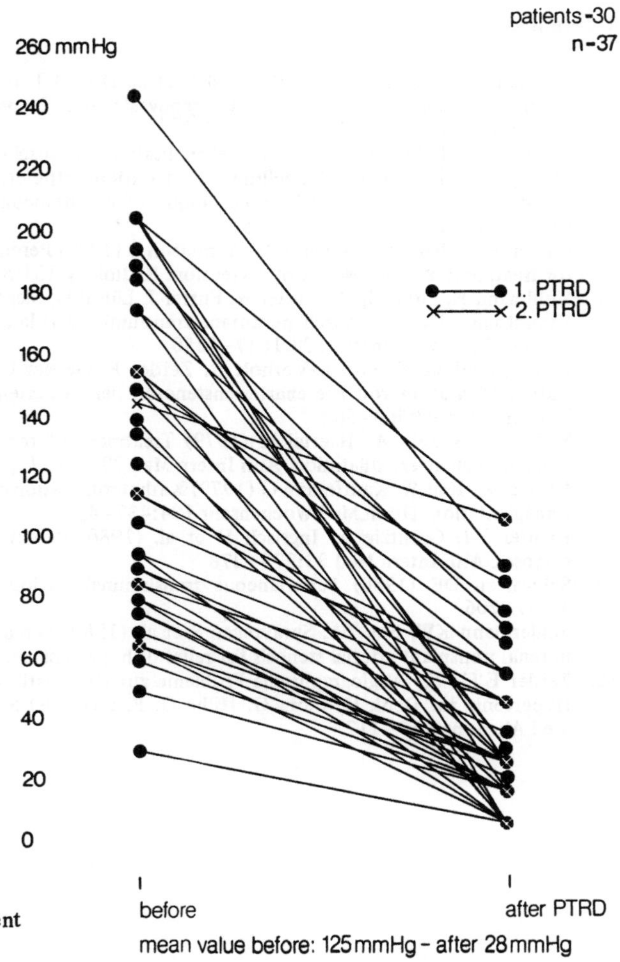

Fig. 2. Change of pressure gradient Δp after PTRD

provable, in 11 further cases function had significantly decreased, and in three cases it remained unchanged. Improvement of tubulosecretory function was objectifiable in 50% of the patients.

Normalization of blood pressure and reduced dependence on antihypertensives are the best test methods which can easily be applied after effective PTRD [1, 6, 10].

When we differentiated between patients younger than 40 years and older than 45 years we found that the pressure values always normalized in younger patients, without medication in four of five cases. In five of the 15 patients older than 45 years (33%) the blood pressure normalized without medicaments, and in a further five additional drug therapy led to normalization. In the remaining five, however, the pressure values remained unchanged. Taking into consideration that these are the results of follow-up controls over a mean observation period of 11 months, it becomes apparent how effective PTRD is. However, more detailed results and follow-up studies are still necessary.

References

1. Bussmann WD, Faßbinder W, Rummel D et al. (1981) Transluminale Dilatation von Nierenarterienstenosen zur Behandlung der renovaskulären Hypertonie. Dtsch Med Wochenschr 106:358–360
2. Grüntzig A (1976) Die perkutane Rekanalisation chronischer arterieller Verschlüsse (Dotter-Prinzip) mit einem neuen doppellumigen Dilatationskatheter. ROEFO 124:80–86
3. Grüntzig A, Kumpe DA (1979) Technique of percutaneous angioplasty with the Grüntzig balloon catheter. AJR 132:547–552
4. Katzen BT, Chang J, Lukowsky G, Abramson E (1979) Percutaneous transluminal angioplasty for treatment of renovascular hypertension. Radiology 131:53–58
5. Kuhlmann H, Grüntzig A, Vetter W, Furrer J, Lütolf U, Siegenthaler W (1978) Renovaskuläre Hypertonie: Therapie durch perkutane transluminale Dilatation von Nierenarterienstenosen. Schweiz Med Wochenschr 108:1847–1850
6. Lux E, Seybold D, Grosse-Vorholt R, Zeitler E, Gessler U (1980) Perkutane transluminale Katheterdilatation von Nierenarterienstenosen bei Patienten mit renovaskulärer Hypertonie. Fortschr Med 98:563–568
7. Mahler F, Krneta A, Haertel M (1979) Treatment of renovascular hypertension by transluminal renal artery dilatation. Ann Intern Med 90:56–57
8. Mathias K, Rau W, Kauffmann G (1979) Katheterdilatation einer Arterienstenose nach Nierentransplantation. Dtsch Med Wochenschr 104:437–438
9. Richter E-I, Grüntzig A, Ingrisch H et al. (1980) Percutaneous dilatation of renal artery stenoses. Ann Intern Med 23:275–278
10. Schwarten DE (1980) Percutaneous transluminal angioplasty of the renal artery. CVIR 3:197–206
11. Snidermann KW, Sos TA, Sprayregen S et al. (1980) Percutaneous transluminal angioplasty in renal transplant arterial stenosis for relief of hypertension. Radiology 135:23–25
12. Zeitler E (1971) Angiographische Probleme zur Diagnostik und Therapie der renovasculären Hypertonie in: Denk H, Flora G, Hilbe G, Piza G (eds) Renovaskuläre Hypertonie. Wiener Med Akad, pp 113–117

Percutaneous Transluminal Angioplasty in the Treatment of Renovascular Hypertension

W.-D. Bussmann, S. Dowinsky, D. Rummel, W. Faßbinder, P. Grützmacher, E. Starke
M. Kaltenbach, W. Schoeppe

Center of Internal Medicine, Department of Cardiology and Nephrology, University Clinic of Frankfurt a.M., Theodor-Stern-Kai 7, 6000 Frankfurt a.M. 70, FRG

Renal artery stenosis remains one of the few curable causes of arterial hypertension. Until recently, such lesions could only be treated surgically. This type of intervention, however, is neither free of risk nor uniformly effective [5]. Since 1978 [4], percutaneous transluminal renal angioplasty (PTRA) using a balloon catheter has been performed successfully in patients with renovascular disease. The objective of this innovative technique lies in reducing the extent of localized vessel narrowing, thereby diminishing the angiotensinogenic component of hypertension. The resulting enhancement in blood flow may also improve impaired renal function or preserve the viability of transplanted kidneys. In this report, we describe our application of the procedure in a series of 12 patients.

Patients

Since February 1980 PTRA has been performed on 12 native renal artery stenoses in 10 hypertensive patients. The two male and eight female patients ranged in age from 20 to 58 years. The two youngest women had fibromuscular dysplasia, whereas the remaining patients had atherosclerotic lesions. Acquired lesions in the arteries of transplanted kidneys were dilated in two additional patients.

Bilateral disease was present in three cases. Angioplasty of the contralateral side was normally attempted during reangiography 3 months after the original procedure. In one case of restenosis, repeat PTRA was also performed at follow-up catheterization. In one transplant patient, multiple redilatation was carried out to preserve the graft.

The selection of patients with native renal artery lesions was based on internationally accepted criteria for the diagnosis of renovascular hypertension amenable to surgery. In addition to angiographic demonstration of the stenoses, selective renal vein renin determinations were made before and after the administration of sodium nitroprusside. A stenosis was judged significant if the ratio between the stenotic and nonstenotic sides was greater than 1.5.

Patients with transplant renal artery stenosis underwent PTRA if blood pressure rose intractably or parameters of renal function indicated that low perfusion was threatening graft survival.

Transluminal Coronary Angioplasty and
Intracoronary Thrombolysis. Ed. by Kaltenbach et al.

Methods

Technique

The procedure corresponds to that described by Grüntzig [3] employing a double-lumen balloon catheter. A femoral approach was used in all cases. As a technical modification, we replaced the standard 9F outer guiding catheter with a more flexible 8F version. No attempt was made to cross the stenosis with a guide wire. Balloons with diameters of 3.7 and 5.0 mm were inflated 2–5 times at 5 atm pressure.

Pressure Determinations

Aortic as well as pre- and poststenotic pressure was measured via the 4F Grüntzig dilatation catheter. Changes in poststenotic pressure following balloon inflation were recorded continuously. In extremely tight lesions, catheter occlusion may have exaggerated the pressure gradient to a certain extent. Aortic pressure following PTRA was also noted during catheter removal.

Laboratory Investigations

Hypertension

Peripheral plasma renin as well as selective renal vein renin activity was determined using a radioimmunoassay technique as modified by Brecht [1]. Normal values at rest in supine position range (mean ± SD) from 3.0 to 7.8 ng angiotensin I/ml · h.

Renal Function

Creatinine clearance and urea levels were determined. Radioisotope renography was carried out before and after PTRA as well as after 3 months.

Blood flow

Iodine-131 hippuran clearance studies were performed before PTRA, immediately after the procedure, and at approximately 3 months.

Premedication

Patients received 1 g acetylsalicylic acid/day to inhibit platelet aggregation, beginning 1 day before PTRA.

Results

Technical Success

Primary dilatation was achieved in all 12 native stenoses and both transplant lesions. In one patient with bilateral disease the balloon could not traverse the stenosis on one side. At 3 months, a virtually complete recurrence in one stenosis could be successfully redilated.

Degree of Stenosis

The extent of vessel narrowing before and after PTRA was estimated in percent. The mean diameter of the stenoses in native arteries was reduced from 83% to 33%. At 3 months, an additional improvement to 27% was noted.

In addition, the stenotic vessel segment was projected on a screen, traced, and measured at the narrowest point. These measurements yielded an increase in the lumen by a factor of 3.1.

Pressure Gradient

The mean systolic blood pressure gradient across the stenosis was reduced from 123 to 22 mmHg (Fig. 1). At follow-up after 3 months, the mean gradient was 7 mmHg. (In one patient after recurrence a second dilatation had to be performed.)

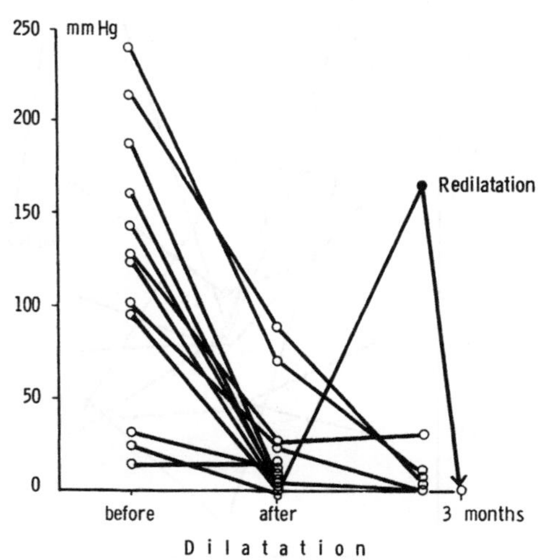

Fig. 1. Pressure gradient across 12 renal artery stenoses in 10 patients before PTRA (123 mmHg), immediately after PTRA (22 mmHg), and 3 months after PTRA (43 mmHg). Following redilatation of a restenosis, the 3-month result was 7 mmHg

Blood Pressure

With a multiple drug regimen, blood pressure in the patients with native lesions was controlled at 162/95 mmHg before PTRA. After the procedure, blood pressure was 141/85 mmHg with a 62% reduction in the dosage of antihypertensive agents (Fig. 2). Two patients required no medication whatsoever. At 3 months, mean pressure was

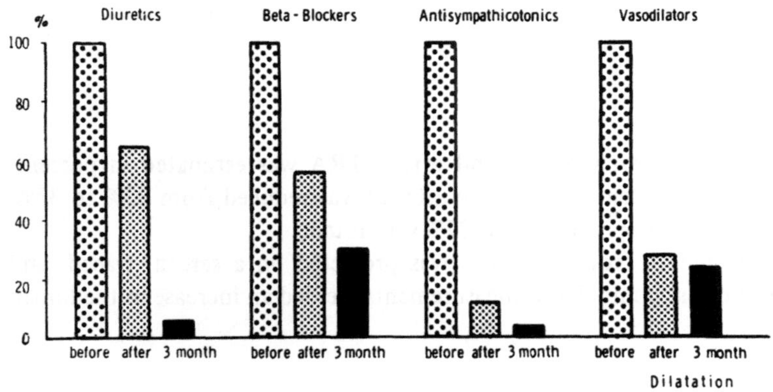

Fig. 2. Dose of antihypertensive agents in seven patients with nine stenoses before PTRA, immediately after PTRA, and 3 months after PTRA. A mean reduction of 62% was achieved following the procedure, with greater reductions for potent antisympathotonic and vasodilator drugs. At 3 months, dosage could be reduced by an additional 13%

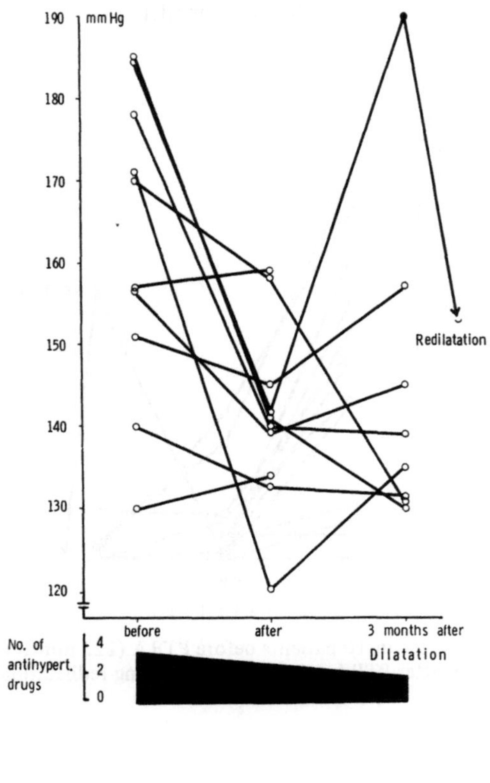

Fig. 3. Systolic blood pressure in eight patients with ten stenoses before PTRA, immediately after PTRA, and 3 months after PTRA. Levels fell from 162 to 140 mmHg and did not increase after 3 months (140 mmHg). Simultaneously, the number of antihypertensive drugs fell from a mean of 3.5 to 2.5, after 3 months to 2.0

virtually unchanged (140/84 mmHg) with a further 13% dose reduction. The mean number of drugs before PTRA was 3.5, after PTRA 2.5, and at 3 months 2.0 (Fig. 3).

Renin Activity

The decline in plasma renin activity following successful PTRA was notable (Fig. 4.). A marked reduction was also seen after dilatation of one side in bilateral disease. Mean plasma renin activity fell from 32.4 to 13.4 ng AI/ml • h. At 3 months, mean renin activity was 15.0 ng AI/ml • h. Selective renal vein renin sampling demonstrated a normalization of renin activity on the treated side. No rise in renin secretion was observed following blood pressure reduction with sodium nitroprusside (Fig. 5).

Renal Function and Blood Flow

Parameters of renal function tended to improve in those patients with previously pathological values. In five such patients, serum creatinine fell from 168 mmol/liter before PTRA to 124 mmol/liter after PTRA. Graft function in the transplant patients recovered markedly following serial PTRA (Fig. 6). The renal blood flow studies produced variable results, showing improvement in four patients.

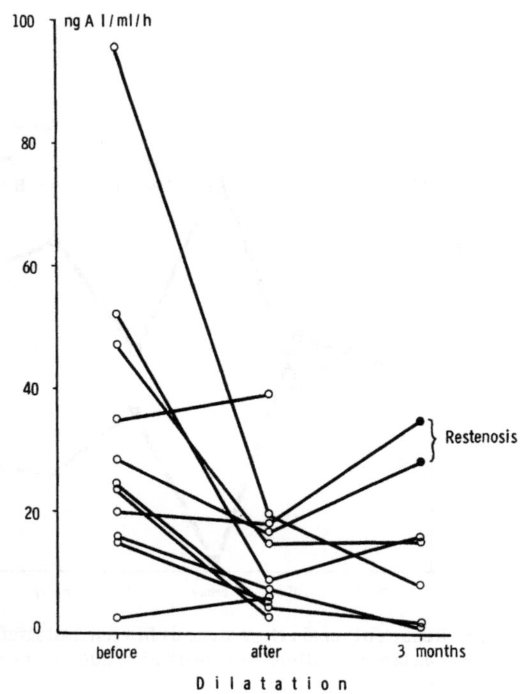

Fig. 4. Plasma renin activity before PTRA, immediately after PTRA, and 3 months after PTRA. Values declined from 32.4 to 13.4 ng AI/ml • h following dilatation and rose only slightly to 15.0 ngAI/ml • h at 3 months

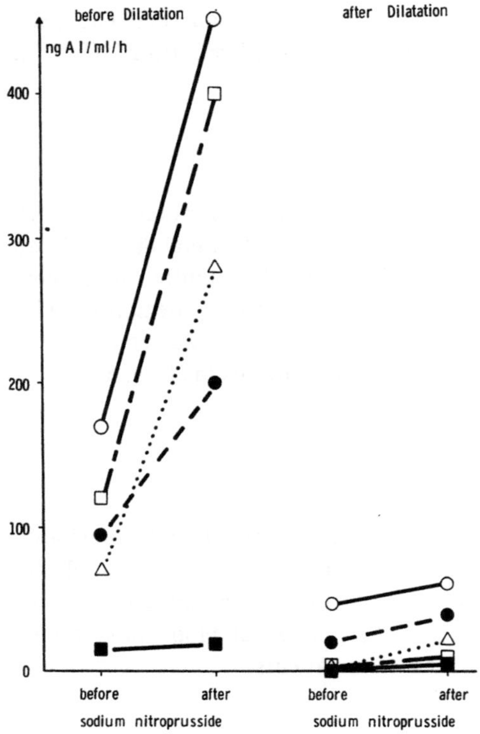

Fig. 5. Selective renin sampling. The pre-PTRA stimulation of renin activity achieved by lowering blood pressure was no longer observable following successful dilatation

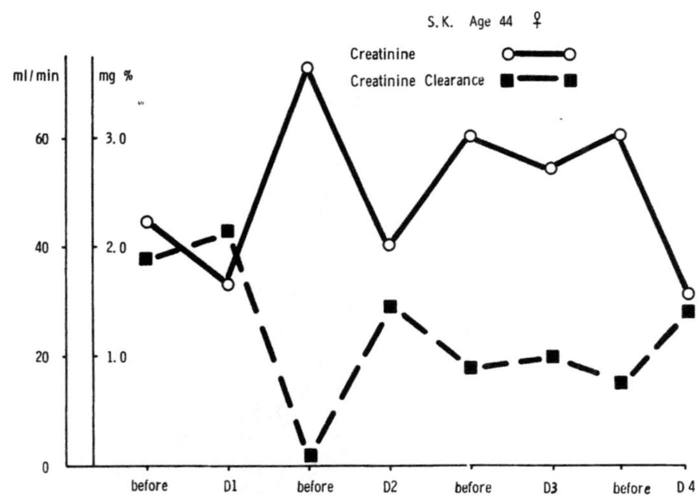

Fig. 6. Recurrent renal artery stenosis in a renal allograft. PTRA was performed four times (D1–D4), in each instance resulting in a marked reduction in serum creatinine and increase in creatinine clearance

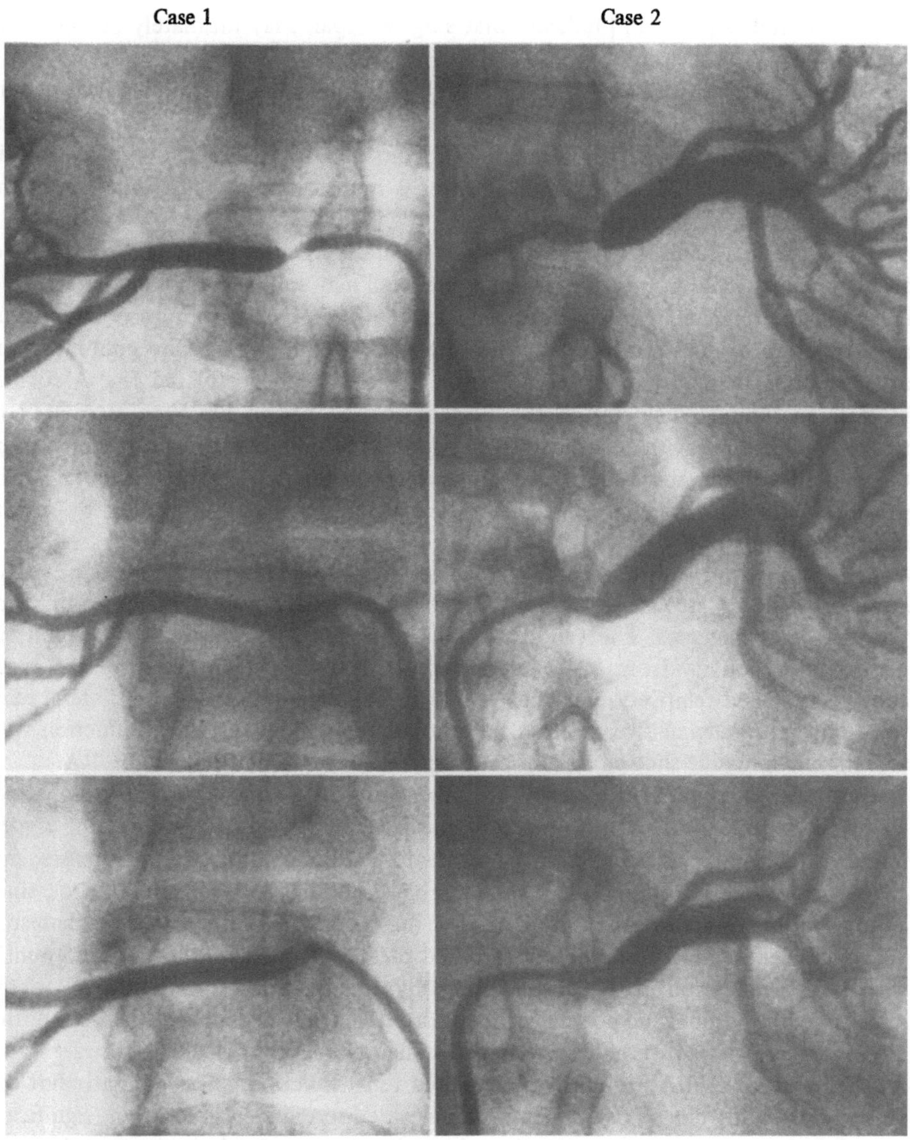

Fig. 7. Selective renal angiography before PTRA (*upper*), immediately after PTRA (*middle*), and at 3 months after PTRA (*lower*) in two cases

Discussion

The correction of functionally significant lesions is of great potential benefit to patients with renovascular hypertension. Until recently, surgery represented the only form of causative therapy, although it has been applied cautiously in the light of not inconsiderable operative morbidity and mortality. The development of PTRA has made available an attractive alternative to revascularization. The results of this and other studies [6, 7, 11] indicate that surgical repair may ultimately become only the treatment of last resort.

The striking ability of PTRA to increase luminal diameter and reduce the pressure gradient across the stenosis is reflected in the angiographic and hemodynamic findings. The mean degree of narrowing was reduced from 83% to 33%, and the trans-stenotic gradient fell from 123 to 22 mmHg. After 3 months the pressure gradient in the follow-up group was 7 mmHg.

The exact mechanism by which balloon dilatation causes the lumen to widen remains unclear. Balloon pressure on the vessel wall may split the atheromatous plaque, enlarging the channel. The elastic media may be freed by the rupture of the plaque and stretch in response to increased pressure [2]. A reduction of fluid content in the atheromatous tissue following compression has also been postulated [8]. A further increase in luminal diameter in the postangioplasty period has been attributed to fibrosis and healing with subsequent retraction of the splits. Medial disruption appears to account for the success of the technique in fibromuscular dysplasia. The repair processes and improvement in results at reangiography have been noted by several investigators [10].

Stringent criteria were used in the selection of patients with lesions of native arteries. Stenoses associated with increased renin activity were thought to enhance the chances of success. The validity of this approach was reflected in a decline in plasma renin activity from 32 to 13 ng AI/ml • h. After PTRA at 3 months, renin activity remained relatively unchanged at 15 ng AI/mg • h. Repeated ipsilateral renal vein renin sampling in five patients before and after blood pressure reduction with sodium nitroprusside showed a significant suppression of renin following PTRA.

Despite these significant changes, only the two young patients with fibromuscular dysplasia became normotensive without medication. It seems clear that the hypertension in the remaining patients is multifactorial. Eliminating the angiotensiogenic component alone is often inadequate to achieve good blood pressure control, since essential or renal parenchymous hypertension may coexist as pathogenetic mechanisms.

Nonetheless, a marked reduction in blood pressure from 162/95 to 141/85 mmHg with a 67% reduction in the dosage of antihypertensive drugs was achieved. At the same time, the number and potency of the agents used could be reduced. After 3 months, blood pressure had not risen despite an additional reduction in medication.

The value of PTRA in improving impaired renal function is less dramatic but can be significant. In four of five patients with elevated serum creatinine levels, significant improvement was noted; in one patient normalization occurred. An improved glomerular filtration rate in three patients was reflected in higher creatinine clearance. Isotope renograms demonstrated faster elimination in four of seven patients. In the two patients with transplant stenosis, allograft function improved with PTRA, although rapid recurrence appears to be a problem in this setting.

The implications of PTRA in the treatment of renovascular hypertension are significant. The technique is capable of widening the stenotic lumen of both fibromuscular and atherosclerotic lesions. Risk and discomfort to the patient appear to be acceptably low, although other authors have reported severe complications [9].

The only problem encountered in this series was a case of transient occlusion at the site of the stenosis; the procedure was nonetheless carried out successfully.

When restenosis does occur, it is usually amenable to redilatation. Although the long-term antihypertensive effects of PTRA are not known, preliminary results compare favorably with other forms of therapy. The exact role of the technique in renal insufficiency remains less clear, although acute intervention to salvage renal allografts has met with modest success.

References

1. Brecht HM (1978) Untersuchungen zur pathologischen Bedeutung des sympathischen Nervensystems, des Renin-Angiotensin-Aldosteron-Systems sowie der Na-Bilanz bei der essentiellen und renoparenchymatösen Hypertonie. Habilitationsschrift, Universität Frankfurt
2. Castaneda-Zunica WR, Formanek M, Tadavarthy M et al. (1980) The mechanism of balloon angioplasty. Radiology 135:565
3. Grüntzig A, Hopff H (1974) Perkutane Rekanalisation chronischer arterieller Verschlüsse mit einem neuen Dilatationskatheter. Modification der Dotter-Technik. Dtsch Med Wochenschr 99:2502
4. Grüntzig A, Kuhlmann U, Vetter W et al. (1978) Treatment of renovascular hypertension with percutaneous transluminal dilatation of a renal-artery stenosis. Lancet 1:801
5. Hunt TC et al. (1974) Renal and renovascular hypertension: a reasoned approach to diagnosis and management. Arch Intern Med 133:988
6. Katzen BT, Chang T, Lukowski GH et al. (1979) Percutaneous transluminal angioplasty for treatment of renovascular hypertension. Radiology 131:53
7. Kuhlmann U, Vetter W, Furrer T et al. (1980) Renovascular hypertension. Treatment by percutaneous transluminal dilatation. Ann Intern Med 92:1
8. Lue H, Grüntzig A (1978) Histopathologic aspects of transluminal recanalization. In: Zeitler E, Grüntzig A, Schoop W (eds) Percutaneous vascular recanalization. Springer, Berlin Heidelberg New York, pp 39
9. Motarjeme AJ, Keifer TW, Zuska AJ (1980) Percutaneous transluminal angioplasty and case selection. Radiology 135:573
10. Schwarten DE, Yune HY, Klatte CE et al. (1980) Clinical experience with percutaneous transluminal angioplasty (PTA) of stenotic renal arteries. Radiology 135:601
11. Tegtmeyer CJ, Oyer R, Teates CD et al. (1980) Percutaneous transluminal dilatation of the renal arteries. Radiology 135:589

Overview

W.-D. Bussmann

Center of Internal Medicine, Department of Cardiology and Nephrology, University Clinic of Frankfurt a.M, Theodor-Stern-Kai 7, 6000 Frankfurt a.M. 70, FRG

Extensive experience exists of transluminal angioplasty and recanalization of leg arteries (Seyferth and Zeitler). In contrast to coronary artery dilatation, the method can be used in peripheral arteries for occlusions up to a length of 10 cm. The success rate in the iliac and femoral-popliteal regions is around 85%. The fate of "no angioplasty" in patients who were considered as possible candidates is discussed by Sörensen and co-workers.

Transluminal angioplasty in the treatment of renovascular hypertension is another important application. Sos, Zeitler, and Bussmann reported their experience in a large number of cases. Until recently surgery was the only form of treatment, although morbidity and mortality had to be considered.

Angioplasty of renal artery stenoses increases the luminal diameter and reduces the pressure gradient across the stenosis. The pressure application may split the atheromatous plaque, enlarge the channel by reduction of fluid content in the atheromatous tissue, or both. Media disruptions appear to account for the success of the technique in fibromuscular disease. Following successful dilatation renin activity declines. A reduction in blood pressure as well as a marked reduction in the dosage of antihypertensive drugs can be achieved. Recurrence of stenosis seems to be in the range of 10%–15%.

Long-term results seem to be reasonable. However, blood pressure may not be normalized in patients with a long-standing history of hypertension.

There is no question that angioplasty is the method of choice for renal artery stenosis, and direct surgery is to be avoided whenever possible.

Transluminal Coronary Angioplasty and
Intracoronary Thrombolysis. Ed. by Kaltenbach et al.

Subject Index

Arterial Hypertension

Pathogenesis, Diagnosis, and Therapy
Translated from the German by T.C. Telger
Editor: J. Rosenthal
1982. 183 figures. XV, 529 pages
ISBN 3-540-90611-8

Beta-Blockers in the Elderly

Editors: E. Lang, F. Sörgel, L. Blaha
With contributions by numerous experts
1982. 29 figures, approx. 22 tables. Approx. 112 pages. ISBN 3-540-11682-6

Catecholamines and the Heart

Recent Advances in Experimental and Clinical Research/Symposium München, May 28–30, 1981
Editors: W. Delius, E. Gerlach, H. Grobecker, W. Kübler
1981. 149 figures, 49 tables. XIX, 383 pages
ISBN 3-540-11119-0

Frontiers in Hypertension Research

Editors: J.H. Laragh, F.R. Bühler, D.W. Seldin
1981. 242 figures. XXXIX, 628 pages
(Proceedings of an International Symposium held May 19–21, 1980 in NewYork and sponsored by USV Pharmaceutical Corporation Revlon Health Care Group)
ISBN 3-540-90557-X

The Heart in Hypertension

Editor: B.E. Strauer
1981. 187 figures, 55 tables. XVI, 464 pages
(International Boehringer Mannheim Symposia - International Symposium, München, Germany, June 13–16, 1979)
ISBN 3-540-10496-8

Microcirculation of the Heart

Theoretical and Clinical Problems
Editors: H. Tillmanns, W. Kübler, H. Zebe
1982. 177 figures. XIV, 353 pages
ISBN 3-540-11346-0

Myocardial Infarction and Psychosocial Risks

Editors: J. Siegrist, M.J. Halhuber
With contributions by numerous experts
1981. 23 figures, 33 tables. X, 152 pages
ISBN 3-540-10386-4

Myocardial Infarction at Young Age

International Symposium Held in Bad Krozingen, January, 30th and 31st, 1981.
Editor: H. Roskamm
1981. 83 figures. XII, 228 pages
ISBN 3-540-11090-9

Nitrates III

Cardiovascular Effects
Editors: P.R. Lichtlen, H.-J. Engel, A. Schrey, H.J.C. Swan
1981. 326 figures. XX, 597 pages
ISBN 3-540-10761-4

Springer-Verlag Berlin Heidelberg NewYork

MIX
Papier aus verantwortungsvollen Quellen
Paper from responsible sources
FSC® C105338

If you have any concerns about our products,
you can contact us on
ProductSafety@springernature.com

In case Publisher is established outside the EU,
the EU authorized representative is:
Springer Nature Customer Service Center GmbH
Europaplatz 3, 69115 Heidelberg, Germany

Printed by Libri Plureos GmbH
in Hamburg, Germany